www.harcourt-international.com

Bringing you products from all Harcourt Health Sciences companies including Baillière Tindall, Churchill Livingstone, Mosby and W.B. Saunders

- ▶ **Browse** for latest information on new books, journals and electronic products

- ▶ **Search** for information on over 20 000 published titles with full product information including tables of contents and sample chapters

...ensive publishing programme ...th eAlert or requesting postal

...rompt delivery, as well as full ...one, fax or post

...promotions

...ng countries, please visit the ...e full details of product ...information

USA: www.harcourthealth.com

Canada: www.harcourtcanada.com

Australia: www.harcourt.com.au

Baillière Tindall   CHURCHILL LIVINGSTONE   Mosby   W.B. SAUNDERS

EMERY'S
ELEMENTS OF
MEDICAL GENETICS

Commissioning Editor: Richard Furn
Project Development Manager: Siân Jarman
Design Direction: Erik Bigland
Project Manager: Nancy Arnott
Illustrator: Robert Britton

ELEVENTH
EDITION

EMERY'S ELEMENTS OF MEDICAL GENETICS

Robert F. Mueller MB BS BSc FRCP

Professor of Clinical Genetics
Department of Clinical Genetics
St James's Hospital
Leeds, UK

Ian D. Young MD MSc FRCP

Visiting Professor
Department of Clinical Genetics
Leicester Royal Infirmary
Leicester, UK

CHURCHILL LIVINGSTONE

EDINBURGH LONDON NEW YORK PHILADELPHIA SYDNEY TORONTO 2001

CHURCHILL LIVINGSTONE
An imprint of Harcourt Publishers Limited

©Harcourt Publishers Limited 2001

⬛ is a registered trademark of Harcourt Publishers Limited

First edition (University of California Press) 1968
Second edition 1971
Third edition 1974
Fourth edition 1975
Fifth edition 1979
Sixth edition 1983
Seventh edition 1988
Eighth edition 1992
Ninth edition 1995
Tenth edition 1998
Eleventh edition 2001
    Reprinted 2001

ISBN 0 443 07125 X

British Library Cataloguing in Publication Data
A catalogue record for this book is available from the British
Library

Library of Congress Cataloging in Publication Data
A catalog record for this book is available from the Library of
Congress

Note
Medical knowledge is constantly changing. As new information
becomes available, changes in treatment, procedures, equipment
and the use of drugs become necessary. The authors and the
publishers have taken care to ensure that the information given in
this text is accurate and up to date. However, readers are strongly
advised to confirm that the information, especially with regard to
drug usage, complies with the latest legislation and standards of
practice.

The
publisher's
policy is to use
**paper manufactured
from sustainable forests**

Printed in Italy by Rotolito Lombarda, Milan

PREFACE

Medical genetics is a fascinating subject, which, after a decade of extraordinary developments in molecular biology, finds itself at the forefront of widespread media and public attention. Rarely a week goes by without news of another major discovery offering new insight into a hitherto poorly understood disease process with a promise of hope for successful treatment. Indeed, it is difficult to think of any area of medical practice in which molecular biology and genetics are not now making a significant impact.

Given this scenario it is not surprising that genetics occupies an increasingly important role in the undergraduate medical curriculum. Unfortunately many students hold a preconceived, and in our view unjustified, view that this is a difficult subject. Consequently in preparing this new edition of the textbook, first conceived with remarkable foresight by Alan Emery over 30 years ago, we have tried once again to focus on basic principles in keeping with the well-earned reputation that *Elements* has gained, as a comprehensive student-friendly introductory text.

At the same time we have tried to convey a flavour of the excitement surrounding recent developments by updating and expanding those sections of the book which review the impact of genetic factors in causing disease. In addition, new developments such as gene therapy and the human genome project are considered at length, with due attention to their associated important and occasionally alarming ethical implications. Thus, while this text continues to be designed primarily for undergraduates confronted by taxing medical examinations on both sides of the Atlantic, it is hoped that it will also find favour with more experienced students, counsellors and practising clinicians, who are keen to keep abreast of progress in this rapidly developing and changing field.

Over the years we have been consistently grateful to the many students who have provided feedback, sometimes positive and sometimes otherwise! Where possible we have incorporated those suggestions which could result in greater clarity and improved understanding, and we look forward to receiving further comments as to how future editions of *Elements* might better fulfil the needs of its readers.

Leeds	R.F.M.
Leicester	I.D.Y.
March 2001	

ACKNOWLEDGEMENTS

We would like to express our sincere gratitude to our many colleagues who have made generous contributions to this new edition. In particular we are grateful to Mr Nigel Smith from the City Hospital, Nottingham, and to both Mr Graham Taylor and Mr Jeff Williams from St James's Hospital, Leeds for providing illustrations, to Mrs Kate Martin for reviewing Chapter 3, and to Mrs Diane Castledine for invaluable secretarial assistance.

This new edition could not have been achieved without the forbearance of our long-suffering wives (Pam and Liz) and children (Katy, Zach, Nick and Andrew) to whom we dedicate this book with gratitude and affection.

CONTENTS

SECTION

B

GENETICS IN MEDICINE

SECTION

C

CLINICAL GENETICS

SECTION

A

PRINCIPLES OF
HUMAN GENETICS

The history and impact of genetics in medicine

Developments in genetics during the twentieth century have been truly spectacular. In 1900 Mendel's principles were awaiting rediscovery, chromosomes were barely visible, and the science of molecular genetics did not exist. By contrast, at the time of writing in the year 2000, over 10 000 single gene disorders or traits have been identified, chromosomes can be analysed to a very high level of sophistication, and the draft sequence of the entire human genome has been reported.

This revolution in scientific knowledge and expertise has led to the realization that genetics is an area of major importance in almost every medical discipline. Recent discoveries impinge not just on rare and esoteric 'small-print' diseases, but also on many of the common acquired disorders of adult life such as cardiovascular disease, psychiatric illness and cancer. Consequently genetics is now widely accepted as being at the forefront of medical science and has become an important and integral component of the undergraduate medical curriculum.

This first chapter starts with a brief overview of some of the most notable milestones in the history of medical genetics. The importance of understanding its role in medicine is then illustrated by reviewing the overall impact of genetic factors in causing disease; finally new developments of major importance are discussed.

EARLY BEGINNINGS

Homo sapiens first appeared on this planet approximately 50 000 years ago and it is reasonable to suppose that man's first thinking ancestors were just as curious as we are about matters of inheritance. For example, engravings in Chaldea in Babylonia (now Iraq) dating back at least 6000 years show pedigrees documenting the transmission of certain characteristics of the mane in horses. However, any early attempts to unravel the mysteries of genetics would have been severely hampered by a total lack of knowledge and understanding of basic processes such as conception and reproduction.

Early Greek philosophers and physicians such as Aristotle and Hippocrates concluded, with typical masculine modesty, that important human characteristics were determined by semen utilizing menstrual blood as a culture medium and the uterus as an incubator. Semen was thought to be produced by the whole body; hence baldheaded fathers would beget baldheaded sons. These ideas prevailed until the seventeenth century, when Dutch scientists such as Leeuwenhoek and de Graaf recognized the existence of sperm and ova, thus explaining how the female could also transmit characteristics to her offspring.

The blossoming of the scientific revolution in the eighteenth and nineteenth centuries saw a revival of interest in heredity by both scientists and physicians among whom two particular names stand out. Pierre de Maupertuis, a French naturalist, studied hereditary traits such as extra digits (polydactyly) and lack of pigmentation (albinism), and showed from pedigree studies that these two conditions were inherited in different ways. Joseph Adams, a British doctor, also recognized that different mechanisms of inheritance existed and published *A Treatise on the Supposed Hereditary Properties of Diseases* which was intended as a basis for genetic counselling.

GREGOR MENDEL AND THE LAWS OF INHERITANCE

Our present understanding of human genetics owes much to the work of the Austrian monk Gregor Mendel who, in 1865, presented the results of his breeding experiments on garden peas to the Natural Science Association in Brünn (now Brno in the Czech Republic). Shortly afterwards Mendel's observations were published by this association in their *Proceedings*, where they remained largely unnoticed until 1900 when their importance was first recognized. In essence Mendel's work can be considered as the discovery of genes and how they are inherited. In acknowledgement of this enormous contribution the term *Mendelian* is now applied both to the different patterns of inheritance shown by single gene characteristics and to disorders found to be the result of defects in a single gene.

In his breeding experiments Mendel studied contrasting characters in the garden pea, using for each experiment varieties which differed in only one characteristic. For example, he noted that when strains which were bred for a feature such as tallness were crossed with plants bred to be short, all the offspring in the first *filial* or F1 generation were tall. If plants in this F1 generation were interbred, then this led to both tall and short plants in a ratio of three to one (Fig. 1.1). Those characteristics which were manifest in the F1 hybrids were referred to as *dominant*, whereas those which reappeared in the F2 generation were described as being *recessive*. On re-analysis it has been suggested that Mendel's results were 'too good to be true', in that the segregation ratios he derived were suspiciously closer to the value of 3:1 than the laws of statistics would predict. One possible explanation is that he may have published only those results which best agreed with his preconceived single gene hypothesis. Whatever the truth of the matter, events have shown that Mendel's interpretation of his results was entirely correct.

Mendel's proposal was that the plant characteristics being studied were each controlled by a pair of factors, one of which was inherited from each parent. A Danish botanist, Johannsen, subsequently coined the term *gene* for these hereditary factors. The pure bred plants, with two identical genes, used in the initial cross would now be referred to as *homozygous*. The hybrid F1 plants, each of which has one gene for tallness and one for shortness, would be referred to as *heterozygous*. The genes responsible

for these contrasting characteristics are referred to as *allelomorphs* or *alleles* for short.

An alternative method for determining *genotypes* in offspring involves the construction of what is known as a Punnett's square (Fig. 1.2). This will be utilized further in Chapter 7 when considering how genes segregate in large populations.

On the basis of Mendel's plant experiments, three main principles were established. These are known as the laws of uniformity, segregation and independent assortment.

THE LAW OF UNIFORMITY

The *law of uniformity* refers to the fact that when two homozygotes with different alleles are crossed, all the offspring in the F1 generation are identical and heterozygous. In other words the characteristics do not blend, as had been believed previously, and can reappear in later generations.

THE LAW OF SEGREGATION

The *law of segregation* refers to the observation that each individual possesses two genes for a particular characteristic, only one of which can be transmitted at any one time. Rare exceptions to this rule can occur when two allelic genes fail to separate because of chromosome non-disjunction at the first meiotic division (p. 44).

THE LAW OF INDEPENDENT ASSORTMENT

The *law of independent assortment* refers to the fact that members of different gene pairs segregate to offspring

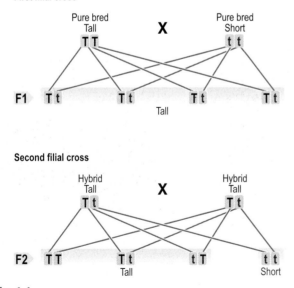

First filial cross

Second filial cross

Fig. 1.1
An illustration of one of Mendel's breeding experiments and how he correctly interpreted the results.

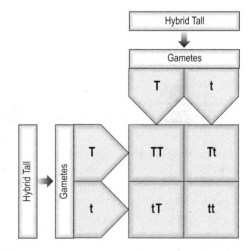

Fig. 1.2
A Punnett's square showing the different ways in which genes can segregate and combine in the second filial cross from Figure 1.1. Construction of a Punnett's square provides a simple method for showing the possible gamete combinations in different matings.

independently of one another. In reality this is not always true as genes which are close together on the same chromosome tend to be inherited together, i.e. they are 'linked' (p. 121).

THE CHROMOSOMAL BASIS OF INHERITANCE

As interest in Mendelian inheritance grew, there was much speculation as to how it actually occurred. At that time it was also known that each cell contains a nucleus within which there are several thread-like structures known as *chromosomes*, so called because of their affinity for certain stains (chroma = colour, soma = body). In 1903, Walter Sutton, an American medical student, and Theodor Boveri, a German biologist, independently proposed that chromosomes carry the hereditary factors, or genes. These suggestions were prompted by the realization that the behaviour of chromosomes at cell division could provide an explanation for how genes could segregate (Fig. 1.3).

When the connection between Mendelian inheritance and chromosomes was first made, it was thought that the normal chromosome number in humans was 48; the correct number of 46 was not established until 1956. Shortly thereafter it was shown that some disorders in humans could be caused by loss or gain of a whole chromosome as well as an abnormality in a single gene. Chromosome disorders are discussed at length in Chapter 17. Some chromosome abnormalities, such as translocations, can run in families (p. 46), and are sometimes said to be segregating in a Mendelian fashion.

THE FRUIT FLY

Before returning to historical developments in human genetics, it is worth a brief diversion to consider the merits of this unlikely creature which has proved to be of great value in genetic research. The fruit fly, *Drosophila*, possesses several distinct advantages for the study of genetics. These are as follows:

1. It can be bred easily in a laboratory.
2. It reproduces rapidly and prolifically at a rate of 20–25 generations per annum.
3. It has a number of easily recognized characteristics such as *curly wings* and *yellow body* which show Mendelian inheritance.
4. *Drosophila melanogaster*, the species most frequently studied, has only four pairs of chromosomes each of which has a distinct appearance so that they can be identified easily.
5. The chromosomes in the salivary glands of *Drosophila* larvae are among the largest known in nature, being at least 100 times bigger than those in other body cells.

In view of these unique properties, fruit flies were used extensively in early breeding experiments. Today their study is still proving of great value in fields such as developmental biology, where knowledge of gene homology throughout the animal kingdom has enabled scientists to identify families of genes which are very important in human embryogenesis (ch. 5). When considering major scientific achievements in the history of genetics it is notable that sequencing of the 180 million base pairs of the *Drosophila melanogaster* genome was completed towards the end of 1999.

Fig. 1.3
Shows chromosomes dividing into two daughter cells at different stages of cell division. A = metaphase; B = anaphase; C = telophase. The behaviour of chromosomes in cell division (mitosis) is described at length in Chapter 3. (Photographs courtesy of Dr K Ocraft, City Hospital, Nottingham.)

THE ORIGINS OF MEDICAL GENETICS

Mention has already been made of the pioneering studies of far-sighted individuals such as Pierre de Maupertuis and Joseph Adams whose curiosity was aroused by familial conditions such as polydactyly and albinism. Others, such as John Dalton of atomic theory fame, observed that some conditions, notably colour blindness and haemophilia, show what is now referred to as *sex-* or *X-linked inheritance*, and to this day colour blindness is still sometimes referred to as *Daltonism*. Inevitably these founders of human and medical genetics could only speculate as to the nature of the mechanisms underlying their observations.

The rediscovery of Mendelism in 1900 marked the real beginning of medical genetics and provided an enormous impetus for the study of inherited disease. Credit for the first recognition of a single gene trait is shared by William Bateson and Archibald Garrod who together proposed that alkaptonuria was a rare recessive disorder. In this relatively benign condition urine turns dark on standing or on exposure to alkali because of an inability on the part of the patient to metabolize homogentisic acid (p. 155). Young children show skin discolouration in the napkin (diaper) area and affected adults are prone to develop arthritis in large joints. Realizing that this was an inherited disorder involving a chemical process, Garrod coined the term *inborn error of metabolism*. Several hundred such disorders have now been identified giving rise to the field of study known as biochemical genetics (ch. 10). The history of alkaptonuria neatly straddles almost the entire twentieth century starting with Garrod's original observations of recessive inheritance in 1902 and culminating in cloning of the relevant gene on chromosome 3 in 1996.

CLASSIFICATION OF GENETIC DISEASE

During the course of the twentieth century it gradually became clear that hereditary factors are implicated in many conditions and that different genetic mechanisms are involved. Traditionally, hereditary conditions have been considered under the headings of single gene, chromosomal and multifactorial. Recent discoveries have shown that a fourth category, consisting of acquired somatic genetic disease, should also be included.

SINGLE GENE DISORDERS

In addition to alkaptonuria, Garrod suggested that albinism and cystinuria could also show recessive inheritance. Soon other examples followed, leading to an explosion in knowledge and disease delineation. By 1966 almost 1500 single gene disorders or traits had been identified prompting the publication by an American physician, Victor McKusick, of a catalogue of all known single gene conditions. By 1998 when the twelfth edition of this catalogue was published, it contained over 8500 entries (Fig. 1.4). Given that there are between 50 000 and 100 000 coding genes in each set of human chromosomes, it is not surprising that the pace of developments in this field, coupled with the need for an up-to-date reference source, has led to the creation of an online version of 'McKusick's catalogue'. This is known formally as *Online Mendelian Inheritance in Man* (OMIM) and can be accessed via the Internet (see appendix). By the beginning of 2000 OMIM contained a total of 11 084 entries.

CHROMOSOME ABNORMALITIES

Improved techniques for studying chromosomes led to the demonstration in 1959 that the presence of an additional number 21 chromosome (*trisomy 21*) results in Down's syndrome. Other similar discoveries followed rapidly. The identification of chromosome abnormalities was further aided by the development of banding techniques in 1970 (p. 31). These enabled reliable identification of individual chromosomes and helped confirm that loss or gain of even a very small segment of a chromosome can have devastating effects on human development (ch. 17).

Most recently it has been shown that several rare conditions featuring mental retardation and abnormal physical features are due to loss of such a tiny amount of chromosome material that no abnormality can be detected using even the most high powered light microscope. These conditions are referred to as microdeletion syndromes (pp. 50, 253) and are diagnosed using a

Fig. 1.4
Histogram showing the rapid increase in recognition of conditions and characteristics (traits) showing single gene inheritance. (Adapted from McKusick 1998 and OMIM — see appendix.)

technique known as FISH (fluorescent in situ hybridization) which combines conventional chromosome analysis (cytogenetics) with much newer DNA diagnostic technology (molecular genetics) (p. 34).

MULTIFACTORIAL DISORDERS

Francis Galton, a cousin of Charles Darwin, had a long-standing interest in human characteristics such as stature, physique and intelligence. Much of his research was based on the study of identical twins in whom differences in these parameters must be the result of environmental influences. Galton introduced to genetics the concept of the *regression coefficient* as a means of estimating the degree of resemblance between various relatives. This concept was later extended to incorporate Mendel's discovery of genes, to try to explain how parameters such as height and skin colour could be determined by the interaction of many genes, each exerting a small additive effect. This is in contrast to single gene characteristics in which the action of one gene is exerted independently, i.e. in a non-additive fashion.

This model of *quantitative inheritance* is now widely accepted and has been adapted to explain the pattern of inheritance observed for many relatively common conditions (ch. 8). These include congenital malformations such as cleft lip and palate and acquired disorders such as hypertension and diabetes mellitus. The prevailing view is that genes at several loci interact to generate a susceptibility to the effects of adverse environmental trigger factors. Recent research has confirmed that many genes are involved in most of these adult onset disorders, although progress in identifying specific susceptibility loci has been disappointingly slow. It has also emerged that in some conditions, such as type I diabetes mellitus, different genes can exert major or minor effects in determining susceptibility (p. 133). Overall multifactorial conditions are now known to make a very major contribution to chronic illness in adult life (ch. 14).

ACQUIRED SOMATIC GENETIC DISEASE

Not all genetic errors are present from conception. Many billions of cell divisions (mitoses) occur in the course of an average human lifetime. During each *mitosis* there is an opportunity for both single gene mutations to occur, because of DNA copy errors, and for numerical chromosome abnormalities to arise as a result of errors in chromosome separation. Accumulating somatic mutations and chromosome abnormalities are now known to play a major role in causing cancer (ch. 13) and they probably also explain the rising incidence with age of many other serious illnesses as well as the ageing process itself.

DEFINITIONS

Before considering the impact of hereditary disease it is necessary to introduce a few definitions.

INCIDENCE

Incidence refers to the rate at which new cases occur. Thus if the birth incidence of a particular condition equals 1 in 1000, then on average 1 in every 1000 newborn infants is affected.

PREVALENCE

This refers to the proportion of a population affected at any one time. The prevalence of a genetic disease will usually be less than its birth incidence, either because life expectancy is reduced or because the condition shows a delayed age of onset.

FREQUENCY

Frequency is a general term which lacks scientific specificity, although this word is often taken as being synonymous with incidence when calculating gene 'frequencies' (ch. 7).

CONGENITAL

Congenital means that a condition is present at birth. Thus cleft palate represents an example of a congenital malformation. Not all genetic disorders are congenital in terms of age of onset (for example, Huntington's disease), nor are all congenital abnormalities genetic in origin (e.g. fetal disruptions as discussed in Chapter 15).

THE IMPACT OF GENETIC DISEASE

During the twentieth century improvements in all areas of medicine, most notably public health and therapeutics, resulted in changing patterns of disease, with increasing recognition of the role of genetic factors in causing illness at all ages. For some parameters, such as perinatal mortality, the actual numbers of cases with exclusively genetic causes have probably remained constant but their *relative* contribution to overall figures has increased as other causes such as infection have declined. For other conditions, such as the chronic diseases of adult life, the overall contribution of genetics has almost certainly increased as greater life expectancy has provided more opportunity for adverse genetic environmental interaction to manifest itself, for example in coronary heart disease and diabetes mellitus.

An indication of the incidence of genetic disorders and their impact on health at all ages can be gauged from the following observations.

SPONTANEOUS MISCARRIAGES

A chromosome abnormality is present in 40–50% of all recognized first-trimester pregnancy loss. Approximately 1 in 6 of all pregnancies results in spontaneous miscarriage, thus around 5–7% of all recognized conceptions are chromosomally abnormal. This figure would almost certainly be much higher if unrecognized pregnancies could also be included.

NEWBORN INFANTS

Of all neonates, 2–3% have at least one major congenital abnormality, at least 50% of which are caused exclusively or partially by genetic factors (ch. 15). The incidences of chromosome abnormalities and single gene disorders in neonates are approximately $\frac{1}{200}$ and $\frac{1}{100}$ respectively.

CHILDHOOD

Genetic disorders account for 50% of all childhood blindness, 50% of all childhood deafness and 50% of all cases of severe mental retardation. Genetic disorders and congenital malformations together also account for 30% of all childhood hospital admissions and 40–50% of all childhood deaths.

ADULT LIFE

Approximately 1% of all malignancy is caused by single gene inheritance, and between 5% and 10% of common cancers such as breast, colon and ovary have a strong genetic component. By the age of 25, 5% of the population will have a disorder in which genetic factors play an important role. Taking into account the genetic contribution to cancer and cardiovascular diseases, such as coronary artery occlusion and hypertension, it has been estimated that over 50% of the older adult population will have a genetically determined medical problem.

MAJOR NEW DEVELOPMENTS

The study of genetics and its role in causing human disease is now widely acknowledged as being among the most exciting and influential areas of medical research. Since 1962 when Francis Crick, James Watson and Maurice Wilkins gained acclaim for their elucidation

of the structure of DNA, the Nobel Prize for Medicine and/or Physiology has been won on 15 occasions by scientists working in human and molecular genetics or related fields (Table 1.1). These pioneering studies have spawned a thriving molecular technology industry with applications as diverse as the development of genetically modified disease-resistant crops, the use of genetically engineered animals to produce therapeutic drugs, and the possible introduction of DNA based vaccines for conditions such as malaria.

THE HUMAN GENOME PROJECT

This has been likened to the Apollo moon mission in terms of its complexity, although in practical terms the benefits are likely to be much more tangible. Essentially

Table 1.1   Genetic discoveries which have led to the award of the Nobel Prize for Medicine and/or Physiology 1962–1999

Year	Prize-winners	Discovery
1962	Francis Crick James Watson Maurice Wilkins	The molecular structure of DNA
1965	Francois Jacob Jacques Monod André Lwoff	Genetic regulation
1966	Peyton Rous	Oncogenic viruses
1968	Robert Holley Gobind Khorana Marshall Nirenberg	Deciphering of the genetic code
1975	David Baltimore Renato Dulbecco Howard Temin	Interaction between tumour viruses and nuclear DNA
1978	Werner Arber Daniel Nathans Hamilton Smith	Restriction endonucleases
1980	Baruj Benacerraf Jean Dausset George Snell	Genetic control of immunological response
1983	Barbara McClintock	Mobile genes (transposons)
1985	Michael Brown Joseph Goldstein	Cell receptors in familial hypercholesterolaemia
1987	Tonegawa Susumu	Genetic aspects of antibodies
1989	Michael Bishop Harold Varmus	Study of oncogenes
1993	Richard Roberts Phillip Sharp	'Split genes'
1995	Edward Lewis Christiane Nüsslein-Volhard Eric Wieschaus	Homeotic and other developmental genes
1997	Stanley Prusiner	Prions
1999	Günter Blobel	Protein transport signalling

it involves a major international collaboration to sequence the 3 billion base pairs that make up the human genome and in so doing to facilitate the isolation of the 50 000–100 000 coding genes which provide the blueprint for human life (p. 321). In the short term improved knowledge of gene structure will enable better diagnosis and counselling for families with a genetic disease. In the longer term an improved understanding of how genes are expressed will inevitably lead to the development of new strategies for the prevention and treatment of both single gene and polygenic disorders. It was initially anticipated that this project would be completed by 2005. However improvements in technology promise a much shorter time frame; by the end of 1999 sequencing of chromosome 22 had been completed and over one-third of the total genome (i.e. 1 billion base pairs!) had been sequenced. The draft DNA sequence of the whole human genome was successfully completed in 2000.

GENE THERAPY

Most genetic disease is resistant to conventional treatment so that the prospect of successfully modifying the genetic code in a patient's cells is extremely attractive. Despite major investment and extensive research success in humans has so far been limited to a few very rare immunological disorders. For more common conditions, such as cystic fibrosis, major problems have been encountered such as targeting the correct cell populations, overcoming the body's natural defence barriers and identifying suitably non-immunogenic vectors. However, the availability of mouse models for genetic disorders such as cystic fibrosis (p. 276) and Duchenne muscular dystrophy (p. 280) has greatly enhanced research opportunities and there is universal optimism that in the short to medium term the prospects for successful gene therapy are good (p. 327).

THE INTERNET

The availability of information in genetics has been greatly enhanced by the development of several excellent online databases, a selection of which are listed in the appendix. These are updated regularly and provide instant access to a vast amount of contemporary information. For the basic scientist facilities such as the Genome Database and GenBank enable rapid determination of whether a particular gene has been cloned, together with details of its sequence, location and pattern of expression. For the clinician OMIM offers a full account of the important genetic aspects of all Mendelian disorders together with pertinent clinical details and extensive references. Although it is unlikely that more traditional

sources of information, such as this textbook, shall become totally obsolete, it is clear that only electronic technology can hope to match the explosive pace of developments in all areas of genetic research.

ELEMENTS

1 A characteristic manifest in a hybrid (heterozygote) is dominant. A recessive characteristic is expressed only in an individual with two copies of the gene, i.e. a homozygote.

2 Mendel proposed that each individual has two genes for each characteristic: one is inherited from each parent and one is transmitted to each child. Genes at different loci act and segregate independently.

3 Chromosome separation at cell division facilitates gene segregation.

4 Genetic disorders are present in at least 2% of all neonates, account for 50% of childhood blindness, deafness, mental retardation and deaths, and affect 5% of the population by the age of 25.

5 Molecular genetics is at the forefront of medical research. The human genome project and the development of gene therapy represent major new initiatives which will revolutionize the management and treatment of genetic diseases.

FURTHER READING

Baird P A, Anderson T W, Newcombe H B, Lowry R B 1988 Genetic disorders in children and young adults: a population study. Am J Hum Genet 42: 677–693
A comprehensive study of the incidence of genetic disease in a large Western urban population.
Dunham I, Shimizu N, Roe B A et al 1999 The DNA sequence of human chromosome 22. Nature 402: 489–495
The first report of the complete sequencing of a human chromosome.
Emery A E H 1989 Portraits in medical genetics — Joseph Adams 1756–1818. J Med Genet 26: 116–118
An account of the life of a London doctor who made remarkable observations about hereditary disease in his patients.
Garrod A E 1902 The incidence of alkaptonuria: a study in chemical individuality. Lancet ii: 1916–1920
A landmark paper in which Garrod proposed that alkaptonuria could show Mendelian inheritance and also noted that 'the mating of first cousins gives exactly the conditions most likely to enable a rare, and usually recessive, character to show itself'.
McKusick V A 1998 Mendelian inheritance in man, 11th edn. Johns Hopkins University Press, Baltimore
An exhaustive three-volume catalogue of all known conditions and traits showing Mendelian inheritance.

On-line mendelian inheritance in man, OMIM (TM). Johns Hopkins University, Baltimore. World Wide Web URL:http://www3.ncbi.nlm.nih.gov/omim/
Regularly updated online version of Mendelian inheritance in man.
Orel V 1995 Gregor Mendel: the first geneticist. Oxford University Press, Oxford

A detailed biography of the life and work of the Moravian monk who was described by his abbot as being 'very diligent in the study of the sciences but much less fitted for work as a parish priest'.
Ouellette F 1999 Internet resources for the clinical geneticist. Clin Genet 56: 179–185
A guide to how to access some of the most useful online databases.

The cellular and molecular basis of inheritance

The hereditary material is present in the nucleus of the cell, while protein synthesis takes place in the cytoplasm. What is the chain of events which leads from the gene to the final product?

This chapter covers basic cellular biology outlining the structure of DNA, the process of DNA replication, the types of DNA sequences, gene structure, the genetic code, the processes of transcription and translation, the various types of mutations, mutagenic agents and DNA repair.

THE CELL

Within each cell of the body, visible with the light microscope, is the *cytoplasm* and a darkly staining body, the *nucleus*, the latter containing the hereditary material in the form of *chromosomes* (Fig. 2.1). The phospholipid bilayer of the plasma membrane protects the interior of the cell but remains selectively permeable and has integral proteins involved in recognition and signalling between cells. The nucleus has a darkly staining area, the *nucleolus*. The nucleus is surrounded by a membrane, the *nuclear envelope*, which separates it from the cytoplasm but still allows communication through *nuclear pores*.

The cytoplasm contains the *cytosol* which is semifluid in consistency containing both soluble elements and cytoskeletal structural elements. In addition, in the cytoplasm there is a complex arrangement of very fine, highly convoluted interconnecting channels, the *endoplasmic reticulum*. The endoplasmic reticulum, in association with the *ribosomes*, is involved in the biosynthesis of proteins and lipids. Also situated within the cytoplasm are other even more minute cellular organelles which can only be visualized with an electron microscope. These include the Golgi apparatus which is responsible for the secretion of cellular products, the mitochondria which are involved in energy production through the oxidative phosphorylation metabolic pathways and the

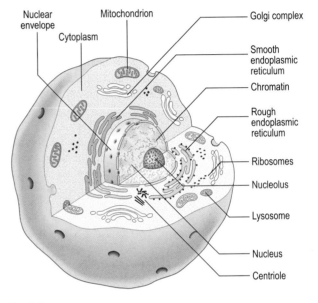

Fig. 2.1
Diagrammatic representation of an animal cell.

peroxisomes and the lysozomes, both of which are involved in the degradation and disposal of cellular waste material and toxic molecules.

DNA: THE HEREDITARY MATERIAL

COMPOSITION

Nucleic acid is composed of a long polymer of individual molecules called *nucleotides*. Each nucleotide is composed of a nitrogenous base, a sugar molecule and a phosphate molecule. The nitrogenous bases fall into two types, *purines* and *pyrimidines*. The purines include adenine and guanine; the pyrimidines include cytosine, thymine and uracil.

There are two different types of nucleic acid, *ribonucleic acid* (RNA) which contains the five carbon sugar ribose and *deoxyribonucleic acid* (DNA) in which the hydroxyl group at the 2′ position of the ribose sugar is replaced by a hydrogen, i.e. an oxygen molecule is lost, hence deoxy. DNA and RNA both contain the purine bases adenine and guanine and the pyrimidine cytosine but thymine occurs only in DNA while uracil is only found in RNA.

RNA is present in the cytoplasm and in particularly high concentrations in the nucleolus of the nucleus. DNA, on the other hand, is found mainly in the chromosomes.

STRUCTURE

For genes to be composed of DNA it is necessary that the latter should have a structure sufficiently versatile to account for the great variety of different genes and yet, at the same time, be able to reproduce itself in such a manner that an identical replica is formed at each cell division. In 1953, Watson and Crick, based on X-ray diffraction studies by themselves and others, proposed a structure for the DNA molecule which fulfilled all the essential requirements. They suggested that the DNA molecule is composed of two chains of nucleotides arranged in a double helix. The backbone of each chain is formed by phosphodiester bonds between the 3′ and 5′ carbons of adjacent sugars, the two chains being held together by hydrogen bonds between the nitrogenous bases which point in towards the centre of the helix. Each DNA chain has a polarity determined by the orientation of the sugar–phosphate backbone. The chain end terminated by the 5′ carbon atom of the sugar molecule is referred to as the 5′ end, and the end terminated by the 3′ carbon atom is called the 3′ end. In the DNA duplex the 5′ end of one strand is opposite the 3′ end of the other, i.e. they have opposite orientations and are said to be *antiparallel*.

The arrangement of the bases in the DNA molecule is not random: a purine in one chain always pairs with a pyrimidine in the other chain with specific pairing of the base pairs: guanine in one chain always pairs with cytosine in the other chain and adenine always pairs with thymine, i.e. this base pairing forming *complementary strands* (Fig. 2.2). For their work Watson and Crick, along with Maurice Wilkins, were awarded the Nobel Prize for Medicine or Physiology in 1962 (p. 8).

REPLICATION

The process of *DNA replication* provides an answer to the question of how genetic information is transmitted from one generation to the next. During nuclear division the

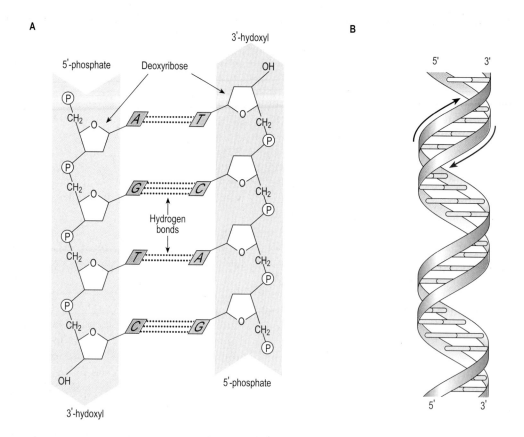

Fig. 2.2
DNA double helix. (A) Sugar–phosphate backbone and nucleotide pairing of the DNA double helix (P = phosphate; A = adenine; T = thymine; G = guanine; C = cytosine). (B) Representation of the DNA double helix.

two strands of the DNA double helix separate through the action of enzyme DNA helicase, each DNA strand directing the synthesis of a complementary DNA strand through specific base pairing, resulting in two daughter DNA duplexes which are identical to the original parent molecule. In this way, when cells divide, the genetic information is conserved and transmitted unchanged to each daughter cell. The process of DNA replication is termed *semiconservative*, as only one strand of each resultant daughter molecule is newly synthesized.

DNA replication, through the action of the enzyme DNA polymerase, takes place at multiple points known as *origins of replication* forming bifurcated Y-shaped structures known as *replication forks*. The synthesis of both complementary antiparallel DNA strands occurs in the 5' to 3' direction. One strand, known as the *leading strand*, is synthesized as a continuous process. The other strand, known as the *lagging strand*, is synthesized in pieces called Okazaki fragments which are then joined together as a continuous strand by the enzyme DNA ligase (Fig. 2.3A).

DNA replication progresses in both directions from these points of origin forming bubble-shaped structures, or *replication bubbles* (Fig. 2.3B). Neighbouring replication origins are approximately 50–300 kb apart and occur in clusters or *replication units* of 20–80 origins of replication. DNA replication in individual replication units takes place at different times in the S phase of the cell cycle (p. 40), adjacent replication units fusing until all the DNA is copied forming two complete identical daughter molecules.

CHROMOSOME STRUCTURE

The idea that each chromosome is composed of a single DNA double helix is an oversimplification. A chromosome is very much wider than the diameter of a DNA double helix. In addition, the amount of DNA in the nucleus of each cell in humans means that the total length of DNA contained in the chromosomes, if fully extended, would be several metres long! In fact the total length of the human chromosome complement is less than half a millimetre.

The packaging of DNA into chromosomes involves several orders of DNA coiling and folding. In addition to the primary coiling of the DNA double helix, there is secondary coiling around spherical *histone* 'beads' forming what are called *nucleosomes*. There is a tertiary coiling of the nucleosomes to form the *chromatin fibres* which form long loops on a scaffold of non-histone acidic proteins, which are further wound in a tight coil to make up the chromosome as visualized under the light microscope (Fig. 2.4), the whole structure making up the the so-called *solenoid model* of chromosome structure.

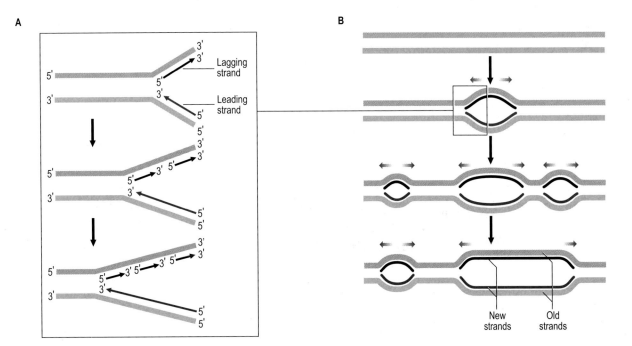

Fig. 2.3
DNA replication. (A) Detailed diagram of DNA replication at the site of origin in the replication fork showing asymmetric strand synthesis with the continuous synthesis of the leading strand and the discontinuous synthesis of the lagging strand with ligation of the Okazaki fragments. (B) Multiple points of origin and semiconservative mode of DNA replication.

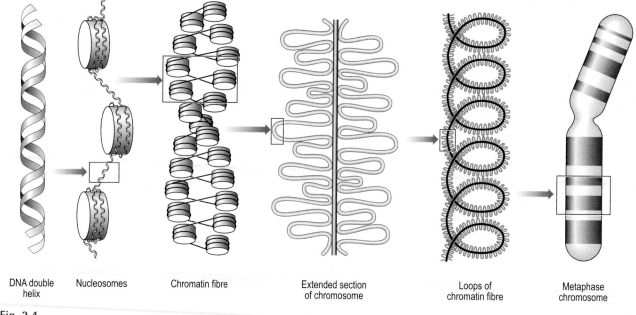

DNA double helix   Nucleosomes   Chromatin fibre   Extended section of chromosome   Loops of chromatin fibre   Metaphase chromosome

Fig. 2.4
Simplified diagram of proposed solenoid model of DNA coiling which leads to the visible structure of the chromosome.

TYPES OF DNA SEQUENCES

DNA, if denatured, will reassociate as a duplex at a rate which is dependent on the proportion of unique and repeat sequences present, the latter occurring more rapidly. Analysis of the results of the kinetics of the reassociation of human DNA have shown that approximately 60–70% of the human *genome* consists of single or low copy number DNA sequences. The remainder of the genome, some 30–40%, consists of either moderately or highly *repetitive DNA* sequences which are not transcribed. This latter portion consists of mainly satellite DNA and interspersed DNA sequences (Table 2.1).

NUCLEAR GENES

It is estimated that there are up to 80 000 genes in the nuclear genome. The distribution of these genes varies greatly between different chromosomes and certain parts of the chromosomes, heterochromatic (p. 30) and centromeric (p. 30) regions containing few, with the majority being located in subtelomeric regions (p. 30).

Unique single copy genes

Most human genes are unique single copy genes coding for polypeptides which are involved in or carry out a variety of cellular functions. These include enzymes, hormones, receptors and structural and regulatory proteins.

Table 2.1   Types of DNA sequences

Nuclear (~3 × 10⁹ bp)
  Genes (50–80 000)
    Unique single copy
    Multigene families
      Classical gene families
      Gene superfamilies
  Extragenic DNA (Unique/low copy number or moderate/highly repetitive)
    Tandem repeat
      Satellite
      Minisatellite
       Telomeric
       Hypervariable
      Microsatellite
    Interspersed
      Short interspersed nuclear elements
      Long interspersed nuclear elements
Mitochondrial (16.6 kb, 37 genes)
  Two rRNA genes
  22 tRNA genes
  13 genes coding for proteins involved in oxidative phosphorylation

Multigene families

Many genes have similar functions, having arisen through gene duplication events with subsequent evolutionary divergence making up what are known as *multigene families*. Some are found physically close together in clusters, e.g. the α- and β-globin gene clusters on chromosomes 16 and 11 (Fig. 2.5), while others are widely dispersed throughout the genome occurring on

Fig. 2.5

Representation of the α- and β-globin regions on chromosomes 16 and 11.

different chromosomes, e.g. the *HOX* homeobox gene family (p. 82).

Multigene families can be split into two types, *classical gene families* which show a high degree of sequence homology and *gene superfamilies* which have limited sequence homology but are functionally related having similar structural domains.

Classical gene families

Examples of classical gene families include the numerous copies of genes coding for the various ribosomal RNAs which are clustered as tandem arrays at the nucleolar organizing regions on the short arms of the five acrocentric chromosomes (p. 30), and the different transfer RNA (p. 18) gene families which are dispersed in numerous clusters throughout the human genome.

Gene superfamilies

Examples of gene superfamilies include the HLA genes on chromosome 6 (p. 181) and the T cell receptor genes which have structural homology with the immunoglobulin (Ig) genes (p. 181). It is believed that these are almost certainly derived from duplication of a precursor gene with subsequent evolutionary divergence forming the Ig superfamily.

Gene structure

The original concept of a gene as a continuous sequence of DNA coding for a protein was turned on its head in the early 1980s by detailed analysis of the structure of

the human β-globin gene. It was revealed that the gene was much longer than necessary to code for the β-globin protein containing non-coding intervening sequences or *introns*, which separate the coding sequences or *exons* (Fig. 2.6). It appears to be the exception for genes in humans to consist of uninterrupted coding sequences (pp. 273, 276, 281). The number and size of introns in various genes in humans are extremely variable, although there is a general trend that the larger the gene, the greater the number and size of the exons. Individual introns can be far larger than the coding sequences and some have been found to contain coding sequences for other genes, i.e. genes occurring within genes (p. 273). Genes in humans do not usually overlap being separated from each other by an average of 30 kb, although some of the genes in the HLA complex (p. 182) have been shown to be overlapping.

Pseudogenes

Particularly fascinating is the occurrence of genes that closely resemble known structural genes but which, in general, are not functionally expressed, so-called *pseudogenes* (p. 141). These are thought to have arisen in two main ways, either by genes undergoing duplication events which are rendered silent through the acquisition of mutations in coding or regulatory elements, or as the result of the insertion of complementary DNA sequences, produced by the action of the enzyme *reverse transcriptase* on a naturally occurring mRNA transcript, which lack the promoter sequences necessary for expression.

EXTRAGENIC DNA

The estimate of 80 000 unique single copy genes in humans, along with the average nuclear gene being 10–15 kb in size, means that they only account for a maximum of one-quarter to one-third of the human genome. The remainder, some 70–75%, of the human genome is made up of repetitive DNA sequences which are predominantly transcriptionally inactive.

There is at present no entirely satisfactory explanation for the vast amount of repetitive DNA sequences in the

Fig. 2.6

Representation of a typical human structural gene.

genome which appears to have little or no obvious function and does not appear to contribute to the *phenotype*. It has even been referred to as *selfish DNA*, the implication being that it preserves itself as a result of selection within the genome.

Tandemly repeated DNA sequences

Tandemly repeated DNA sequences consist of blocks of tandem repeats of non-coding DNA which can be either highly dispersed or restricted in their location in the genome. Tandemly repeated DNA sequences can be divided into three subgroups: satellite, minisatellite and microsatellite DNA.

Satellite DNA

Satellite DNA accounts for approximately 10–15% of the repetitive DNA sequences of the human genome and consists of very large series of simple or moderately complex short tandemly repeated DNA sequences which are transcriptionally inactive and are clustered around the centromeres of certain chromosomes. This class of DNA sequences can be separated on density-gradient centrifugation as a shoulder, or 'satellite', to the main peak of genomic DNA and has therefore been referred to as satellite DNA.

Minisatellite DNA

Minisatellite DNA consists of two families of tandemly repeated short DNA sequences, telomeric and hypervariable minisatellite DNA sequences which are transcriptionally inactive.

Telomeric DNA
The terminal portion of the telomeres of the chromosomes (p. 30) contains 10–15 kb of tandem repeats of a 6 bp DNA sequence, known as *telomeric DNA*. The telomeric repeat sequences are necessary for chromosomal integrity in replication and are added to the chromosome by a specialized enzyme known as telomerase (p. 30).

Hypervariable minisatellite DNA
Hypervariable minisatellite DNA is made up of highly polymorphic DNA sequences consisting of short tandem repeats of a common core sequence, the highly variable number of repeat units in different hypervariable minisatellites forming the basis of DNA fingerprinting used in forensic and paternity testing (p. 67). Although often located near the telomeres, hypervariable minisatellite DNA also occurs at other locations in the chromosomes.

Microsatellite DNA

Microsatellite DNA consists of tandem single, di-, tri- and tetranucleotide repeat base pair sequences located throughout the genome. Microsatellite repeats rarely occur within coding sequences but trinucleotide repeats in or near genes are associated with certain inherited disorders (p. 22).

DNA microsatellites are highly polymorphic (p. 120), i.e. the number of CA repeats vary between persons, and can be used in linkage studies in gene mapping (p. 67). This variation in repeat number is thought to arise by incorrect pairing of the tandem repeats of the two complementary DNA strands during DNA replication or what is known as *slipped strand mispairing*. Duplications or deletions of longer sequences of tandemly repeated DNA are thought to arise through unequal cross-over of non-allelic DNA sequences on chromatids of homologous chromosomes or sister chromatids (p. 21).

Highly repeated interspersed repetitive DNA sequences

Approximately one-third of the human genome is made up of two main classes of short and long repetitive DNA sequences which are interspersed throughout the genome.

Short interspersed nuclear elements

About 5% of the human genome consists of some 750 000 copies of *short interspersed nuclear elements* or *SINEs*. The most common are DNA sequences of approximately 300 bp which have sequence similarity to a signal recognition particle involved in protein synthesis. They are called *Alu repeats* because they contain an *AluI* restriction enzyme recognition site.

Long interspersed nuclear elements

About 5% of the DNA of the human genome is made up of *long interspersed nuclear elements* or *LINEs*. The most commonly occurring LINE, known as LINE-1 or an L1 element, consists of over 100 000 copies of a slightly longer DNA sequence of approximately 6000 bp which occurs approximately once every 50 kb and encodes a reverse transcriptase.

The function of these interspersed repeat sequences is not clear at present. Members of the *Alu* repeat family are flanked by short direct repeat sequences and therefore resemble unstable DNA sequences called transposable elements or *transposons*. Transposons, originally identified in maize by Barbara McClintock (p. 8), move spontaneously throughout the genome from one chromosome location to another and appear to be ubiquitous in the plant and animal kingdoms. It is postulated that

Alu repeats could promote unequal recombination which could lead to pathogenic mutations (p. 21) or provide selective advantage in evolution by gene duplication. Both *Alu* and LINE-1 repeat elements have been implicated as a cause of mutation in inherited human disease (p. 70).

MITOCHONDRIAL DNA

In addition to nuclear DNA, the several thousand mitochondria of each cell possess their own 16.6 kb circular double stranded DNA, *mitochondrial DNA* or mtDNA. The mitochondrial DNA genome is very compact containing little repetitive DNA and codes for 37 genes which include two types of ribosomal RNA, 22 transfer RNAs (p. 18) and 13 protein subunits for enzymes, such as cytochrome b and cytochrome oxidase, which are involved in the energy producing oxidative phosphorylation pathways. The genetic code of the mtDNA differs slightly from nuclear DNA.

The mitochondria of the fertilized zygote are inherited exclusively from the oocyte leading to the maternal pattern of inheritance of mitochondrially inherited disorders (p. 110).

TRANSCRIPTION

The process whereby genetic information is transmitted from DNA to RNA is called *transcription*. The information stored in the genetic code is transmitted from the DNA of a gene to *messenger RNA* or mRNA. Every base in the mRNA molecule is complementary to a corresponding base in the DNA of the gene but with uracil replacing thymine in mRNA. mRNA is single stranded being synthesized by the enzyme RNA polymerase which adds the appropriate complementary ribonucleotide to the 3' end of the RNA chain.

In any particular gene only one DNA strand of the double helix acts as the so-called *template strand*. The transcribed mRNA molecule is a copy of the complementary strand or what is called the *sense strand* of the DNA double helix. The template strand is sometimes called the *antisense strand*. The particular strand of the DNA double helix used for RNA synthesis appears to differ throughout different regions of the genome.

POST-TRANSCRIPTIONAL PROCESSING

Before the primary mRNA molecule leaves the nucleus, it undergoes a number of modifications or what is known as *post-transcriptional processing*.

mRNA splicing

After transcription, the non-coding introns in the primary mRNA are excised, and the non-contiguous coding exons are spliced together to form a shorter mature mRNA before its transportation to the ribosomes in the cytoplasm for translation. The process is known as *mRNA splicing* (Fig. 2.7). The boundary between the

Fig. 2.7

Transcription, post-transcriptional processing, translation and post-translational processing.

introns and exons consists of a 5′ donor GT dinucleotide and a 3′ acceptor AG dinucleotide. These, along with surrounding short *splicing consensus sequences*, another intronic sequence known as the *splicing branch site*, *small nuclear RNA molecules* and associated proteins are necessary for the splicing process.

5′ capping

Shortly after transcription the nascent mRNA is modified by the addition of a methylated guanine nucleotide to the 5′ end of the molecule by an unusual 5′ to 5′ phosphodiester bond, the so-called *5′ cap*. The 5′ cap is thought to facilitate transport of the mRNA to the cytoplasm and attachment to the ribosomes as well as protect the RNA transcript from degradation by endogenous cellular exonucleases.

Polyadenylation

The cleavage of the 3′ end of the mRNA molecule from the DNA involves the addition of approximately 200 adenylate residues, the so-called *poly(A) tail*, after cleavage of the RNA transcript at a site downstream from a specific six nucleotide sequence. The addition of the poly(A) tail is thought to facilitate transport of the mRNA to the cytoplasm and translation.

TRANSLATION

Translation is the transmission of the genetic information from mRNA to protein. Newly processed mRNA is transported from the nucleus to the cytoplasm where it becomes associated with the *ribosomes* which are the site of protein synthesis. Ribosomes are made up of two different sized subunits which consist of four different types of *ribosomal RNA* (rRNA) molecules, and a large number of ribosomal specific proteins. Groups of ribosomes associated with the same molecule of mRNA are referred to as *polyribosomes* or *polysomes*. In the ribosomes the mRNA forms the template for producing the specific sequence of amino acids of a particular *polypepetide*.

TRANSFER RNA

In the cytoplasm there is another form of RNA called *transfer RNA* or tRNA. The incorporation of amino acids into a *polypeptide* chain requires the amino acids to be covalently bound by reacting with ATP to the specific tRNA molecule by the activity of the enzyme aminoacyl tRNA synthetase. The ribosome, with its associated rRNAs, moves along the mRNA, the amino acids linking

up by the formation of peptide bonds through the action of the enzyme peptidyl transferase to form a polypeptide chain (Fig. 2.8).

POST-TRANSLATIONAL MODIFICATION

Many proteins, before they attain their normal structure or functional activity, undergo *post-translational modification* which can include chemical modification of amino acid side-chains (e.g. hydroxylation, methylation, etc.), addition of carbohydrate or lipid moieties (e.g. glycosylation) or proteolytic cleavage of polypeptides (e.g. the conversion of proinsulin to insulin).

This post-translational modification, along with certain short amino acid sequences known as *localization sequences* in the newly synthesized proteins, results in transport to specific cellular locations, e.g. the nucleus, or their secretion.

THE GENETIC CODE

Twenty different amino acids are found in proteins and, as DNA is composed of four different nitrogenous bases, then obviously a single base cannot specify one amino acid. If two bases were to specify one amino acid, there would only be 4^2 or 16 possible combinations. If, however, three bases specified one amino acid then the possible number of combinations of the four bases would be 4^3 or 64. This is more than enough to account for all the 20 known amino acids and is known as the *genetic code*.

TRIPLET CODONS

The triplet of nucleotide bases in the mRNA which codes for a particular amino acid is called a *codon*. Each triplet codon in sequence codes for a specific amino acid in sequence and so the genetic code is non-overlapping. The order of the triplet codons in a gene is known as the translational *reading frame*. However, some amino acids are coded for by more than one triplet and so the code is said to be *degenerate* (Table 2.2). Each tRNA species for a particular amino acid has a specific trinucleotide sequence called the *anticodon* which is complementary to the codon of the mRNA. Although there are 64 codons, there are only 30 cytoplasmic tRNAs, the anitcodons of a number of the tRNAs recognizing codons which differ at the position of the third base with guanine being able to pair with uracil as well as cytosine. Termination of translation of the mRNA is signalled by the presence of one of the three *stop* or *termination codons*.

The genetic code of mtDNA differs from the nuclear genome. Eight of the 22 tRNAs are able to recognize

Fig. 2.8
Representation of the way in which genetic information is translated into protein.

codons which differ only at the third base of the codon, 14 can recognize pairs of codons which are identical at the first two bases with either a purine or pyrimidine for the third base, the other four codons acting as stop codons (Table 2.2).

REGULATION OF GENE EXPRESSION

Many cellular processes and therefore the genes that are expressed are common to all cells, for example ribosomal, chromosomal and cytoskeleton proteins, constituting what are called the *housekeeping genes*. Some cells express large quantities of a specific protein in certain tissues or at specific times in development, e.g. haemoglobin in red blood cells (p. 139). This differential control of gene expression can occur at a variety of stages.

CONTROL OF TRANSCRIPTION

The control of transcription can be affected permanently or reversibly by a variety of factors, both environmental (e.g. hormones) and genetic (cell signalling). This occurs through a number of different mechanisms which include signalling molecules which bind to regulatory sequences in the DNA known as *response elements*, intracellular

Table 2.2   The genetic code of the nuclear and mitochondrial genome. (Differences in mitochondrial genetic code are in *italics*.)

1st base	2nd base U	C	A	G	3rd base
U	Phenylalanine	Serine	Tyrosine	Cysteine	U
	Phenylalanine	Serine	Tyrosine	Cysteine	C
	Leucine	Serine	Stop	Stop (*Tryptophan*)	A
	Leucine	Serine	Stop	Tryptophan	G
C	Leucine	Proline	Histidine	Arginine	U
	Leucine	Proline	Histidine	Arginine	C
	Leucine	Proline	Glutamine	Arginine	A
	Leucine	Proline	Glutamine	Arginine	G
A	Isoleucine	Threonine	Asparagine	Serine	U
	Isoleucine	Threonine	Asparagine	Serine	C
	Isoleucine (*Methionine*)	Threonine	Lysine	Arginine (*Stop*)	A
	Methionine	Threonine	Lysine	Arginine (*Stop*)	G
G	Valine	Alanine	Aspartic acid	Glycine	U
	Valine	Alanine	Aspartic acid	Glycine	C
	Valine	Alanine	Glutamic acid	Glycine	A
	Valine	Alanine	Glutamic acid	Glycine	G

receptors known as *hormone nuclear receptors* and receptors for specific ligands on the cell surface involved in the process of *signal transduction*.

All these mechanisms affect transcription through the binding of transcription factors to short specific DNA promoter elements which are located within 200 bp 5′ or *upstream* of most eukaryotic genes in the so-called *promoter region* which leads to activation of RNA polymerase (Fig. 2.9). This includes the TATA (or Hogness), the GC (or GGGCGGG *consensus sequence*) and the CAAT boxes. The TATA box which is about 25 bp upstream of the transcription start site is involved in the initiation of transcription at a basal constitutive level and mutations in it can lead to alteration of the transcription start site. The GC box which is about 80 bp upstream and the CAAT box increase the basal level of transriptional activity of the TATA box.

The regulatory elements in the promoter region are said to be *cis-acting*, that is, they only affect the expression of the adjacent gene on the same DNA duplex, while the transcription factors are said to be *trans-acting*, acting on both copies of a gene on each chromosome being synthesized from genes which are located at a distance. DNA sequences which increase transcriptional activity, such as the GC and CAAT boxes, are known as *enhancers*. There are also negative regulatory elements or *silencers* which inhibit transcription. In addition, there are short sequences of DNA, usually 500 bp to 3 kb in size, which are known as *boundary elements*, which block or inhibit the influence of regulatory elements of adjacent genes.

TRANSCRIPTION FACTORS

An increasing number of genes are being identified which code for gene regulatory proteins, which have DNA binding activity to short nucleotide sequences usually mediated through α helical protein motifs, constituting what are known as *transcription factors*. These gene regulatory proteins have a transcriptional activation domain and one of four main types of DNA binding domains. The most common type of gene regulatory proteins are the *helix-turn-helix proteins*, so named because they are made up of two α helices connected by a short chain of amino acids which make up the 'turn'.

Perhaps not surprisingly, structural analysis of the homeodomain sequence of the homeotic genes (p. 82) has revealed that they contain a helix-turn-helix motif. Analysis of other gene regulatory proteins has shown them to contain one of three other types of DNA binding motifs which include the *zinc finger*, *leucine zipper* or *helix-loop-helix* motifs, so named as a result of specific structural features (p. 85).

POST-TRANSCRIPTIONAL CONTROL OF GENE EXPRESSION

Regulation of expression of most genes occurs at the level of regulation of transcription but can also occur at the levels of RNA processing, RNA transport, mRNA degradation and translation. While examples of control of gene expression occurring at the level of RNA processing through either alternative RNA splicing or editing have been reported, e.g. the HLA class I and II genes (p. 181) and Wilms' tumour gene (p. 254), examples of the latter three mechanisms are, at present, less well documented.

RNA-DIRECTED DNA SYNTHESIS

The process of the transfer of the genetic information from DNA to RNA to protein has been called the *central dogma*. It was initially believed that genetic information was only transferred from DNA to RNA and thence translated into protein. However, there is evidence from the study of certain types of virus — retroviruses — that genetic information can occasionally flow in the reverse direction, i.e. from RNA to DNA (p. 191). This is referred to as *RNA-directed DNA synthesis*. It has been suggested that regions of DNA in normal cells serve as templates for the synthesis of RNA which in turn then acts as a template for the synthesis of DNA which later becomes integrated into the nuclear DNA of other cells. Homology between human and retroviral oncogene sequences could reflect this process (p. 191) which could be an important therapeutic approach for the treatment of inherited disease in humans (p. 325).

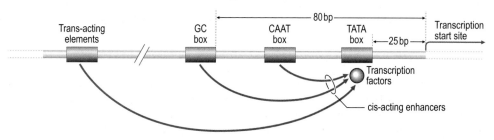

Fig. 2.9
Diagrammatic representation of the factors regulating gene expression.

MUTATIONS

A *mutation* is defined as a heritable alteration or change in the genetic material. Mutations are usually harmful. Mutations can arise through exposure to mutagenic agents (p. 24) but the vast majority occur spontaneously through errors in DNA replication and repair. In humans, although mutations can occur either in non-coding or coding sequences, it is only when they occur in the latter that they are recognized through the deleterious consequences commonly recognized as an inherited disorder or disease.

A mutation arising in a *somatic cell* cannot be transmitted to offspring, whereas if it occurs in *gonadal tissue* or a *gamete* it can be transmitted to future generations. It is estimated that each individual carries up to six lethal or semilethal recessive mutant alleles which in the homozygous state would have very serious effects. These are conservative estimates and the actual figure could be many times greater. Harmful alleles of all kinds constitute the so-called *genetic load* of the population.

TYPES OF MUTATIONS

Although mutations can traditionally be considered in two main groups, either microscopically detectable gross structural chromosomal changes (p. 46) or submicroscopic alterations involving one or a small number of nucleotides, they can also be considered in two main classes according to how they are transmitted (Table 2.3). Until recently, mutations had been considered to be transmitted unaltered as what are termed *fixed* or *stable mutations*. More recently a new class of mutations, known as *dynamic* or *unstable mutations*, have been demonstrated to undergo further alteration as they are transmitted in families, providing an explanation for unusual phenomena in certain patterns of inheritance within families.

Fixed/stable mutations

Fixed/stable point mutations can be classified according to the specific molecular changes at the DNA level. These include single base pair substitutions, insertions, deletions or duplications of part of a gene or DNA sequence.

Substitutions

A *substitution* is the replacement of a single nucleotide by another. These are the most common type of mutation. If the substitution involves replacement by the same type of nucleotide, i.e. a pyrimidine for a pyrimidine (C for T

Table 2.3   The main classes, groups and types of mutations and effects on protein product

Class	Group	Type	Effect on protein product
Stable/fixed	Synonymous	Substitution	Silent — same amino acid
	Non-synonymous	Substitution	
		Missense	Altered amino acid
		Non-conservative	Altered activity, function or stability
		Conservative	No effect
		Nonsense	Stop codon — premature termination with loss-of-function/activity/stability
		Deletion/insertion	
		Multiple of 3 (codon)	Deletion/insertion of one or more amino acid(s) in protein — altered activity/function/stability
		Not multiple of 3	Altered reading frame or frameshift, premature termination of protein — altered amino acid sequence, loss-of-function/activity/stability
Dynamic/unstable	Triplet repeat	Expansion	Altered gene expression, reduced transcription or translation, altered transcript — altered function/activity/stability

or vice versa) or a purine for a purine (A for G or vice versa), this is termed a *transition*. Substitution of a pyrimidine by a purine or vice versa is termed a *transversion*. Transitions occur more frequently than transversions. This could be accounted for by the relatively high frequency of C to T transitions which is likely to be the result of the nucleotides cytosine and gunanine occurring together, or what are known as *CpG dinucleotides* (p represents the phosphate) frequently being methylated in genomic DNA with spontaneous deamination of cytosine converting them to thymine. CpG dinucleotides have been termed 'hot spots' for mutation.

Deletions

A *deletion* involves the loss of one or more nucleotides. If it occurs in coding sequences and involves one, two or more nucleotides which are not a multiple of three, it will disrupt the reading frame (p. 18).

Insertions

An *insertion* involves the addition of one or more nucleotides into a gene. Again, if an insertion occurs in a coding sequence and involves one, two or more nucleotides which are not a multiple of three, it will disrupt the reading frame (p. 18).

Dynamic/unstable mutations

A new class of mutation has recently been identified which has emerged as an important and unexpected cause of inherited disease in humans. These have been called *unstable* or *dynamic mutations* and consist of triplet repeat sequences which, in affected persons, occur in increased copy number when compared to the general population. Increase in the copy number of triplet repeat sequences, which is referred to as *triplet amplification or expansion*, has been identified as the mutational basis for a number of different single gene disorders including Huntington's disease (p. 266), Fragile X mental retardation (p. 258) and myotonic dystrophy (p. 269) (Table 2.4).

The mechanism by which amplification or expansion of the triplet repeat sequence occurs is not clear at present. Triplet repeats below a certain length for each disorder are faithfully transmitted in mitosis and meiosis. Above a certain repeat number for each disorder they are more likely to be transmitted unstably, usually with an increase or decrease in repeat number. A variety of possible explanations have been offered as to how the increase in triplet repeat number occurs. These include unequal cross-over or unequal sister chromatid exchange (pp. 41, 263) in non-replicating DNA and slipped strand mispairing and polymerase slippage in replicating DNA.

Triplet repeat expansions usually take place over a number of generations within a family, providing an explanation for some unusual aspects of patterns of inheritance (p. 106) as well as possibly being the basis of the previously unexplained phenomenon of *anticipation* (p. 107). There is, at present, no convincing explanation of how such triplet expansions lead to the disease features in any of these disorders, the triplet expansions in some disorders occurring within the coding sequence and in others 5' or 3' to the gene, although in Fragile X mental retardation the triplet expansion results in methylation which leads to inactivation of the gene. It is of interest that to date all the disorders which are caused by triplet repeat expansion appear to be neurological disorders or have serious central nervous system involvement.

STRUCTURAL EFFECTS OF MUTATIONS ON THE PROTEIN

Mutations can also be subdivided into two main groups according to the effect on the polypeptide sequence of the encoded protein, being either synonymous or non-synonymous.

Synonymous/silent mutations

If a mutation does not alter the polypeptide product of the gene, this is termed a *synonymous* or *silent mutation*. A single base pair substitution, particularly if it occurs in the third position of a codon because of the degeneracy of the genetic code, will often result in another triplet which codes for the same amino acid with no alteration in the properties of the resulting protein.

Table 2.4 Diseases arising from triplet repeat expansion

Disease	Repeat sequence	Repeat number	Mutation number	Repeat location
Huntington's disease (HD)	CAG	9–35	37–100	Coding
Myotonic dystrophy (DM)	CTG	5–35	50–4000	3' UTR
Fragile X site A (FRAXA)	CGG	10–50	200–2000	5' UTR
Kennedy disease (SBMA)	CAG	17–24	40–55	Coding
Spino-cerebellar ataxia 1 (SCA1)	CAG	19–36	43–81	Coding
Spino-cerebellar ataxia 2 (SCA2)	CAG	15–24	35–39	Coding
Machado–Joseph disease (MJD, SCA3)	CAG	12–36	67–>79	Coding
Spino-cerebellar ataxia 6 (SCA6)	CAG	4–16	21–27	Coding
Spino-cerebellar ataxia 7 (SCA7)	CAG	7–35	37–200	Coding
Spino-cerebellar ataxia 8 (SCA8)	CTG	16–37	100–>500	UTR
Dentatorubral-pallidoluysian atrophy (DRPLA)	CAG	7–23	49–>75	Coding
Friedreich's ataxia (FA)	GAA	17–22	200–900	Intronic
Fragile X site E (FRAXE)	CCG	6–25	>200	Promoter
Fragile X site F (FRAXF)	GCC	6–29	>500	?
Fragile 16 site A (FRA16A)	CCG	16–49	1000–2000	?

UTR = untranslated region.

Non-synonymous mutations

If a mutation leads to an alteration in the encoded polypeptide, it is known as a *non-synonymous mutation*. Non-synonymous mutations are observed to occur less frequently than synonymous mutations. Synonymous mutations will be selectively neutral, while alteration of the amino acid sequence of the protein product of a gene is likely to result in abnormal function which is usually associated with disease or lethality which has an obvious selective disadvantage.

Non-synonymous mutations can occur in one of three main ways.

Missense

A single base pair substitution can result in coding for a different amino acid and the synthesis of an altered protein, a so-called *missense mutation*. If the mutation codes for an amino acid which is chemically dissimilar, e.g. a different charge, the structure of the protein will be altered. This is termed a *non-conservative substitution* and can lead to a gross reduction, or even a complete loss, of biological activity. Single base pair mutations can lead to qualitative rather than quantitative changes in the function of a protein such that it retains its normal biological activity (e.g. enzyme activity) but differs in characteristics such as its mobility on electrophoresis, its pH optimum, or its stability so that it is more rapidly broken down in vivo. Many of the abnormal haemo-globins (p. 142) are the result of missense mutations.

Some single base pair substitutions, although resulting in the replacement by a different amino acid if it is chemically similar, will often have no functional effect. These are termed *conservative substitutions*.

Nonsense

A substitution which leads to the generation of one of the stop codons (Table 2.2) will result in premature termination of translation of a peptide chain or what is termed a *nonsense mutation*. In most cases the shortened chain is unlikely to retain normal biological activity, particularly if the termination codon results in the loss of an important functional domain(s) of the protein.

Frameshift

If a mutation involves the insertion or deletion of nucleotides which are not a multiple of three, it will disrupt the reading frame and constitute what is known as a *frameshift mutation*. The amino acid sequence of the protein subsequent to the mutation bears no resemblance to the normal sequence and is likely to affect its function adversely. In addition, it is not unusual for a frameshift mutation to also result in a stop codon downstream to the mutation leading to premature termination of the encoded polypeptide.

Mutations in non-coding DNA

Mutations in non-coding DNA, in general, would not be expected to have a phenotypic effect unless they occur in the DNA sequences involved in gene regulation, e.g. the TATA box (p. 20), or in the splicing of introns, e.g. the highly conserved GT and AG dinucleotides at the end of introns (p. 18). Mutations in regulatory elements can affect the level of gene expression while mutations in splice junctions can result in coding sequences being lost or intronic sequences being added to the mRNA molecule. Splice junction mutations appear to occur relatively commonly in the collagen genes, some of which are responsible for osteogenesis imperfecta (p. 70).

FUNCTIONAL EFFECTS OF MUTATIONS ON THE PROTEIN

Mutations exert their phenotypic effect in one of two ways, either through loss- or gain-of-function.

Loss-of-function

Loss-of-function mutations can result in either reduced activity or complete loss of the gene product. The former can be the result of either reduced activity or of decreased stability of the gene product and is known as a *hypomorph*, the latter being known as a *null allele* or *amorph*. Loss-of-function mutations in the heterozygous state would, at worst, be associated with half normal levels of the protein product. Loss-of-function mutations involving enzymes will usually be inherited in an autosomal or X-linked recessive manner, because the catalytic activity of the product of the normal allele is more than adequate to carry out the reactions of most metabolic pathways.

Haploinsufficiency

Loss-of-function mutations in the heterozygous state in which half normal levels of the gene product result in phenotypic effects are termed *haploinsufficiency mutations*. The phenotypic manifestations sensitive to gene dosage are a result of mutations occurring in genes which code for either receptors or more rarely enzymes, the functions of which are rate limiting, e.g. familial hypercholesterol-aemia (p. 160) and acute intermittent porphyria (p. 165)

There are a number of autosomal dominant disorders where the mutational basis of the functional abnormality is the result of haploinsufficiency, in which, not surprisingly, homozygous mutations result in more severe phenotypic effects, e.g. angioneurotic oedema (p. 183) and familial hypercholesterolaemia (p. 160).

Gain-of-function mutations

Gain-of-function mutations, as the name suggests, result in either increased levels of gene expression or the development of a new function(s) of the gene product. Increased expression levels due to activating point mutations or increased gene dosage are responsible for one type of Charcot–Marie–Tooth disease, hereditary motor and sensory neuropathy type Ia (p. 271). The expanded triplet repeat mutations in the Huntington gene cause qualitative changes in the gene product, which results in its aggregation in the central nervous system leading to the classical clinical features of the disorder (p. 267).

Mutations which alter the timing or tissue specificity of the expression of a gene can also be considered to be gain-of-function mutations. Examples include the chromosomal rearrangments which result in the combination of sequences from two different genes seen with specific tumours (p. 192). The novel function of the resulting chimeric gene causes the neoplastic process.

Gain-of-function mutations are dominantly inherited and the rare instances of gain-of-function mutations occurring in the homozygous state are associated with a much more severe phenotype, which is often a prenatally lethal disorder, e.g. homozygous achondroplasia (p. 86) or Waardenburg's syndrome type I (p. 84).

Dominant-negative mutations

A *dominant-negative mutation* is one in which a mutant gene in the heterozygous state results in the loss of protein activity/function, as a consequence of the mutant gene product interfering with the function of the normal gene product of the corresponding allele. Dominant-negative mutations are particularly common in proteins which are dimers or multimers, e.g. structural proteins such as the collagens, mutations in which can lead to osteogeneis imperfecta (p. 70).

GENOTYPE–PHENOTYPE CORRELATION

Many genetic disorders are well recognized as being very variable in the severity of involvement (p. 99) or in the particular features a person with the disorder will manifest (p. 98). Developments in molecular genetics (p. 64) increasingly allow identification of the mutational basis of the specific features which occur in a person with a particular inherited disease, or what is known as the *phenotype*. This has resulted in attempts to correlate the presence of a particular mutation, which is often called the *genotype*, with the specific features seen in a

person with an inherited disorder, this being referred to as *genotype–phenotype correlation*. This can be important in the management of a patient. One example includes the association of mutations in the *BRCA1* gene with the risk of developing ovarian cancer as well as breast cancer (p. 201). Particularly striking examples are mutations in the receptor tyrosine kinase gene *RET* which, depending on their location, can lead to four different syndromes which differ in the functional mechanism and clinical phenotype. Loss-of-function nonsense mutations lead to lack of migration of neural crest derived cells to form the ganglia of the myenteric plexus of the large bowel leading to Hirshsprung's disease, while gain-of-function missense mutations result in familial medullary thyroid carcinoma or one of the two types of multiple endocrine neoplasia type II (pp. 86, 88).

MUTAGENS AND MUTAGENESIS

Naturally occurring mutations are referred to as *spontaneous mutations* and are thought to arise through chance errors in chromosomal division or DNA replication. Environmental agents which cause mutations are known as *mutagens*.

MUTAGENS

These include natural or artificial ionizing radiation and chemical or physical mutagens.

Ionizing radiation

Ionizing radiation includes electromagnetic waves of very short wavelength (X-rays and gamma rays), and high energy particles (α particles, β particles and neutrons). X-rays, gamma rays and neutrons have great penetrating power but alpha particles can penetrate soft tissues to a depth of only a fraction of a millimetre and beta particles only up to a few millimetres.

Measures of radiation

The amount of radiation received by irradiated tissues is often referred to as the 'dose' of radiation, which is measured in terms of the *radiation absorbed dose* or *rad*. The rad is a measure of the amount of any ionizing radiation which is actually absorbed by the tissues, 1 rad being equivalent to 100 ergs of energy absorbed per gram of tissue. The biological effects of ionizing radiation depend on the volume of tissue exposed. In humans, irradiation of the whole body with a dose of 300–500 rads is usually fatal, but as much as 10 000 rads can be given to a small volume of tissue in the treatment of malignant tumours without serious effects.

Humans can be exposed to a mixture of radiation and the *rem* (<u>r</u>oentgen <u>e</u>quivalent for <u>man</u>) is a convenient unit as it is a measure of any radiation in terms of X-rays. A rem of radiation is that absorbed dose which produces in a given tissue the same biological effect as 1 rad of X-rays. Expressing doses of radiation in terms of rems permits us to compare the amounts of different types of radiation to which humans are exposed. A millirem (mrem) is one-thousandth of a rem. 100 rem is equivalent to 1 *sievert* (Sv), and 100 rad is equivalent to 1 *gray* (Gy) in SI units. For all practical purposes, sieverts and grays are approximately equal. In this discussion sieverts and millisieverts (mSv) will be used as the units of measure.

Dosimetry

Dosimetry is the measurement of radiation. The dose of radiation is expressed in relation to the amount received by the gonads because it is the effects of radiation on germ cells rather than somatic cells which are important as far as transmission of mutations to future progeny is concerned. The *gonad dose* of radiation is often expressed as the amount received in 30 years. This period of time has been chosen because it corresponds roughly to the generation time in humans.

Sources of radiation

The various sources and average annual doses of the different types of natural and artificial ionizing radiation are listed in Table 2.5. Natural sources of radiation include cosmic rays, external radiation from radioactive materials in certain rocks and internal radiation from radioactive materials in tissues. Artificial sources include diagnostic and therapeutic radiology, occupational exposure and fallout from nuclear explosions.

The average gonad dose of ionizing radiation from radioactive fallout resulting from the testing of nuclear weapons is less than that from any of the sources of background radiation. However, the possibility of serious accidents involving nuclear reactors, as occurred at Three Mile Island in the United States in 1979 and at Chernobyl in the Soviet Union in 1986 with widespread effects, always has to be kept in mind.

Genetic effects

Experiments with animals and plants have shown that the number of mutations produced by irradiation is proportional to the dose; the larger the dose the more mutations produced. It is believed that there is no threshold below which irradiation has no effect — even the smallest dose of radiation can result in a mutation. The genetic effects of ionizing radiation are also cumulative, so that each time a person is exposed to radiation, the dose received has to be added to the amount of radiation already received. The total number of radiation-induced mutations is directly proportional to the total gonad dose.

Atomic radiation

Neel and Schull tackled the problem of trying to demonstrate the genetic effects of radiation by comparing the offspring of parents exposed to atomic radiation at the time Hiroshima and Nagasaki were bombed with those of parents who were not similarly exposed to this source of radiation. Analysis of several thousand births revealed no significant differences in the incidence of stillbirths, congenital malformations or neonatal deaths. This does not mean, however, that there are no genetic consequences of ionizing radiation.

The genetic effects of radiation are not easy to assess for they will not manifest in the generation which is exposed to radiation but only in subsequent generations. If a dominant mutation is produced then it will be manifest in the next generation, but a recessive mutation will only be manifest if two heterozygotes with a mutation in the same gene have children. If a recessive mutant allele is very rare then the chance of this happening will be small. It was argued, however, that recessive mutations induced on the X chromosome would be immediately manifest in hemizygous (p. 102) male offspring of mothers who had been irradiated. If these mutants were lethal then the number of male births would be diminished; the sex ratio (number of

Table 2.5 Approximate average doses of ionizing radiation from various sources to the gonads of the general population

Source of radiation	Average dose per year (mSv)	Average dose per 30 years (mSv)
Natural		
Cosmic radiation	0.25	7.5
External gamma radiation*	1.50	45.0
Internal gamma radiation	0.30	9.0
Artificial		
Medical radiology	0.30	9.0
Radioactive fallout	0.01	0.3
Occupational and miscellaneous	0.04	1.2
Total	2.40	72.0

*Including radon in dwelling.
(Data from Clarke R H, Southwood T R E 1989 Risks from ionizing radiation. Nature 338: 197–198)

male births divided by the number of female births) would be reduced. This is what would be expected if lethal recessive X-linked mutations were produced in gonadal tissue of a woman who has been irradiated. If X-linked dominant lethal mutations were produced then there would be an equal chance of both male and female babies being eliminated and the sex ratio would remain unchanged. Recessive X-linked lethal mutations induced in the paternal gonads would have no effect on the sex ratio, but dominant X-linked lethal mutations would lead to an excess of live male births with a resultant increase in the sex ratio. In other words, if a large enough sample was studied, one would expect that in the case of fathers exposed to radiation the sex ratio of their offspring would be increased whereas in the case of mothers exposed to radiation the sex ratio of their offspring would be decreased.

In the study of parents who had been exposed to atomic radiation in Japan, evidence was obtained by Neel and Schull of slight changes in the sex ratio which could be interpreted as being due to the production of X-linked mutations. In non-irradiated parents the sex ratio was 0.5209 but in those parents who had received a dose of about 200 rad the sex ratio was 0.5272 when the father had been irradiated and 0.5119 when the mother had been irradiated.

However, in an extension of this study published in 1966, it was not possible to confirm the effects of radiation on the sex ratio. In fact, careful studies have revealed no higher incidence of abnormality among survivors' offspring than among the normal population and the practice of giving Green Cards to survivors' children, which gave certain medical and financial privileges, was abandoned in 1966.

The results of both these studies have to be considered with caution because many factors other than radiation can influence the sex ratio. For instance, the sex ratio is affected by paternal age and birth order, the proportion of males being highest in first births and decreasing with successive births.

Medical radiation

Similar results were obtained in studies looking at the offspring of parents who received pelvic radiotherapy. These showed a slight increase in the sex ratio when the father was irradiated and a slight decrease when the mother was irradiated.

Other attempts to detect genetic damage resulting from radiation have been made by comparing the incidence of abortions, stillbirths and congenital malformations in the offspring of radiologists and in the offspring of other medical specialists, the assumption being that radiologists are exposed to more radiation than other physicians. The results of these studies showed that there were slightly more abortions, stillbirths and congenital malformations in the offspring of radiologists but the differences were not statistically significant.

Occupational radiation

A carefully controlled study of fathers working at the nuclear power plant at Sellafield in West Cumbria, UK, has revealed a significantly increased number of cases of leukaemia among their children. The results suggested that exposure to ionizing radiation in some way led to leukaemia, possibly by inducing mutations in the germ cells of the fathers, though leukaemia is not thought of as a genetic disorder. It will be instructive to see if in future there is any increase of genetic disorders in the offspring of such fathers, though so far there is no evidence of this.

Permissible dose

In summary, attempts to demonstrate that radiation causes genetic damage in humans have not been very convincing. This does not mean, however, that radiation does not cause genetic damage in humans; experiments on other organisms have shown quite clearly that ionizing radiation does cause mutations, the vast majority of which are harmful. The hazard from mutations induced in humans is not so much to ourselves as to our descendants. Unfortunately, in humans we do not have any easy way to demonstrate genetic damage caused by mutagens. Nevertheless the International Commission of Radiological Protection (ICRP), working in close liaison with various agencies of the United Nations (WHO, UNESCO, IAEA, etc.), has been mainly responsible for defining what is referred to as the maximum *permissible dose* of radiation. This is an arbitrary safety limit and is probably very much less than that which would cause any significant effect on the frequency of harmful mutations within the population. It has been recommended that occupational exposure should not exceed 50 mSv in a year. However, there is currently much controversy over exactly what the permissible dose should be and some countries, such as the United States, set the upper limit significantly lower than many others. In the UK the National Radiological Protection Board advises that occupational exposure should not in fact exceed 15 mSv in a year. To put this into perspective, 1 mSv is roughly 50 times the dose received in a single chest X-ray and 100 times the dose incurred in flying from the UK to Spain in a jet aircraft!

There is no doubting the potential dangers, both somatic and genetic, of exposure to ionizing radiation. In the case of medical radiology the dose of radiation resulting from a particular procedure has to be weighed against the ultimate beneficial effect to the patient. In the case of occupational exposure to radiation, the answer lies in defining the risks and introducing and enforcing adequate legislation. With regard to the dangers from fallout from nuclear accidents and explosions the solution would seem obvious.

Chemical and physical mutagens

In humans, chemical mutagenesis could, in fact, be more important than radiation in producing genetic damage. Experiments have shown that certain chemicals such as mustard gas, formaldehyde, benzene, some basic dyes and even caffeine are mutagenic in animals. Many of these mutagenic substances are present in various agricultural, industrial and pharmaceutical chemicals in common use today. Consideration of animal data on the effects of chemicals on the induction of mutations makes it seem likely to be relevant in humans. High temperature is also known to increase the mutation rate in animals, but again the relevance of this to humans is conjectural.

Concern over exposure to environmental chemicals with potential mutagenicity is receiving increasing attention although, again, formal proof of the consequences of such exposures is difficult to obtain.

DNA REPAIR

The occurrence of mutations in DNA, if left unrepaired, would have serious consequences both for the individual and subsequent generations. The stability of DNA is dependent upon continuous *DNA repair* by a number of different mechanisms. This usually involves removal of the damaged nucleotides, cleavage of the DNA strand by an endonuclease, removal of a number of adjacent nucleotides by an exonuclease, resynthesis of the missing nucelotides and the gap in the DNA molecule being filled in by the enzyme DNA polymerase, the break in the damaged strand being sealed by the enzyme DNA ligase.

Defects in the genes involved in the DNA repair processes result in a variety of disorders which include two of the chromosomal breakage syndromes, xeroderma pigmentosum and Bloom's syndrome (p. 263) as well as

one of the forms of inherited familial cancer syndromes causing bowel cancer, hereditary non-polyposis colorectal cancer (p. 200).

FURTHER READING

Alberts B, Bray D, Lewis J et al 1995 Molecular biology of the cell, 3rd edn. Garland, London
Very accessible, well written and lavishly illustrated comprehensive text of molecular biology with accompanying problems book and CD ROM using multimedia review and self-assessment.
Alberts B, Bray D, Johnson A et al 1997 Essential cell biology: an introduction to the molecular biology of the cell. Garland, London
An excellent introductory textbook with full colour illustrations.
Beir V 1990 Health effects of exposure to low levels of ionizing radiation. National Academy Press, Washington
The fifth report of the National Research Council's Committee on the Biological Effects of Ionizing Radiation.
Dawkins R 1989 The selfish gene, 2nd edn. Oxford University Press, Oxford
An interesting controversial concept.
Lewin B 2000 Genes VII, 7th edn. Oxford University Press, Oxford
The seventh edition of this excellent textbook of molecular biology with colour diagrams and figures. Hard to improve upon.
Lodisch H, Berk A, Zipursky S L et al 1999 Molecular cell biology, 2nd edn. W H Freeman, London
A revised and updated edition of the 1st edn, clearly written with excellent diagrams.
Mettler F A, Moseley R D 1985 Medical effects of ionising radiation. Grune & Stratton, London
Good overview of all aspects of the medical consequences of ionizing radiation.
Schull W J, Neel J V 1958 Radiation and the sex ratio in man. Sex ratio among children of survivors of atomic bombings suggests induced sex-linked lethal mutations. Science 228: 434–438
The original report of possible evidence of the effects of atomic radiation.
Strachan T, Read A P 1999 Human molecular genetics 2nd edn. βios Scientific, Oxford
An up-to-date, comprehensive textbook of all aspects of molecular and cellular biology as it relates to inherited disease in humans.
Turner J E 1995 Atoms, radiation and radiation protection. John Wiley, London
Basis of the physics of radiation, applications and harmful effects.
Watson J D, Crick F H C 1953 Molecular structure of nucleic acids — a structure for deoxyribose nucleic acid. Nature 171: 737–738
The concepts in this paper, presented in just over one page, resulted in the authors receiving the Nobel Prize!
Weaver R F 1998 Molecular biology. WCB/McGraw-Hill, London
Well written and illustrated textbook covering the breadth of molecular biology.

ELEMENTS

❶ Genetic information is stored in DNA (deoxyribonucleic acid) as a linear sequence of two types of nucleotides, the purines (adenine [A] and guanine [G]) and the pyrimidines (cytosine [C] and thymine [T]), linked by a sugar–phosphate backbone.

❷ A molecule of DNA consists of two antiparallel strands held in a double helix by hydrogen bonds between the complementary G–C and A–T base pairs.

3 DNA replication has multiple sites of origin and is semiconservative, each strand acting as a template for synthesis of a complementary strand.

4 Genes coding for proteins in higher organisms (eukaryotes) consist of coding (exons) and non-coding (introns) sections.

5 Transcription is the synthesis of a single stranded complementary copy of one strand of a gene which is known as messenger RNA (mRNA). RNA (ribonucleic acid) differs from DNA in containing the sugar ribose and the base uracil instead of thymine.

6 mRNA is processed during transport from the nucleus to the cytoplasm, eliminating the non-coding sections. In the cytoplasm it becomes associated with the ribosomes where translation, i.e. protein synthesis, occurs.

7 The genetic code is 'universal' and consists of triplets (codons) of nucleotides, each of which codes for an amino acid or termination of peptide chain synthesis. The code is degenerate, i.e. all but two amino acids are specified by more than one codon.

8 The major control of gene expression is at the level of transcription by DNA regulatory sequences in the 5' flanking promoter region of structural genes in eukaryotes. General and specific transcription factors are also involved in the regulation of genes.

9 Mutations occur both spontaneously and as a result of exposure to mutagenic agents such as ionizing radiation. Mutations are continuously corrected by DNA repair enzymes.

Chromosomes and cell division

At the molecular or submicroscopic level DNA can be regarded as the basic template which provides a blueprint for the formation and maintenance of an organism. DNA is packaged into *chromosomes* and at a very simple level these can be considered as being made up of tightly coiled long chains of genes. Unlike DNA, chromosomes can be visualized during cell division using a light microscope, under which they appear as thread-like structures or 'coloured bodies'. The word chromosome is derived from the Greek *chroma* (= colour) and *soma* (= body).

Chromosomes are the factors which distinguish one species from another and which enable transmission of genetic information from one generation to the next. Their behaviour at somatic cell division in *mitosis* provides a means of ensuring that each daughter cell retains its own complete genetic complement. Similarly their behaviour during gamete formation in *meiosis* enables each mature ovum and sperm to contain a unique single set of parental genes. Chromosomes are quite literally the vehicles which facilitate reproduction and the maintenance of a species.

The study of chromosomes and cell division is referred to as *cytogenetics*. Prior to the 1950s it was believed, incorrectly, that each human cell contained 48 chromosomes and that human sex was determined by the number of X chromosomes present at conception. Following the development in 1956 of more reliable techniques for studying human chromosomes it was realized that the correct chromosome number in humans is 46 and that maleness is determined by the presence of a Y chromosome regardless of the number of X chromosomes present in each cell. It was also realized that abnormalities of chromosome number and structure could seriously disrupt normal growth and development.

DNA, which has been likened to the tightly coiled network of wiring seen in a solenoid (p. 13). Under the electron microscope chromosomes can be seen to have a rounded and rather irregular morphology (Fig 3.1). However most of our knowledge of chromosome structure has been gained using light microscopy. Special stains selectively taken up by DNA have enabled each individual chromosome to be identified. These are best seen during cell division when the chromosomes are maximally contracted and the constituent genes can no longer be transcribed.

At this time each chromosome can be seen to consist of two identical strands known as *chromatids*, or *sister chromatids*, which are the result of DNA replication having

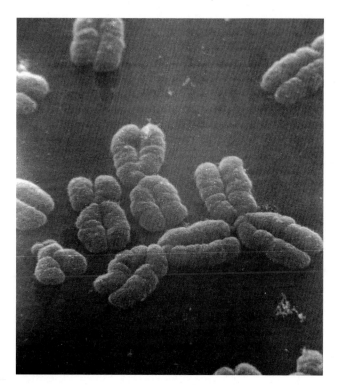

Fig. 3.1
Electron micrograph of human chromosomes showing the centromeres and well-defined chromatids. (Courtesy of Dr Christine Harrison. Reproduced from Cytogenetics and Cell Genetics 1983, 35: 21–27 with permission of the publisher, S Karger A G, Basel.)

HUMAN CHROMOSOMES

MORPHOLOGY

At the submicroscopic level chromosomes consist of an extremely elaborate complex, made up of supercoils of taken place during the S (synthesis) phase of the cell cycle (p. 40). These sister chromatids can be seen to be joined at a primary constriction known as the *centromere*. Centromeres consist of several hundred kilobases of repetitive DNA and are responsible for the movement of chromosomes at cell division. Each centromere divides the chromosome into short and long arms designated p (= petite) and q ('g' = grande) respectively.

The tip of each chromosome arm is known as the *telomere*. Telomeres play a crucial role in sealing the ends of chromosomes and maintaining their structural integrity. Telomeres have been highly conserved throughout evolution and in humans they consist of many tandem repeats of a TTAGGG sequence. During DNA replication an enzyme known as *telomerase* replaces the 5' end of the long strand (p. 16), which would otherwise become progressively shorter until a critical length is reached when the cell can no longer divide and thus becomes senescent. This is in fact part of the normal cellular ageing process with most cells being unable to undergo more than 50–60 divisions. However in some tumours increased telomerase activity has been implicated as a cause of abnormally prolonged cell survival.

Morphologically chromosomes are classified according to the position of the centromere. If this is located centrally, the chromosome is *metacentric*, if terminal it is *acrocentric*, and if the centromere is in an intermediate position the chromosome is *submetacentric* (Fig. 3.2). Acrocentric chromosomes sometimes have stalk-like appendages called *satellites* which form the nucleolus of the resting interphase cell and contain multiple repeat copies of the genes for ribosomal RNA.

CLASSIFICATION

Individual chromosomes differ not only in the position of the centromere but also in their overall length. Based on the three parameters of length, position of the centromere and the presence or absence of satellites, early pioneers of cytogenetics were able to identify most individual chromosomes or at least subdivide them into groups labelled A–G on the basis of overall morphology (A = 1–3, B = 4–5, C = 6–12 + X, D = 13–15, E = 16–18, F = 19–20, G = 21–22 + Y). In humans the normal cell nucleus contains 46 chromosomes, made up of 22 pairs of *autosomes* and a single pair of sex chromosomes — XX in the female and XY in the male. One member of each of these pairs is derived from each parent. Somatic cells are said to have a *diploid* complement of 46 chromosomes whereas gametes (i.e. ova and sperm) have a *haploid* complement of 23 chromosomes. Members of a pair of chromosomes are known as *homologues*.

The development of chromosome banding (p. 31) enabled very precise recognition of individual chromosomes and the detection of subtle chromosome

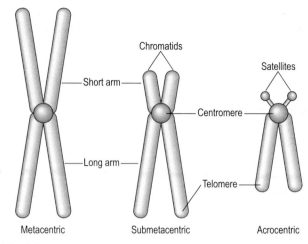

Fig. 3.2
Morphologically chromosomes are divided into metacentric, submetacentric and acrocentric depending on the position of the centromere.

abnormalities. This technique also revealed that *chromatin*, the combination of DNA and histone proteins of which chromosomes are made, exists in two main forms. *Euchromatin* stains lightly and consists of genes which are actively expressed. In contrast *heterochromatin* stains darkly and is made up largely of inactive unexpressed repetitive DNA.

The total number of chromosomes in different organisms varies considerably but is constant for any particular species. Whereas the marmoset and certain monkeys resemble man in having 46 chromosomes, higher primates more closely related to humans, such as the chimpanzee, gorilla and orangutan, have 48 chromosomes. Among these primates the chromosomes of the chimpanzee most closely resemble those of humans. This is consistent with the fact that there is a difference of only 1% between human and chimpanzee DNA. There is general agreement that the human number 2 chromosome is the product of the fusion of two chimpanzee chromosomes, with many other differences between the chromosome complements in the two species being due to paracentric and pericentric inversions (p. 50). These observations have been exploited by molecular biologists to help map and clone genes in humans (p. 73).

THE SEX CHROMOSOMES

The X and Y chromosomes are known as the sex chromosomes because of their crucial role in sex determination. The X chromosome was originally labelled as such because of uncertainty as to its function when it was realized that in some insects this chromosome is present in some gametes but not in others. In these insects the male has only one sex chromosome (X) whereas the female has two (XX). In humans, and in most mammals, both the male and the female have two sex chromosomes —XX in the female and XY in the male. The Y chromosome is much smaller than the X and carries only a few genes of functional importance, most notably the testis determining factor known as *SRY* (p. 90). Other genes on the Y chromosome are known to be important in maintaining spermatogenesis.

In the female each ovum carries an X chromosome, whereas in the male each sperm carries either an X or a Y chromosome. As there is a roughly equal chance of either an X-bearing sperm or a Y-bearing sperm fertilizing an ovum, the numbers of male and female conceptions are approximately equal (Fig. 3.3). In fact slightly more male babies are born than females, although during childhood and adult life the sex ratio evens out at 1:1.

The process of sex determination will be considered in detail later (p. 90).

METHODS OF CHROMOSOME ANALYSIS

It was generally believed that each cell contained 48 chromosomes until 1956 when Tjio and Levan correctly concluded on the basis of their studies that the normal human somatic cell contains only 46 chromosomes. The methods they used, with certain modifications, are now universally employed in cytogenetic laboratories to analyse the chromosome constitution of an individual which is known as a *karyotype*. This term is also used to describe a photomicrograph of an individual's chromosomes, arranged in a standard manner.

CHROMOSOME PREPARATION

Any tissue with living nucleated cells which undergo division can be used for studying human chromosomes.

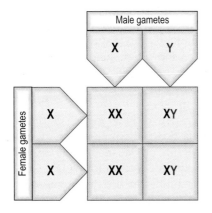

Fig. 3.3
Punnett's square showing sex chromosome combinations for male and female gametes.

Most commonly circulating lymphocytes from peripheral blood are used, although samples for chromosomal analysis can be prepared relatively easily using skin, bone marrow, chorionic villi or cells from amniotic fluid (amniocytes).

In the case of peripheral (venous) blood, a sample is added to a small volume of nutrient medium containing phytohaemagglutinin, which stimulates T lymphocytes to divide. The cells are cultured under sterile conditions at 37°C for about 3 days, during which they divide and colchicine is then added to each culture. This drug has the extremely useful property of preventing formation of the spindle, thereby arresting cell division during metaphase, the time when the chromosomes are maximally condensed and therefore most easily visible. Hypotonic saline is then added which causes the red blood cells to lyse and results in spreading of the chromosomes which are then fixed, mounted on a slide and stained ready for analysis (Fig. 3.4).

CHROMOSOME BANDING

Several different staining methods can be utilized to identify individual chromosomes.

G (Giemsa) banding

This is the method most commonly used. The chromosomes are treated with trypsin which denatures their protein content and then stained with a DNA binding dye known as Giemsa which gives each chromosome a characteristic and reproducible pattern of light and dark bands (Fig. 3.5).

Q (Quinacrine) banding

This gives a banding pattern similar to that obtained with Giemsa, and requires examination of the chromosomes with an ultraviolet fluorescent microscope.

R (Reverse) banding

The chromosomes are heat-denatured before staining with Giemsa, yielding light and dark bands which are the reverse of those obtained using conventional G banding (Fig. 3.6).

C (Centromeric heterochromatin) banding

If the chromosomes are pretreated with acid followed by alkali prior to G banding, the centromeres and other heterochromatic regions containing highly repetitive DNA sequences are preferentially stained.

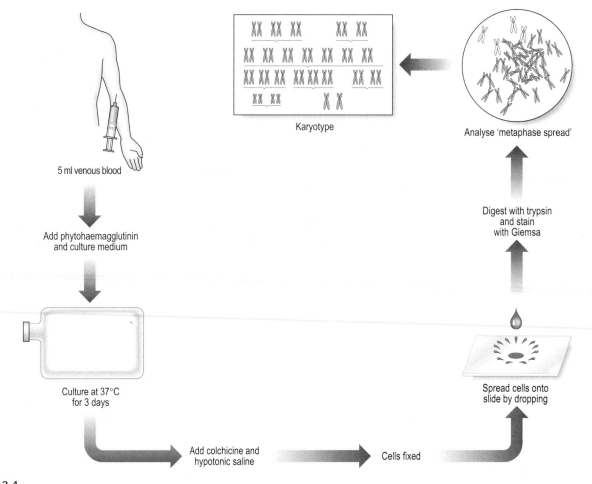

Fig. 3.4
Preparation of a karyotype.

High resolution banding

G banding generally provides high quality chromosome analysis with approximately 400–500 bands per haploid set. Each of these bands corresponds on average to approximately 6000–8000 kb (i.e. 6–8 megabases) of DNA. High resolution banding of the chromosomes at an earlier stage of mitosis such as prophase or prometaphase provides greater sensitivity with up to 800 bands per haploid set but is much more demanding technically. This involves first inhibiting cell division with an agent such as methotrexate or thymidine. Folic acid or deoxy-cytidine is added to the culture medium which releases the cells into mitosis. Colchicine is then added at a specific time interval, when a higher proportion of cells will be in prometaphase and the chromosomes will not be fully contracted, giving a more detailed banding pattern.

KARYOTYPE ANALYSIS

The next stage in chromosome analysis involves first counting the number of chromosomes present in a specified number of cells, sometimes referred to as *metaphase spreads*, followed by careful analysis of the banding pattern of each individual chromosome in selected cells. Usually the total chromosome count is determined in 10–15 cells, but if mosaicism is suspected then 30 or more cell counts will be undertaken. Detailed analysis of the banding pattern of the individual chromosomes is carried out on both members of each pair of homologues in approximately 3–5 metaphase spreads which show high quality banding.

The banding pattern of each chromosome is specific and can be shown in the form of a stylized ideal karyotype known as an *idiogram* (Fig. 3.7). The cytogeneticist analyses each pair of homologous chromosomes, either while looking down the microscope or, less commonly, on a photograph of the metaphase spread which can now be produced electronically (Fig. 3.8). Until the advent of banding in 1971, chromosomes could be classified only on the basis of their overall morphology. Now a formally presented karyotype or *karyogram* will show each chromosome pair in descending order of size.

Fig. 3.5
A normal G banded male karyotype.

Fig. 3.7
An idiogram showing the banding patterns of individual chromosomes as revealed by fluorescent and Giemsa staining.

Fig. 3.6
A normal R banded male karyotype.
(Courtesy of H. J. Evans.)

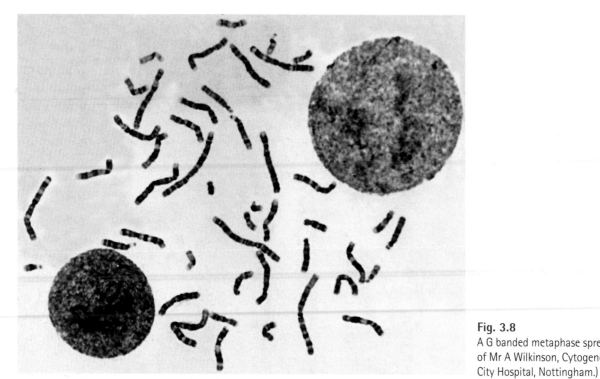

Fig. 3.8
A G banded metaphase spread. (Courtesy of Mr A Wilkinson, Cytogenetics Unit, City Hospital, Nottingham.)

MOLECULAR CYTOGENETICS

FLUORESCENT IN SITU HYBRIDIZATION (FISH)

This relatively new diagnostic tool combines conventional cytogenetics with molecular genetic technology. It is based on the unique ability of a portion of single stranded DNA, i.e. a probe (p. 60), to anneal with its complementary target sequence wherever it is located on a metaphase spread. Unlike most other methods used for chromosome analysis, FISH can also be used to study chromosomes in cells which are resting between cell division in the interval known as *interphase*. Hence this area of study is sometimes referred to as *interphase cytogenetics*.

In this technique the DNA probe is conjugated with modified nucleotides which, after hybridization with the patient sample, allows the region where hybridization has occurred to be visualized under ultraviolet light. FISH is now used widely for clinical diagnostic purposes and has a major advantage in that results are usually obtained very rapidly.

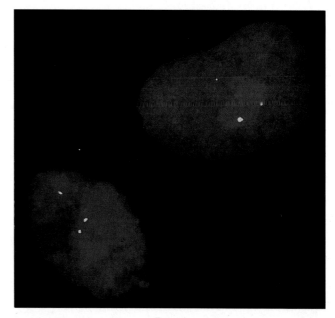

Fig. 3.9
Fluorescent in situ hybridization (FISH) of interphase nuclei with a chromosome 21 centromeric probe (CAMBIO) showing three signals consistent with trisomy 21. (Courtesy of Nigel Smith, City Hospital, Nottingham.)

Different types of FISH probes

Centromeric probes

These consist of repetitive DNA sequences found in and around the centromere of a specific chromosome. They are suitable for making a rapid diagnosis of one of the common aneuploidy syndromes (trisomy 13, 18, 21 — see p. 250) using non-dividing cells in interphase obtained from a prenatal diagnostic sample of chorionic villi (Fig. 3.9). Some centres are exploring the use of a set of centromere specific probes for chromosomes 13, 18, 21, X and Y as an adjunct to provide rapid prenatal diagnosis for some of the more common numerical chromosomal abnormalities (p. 303).

Chromosome-specific unique sequence probes

These are specific for a particular single locus. They are particularly useful for identifying tiny submicroscopic deletions and duplications (Fig. 3.10). The group of disorders referred to as the *microdeletion syndromes* are described in Chapter 17. Unique sequence probes are used widely in gene mapping studies (p. 72).

Telomeric probes

A complete set of telomeric probes has been developed for all 24 chromosomes (i.e. autosomes 1–22 plus X and Y). Using these a method has been devised which enables the simultaneous analysis of the subtelomeric region of every chromosome using only a single microscope slide per patient. This has proved to be a particularly useful technique for identifying tiny 'cryptic' subtelomeric abnormalities, such as deletions and translocations, in a small but significant proportion of children with unexplained mental retardation.

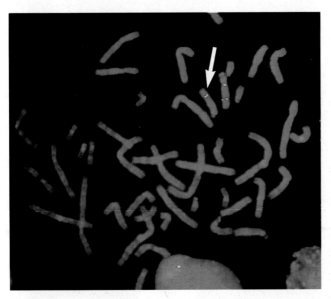

Fig. 3.10
Shows FISH demonstration of a microdeletion in one number 15 chromosome in a child with Prader–Willi syndrome using chromosome 15 locus specific probes (ONCOR). The arrow indicates the deleted chromosome which shows only the signal generated by the chromosome 15 marker probe. (Courtesy of Meg Heath, City Hospital, Nottingham.)

Whole chromosome paint probes

These consist of a cocktail of probes obtained from different parts of a particular chromosome. When this mixture of probes is used together in a single hybridization, the entire relevant chromosome fluoresces, i.e. is 'painted'. Chromosome painting is extremely useful for characterizing complex rearrangements such as subtle translocations (Fig. 3.11) and for identifying the origin of additional chromosome material such as small supernumerary markers or rings (Fig. 3.12).

Fig. 3.11
Chromosome painting showing a subtle reciprocal translocation involving chromosomes 1 (white) and 9 (purple). The small translocated segments are indicated. (Courtesy of Meg Heath, City Hospital, Nottingham.)

Fig. 3.12
Chromosome painting showing two normal number 17 chromosomes and a small ring 17 chromosome (arrowed) (paint provided by CAMBIO). (Courtesy of Nigel Smith, City Hospital, Nottingham.)

Reverse painting

In this procedure a portion of unidentified chromosome material, such as a small supernumerary marker or ring, is used as a paint for hybridization to a normal metaphase spread. The unidentified chromosome is obtained using a fluorescent activated cell sorter (see below) and is then amplified using the polymerase chain reaction (p. 58) to prepare the labelled paint. The origin of the unidentified chromosome segment is then revealed by identifying the chromosome(s) to which it hybridizes. In practice this technique is mainly used on a research basis only, because it is very labour intensive.

Multicolour spectral karyotyping (SKY) and multicolour FISH (M–FISH)

These latest developments in FISH technology utilize pools of whole human chromosome paint probes to provide a multicolour human karyotype in which each pair of homologous chromosomes can be identified on the basis of its unique colour when studied using a computer based image analysis (Fig. 3.13). These approaches have proved to be extremely useful for detecting subtle chromosome rearrangements, such as deletions and translocations, and for identifying small supernumerary markers and ring chromosomes.

COMPARATIVE GENOMIC HYBRIDIZATION (CGH)

This ingenious modification of reverse painting is used widely in cancer genetics to detect regions of allele loss and gene amplification (p. 196). Tumour or 'test' DNA is labelled with a green paint and control normal DNA is labelled with a red paint. The two samples are mixed and hybridized competitively to normal metaphase chromosomes photographed using a fluorescence microscope (Fig. 3.14). If the test sample contains more DNA

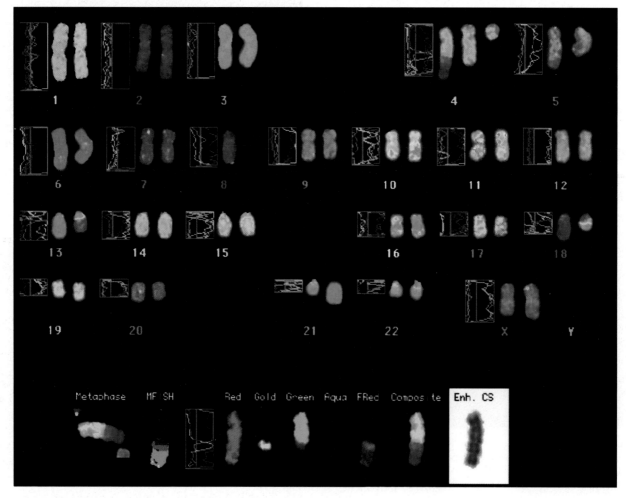

Fig. 3.13
M-FISH showing complex chromosome rearrangement involving chromosomes 4, 8, 13, 18 and 21 as observed in cultured blood lymphocytes. (Courtesy of Dr Rhona Anderson, Radiation and Genome Stability Unit, MRC Harwell, Oxon, UK and Applied Imaging.)

Fig. 3.14
Comparative genomic hybridization (CGH) analysis showing areas of gene amplification and reduction (deletion) in tumour DNA. (Courtesy of Dr Peter Lichter, DKFZ, Heidelberg and Applied Imaging.)

from a particular chromosome region than the control sample, then that region is identified by an increase in the green to red fluorescence ratio (Fig. 3.15). Similarly a deletion in the test sample is identified by a reduction in the green to red fluorescence ratio.

FLOW CYTOMETRY

Because of their differing size and DNA composition chromosomes bind different amounts of fluorescent dyes, some of which bind specifically to GC ('gene-rich') sequences and others to AT ('gene-poor') sequences. This property of differential binding allows chromosomes to be separated by the process of *flow cytometry* or *fluorescent activated cell sorting* (FACS). This involves staining metaphase chromosomes with a fluorescent DNA-binding dye and then projecting them in a fine jet of droplets across a focused laser beam which excites the chromosomes to fluoresce. The fluorescence intensity is measured by a photomultiplier and the results are analysed by a computer which draws up a distribution histogram of chromosome size. This is referred to as a *flow karyotype*.

Flow cytometry can be used to analyse an individual's chromosomes but its clinical application is severely limited at present by its expense and by the relatively poor separation achieved for certain chromosomes, most noticeably those in the C group. It finds greater application in separating preparations of single chromosomes for the construction of chromosome-specific DNA libraries and in the manufacture of chromosome paints for FISH.

CHROMOSOME NOMENCLATURE

By convention each chromosome arm is divided into regions and each region is subdivided into bands numbering always from the centromere outwards (Fig. 3.16). A given point on a chromosome is designated by the chromosome number, the arm (p or q), the region and the band, e.g. 15q12. Sometimes the word region is omitted so that 15q12 would be referred to simply as band 12 on the long arm of chromosome 15.

A shorthand notation system exists for the description of chromosome abnormalities (Table 3.1). Normal male and female karyotypes are depicted as 46,XY and 46,XX respectively. A male with Down's syndrome as a result of trisomy 21 would be represented as 47,XY,+21, whereas a female with a deletion of the short arm of one number 5

Fig. 3.15

CGH ratio profiles for the CGH analysis shown in Fig. 3.14. The vertical lines adjacent to each chromosome show fluorescence ratios of 0.5 to 1.5 between test and control DNA. (Courtesy of Dr Peter Lichter, DKFZ, Heidelberg and Applied Imaging.)

Table 3.1 Symbols used in describing a karyotype

Term	Explanation
p	Short arm
q	Long arm
cen	Centromere
del	Deletion, e.g. 46,XX,del(1)(q21)
dup	Duplication, e.g. 46,XY,dup(13)(q14)
fra	Fragile site
i	Isochromosome, e.g. 46,X,i(Xq)
inv	Inversion, e.g. 46XX,inv(9)(p12q12)
ish	In situ hybridization
r	Ring, e.g. 46,XX,r(21)
t	Translocation, e.g. 46,XY,t(2;4)(q21;q21)
ter	terminal or end, i.e. tip of arm, e.g. pter or qter
/	Mosaicism, e.g. 46,XY/47,XXY
+ or –	Sometimes used after a chromosome arm in text to indicate gain or loss of part of that chromosome, e.g. 46,XX,5p–

a reciprocal translocation involving the short arm of chromosome 2 at region 2 band 3 and the long arm of chromosome 4 at region 2 band 5.

This system of karyotype nomenclature has been extended to include the results of FISH studies. For example a karyotype which reads 46,XX.ish del(15) (q11.2q11.2)(D15S10–) refers to a female with a microdeletion involving 15q11.2 identified by in situ hybridization analysis using a probe for the D15S10 locus (D15S10 = DNA from chromosome 15 site 10). This individual will have either the Prader–Willi or Angelman syndrome as discussed in Chapter 17.

CELL DIVISION

MITOSIS

At conception the human zygote consists of a single cell. This undergoes rapid division leading ultimately to the mature human adult, consisting of approximately 1 X

chromosome (Cri du chat syndrome, p. 253) would be represented as 46,XX,del(5p). A chromosome report reading 46,XY,t(2;4)(p23;q25) would indicate a male with

Fig. 3.16
An X chromosome showing the short and long arms each subdivided into regions and bands.

10^{14} cells in total. In most organs and tissues, such as bone marrow and skin, cells continue to divide throughout life. This process of somatic cell division, during which the nucleus also divides, is known as *mitosis*. During mitosis each chromosome divides into two daughter chromosomes one of which segregates into each daughter cell. Consequently the number of chromosomes per nucleus remains unchanged.

Prior to a cell entering mitosis, each chromosome consists of two identical sister chromatids as a result of DNA replication having taken place during the S phase of the cell cycle (p. 40). Mitosis is the process whereby each of these pairs of chromatids separates and disperses into separate daughter cells.

Mitosis is a continuous process which usually lasts 1–2 hours, but for descriptive purposes it is convenient to distinguish five distinct stages. These are prophase, prometaphase, metaphase, anaphase and telophase (Fig. 3.17).

Prophase

During the initial stage of *prophase* the chromosomes condense and the mitotic spindle begins to form. Two *centrioles* form in each cell from which *microtubules* radiate as the centrioles move towards opposite poles of the cell.

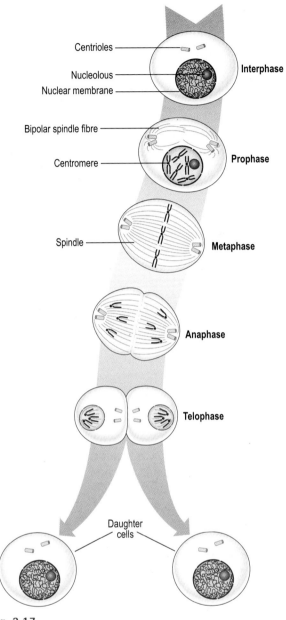

Fig. 3.17
Stages of mitosis.

Prometaphase

During *prometaphase* the nuclear membrane begins to disintegrate allowing the chromosomes to spread around the cell. Each chromosome becomes attached at its centromere to a microtubule of the mitotic spindle.

Metaphase

In *metaphase* the chromosomes become aligned along the equatorial plane or plate of the cell, where each chromosome is attached to the centriole by a microtubule forming the mature spindle. At this point the chromosomes are maximally contracted and therefore most easily visible. Each chromosome resembles the letter X in shape as the chromatids of each chromosome have separated longitudinally but remain attached at the centromere which has not yet undergone division.

Anaphase

In *anaphase* the centromere of each chromosome divides longitudinally and the two daughter chromatids separate to opposite poles of the cell.

Telophase

By *telophase* the chromatids, which are now independent chromosomes consisting of a single double helix, have separated completely and the two groups of daughter chromosomes each become enveloped in a new nuclear membrane. The cell cytoplasm also separates (*cytokinesis*) resulting in the formation of two new daughter cells each of which contains a complete diploid chromosome complement.

THE CELL CYCLE

The period between successive mitoses is known as the *interphase* of the cell cycle (Fig. 3.18). In rapidly dividing cells this lasts for between 16 and 24 hours. Interphase commences with the G_1 (G = gap) phase during which the chromosomes become thin and extended. This phase of the cycle is very variable in length and is responsible for the variation in generation time between different cell populations. Cells which have stopped dividing,

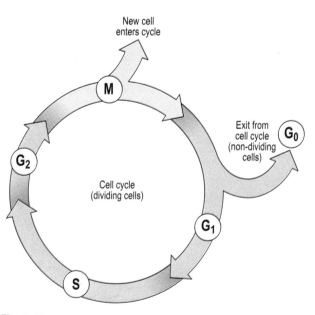

Fig. 3.18
Stages of the cell cycle. G_1 and G_2 are the first and second 'resting' stages of interphase. S is the stage of DNA replication. M = mitosis.

such as neurones, usually arrest in this phase and are said to have entered a non-cyclic stage known as G_0.

The G_1 phase is followed by the S phase (S = synthesis), when DNA replication occurs and the chromatin of each chromosome is replicated. This results in the formation of two chromatids which give each chromosome its characteristic X-shaped configuration. The process of DNA replication commences at multiple points on a chromosome (p. 13).

Usually homologous pairs of chromosomes replicate in synchrony. However one of the X chromosomes is always late replicating. This is the inactive X chromosome (p. 92) which forms the *sex chromatin*, or the so-called *Barr body*, which can be visualized in interphase in female somatic cells. This used to be the basis of a rather unsatisfactory means of sex determination based on analysis of cells obtained by scraping the buccal mucosa — a 'buccal smear'.

Interphase is completed by a relatively short G_2 phase during which the chromosomes begin to condense in preparation for the next mitotic division.

MEIOSIS

Meiosis is the process of nuclear division which occurs during the final stage of gamete formation. Meiosis differs from mitosis in three fundamental ways:

1. Mitosis results in each daughter cell having a diploid chromosome complement (46). During meiosis the diploid count is halved so that each mature gamete receives a haploid complement of 23 chromosomes.

2. Mitosis takes place in somatic cells and during the early cell divisions in gamete formation. Meiosis occurs only at the final division of gamete maturation.

3. Mitosis occurs as a single one-step process. Meiosis can be considered as two cell divisions known as meiosis I and meiosis II, each of which can be considered as having prophase, metaphase, anaphase and telophase stages as in mitosis (Fig. 3.19).

Meiosis I

This is sometimes referred to as the reduction division because it is during the first meiotic division that the chromosome number is halved.

Prophase I

Chromosomes enter this stage already split longitudinally into two chromatids joined at the centromere. Homologous chromosomes pair, and with the exception of the X and Y chromosomes in male meiosis, exchange of homologous segments occurs between non-sister chromatids, that is, chromatids from each of the pair of homologous chromosomes. This exchange of homologous segments

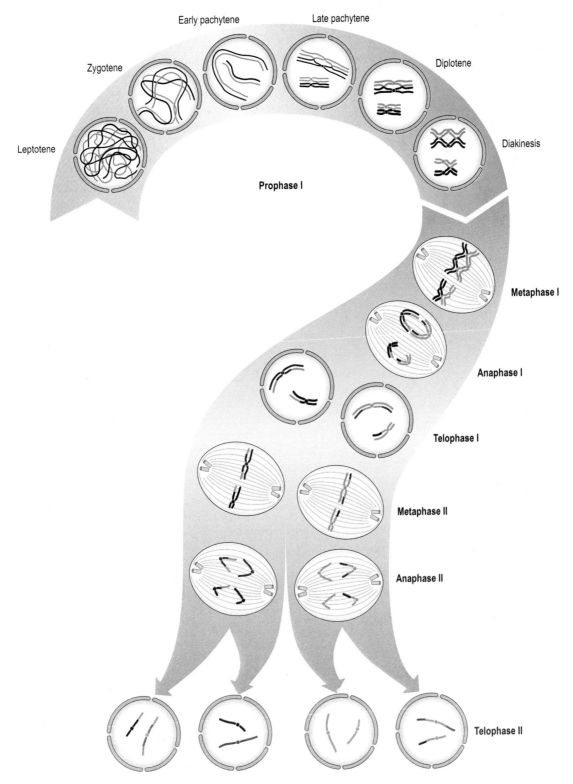

Fig. 3.19
Stages of meiosis.

between chromatids occurs as a result of a process known as *crossing over* or *recombination*. The importance of crossing over in linkage analysis and risk calculation is considered later (pp. 121, 299).

During prophase I in the male pairing occurs between homologous segments of the X and Y chromosomes at the tip of their short arms, with this portion of each chromosome being known as the *pseudoautosomal* region (p. 105).

The prophase stage of meiosis I is relatively lengthy and can be subdivided into five stages.

Leptotene
The chromosomes become visible as they start to condense.

Zygotene
Homologous chromosomes align directly opposite each other, a process known as *synapsis*, and are held together at several points along their length by filamentous structures known as *synaptonemal complexes*.

Pachytene
Each pair of homologous chromosomes, known as a *bivalent*, becomes tightly coiled. Crossing over occurs during which homologous regions of DNA are exchanged between chromatids.

Diplotene
The homologous recombinant chromosomes now begin to separate but remain attached at the points where crossing over has occurred. These are known as *chiasmata*. On average small, medium and large chromosomes have one, two and three chiasmata respectively, giving an overall total of approximately 40 recombination events per meiosis per gamete.

Diakinesis
Separation of the homologous chromosome pairs proceeds as the chromosomes become maximally condensed.

Metaphase I
The nuclear membrane disappears and the chromosomes become aligned on the equatorial plane of the cell where they have become attached to the spindle as in metaphase of mitosis.

Anaphase I
The chromosomes now separate to opposite poles of the cell as the spindle contracts.

Telophase I
Each set of haploid chromosomes has now separated completely to opposite ends of the cell which cleaves into two new daughter gametes, so-called *secondary spermatocytes* or *oocytes*.

Meiosis II
This is essentially similar to an ordinary mitotic division. Each chromosome, which exists as a pair of chromatids, becomes aligned along the equatorial plane and then splits longitudinally leading to the formation of two new daughter gametes, known as *spermatids* or *ova*.

The consequences of meiosis
When considered in terms of reproduction and the maintenance of the species, meiosis achieves two major objectives. Firstly it facilitates halving of the diploid number of chromosomes so that each child receives half of its chromosome complement from each parent. Secondly it provides an extraordinary potential for generating genetic diversity. This is achieved in two ways:

1. When the bivalents separate during prophase of meiosis I, they do so independently of one another. This is consistent with Mendel's third law (p. 4). Consequently each gamete receives a selection of parental chromosomes. The likelihood that any two gametes from an individual will contain exactly the same chromosomes equals 1 in 2^{23}, i.e. approximately 1 in 8 million.

2. As a result of crossing over, each chromatid will usually contain portions of DNA derived from both parental homologous chromosomes. A large chromosome will typically consist of three or more segments of alternating parental origin. The ensuing probability that any two gametes will have an identical genome is therefore infinitesimally small. This dispersion of DNA into different gametes is sometimes referred to as 'gene shuffling'.

GAMETOGENESIS

The process of gametogenesis shows fundamental differences in males and females (Table 3.2). These have quite distinct clinical consequences if errors occur.

Table 3.2 Differences in gametogenesis in male and female

	Male	Female
Commences	Puberty	Early embryonic life
Duration	60–65 days	10–50 years
Numbers of mitoses in gamete formation	30–500	20–30
Gamete production per meiosis	4 spermatids	1 ovum + 3 polar bodies
Gamete production	100–200 million per ejaculate	1 ovum per menstrual cycle

OOGENESIS

Mature ova develop from oogonia by a complex series of intermediate steps. Oogonia themselves originate from primordial germ cells by a process involving 20–30 mitotic divisions which occur during the first few months of embryonic life. By the completion of embryogenesis at 3 months of intra-uterine life, the oogonia have begun to mature into primary oocytes which start to undergo meiosis. At birth all of the primary oocytes have entered a phase of maturation arrest, known as *dictyotene*, in which they remain suspended until meiosis I is completed at the time of ovulation when a single secondary oocyte is formed. This receives most of the cytoplasm. The other daughter cell from the first meiotic division consists largely of a nucleus and is known as a polar body. Meiosis II then commences during which fertilization can occur. This second meiotic division results in the formation of a further polar body (Fig. 3.20).

It is probable that the very lengthy interval between the onset of meiosis and its eventual completion, up to 50 years later, accounts for the well-documented increased incidence of chromosome abnormalities in the offspring of older mothers (p. 44). The accumulating effects of wear and tear on the primary oocyte during the dictyotene phase probably damage the cell's spindle formation and repair mechanisms thereby predisposing to non-disjunction (p. 44).

SPERMATOGENESIS

In contrast, spermatogenesis is a relatively rapid process with an average duration of 60–65 days. At puberty spermatogonia, which will already have undergone approximately 30 mitotic divisions, begin to mature into primary spermatocytes which enter meiosis I and emerge as haploid secondary spermatocytes. These then undergo the second meiotic division to form spermatids, which in turn develop without any subsequent cell division into mature spermatozoa, of which 100–200 million are present in each ejaculate.

Spermatogenesis is a continuous process involving many mitotic divisions, possibly as many as 20–25 per annum, so that mature spermatozoa produced by a man of 50 years or older could well have undergone several hundred mitotic divisions. The observed paternal age effect for new dominant mutations (p. 100) is consistent

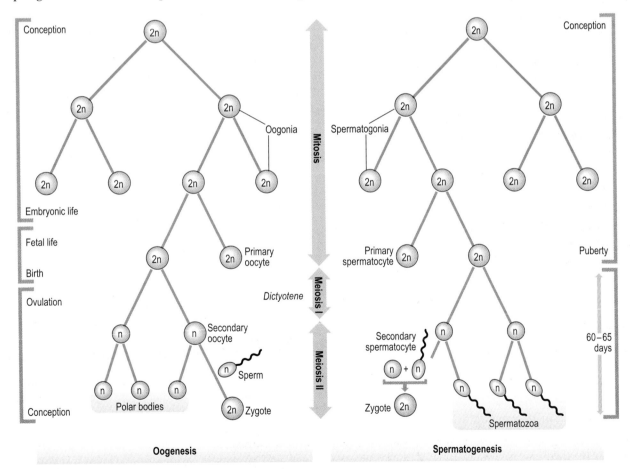

Fig. 3.20
Stages of oogenesis and spermatogenesis. n = haploid number.

with the concept that many mutations arise as a consequence of DNA copy errors occurring during mitosis.

CHROMOSOME ABNORMALITIES

Specific disorders caused by chromosome abnormalities are considered in Chapter 17. In this section discussion will be restricted to a review of the different types of abnormality which can occur. These can be divided into numerical and structural, with a third category consisting of different chromosome constitutions in two or more cell lines (Table 3.3).

NUMERICAL ABNORMALITIES

Numerical abnormalities involve the loss or gain of one or more chromosomes, which is referred to as *aneuploidy*, or the addition of one or more complete haploid complements, which is known as *polyploidy*. Loss of a single chromosome results in *monosomy*. Gain of one or two homologous chromosomes is referred to as *trisomy* and *tetrasomy* respectively.

Trisomy

The presence of an extra chromosome is referred to as trisomy. Most cases of Down's syndrome are due to the presence of an additional number 21 chromosome, hence Down's syndrome is often known as trisomy 21. Other autosomal trisomies which are compatible with survival to term are Patau's syndrome (trisomy 13) (p. 252) and Edwards' syndrome (trisomy 18) (p. 252). Most other autosomal trisomies result in early pregnancy loss with trisomy 16 being a particularly common finding in first trimester spontaneous miscarriages. The presence of an additional sex chromosome (X or Y) has only mild phenotypic effects (pp. 256, 258).

Trisomy 21 is usually caused by failure of separation of one of the pairs of homologous chromosomes during anaphase of maternal meiosis I. This failure of the bivalent to separate is called *non-disjunction*. Less often, trisomy can be caused by non-disjunction occurring during meiosis II when a pair of sister chromatids fail to separate. Either way the gamete receives two homologous chromosomes (*disomy*), and if subsequent fertilization occurs a trisomic conceptus results (Fig. 3.21).

The origin of non-disjunction

The consequences of non-disjunction in meiosis I and meiosis II differ in the chromosomes found in the gamete. An error in meiosis I leads to the gamete containing both homologues of one chromosome pair. In

Table 3.3   Types of chromosome abnormality

Numerical	
Aneuploidy	— Monosomy
	— Trisomy
	— Tetrasomy
Polyploidy	— Triploidy
	— Tetraploidy
Structural	
Translocations	— Reciprocal
	— Robertsonian
Deletions	
Insertions	
Inversions	— Paracentric
	— Pericentric
Rings	
Isochromosomes	
Different cell lines (mixoploidy)	
Mosaicism	
Chimerism	

Table 3.4   Parental origin of meiotic error leading to aneuploidy

Chromosome abnormality	Paternal (%)	Maternal (%)
Trisomy 13	15	85
Trisomy 18	10	90
Trisomy 21	5	95
45,X	80	20
47,XXX	5	95
47,XXY	45	55
47,XYY	100	0

contrast, non-disjunction in meiosis II results in the gamete receiving two copies of one of the homologues of the chromosome pair. Studies using DNA markers have shown that most children with an autosomal trisomy have inherited their additional chromosome as a result of non-disjunction occurring during one of the maternal meiotic divisions (Table 3.4).

Non-disjunction can also occur during an early mitotic division in the developing zygote. This results in the presence of two or more different cell lines, a phenomenon known as mosaicism (p. 52).

The cause of non-disjunction

The cause of non-disjunction is uncertain. The most favoured explanation is that of an ageing effect on the primary oocyte which can remain in a state of suspended inactivity for up to 50 years (p. 43). This is based on the well-documented association between advancing maternal age and increased incidence of Down's syndrome in offspring (Table 17.4, p. 250). A maternal age effect has also been noted for trisomies 13 and 18.

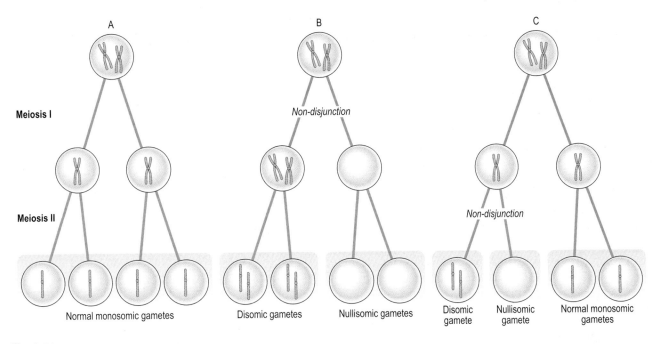

Fig. 3.21
Segregation at meiosis of a single pair of chromosomes in (A) normal meiosis, (B) non-disjunction in meiosis I and (C) non-disjunction in meiosis II.

It is not known how or why advancing maternal age predisposes to non-disjunction, although research has shown that absence of recombination in prophase of meiosis I predisposes to subsequent non-disjunction. This is not surprising as the chiasmata which are formed after recombination are responsible for holding each pair of homologous chromosomes together until subsequent separation occurs in diakinesis. Thus failure of chiasmata formation could allow each pair of homologues to separate prematurely and then segregate randomly to daughter cells. In the female, however, recombination occurs before birth whereas the non-disjunctional event occurs any time between 15 and 50 years later. This suggests that at least two factors can be involved in causing non-disjunction, the first being an absence of recombination between homologous chromosomes in the fetal ovary and the second an abnormality in spindle formation many years later.

An alternative explanation for the association of advancing maternal age with increased risk of autosomal trisomy is that survival of trisomic embryos could be the result of an age-related reduction in 'immunological' competence. Firm evidence for this theory is limited.

Other factors which have been implicated in causing non-disjunction include radiation and delayed fertilization after ovulation. In animals it has been shown that an increased incidence of aneuploid embryos can result from lengthening of the interval between ovulation and fertilization. It has been suggested that this could account for the relationship between maternal age and the incidence of Down's syndrome, as with increasing age intercourse is likely to occur less frequently, with delayed

fertilization therefore being more likely. The story is further complicated by the fact that in some species such as *Drosophila*, non-disjunction is under genetic control. This could account for those occasional families which seem to be prone to recurrent non-disjunction.

Monosomy

The absence of a single chromosome is referred to as monosomy. Monosomy for an autosome is almost always incompatible with survival to term. Lack of contribution of an X or a Y chromosome results in a 45,X karyotype which causes the condition known as Turner's syndrome (p. 257).

As with trisomy, monosomy can result from non-disjunction in meiosis. If one gamete receives two copies of a homologous chromosome (*disomy*), the other corresponding daughter gamete will have no copy of the same chromosome (*nullisomy*). Monosomy can also be caused by loss of a chromosome as it moves to the pole of the cell during anaphase, an event known as 'anaphase lag'.

Polyploidy

Polyploid cells contain multiples of the haploid number of chromosomes such as 69, *triploidy*, or 92, *tetraploidy*. In humans triploidy is found relatively often in material grown from spontaneous miscarriages but survival beyond mid-pregnancy is rare. Only a few triploid live births have been described and all have died soon after birth.

Triploidy can be caused by failure of a maturation meiotic division in an ovum or sperm, leading, for example, to retention of a polar body or to the formation of a diploid sperm. Alternatively it can be caused by fertilization of an ovum by two sperm: this is known as *dispermy*. When triploidy results from the presence of an additional set of paternal chromosomes, the placenta is usually swollen with what are known as hydatidiform changes (p. 89). In contrast when triploidy results from an additional set of maternal chromosomes, the placenta is usually small. Triploidy usually results in early spontaneous miscarriage (Fig. 3.22).

STRUCTURAL ABNORMALITIES

Structural chromosome rearrangements result from chromosome breakage with subsequent reunion in a different configuration. They can be balanced or unbalanced. In balanced rearrangements the chromosome complement is complete with no loss or gain of genetic material. Consequently, balanced rearrangements are generally harmless with the exception of rare cases in which one of the break-points damages an important functional gene. However, carriers of balanced rearrangements are often at risk of producing children with an unbalanced chromosomal complement.

When a chromosome rearrangement is unbalanced the chromosomal complement contains an incorrect amount of chromosome material and the clinical effects are usually very serious.

Translocations

A *translocation* refers to the transfer of genetic material from one chromosome to another. A *reciprocal translocation* is formed when a break occurs in each of two chromosomes with the segments being exchanged to form two new derivative chromosomes. A *Robertsonian translocation* is a particular type of reciprocal translocation in which the break-points are located at or close to the centromeres of two acrocentric chromosomes (Fig. 3.23).

Reciprocal translocations

A reciprocal translocation involves breakage of at least two chromosomes with exchange of the fragments. Usually the chromosome number remains at 46, and if the exchanged fragments are of roughly equal size, a reciprocal translocation can only be identified with detailed chromosomal banding studies or FISH (see Fig. 3.11). In general reciprocal translocations are unique to a particular family, although, for reasons which are unknown, a particular balanced reciprocal translocation involving the long arms of chromosomes 11 and 22 is relatively common. The overall incidence of reciprocal translocations in the general population is approximately 1 in 500.

Segregation at meiosis
The importance of balanced reciprocal translocations lies in their behaviour at meiosis when they can segregate to generate significant chromosome imbalance. This can

Fig. 3.22
Karyotype from products of conception of a spontaneous miscarriage showing triploidy.

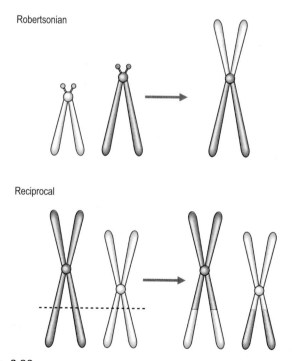

Fig. 3.23
Types of translocation.

lead to early pregnancy loss or to the birth of an infant with multiple abnormalities. Problems arise at meiosis because the chromosomes involved in the translocation cannot pair normally to form bivalents. Instead they form a cluster known as a *pachytene quadrivalent* (Fig. 3.24). The key point to note is that each chromosome aligns with homologous material in the quadrivalent.

2:2 segregation When the constituent chromosomes in the quadrivalent separate during the later stages of meiosis I they can do so in several different ways (Table 3.5). If alternate chromosomes segregate to each gamete, then the gamete will carry a normal or balanced haploid complement (Fig. 3.25) and with fertilization the embryo will either have normal chromosomes or carry the balanced rearrangement. If, however, adjacent chromosomes segregate together, this will invariably result in the gamete acquiring an unbalanced chromosome complement. For example, in Figure 3.24 if the gamete inherits the normal number 11 chromosome (A) and the derivative number 22 chromosome (C), then fertilization will result in an embryo with monosomy for the distal long arm of chromosome 22 and trisomy for the distal long arm of chromosome 11.

3:1 segregation Another possibility is that three chromosomes segregate to one gamete with only one chromosome in the other gamete. If, for example, in Figure 3.24 chromosomes 11 (A), 22 (D) and the derivative 22 (C) segregate together to a gamete which is subsequently fertilized, this will result in the embryo being trisomic for the material present in the derivative 22 chromosome. This is sometimes referred to as *tertiary trisomy*. Experience has shown that with this particular reciprocal translocation, tertiary trisomy for the derivative 22 chromosome is the only viable unbalanced product. All other patterns of malsegregation lead to early pregnancy loss. Unfortunately tertiary trisomy for the derivative 22 chromosome is a

Pachytene
quadrivalent

1 Alternate segregation yields normal or balanced haploid complement

2 Adjacent–1 segregation yields unbalanced haploid complement

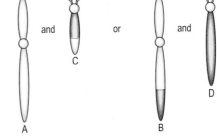

3 Adjacent–2 segregation yields unbalanced haploid complement

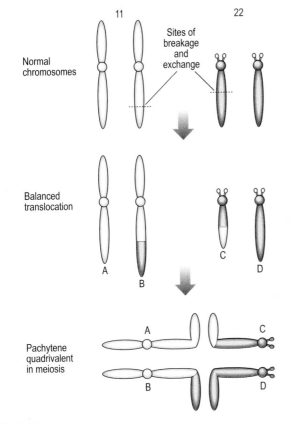

11   22

Sites of
breakage
and
exchange

Normal
chromosomes

Balanced
translocation

Pachytene
quadrivalent
in meiosis

Fig. 3.24
Shows how a balanced reciprocal translocation involving chromosomes 11 and 22 leads to the formation of a quadrivalent at pachytene in meiosis I. The quadrivalent is formed to maintain homologous pairing.

Fig. 3.25
Shows the different patterns of 2:2 segregation which can occur from the quadrivalent shown in Figure 3.24. See Table 3.5.

Table 3.5 Patterns of segregation of a reciprocal translocation (see Figs 3.24 and 3.25)

Pattern of segregation	Segregating chromosomes	Chromosome constitution in gamete
2:2 Alternate		
	A + D	Normal
	B + C	Balanced translocation
Adjacent—1 (non-homologous centromeres segregate together)	A + C or B + D	Unbalanced leading to a combination of partial monosomy and partial trisomy in the zygote
Adjacent—2 (homologous centromeres segregate together)	A + B or C + D	
3:1 Three chromosomes	A + B + C A + B + D A + C + D B + C + D	Unbalanced leading to trisomy in the zygote
One chromosome	A B C D	Unbalanced leading to monosomy in the zygote

serious condition in which affected children have multiple congenital abnormalities and severe learning difficulties.

Risks in reciprocal translocations

When counselling a carrier of a balanced translocation it is necessary to consider the particular rearrangement to determine whether it could result in the birth of an abnormal baby. This risk will usually lie somewhere between 1% and 10%. For carriers of the 11;22 translocation discussed, the risk has been shown to be 5%.

Robertsonian translocations

A Robertsonian translocation results from breakage of two acrocentric chromosomes (numbers 13, 14, 15, 21 and 22) at or close to their centromeres, with subsequent fusion of their long arms (see Fig. 3.23). This is also referred to as *centric fusion*. The short arms of each chromosome are lost, this being of no clinical importance as they contain only genes for ribosomal RNA for which there are multiple copies on the various other acrocentric chromosomes. The total chromosome number is reduced to 45. Since there is no loss or gain of important genetic material this is a functionally balanced rearrangement. The overall incidence of Robertsonian translocations in the general population is approximately 1 in 1000, with by far the most common being fusion of the long arms of chromosomes 13 and 14 (i.e. 13q14q).

Segregation at meiosis

As with reciprocal translocations, the importance of Robertsonian translocations lies in their behaviour at meiosis. For example, a carrier of a 14q21q translocation can produce gametes with (Fig. 3.26):

1. A normal chromosome complement, i.e. a normal 14 and a normal 21.

2. A balanced chromosome complement, i.e. a 14q21q translocation chromosome.

3. An unbalanced chromosome complement possessing both the translocation chromosome and a normal 21. This will result in the fertilized embryo having Down's syndrome.

4. An unbalanced chromosome complement with a normal 14 and a missing 21.

5. An unbalanced chromosome complement with a normal 21 and a missing 14.

6. An unbalanced chromosome complement with the translocation chromosome and a normal 14 chromosome.

The last three combinations will result in zygotes with monosomy 21, monosomy 14 and trisomy 14 respectively. All of these combinations are incompatible with survival beyond early pregnancy.

Translocation Down's syndrome

The major practical importance of Robertsonian translocations is that they can predispose to the birth of babies with Down's syndrome as a result of the embryo inheriting two normal number 21 chromosomes (one from each parent) plus a translocation chromosome involving a number 21 chromosome (Fig. 3.27). The clinical consequences are exactly the same as those seen in pure trisomy 21. However unlike trisomy 21, the parents of a child with translocation Down's syndrome have a relatively high risk of having further affected children if one of them carries the rearrangement in a balanced form.

Consequently the importance of performing a chromosome analysis in a child with Down's syndrome lies not only in confirmation of the diagnosis, but also in identification of those children with a translocation. In roughly two-thirds of these latter children with Down's syndrome, the translocation will have occurred as a new (de novo) event in the child, but in the remaining one-third one parent will be a carrier. Other relatives can also be carriers. Therefore it is regarded as essential that efforts are made to identify all adult translocation carriers in a family so that they can be alerted to possible risks to future offspring. This is sometimes referred to as translocation tracing or 'chasing'.

Risks in Robertsonian translocations

Studies have shown that the female carrier of either a 13q21q or a 14q21q Robertsonian translocation runs a risk of approximately 10% for having a baby with Down's

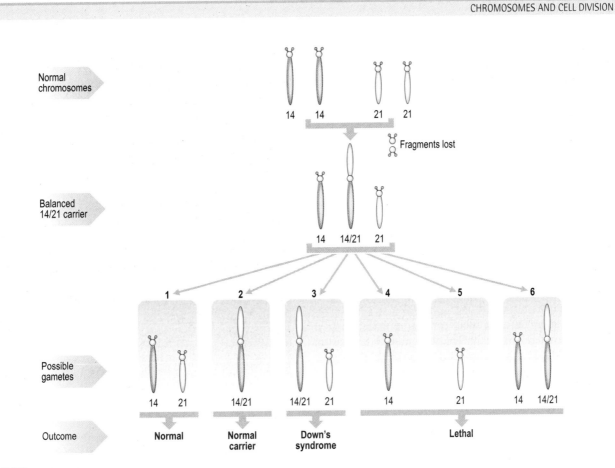

Fig. 3.26
Formation of a 14q21q Robertsonian translocation and the possible gamete chromosome patterns which can be produced at meiosis.

Fig. 3.27
Chromosome painting showing a 14q21q Robertsonian translocation in a child with Down's syndrome. Chromosome 21 is shown in blue and chromosome 14 in yellow. (Courtesy of Meg Heath, City Hospital, Nottingham.)

syndrome, whereas for male carriers the risk is 1–3%. It is worth sparing a thought for the unfortunate carrier of

a 21q21q Robertsonian translocation. All gametes will be either nullisomic or disomic for chromosome 21. Consequently all pregnancies will end either in spontaneous miscarriage or in the birth of a child with Down's syndrome. This is one of the very rare situations in which offspring are at a risk of greater than 50% for having an abnormality. Other examples are the children of a mother with untreated phenylketonuria (p. 236) and of parents who are both heterozygous for the same autosomal dominant disorder (p. 100).

Deletions

A *deletion* involves loss of part of a chromosome and results in monosomy for that segment of the chromosome. Usually a very large deletion will be incompatible with survival to term and as a general rule any deletion resulting in loss of more than 2% of the total haploid genome will have a lethal outcome.

Deletions are now recognized as existing at two levels. A 'large' chromosomal deletion can be visualized under the microscope. Several deletion syndromes have been described such as the Wolf–Hirschhorn and Cri du chat syndromes which involve loss of material from the short arms of chromosomes 4 and 5 respectively (p. 253). More recently submicroscopic microdeletions have been identified with the help of high resolution prometaphase cytogenetics augmented by fluorescent in situ hybridization studies (p. 35). For example it has been shown that several previously unexplained conditions such as the Prader–Willi and Angelman syndromes can be caused by microdeletions (p. 254).

Insertions

An *insertion* occurs when a segment of one chromosome becomes inserted into another chromosome (Figs 3.28 and 3.29). If the inserted material has moved from elsewhere in another chromosome then the karyotype is balanced. Otherwise an insertion causes an unbalanced chromosome complement. Carriers of a balanced deletion–insertion rearrangement are at a 50% risk of producing unbalanced gametes as random chromosome segregation at meiosis will result in 50% of the gametes inheriting either the deletion or the insertion but not both.

Inversions

An inversion is a two-break rearrangement involving a single chromosome in which a segment is reversed in position, i.e. inverted. If the inversion segment involves the centromere it is termed a *pericentric inversion* (Fig. 3.30A). If it involves only one arm of the chromosome it is known as a *paracentric inversion* (Fig. 3.30B).

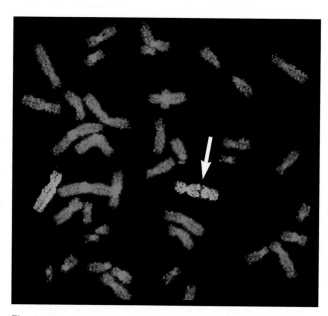

Fig. 3.28
Chromosome painting using chromosome 5 paint (CAMBIO) showing a small portion of chromosome 5 (arrowed) which marks the site of an insertion from chromosome 13. See Fig. 3.29. (Courtesy of Meg Heath, City Hospital, Nottingham.)

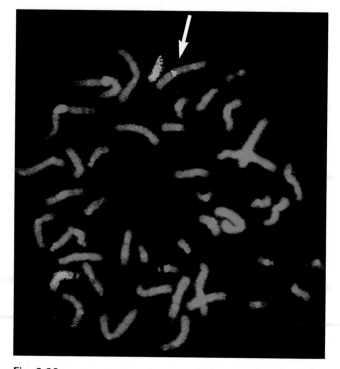

Fig. 3.29
Chromosome painting using chromosome 13 paint (CAMBIO) showing material of chromosome 13 origin inserted into chromosome 5 (arrowed). (Courtesy of Meg Heath, City Hospital, Nottingham.)

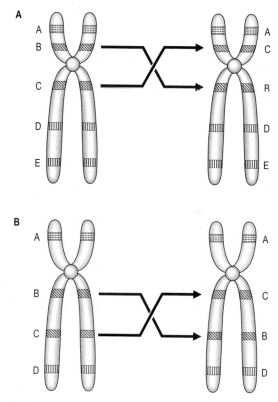

Fig. 3.30
A pericentric (A) and a paracentric (B) inversion. (Courtesy of Dr J Delhanty, Galton Laboratory, London.)

Inversions are balanced rearrangements which rarely cause problems in carriers unless one of the break-points has disrupted an important gene. A pericentric inversion involving chromosome number 9 occurs as a common structural variant or polymorphism (p. 120), also known as a *heteromorphism*, and is not thought to be of any functional importance. However, other inversions, while not causing any clinical problems in balanced carriers, can lead to significant chromosome imbalance in offspring with important clinical consequences.

Segregation at meiosis

Pericentric inversions

An individual who carries a pericentric inversion can produce unbalanced gametes if a cross-over occurs within the inversion segment during meiosis I, when an inversion loop forms as the chromosomes attempt to maintain homologous pairing at synapsis. For a pericentric inversion a cross-over within the loop will result in two complementary recombinant chromosomes, one with duplication of the distal non-inverted segment and deletion of the other end of the chromosome, and the other having the opposite arrangement (Fig. 3.31A).

If a pericentric inversion involves only a small proportion of the total length of a chromosome then, in the event of crossing over within the loop, the duplicated and deleted segments will be relatively large. The larger these are then the more likely it is that their effects on the embryo will be so severe that miscarriage ensues. For a large pericentric inversion the duplicated and deleted segments will be relatively small so that survival to term and beyond becomes more likely. Thus in general, the larger the size of a pericentric inversion then the more likely it becomes that it will result in the birth of an abnormal infant.

The pooled results of several studies have shown that a carrier of a balanced pericentric inversion runs a risk of approximately 5–10% for having a child with viable imbalance if that inversion has already resulted in the birth of an abnormal baby. The risk is nearer 1% if the inversion has been ascertained because of a history of recurrent miscarriage.

Paracentric inversions

If a cross-over occurs in the inverted segment of a paracentric inversion this will result in recombinant chromosomes which are either acentric or dicentric (Fig. 3.31B).

Fig. 3.31
Mechanism of production of recombinant unbalanced chromosomes from a pericentric (A) and paracentric (B) inversion by crossing over in an inversion loop. (Courtesy of Dr J Delhanty, Galton Laboratory, London.)

Acentric chromosomes, which strictly speaking should be known as *chromosomal fragments*, cannot undergo mitotic division so that survival of an embryo with such a rearrangement is extremely uncommon. Dicentric chromosomes are inherently unstable during cell division and are therefore also unlikely to be compatible with survival of the embryo. Thus overall the likelihood that a balanced parental paracentric inversion will result in the birth of an abnormal baby is extremely low.

Ring chromosomes

A *ring chromosome* is formed when a break occurs on each arm of a chromosome leaving two 'sticky' ends on the central portion which reunite as a ring (Fig. 3.32). The two distal chromosomal fragments are lost so that, if the involved chromosome is an autosome, the effects are usually very serious.

Ring chromosomes are often unstable in mitosis so that it is common to find a ring chromosome in only a proportion of cells. The other cells in the individual are usually monosomic because of the absence of the ring chromosome.

Isochromosomes

An isochromosome shows loss of one arm with duplication of the other. The most probable explanation for the formation of an isochromosome is that the centromere has divided transversely rather than longitudinally. The most commonly encountered isochromosome is that which consists of two long arms of the X chromosome. This accounts for approximately 15% of all cases of Turner's syndrome (p. 257).

MOSAICISM AND CHIMERISM (MIXOPLOIDY)

Mosaicism

Mosaicism can be defined as the presence in an individual or in a tissue of two or more cell lines which differ in their genetic constitution but are derived from a single zygote, i.e. they have the same genetic origin. Chromosome mosaicism usually results from non-disjunction occurring in an early embryonic mitotic division with the persistence of more than one cell line. If, for example, the two chromatids of a number 21 chromosome failed to separate at the second mitotic division in a human zygote (Fig. 3.33) this would result in the four-cell zygote having two cells with 46 chromosomes, one cell with 47 chromosomes (trisomy 21) and one cell with 45 chromosomes (monosomy 21). The ensuing cell line with 45 chromosomes would probably not survive so that the resulting embryo would be expected to show approximately 33% mosaicism

9   r(9)

Fig. 3.32
Partial karyotype showing a ring chromosome 9. (Courtesy of Meg Heath, City Hospital, Nottingham.)

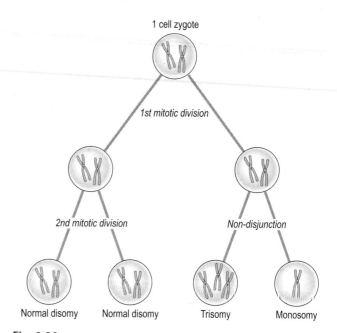

Fig. 3.33
Generation of somatic mosaicism caused by mitotic non-disjunction.

for trisomy 21. Mosaicism accounts for 1–2% of all clinically recognized cases of Down's syndrome.

Mosaicism can also exist at a molecular level if a new mutation arises in a somatic or early germ line cell division. The possibility of germ line or gonadal mosaicism is a particular concern when counselling the parents of a child who is an isolated case of a condition such as Duchenne muscular dystrophy (p. 280).

Chimerism

Chimerism can be defined as the presence in an individual of two or more genetically distinct cell lines derived from more than one zygote, i.e. they have a different genetic origin. The word chimera is derived from the mythological Greek monster which had the head of a lion, the body of a goat and the tail of a dragon. In humans chimeras are of two kinds: *dispermic chimeras* and *blood chimeras*.

Dispermic chimeras

These are the result of double fertilization whereby two genetically different sperm fertilize two ova and the resulting two zygotes fuse to form one embryo. If the two zygotes are of different sex, the chimeric embryo can develop into an individual with true *hermaphroditism* (p. 261) and an XX/XY karyotype. Mouse chimeras of this type can now be produced experimentally in the laboratory to facilitate the study of gene transfer.

Blood chimeras

Blood chimeras result from an exchange of cells, via the placenta, between non-identical twins in utero. For example, 90% of one twin's cells can have an XY karyotype with red blood cells showing predominantly blood group B, whereas the other twin can have 90% of cells showing an XX karyotype with red blood cells showing predominantly blood group A. It has long been recognized that when twin calves of opposite sex are born, the female can have ambiguous genitalia. It is now believed that this is because of gonadal chimerism in the female calves which are known as *freemartins*.

FURTHER READING

Barch M J, Knutsen T, Spurbeck J L (eds) 1997 The AGT cytogenetics laboratory manual, 3rd edn. Lippincott-Raven, Philadelphia
A large multiauthor laboratory handbook produced by the Association of Genetic Technologists.
Gersen S L, Keagle M B (eds) 1999 The principles of clinical cytogenetics. Humana Press, Totowa, New Jersey
A detailed multiauthor guide to all aspects of laboratory and clinical cytogenetics.
ISCN 1995 Mitelman F (ed) An international system for human cytogenetic nomenclature. Karger, Basel
An updated report giving details of how chromosome abnormalities including the results of FISH studies should be described.
Jalal S M, Law M E 1999 Utility of multicolor fluorescent in situ hybridization in clinical cytogenetics. Genet Med 1 181–186
A contemporary account of how this new technique can be used to identify subtle and complex chromosome abnormalities.
Rooney D E, Czepulkowski B H 1997 Human chromosome preparation. Essential techniques. John Wiley, Chichester
A laboratory handbook describing the different methods available for chromosome analysis.
Therman E, Susman M 1993 Human chromosomes. Structure, behaviour and effects, 3rd edn. Springer-Verlag, New York
A useful and comprehensive introduction to human cytogenetics.
Tjio J H, Levan A 1956 The chromosome number of man. Hereditas 42: 1–6
A landmark paper which described a reliable method for studying human chromosomes and gave birth to the subject of clinical cytogenetics.
Vogel F, Motulsky A G 1997 Human genetics, problems and approaches, 3rd edn. Springer-Verlag, Berlin
An extremely comprehensive textbook of human genetics with a large section devoted to cytogenetics and cell division.

ELEMENTS

1 The normal human karyotype is made up of 46 chromosomes consisting of 22 pairs of autosomes and a pair of sex chromosomes, XX in the female and XY in the male.

2 Each chromosome consists of a short (p) and long (q) arm joined at the centromere. Chromosomes are analysed using cultured cells and specific banding patterns can be identified using special staining techniques. Newly developed molecular cytogenetic techniques, such as fluorescent in situ hybridization (FISH) and comparative genomic hybridization (CGH), can be used to detect and characterize subtle chromosome abnormalities.

3 During mitosis in somatic cell division, the two sister chromatids of each chromosome separate with one chromatid passing to each daughter cell. During meiosis, which occurs during the final stage of gametogenesis, homologous chromosomes pair, exchange segments, and then segregate independently to the mature daughter gametes.

4 Chromosome abnormalities can be structural or numerical. Numerical abnormalities include trisomy and polyploidy. In trisomy a single extra chromosome is present, usually as a result of non-disjunction in the first or second meiotic division. In polyploidy, three or more complete haploid sets are present instead of the usual diploid complement.

5 Structural abnormalities include translocations, inversions, insertions, rings and deletions. Translocations can be balanced or unbalanced. Carriers of balanced translocations are at risk of having children with unbalanced rearrangements who will usually be physically and mentally handicapped.

DNA technology and applications

In the history of medical genetics, the 'chromosome breakthrough' in the mid-1950s was revolutionary. In the last two decades, DNA technology has had a profound effect, not only in medical genetics (Fig. 4.1), but also in many areas of biological science (Table 4.1).

The identification of restriction endonucleases, the development of the DNA cloning vectors, the introduction of the Southern blot technique in the 1970s and the more recent development of the polymerase chain reaction rank as seminal developments in the field.

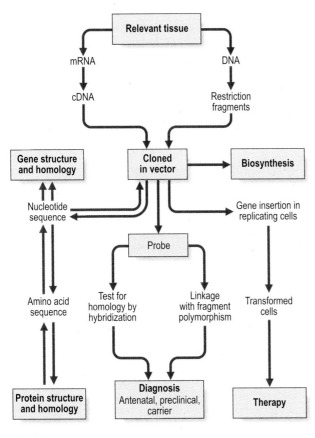

Fig. 4.1
Some of the applications of DNA technology in medical genetics.

PRINCIPLES OF DNA TECHNOLOGY

DNA technology can be split into two main areas: DNA cloning and methods of DNA analysis.

DNA CLONING

DNA cloning is the selective amplification of a specific DNA fragment or sequence to produce relatively large amounts of a homogeneous DNA fragment which allows its structure and function to be analysed in detail.

DNA cloning falls into two main types: techniques which use natural in vivo cell-based mechanisms of DNA replication and the more recently developed cell-free or in vitro polymerase chain reaction.

In vivo cell–based DNA cloning

There are six basic steps in in vivo cell-based DNA cloning.

Generation of DNA fragments

Although fragments of DNA can be produced by mechanical shearing techniques, this is a very haphazard

Table 4.1 Applications of DNA technology

Gene structure/mapping/function
Population genetics
Clinical genetics
   Prenatal diagnosis
   Presymptomatic diagnosis
   Carrier detection
Diagnosis and pathogenesis of disease
   Genetic
   Acquired — infective, malignant
Biosynthesis
   e.g. insulin, growth hormone, interferon, immunization
Treatment of genetic disease
Gene therapy
Agriculture
   e.g. nitrogen fixation

process producing fragments which vary in size. In the early 1970s it was recognized that certain microbes contained enzymes which cleave double stranded DNA in or near a particular sequence of nucleotides. These enzymes restrict the entry of foreign DNA into bacterial cells and were therefore called *restriction enzymes*. They recognize a palindromic nucleotide sequence of DNA between 4–8 nucleotides in length, i.e. the same sequence of nucleotides occurring on the two complementary DNA strands when read in one direction of polarity, e.g. 5′ to 3′ (Table 4.2). The longer the nucleotide recognition sequence of the restriction enzyme, the less frequently that particular nucleotide sequence will occur by chance and therefore the bigger average size of the DNA fragments generated.

Well over 300 different restriction enzymes have been isolated from various bacterial organisms. Restriction endonucleases are named according to the organism from which they are derived, e.g. *Eco RI* is from *E. coli* and was the first restriction enzyme isolated from that organism.

The complementary pairing of bases in the DNA molecule means that cleavage of double stranded DNA by a restriction endonuclease always creates double stranded breaks, which, depending on the cleavage points of the particular restriction enzyme used, results in either a staggered or a blunt end (Fig. 4.2).

Digesting DNA from a specific source with a particular restriction enzyme will produce the same reproducible collection of DNA fragments each time the process is carried out.

Recombination of DNA fragments

DNA from any source, when digested with the same restriction enzyme, will produce DNA fragments with identical complementary ends or termini. When DNA has been cleaved by a restriction enzyme which produces staggered termini, these are referred to as being 'sticky'

Fig. 4.2
The staggered and blunt ends generated by restriction digest of double stranded DNA by *EcoRI* and *SmaI*. Sites of cleavage of the DNA strands are indicated by arrows.

or 'cohesive' since they will unite under appropriate conditions with complementary sequences produced by the same restriction enzyme on DNA from any source. Initially the cohesive termini are held together by hydrogen bonding but are covalently attached with the enzyme called *DNA ligase*. The union of two DNA fragments from different sources produces what is referred to as a *recombinant DNA molecule*.

Vectors

A *vector*, or *replicon*, is the term for the carrier DNA molecule used in the cloning process which, through its own independent replication within a host organism, will allow production of multiple copies of itself. The incorporation of the *foreign* or *target DNA* into a vector allows production of large amounts of that DNA fragment.

In order for naturally occurring vectors to be used for DNA cloning, they need to be modified to ensure that the foreign DNA is inserted at a specific location and that recombinant vectors containing foreign inserted DNA can be detected. Many of the early vectors were constructed so that insertion of the foreign DNA in a gene for antibiotic resistance resulted in loss of that function (Fig. 4.3).

There are five main types of vectors commonly used which include *plasmids, bacteriophages, cosmids, bacterial* and *yeast artificial chromosomes*. The choice of vector used in cloning depends on a number of factors, such as the particular restriction enzyme being used and the size of the foreign DNA to be inserted. Some of the early vectors, such as plasmids and bacteriophages, were severely limited in the size of the foreign DNA fragment which could be inserted. Later generations of vectors, such as

Table 4.2 Some examples of restriction endonucleases with their nucleotide recognition sequence and cleavage sites			
Enzyme	**Organism**	**Cleavage site**	
		5′	**3′**
*Bam*HI	*Bacillus amyloliquefaciens* H	G • G A T C C	
*Eco*RI	*Escherichia coli* RY 13	G • A A T T C	
*Hae*III	*Haemophilus aegyptius*	G G • C C	
*Hind*III	*Haemophilus influenzae* Rd	A • A G C T T	
*Hpa*I	*Haemophilus parainfluenzae*	G T T • A A C	
*Pst*I	*Providencia stuartii*	C T G C A • G	
*Sma*I	*Serratia marcescens*	C C C • G G G	
*Sal*I	*Streptomyces albus* G	G • T C G A C	

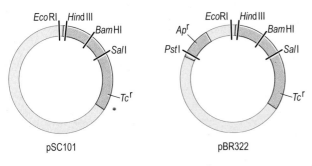

Fig. 4.3
Two plasmids originally used in recombinant DNA technology showing drug resistance genes (Ap^r = ampicillin resistance; Tc^r = tetracycline resistance) and cleavage sites of restriction endonucleases which are present in the DNA only once for use as a cloning site.

cosmids, can take inserts up to approximately 50 kb in size. A cosmid is essentially a plasmid which has had all but the minimum vector DNA necessary for propagation removed, i.e. the cos sequence, to enable insertion of the largest possible foreign DNA fragment and still allow replication.

More recently, the development of *bacterial* and *yeast artificial chromosomes* (*BACs* and *YACs*) allows the possibility of cloning DNA fragments between 300 kb and up to 1000 kb in size. A yeast artificial chromosome consists of a plasmid which contains within it the minimum DNA sequences necessary for centromere and telomere formation plus DNA sequences known as *autonomous replication sequences*, all of which are necessary for accurate replication within yeast. YACs have the advantage that they can incorporate DNA fragments up to 1000 kb in size as well as allow replication of eukaryotic DNA with repetitive DNA sequences which often cannot take place in bacterial cells. Many eukaryotic genes are very large, being up to 2 000 000–3 000 000 bp in length (p. 267). YACs allow detailed mapping of genes of this size and their flanking regions whereas using conventional vectors would require an inordinate number of overlapping clones.

Transformation of the host organism

After introduction of the foreign DNA fragment into the vector, the recombinant vector is introduced into specially modified bacterial or yeast host cells. The bacterial cell membrane is not normally permeable to large molecules such as DNA fragments but can be made permeable by a variety of different methods including exposure to certain salts or high voltage, or what is known as becoming *competent*. Usually only a single DNA molecule will be taken up by a host cell undergoing the process known as *transformation*. If the transformed cells are allowed to multiply, large quantities of identical copies of the original single target DNA or *clones* will be produced (Fig. 4.4).

Screening for recombinant vectors

After the transformed cells have multiplied in culture medium, they are plated out on a master plate of nutrient agar in a Petri dish. Recombinant vectors can be screened for by a detection system, e.g. loss of antibiotic resistance which can be screened for by replica plating on agar which contains the appropriate antibiotic (see Fig. 4.3). Thus, if the enzyme *Pst*I were used to generate DNA fragments and to cut the plasmid pBR322, any recombinant plasmids produced would make the bacterial host cells they transform sensitive to ampicillin, since this gene would no longer be functional, but they would remain resistant to tetracycline. Replica plating of the master plates from the cultures allows identification of individual specific recombinant clones.

Selection of specific clones

A number of techniques have been developed to detect the presence of clones with specific DNA sequence inserts. The most widely used method is by nucleic acid hybridization (p. 60). Colonies of transformed host bacteria with recombinant clones are used to make replica plates which are lysed and then blotted on to a nitrocellulose filter to which nucleic acid binds. The DNA of the replica blot is then denatured to make the DNA single stranded which will allow it to hybridize with single stranded, radioactively labelled DNA or RNA probes (p. 60) which can then be detected by exposure to an X-ray film, or what is known as *autoradiography*. In this way a transformed host bacterial colony containing a sequence complementary to the probe can be detected and from its position on the replica plate, the colony containing that clone can be identified on the master plate, 'picked' and cultured separately (Fig. 4.5).

Alternatively, if an antibody is available to a protein and an expression vector is used for the DNA cloning, then the replica filter clones can be screened for by the presence or absence of binding of the antibody to detect clones containing recombinant vectors with the DNA fragment containing the gene (or part of) of interest.

DNA libraries

Different sources of DNA can be used to make recombinant DNA molecules. DNA from nucleated cells is termed *total* or *genomic DNA*. DNA made by the action of the enzyme reverse transcriptase on mRNA is called *complementary DNA* or *cDNA*. It is possible to enrich for DNA sequences of particular interest by using a specific tissue or cell type as a source of mRNA, e.g. immature red blood cells (reticulocytes) containing predominantly globin mRNA resulted in cloning of the genes for the globin chains of haemoglobin (p. 140).

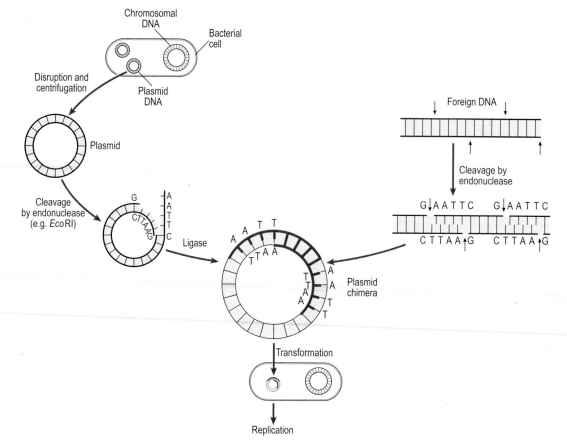

Fig. 4.4
Generation of a recombinant plasmid using *Eco*RI and transformation of the host bacterial organism. (From Emery A E H 1981 Lancet ii: 1406, with permission.)

The collection of recombinant DNA molecules generated from a specific source is referred to as a *DNA library*, e.g. a genomic or cDNA library. A DNA library of the human genome using plasmids as a vector would need to consist of several hundred thousand clones to be likely to contain the whole of the human genome. The use of YACs as cloning vectors with DNA digested by infrequently cutting restriction enzymes means that the whole of the human genome can be contained in a library of 13 000–14 000 clones.

Cell-free DNA cloning

One of the most revolutionary developments in DNA technology is the technique which was originally called DNA sequence amplification when it was first developed in the mid-1980s but is now commonly known as the *polymerase chain reaction* or *PCR*. PCR can be used to produce vast quantities of a target DNA fragment provided that the base pair sequence of that region is known or can be inferred from the amino acid sequence of a protein.

The polymerase chain reaction

PCR involves synthesizing two oligonucleotide primers of approximately 20 bp in length complementary to the DNA sequences flanking the target DNA fragment. The primers when added to denatured DNA will bind to the complementary DNA sequences which, with the action of DNA polymerase, will result in extension of the primer DNA on the single stranded DNA template in the presence of the deoxynucleotide triphosphates (dATP, dCTP, dGTP and dTTP) to synthesize the complementary DNA sequence. Subsequent heat denaturation of the double stranded DNA, followed by annealing of the same primer sequences to the resulting single stranded DNA will result in synthesis of further copies of the target DNA. 20–30 successive repeated cycles results in a 10^5–10^6-fold increase in the amount of the target DNA fragment, sufficient quantities of the target DNA for direct visualization by ultraviolet fluorescence after ethidium bromide staining, without the need to use indirect detection techniques (Fig. 4.6).

PCR allows analysis of DNA from any cellular source containing nuclei which, in addition to blood, can

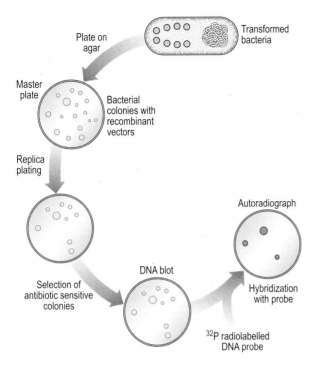

Fig. 4.5

Identification of recombinant DNA clones with specific DNA inserts by loss of antibiotic resistance, nucleic acid hybridization and autoradiography.

Fig. 4.6

Diagram of the polymerase chain reaction showing serial denaturation of DNA, primer annealing and extension with doubling of the target DNA fragment numbers in each cycle.

include less invasive samples such as buccal scrapings or pathological archival material. It is also possible to start with quantities of DNA as small as that from a single cell! Great care has to be taken with PCR, however, since DNA from a contaminating extraneous source such as desquamated skin from a laboratory worker, will also be amplified. This can lead to false-positive results unless the appropriate control studies are used to detect this possible source of error.

Another advantage of PCR is the rapid turn-round time of samples for analysis. Initially the PCR amplification cycles had to be carried out manually. In addition, the high temperatures required to denature the double stranded DNA for primer annealing resulted in the inactivation of the enzyme DNA polymerase I which was used for primer extension. This meant that further aliquots of DNA polymerase had to be added manually in each cycle of the amplification process. Human ingenuity and nature combined to overcome these difficulties by automation of the temperature cycling, aided by the use of heat-stable DNA polymerase isolated from the bacterium *Thermophilus aquaticus* which grows naturally in hot springs! This means that PCR products can be produced in a matter of hours rather than the days or weeks required for cell-based in vivo DNA cloning techniques.

DNA cloning by PCR, in contrast to in vivo cell-based techniques, has the disadvantage that it requires knowledge of the nucleotide sequence of the target DNA fragment and usually is best used to clone DNA fragments up to 1 kb, although long range PCR allows amplification of bigger DNA fragments in the range of 1–2 kb.

TECHNIQUES OF DNA ANALYSIS

Many methods of DNA analysis involve the use of nucleic acid probes and the process of nucleic acid hybridization.

NUCLEIC ACID PROBES

Nucleic acid probes are usually single stranded DNA sequences which have been radioactively or non-radioactively labelled and can be used to detect DNA or RNA fragments with sequence homology. DNA probes can come from a variety of sources including random genomic DNA sequences, specific genes, cDNA sequences or oligonucleotide DNA sequences produced synthetically based on knowledge of the protein amino acid sequence. A DNA probe can be labelled by a variety of processes, including isotopic labelling with ^{32}P and non-isotopic methods using modified nucleotides containing fluorophores, e.g. fluorescein or rhodamine. Hybridization of a radioactively labelled DNA probe with complementary DNA sequences on a nitrocellulose filter can be detected by autoradiography while DNA fragments which are fluorescently labelled can be detected by exposure to the appropriate wavelength of light, e.g. fluorescent in situ hybridization (p. 34).

NUCLEIC ACID HYBRIDIZATION

Nucleic acid hybridization involves mixing DNA from two sources which have been denatured by heat or alkali to make them single stranded and then, under the appropriate conditions, allowing complementary base pairing of homologous sequences. If one of the DNA sources has been labelled in some way, i.e. is a DNA probe, this allows identification of specific DNA sequences in the other source. The two main methods of nucleic acid hybridization most commonly used are Southern and Northern blotting.

Southern blotting

Southern blotting, named after Edwin Southern who developed the technique, involves digesting DNA by a restriction enzyme which is then subjected to electrophoresis on an agarose gel. This separates the DNA or restriction fragments by size, the smaller fragments migrating faster than the larger ones. The DNA fragments in the gel are then denaturated with alkali, making them single stranded. A 'permanent' copy of these single stranded fragments is made by transferring them on to a nitrocellulose filter which binds the single-stranded DNA, the so-called *Southern blot*. A particular target DNA fragment of interest from the collection on the filter can be visualized by adding a single stranded ^{32}P radioactively

labelled DNA probe which will hybridize with homologous DNA fragments in the Southern blot which can then be detected by autoradiography (Fig. 4.7).

Northern blotting

Northern blotting differs from Southern blotting by the use of mRNA as the target nucleic acid in the same

Fig. 4.7

Diagram of the Southern blot technique showing size fractionation of the DNA fragments by gel electrophoresis, denaturation of the double stranded DNA to become single stranded and transfer to a nitrocellulose filter which is hybridized with a ^{32}P radioactively labelled DNA probe.

procedure; mRNA is very unstable because of intrinsic cellular ribonucleases. Use of ribonuclease inhibitors allows isolation of mRNA which, if run on an electrophoretic gel, can be transferred to a filter. Hybridizing the blot with a radiolabelled DNA probe allows determination of the size and quantity of the mRNA transcript, a so-called *Northern blot* (Fig. 4.8). In a gene disorder in which a mutation has not been identified in the coding sequences, an alteration in the size of the mRNA transcript suggests the possibility of a mutation in a non-coding region of the gene such as the splice junction of the intron–exon border. Northern blotting can also be used to demonstrate the differential pattern of expression of a gene in different tissues or at different times of development.

RESTRICTION MAPPING

Hybridizing a specific DNA probe to Southern blots prepared from a particular source of DNA digested by a variety of different restriction enzymes, used in combination, allows detailed mapping of a DNA fragment or region. This enables what is termed a *restriction map* of the region to be constructed (Fig. 4.9).

DNA SEQUENCING

The cloning and amplification of a target DNA fragment allows its nucleotide sequence to be determined by *DNA sequencing*. The most commonly used technique is the dideoxy chain termination method. This involves making single stranded DNA templates of the DNA fragment using a special phage vector and then adding an aliquot of this template DNA to four different reaction mixtures which include DNA polymerase, the four deoxynucleotides,

Fig. 4.8
Representation of a Northern blot analysis of the ubiquitin conjugating enzyme gene UBE2L3 probed with cDNA to the human gene showing expression of 3 transcripts of approximately 2.7, 1.5 and 0.5 kb in multiple tissues with the 0.5 kb transcript being more abundantly expressed in testis (courtesy of Dr T Moynihan, Dept of Molecular Medicine, St. James's Hospital, Leeds).

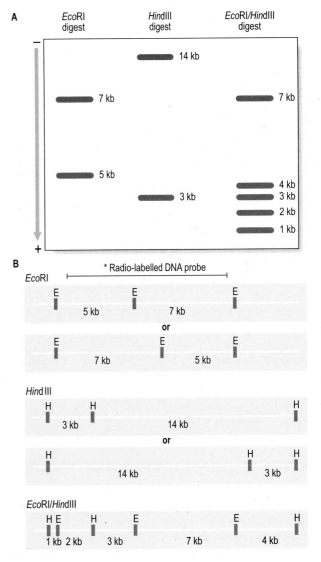

Fig. 4.9
Diagram of restriction mapping. (A) Representation of a Southern blot of *Eco*RI and *Hind*III digests and *Eco*RI/*Hind*III double digests of a DNA fragment. (B) The possible *Eco*RI and *Hind*III restriction maps and the consequent combined *Eco*RI/*Hind*III double digest restriction map.

a proportion of which have been radiolabelled, and a short primer sequence. A small amount of one of the four

respective dideoxynucleotides is added to one of each of the four separate reaction mixtures. The dideoxynucleotides lack a hydroxyl group at the 3' carbon position preventing phosphodiester bonding resulting in each reaction container consisting of a mixture of DNA fragments of different lengths which terminate in their respective dideoxynucleotide, due to chain termination occurring at random in each reaction mixture at the respective nucleotide.

When the reaction products are run on a polyacrylamide gel, a ladder of DNA sequences of differing lengths is produced. The DNA sequence complementary to the single stranded DNA template can be read directly from an autoradiograph of the gel (Fig. 4.10). Use of fluorescently labelled primers or nucleotides, which can be detected by a computerized laser detection system, allows rapid, accurate, automated sequencing which has found ready use in the sequencing of the human genome (p. 322) and in mutation detection for single gene disorders which are mutationally heterogeneous (Fig. 4.11).

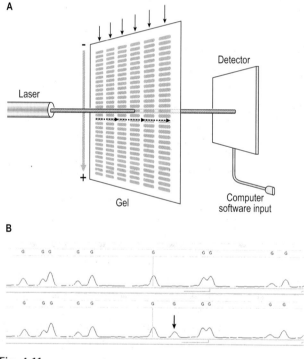

Fig. 4.11
Automated DNA sequencing using fluorescent primers. (A) Diagram of the principle of automated DNA sequencing. Different coloured fluorochromes are used for each ddNTP so that as individual DNA fragments migrate past the laser beam, they fluoresce and are detected. (B) An example of a fluorescent DNA sequencing output. The nucleotide sequence can be read by the various peaks of the coloured fluorochromes with green for adenine, red for thymine, blue for cytosine and black for guanine. The two traces are two different DNA sequences for the same portion of a gene, differing with the thymine being present in the upper trace and guanine in the lower trace at the position arrowed.

Fig. 4.10
Representation of the dideoxy method of DNA sequencing. (A) The reagents added to a single stranded DNA template and the resulting DNA sequences of different lengths ending in their respective dideoxynucleotides in the different reaction aliquots in the dideoxy method of DNA sequencing. (B) A portion of a sequencing gel from which the nucleotide sequence of the single stranded DNA template can be read as arrowed. (Courtesy of Dr G Taylor, Yorkshire Regional DNA Laboratory, St James's Hospital, Leeds.)

DNA microarrays

Short oligonucleotides, usually 7–8 nucleotides in length, which have been fluorescently labelled and attached to a high density gridded *microarray* can be used to detect hybridization of target DNA under appropriate conditions. Manufacture of DNA microarrays, or what are known as *DNA chips*, with the appropriate computerized software will allow rapid, automated high-throughput DNA sequencing.

MUTATION SCREENING TECHNIQUES

Although sequencing a gene can be used to identify mutations, many genes in humans are several hundred thousand or even million base pairs in length and are often mutationally heterogeneous, making this a daunting task. There are a number of techniques which can be used to screen for mutations which differ in their ease of use and reliability. Identification of a possible sequence variant by one of the mutation screening methods requires confirmation by DNA sequencing.

Denaturing gradient gel electrophoresis

Denaturing gradient gel electrophoresis, or *DGGE*, involves mixing a radiolabelled single stranded DNA probe with the double stranded DNA being screened, which has been heated to make it single stranded. This mixture is electrophoresed on a denaturing gradient gel. DNA which is identical with the sequence of the DNA probe will form a homoduplex, which, under the denaturing conditions of the gel, will remain hybridized. Any mismatches between the DNA being screened and the DNA probe will result in the formation of a heteroduplex which, as it is run down the denaturing gradient of the gel, will 'melt' becoming single stranded at a certain point resulting in a branched structure which has decreased mobility compared to the homoduplex. This can be detected on an autoradiograph. When screening DNA from males with X-linked disorders and individuals who are likely to be homozygous for autosomal recessive disorders, e.g. offspring of consanguineous matings, DNA from a normal individual will need to be used.

Single stranded conformational polymorphism

Radiolabelled PCR products of double stranded DNA, if made single stranded, fold up making a three-dimensional structure. An alteration in the DNA sequence can result in a different conformation which, under appropriate gel conditions, results in a different electrophoretic mobility, a so-called *single stranded conformational polymorphism*, or *SSCP* (Fig. 4.12).

Fig. 4.12
An autoradiograph of a gel using single stranded conformational polymorphisms to detect known mutations in the cystic fibrosis gene. (Courtesy of Dr G Taylor, Yorkshire Regional DNA Laboratory, St James's Hospital, Leeds.)

Chemical cleavage mismatch

Chemical cleavage mismatch, or *CCM*, involves the addition of the chemicals hydroxylamine and osmium tetroxide which react with free cytosine and thymine nucleotides respectively. By denaturing the double stranded DNA being screened and allowing it to hybridize with a single stranded radiolabelled DNA probe, any mismatched cytosine or thymine nucleotides will be exposed and therefore be susceptible to reaction with the hydroxylamine and osmium tetroxide. The addition of piperidine results in cleavage of the DNA being screened at any such sites. CCM identifies mismatches on either strand indirectly detecting adenine and guanine mismatches through their complementary nucleotides on the other strand and has the advantage that it can detect mutations in relatively larger DNA fragments up to 1 kb in size. In addition, although SSCP and DGGE do not provide information about the location in the DNA fragment being screened of any sequence variant identified, CCM has the advantage that analysis of the size of the fragments generated allows the location of the mutation in the DNA fragment to be determined.

Protein truncation test

In the *protein truncation test*, or *PTT*, cDNA is made from RNA by use of the technique known as *reverse transcriptase PCR*, or *RT-PCR*. This involves using a special primer which contains a promoter and translation initiator sequence. The resulting cDNA is then translated in a specially designed transcription–translation system with the resulting protein product being analysed on a gel. A truncated protein product will only occur with a nonsense, frameshift or splice site mutation and therefore PTT is used in disorders where these types of mutations most commonly occur, e.g. familial adenomatous polyposis (p. 200) and familial breast cancer arising from mutations in the *BRCA1* gene (p. 20).

DNA chip microarrays

DNA chip microarrays hold the promise of rapid mutation testing. They involve synthesizing custom-designed 20–25 base pair oligonucleotide sequences for both the normal DNA sequence and known and/or possible single nucleotide substitutions of a gene. These are attached to a 'chip' in a structured arrangement in what is known as a microarray. The sample DNA being screened for a mutation is amplified by PCR, fluorescently labelled and hybridized with the oligonucleotides in the microarray in competition with normal DNA which is labelled with a different coloured fluorochrome. Analysis of the colour pattern of the microarray generated after hybridization by a computer allows rapid automated mutation testing. The prospect of gene-specific DNA chip microarrays is likely to lead to a revolution in the speed and reliability of mutation screening, providing the technology is affordable and the technique can be demonstrated to be robust.

SITE-DIRECTED MUTAGENESIS

Site-directed mutagenesis is used to alter or modify DNA sequences in a directed fashion to produce 'tailor-made' mutations to acquire a greater understanding of the relationship between structure and function in proteins and has also enabled analysis of the controlling sequences in the flanking regions of eukaryotic structural genes. A number of different techniques can be used to introduce mutations. These include homologous recombination in which one DNA sequence is replaced by another with close similarity but known specific differences and the use of modified PCR primers which can alter or insert nucleotides into target DNA sequences. Site-directed mutagenesis has been used for the targeted introduction of mutations in genes for the production of transgenic animal models for inherited human disease (p. 69).

APPLICATIONS OF THE TECHNIQUES OF DNA ANALYSIS

DNA technology has allowed an understanding of the structure of genes and the mutational basis of many single gene disorders in humans.

ANALYSIS OF GENE STRUCTURE

Restriction mapping can reveal details of the structure of a gene and adjacent regions, as in the β-globin gene region which has allowed the ordering of the β-like globin genes (Fig. 4.13). Each globin gene, including introns, is about 1.5 kb in length and the total length of the complex is about 50 kb including the intergenic DNA. Interestingly, the physical order of the β-like globin genes corresponds to the order of expression of these genes during development (p. 142).

MUTATIONAL ANALYSIS OF SINGLE GENE DISORDERS

Mutational analysis of single gene disorders can be divided into direct mutation detection and mutation tracking methods.

Direct mutation detection methods

There are a number of ways in which a mutation in a gene can be directly detected.

Deletion detection

One of the first examples of the use of this approach was in the haemoglobinopathies (p. 144). Reticulocytes, immature red blood cells, contain only globin mRNA, from which a radioactive cDNA probe for globin genes can be produced. This probe can then be used to identify and localize DNA fragments which contain the globin genes in an autoradiograph of a Southern blot. In the case of δβ thalassaemia (p. 148), the DNA probe complementary to the β-globin gene does not hybridize with the same number and size of DNA fragments as in normal individuals. Differences in the size of DNA restriction fragments seen after digestion with a single restriction enzyme could be due to a random DNA polymorphism occurring within the nucleotide recognition sequence of that particular restriction enzyme. Demonstration of a difference in the DNA restriction fragment pattern when the DNA is digested with another restriction enzyme with a different nucleotide recognition sequence is consistent with a deletion being the probable cause of the disorder (Fig. 4.14).

Fig. 4.13

Representation of the human β-globin gene region (ψ represents the position of pseudogenes).

Mutation specific RFLPs

In some single gene disorders the mutation responsible eliminates a restriction enzyme recognition site. This direct approach has been used in sickle-cell disease using the restriction enzyme *Mst*II (Fig. 4.15). This approach is of limited use clinically as it is relatively rare for mutations to occur within the nucleotide recognition sequences of restriction endonucleases.

Fig. 4.14

Alteration in the *Eco*RI and *Hind*III restriction fragments in DNA from persons with δβ thalassaemia with a DNA probe from the δ- and β-globin genes compared with DNA from persons with two copies of the normal DNA sequence in the region of the δ- and β-globin genes consistent with δβ thalassaemia being the result of a deletion.

Fig. 4.15

Detection of the sickle-cell mutation by loss of a restriction enzyme nucleotide recognition sequence. (A) The single base pair difference of thymine for adenine in the second nucleotide of the sixth codon of the β-globin gene between HbA and HbS, resulting in the substitution of valine for glutamic acid along with the recognition site nucleotide sequence of the restriction enzyme *Mst*I. (B) Representation of the two different sized DNA restriction fragments of 1.3 kb in persons with the sickle-cell allele (HbS) and 1.1 kb with the normal β-globin allele (HbA) consequent upon loss of the *Mst*I restriction site (*) due to A to T mutation in the first exon in persons with the sickle-cell allele.

Allele specific oligonucleotides

If the mutational basis of a single gene disorder is a point mutation, it is possible to make short synthetic oligo-nucleotide DNA sequences corresponding to the normal and mutant sequences. By using appropriate reaction conditions, the normal and mutant DNA can be distinguished by demonstrating differential hybridization of the normal and mutant oligonucleotide sequences to the normal and mutant DNA sequences (Fig. 4.16).

Mutation tracking

If a gene has been mapped by linkage studies (p. 131) but not yet cloned so that mutation screening or direct mutation detection is not available, it is still possible to use inherited DNA sequence variation to track or follow

Fig. 4.16

Use of allele specific oligonucleotide probes to detect a single base pair mutation. (A) The formation of homo- and heteroduplexes between target mutant and normal DNA sequences and allele specific oligonucleotides for the normal and mutant DNA sequences. (B) The resulting electrophoretic gel of homoduplexes and heteroduplexes of DNA from persons heterozygous and homozygous for the normal and mutant sequences with allele specific oligonucleotides for the normal and mutant β-globin sequence.

a mutation within a family by following the pattern of inheritance of DNA sequence variants which are closely linked to the disease locus. There are a number of different types of *DNA sequence variants* or *polymorphisms* which can be used in *mutation tracking*.

DNA sequence polymorphisms

There is an enormous amount of DNA sequence variation in the human genome (p. 14). Two main types, restriction fragment length polymorphisms and hypervariable tandem repeat DNA length polymorphisms (p. 14), are predominately used in mutation tracking.

Restriction fragment length polymorphisms

Variation in the nucleotide sequence of the human genome is common, occurring approximately once every 200 bp. These single base pair differences in DNA nucleotide sequences are inherited in a Mendelian codominant manner and have no phenotypic effects as they usually occur in intergenic non-coding DNA. If a difference in DNA sequence occurs within the nucleotide recognition sequence of a restriction enzyme, the DNA fragments produced by that restriction enzyme will be of different lengths in different people. This can be recognized by the altered mobility of the restriction fragments on gel electrophoresis, so-called *restriction fragment length polymorphisms, RFLPs*.

Hypervariable tandem repeat DNA length polymorphisms

The different classes of tandemly repeated DNA sequences in the human genome, particularly DNA microsatellites (p. 14), have proven to be useful clinically in indirect methods of mutation detection or mutation 'tracking'.

Variable number tandem repeats

Variable number tandem repeats (VNTRs) are highly polymorphic and are due to the presence of variable numbers of tandem repeats of a short DNA sequence which have been shown to be inherited in a Mendelian codominant fashion (p. 100). VNTRs are very highly polymorphic when compared to RFLPs and have the advantage that they can be demonstrated using any restriction enzyme provided it does not cleave within the DNA sequence of the repeat unit (Fig. 4.17).

The first two examples of this type of DNA sequence polymorphism demonstrated in humans were close to the human insulin gene on chromosome 11 and the α-globin locus on chromosome 16. The latter was shown to be linked to the major locus for adult onset polycystic kidney disease and could be used in presymptomatic

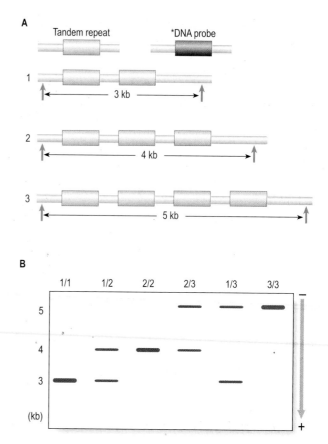

Fig. 4.17

Representation of variable number tandem repeat DNA sequences. (A) The physical arrangement of different length DNA sequence variants due to variable number of tandem repeats. (B) Representation of an autoradiograph of electrophoretic gel of variable number tandem repeats hybridized to a probe to the tandem repeat sequence.

diagnosis in persons from families at risk for this late onset autosomal dominant disorder (p. 290).

Minisatellites

Jeffreys identified a short 10–15 bp 'core' sequence with homology to many highly variable loci spread throughout the human genome (p. 14). Using a probe containing tandem repeats of this core sequence, a pattern of hyper-variable DNA fragments is identified. The multiple variable size repeat sequences identified by the core sequence are known as *minisatellites*.

It was hoped that minisatellite sequences would be useful in mutation tracking or linkage studies (p. 131) of disease loci by enabling simultaneous analysis of many more loci than is possible using conventional RFLPs. Unfortunately, even if an individual family is large enough to demonstrate linkage of a specific disease locus to a particular hypervariable DNA fragment, the data from different families cannot be collated as the genomic localization of each individual fragment is unknown.

Techniques are available, however, which allow the identification of the unique DNA sequences immediately flanking minisatellites. Using the entire minisatellite in high stringency hybridization conditions it is possible to develop locus specific probes which can be used in mutation tracking and allow its location in the human genome to be identified enabling its use in linkage studies.

DNA minisatellites are sufficiently polymorphic, however, to be unique and specific to an individual forming what is called a *DNA fingerprint*, which is now widely used in paternity testing (p. 247) (Fig. 4.18) and for forensic purposes.

Microsatellites

The human genome contains some 50 000–100 000 blocks of a variable number of tandem repeats of the dinucleotide CA:GT, so-called *CA repeats* or *microsatellites* (p. 14). The difference in the number of CA repeats at any one site between individuals is very highly polymorphic and these have been shown to be inherited in a Mendelian codominant manner (Fig. 4.19). In addition, highly polymorphic tri- and tetranucleotide repeats have also been identified, which can be used in a similar way.

Single nucleotide polymorphisms

Single nucleotide DNA sequence variation occurs, on average, approximately every 200 base pairs in the human genome. If this sequence variation is polymorphic, which is estimated to occur every $\frac{1}{500}$ to $\frac{1}{1200}$ base pairs, then there are likely to be in excess of 10^6 in the human genome. This DNA sequence variation, known as *single nucleotide polymorphisms* (SNPs), although only diallelic, has the advantage that it can be detected on solid state microarrays. This will allow high-throughput automated analysis of this polymorphic variation which can be used for genome searches for linkage studies in mapping single gene disorders (p. 70) and association studies in common diseases (p. 211).

Fig. 4.18
An autoradiograph of a minisatellite DNA fingerprint of two parents, their two offspring and an unrelated individual. Each band in the two offspring is present in one of the two parents and the differing pattern seen in the two male children demonstrates that they are non-identical twins. (Courtesy of Professor A Markham, St James's Hospital, Leeds.)

Fig. 4.19
An autoradiograph of a closely linked polymorphic CA repeat microsatellite cosegregating in a family with a dominant disorder. Allele 1 is segregating with the disorder in the affected members of the family. (Courtesy of Dr G Taylor, Yorkshire Regional DNA Laboratory, St James's Hospital, Leeds.)

Clinical applications of mutation tracking

There are a number of ways in which mutation tracking is used clinically.

Locus linked DNA sequence variants

If a locus for a genetic disorder is shown to be linked to a DNA sequence variant or polymorphism, this can be used for prenatal diagnosis (p. 303), to detect the presence of a gene in a person before the onset of symptoms or what is known as presymptomatic diagnosis (p. 290) and to identify female carriers of X-linked disorders (p. 288). The advantage of the use of DNA sequence polymorphisms in these clinical situations is that knowledge of the basic biochemical defect or the nature of the mutation responsible is not required, nor is it necessary to have access to a tissue in which the gene is expressed (Fig. 4.20).

Allele specific DNA sequence variants

Certain DNA sequence variants have been shown to occur in association with specific disease mutations more commonly than would be predicted by their individual frequencies in a population. In blacks of Afro-Caribbean origin with haemoglobin A, the normal β-globin gene usually occurs in a 7.6 or 7.0 kb DNA fragment of a *Hpa*I restriction enzyme digest. On the other hand, the sickle-cell globin gene is found in a 13.0 kb *Hpa*I fragment nearly 90% of the time (Fig. 4.21). This particular type of RFLP can be termed an allele specific DNA sequence variant and is said to be in linkage disequilibrium (p. 124) with the mutation.

DNA haplotypes

If closely linked DNA sequence polymorphisms are being used for carrier testing, presymptomatic or prenatal diagnosis, there can be families in which the results remain uninformative. In other words, the family does not possess the necessary variation at closely linked polymorphic sites to determine on which chromosome the disease allele is located. It is often possible, however, by looking at a number of different closely linked DNA sequence polymorphisms, for the family to be made informative by establishing what is known as a *DNA haplotype*, i.e. the pattern of DNA sequence polymorphisms flanking the disease and normal alleles in that particular family.

This principle can be illustrated in an example (Fig. 4.22). In the pedigree shown the male child (II₁) is affected with the autosomal recessive disorder cystic fibrosis. If the DNA sequence polymorphisms A and B are closely linked markers flanking the cystic fibrosis locus, then in each parent marker allele 2 must be on the

Fig. 4.20

Use of linked polymorphic DNA markers. The *Hsu*II-linked RFLPs in the ^Gγ- and ^Aγ- globin structural genes are closely linked to the β-globin gene in which the mutation responsible for β thalassaemia occurs. Analysis of the pattern of inheritance of these polymorphisms in the affected child and the pattern in the parents confirms that the female sib (II₂) of the male with β thalassaemia is heterozygous for β thalassaemia, having inherited the β thalassaemia gene from her mother and the normal β-globin gene from her father. N = normal; D = disease.

Fig. 4.21

An example of an allele-linked DNA polymorphism which is in linkage disequilibrium with a mutation. (A) The normal β-globin gene occurs most commonly in a 7.0 or 7.6 *Hpa*I DNA fragment. (B) The sickle-cell mutation is in linkage disequilibrium with *Hpa*I restriction site polymorphism to the 3′ side of the β-globin gene producing a 13.0 kb fragment.

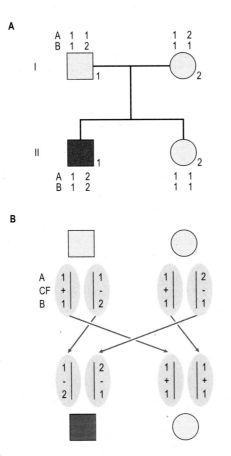

Fig. 4.22
Establishment of a DNA haplotype. (A) A two-generation family with a child affected with the autosomal recessive disorder, cystic fibrosis, with DNA sequence polymorphisms at flanking loci A and B. Neither marker on its own is fully informative. Together they produce a haplotype which is fully informative. (B) Inferred DNA sequence haplotypes at the cystic fibrosis and flanking loci which allow one to infer II₂ is homozygous normal for the cystic fibrosis gene.

same chromosome as the cystic fibrosis mutation. One can then infer that the normal cystic fibrosis gene is flanked by marker allele 1 at both sites in each parent. Analysis of the marker alleles in the affected child's sister (II$_2$) would predict her to be homozygous for the normal gene at that locus.

In some single gene diseases certain DNA haplotypes occur more frequently with particular mutations than would be predicted by their individual frequency in the population, i.e. they are in linkage disequilibrium (p. 124) with the mutation.

MOLECULAR PATHOLOGY

There are now more than 8000 recognized Mendelian characteristics in humans, many of which are associated with disease. In a rapidly increasing number the gene has been cloned and the mutational basis has been identified. As a consequence any list of genes and their mutations,

although of interest, will be of limited practical value as it will rapidly be out of date (Table 4.3). The best way to obtain up-to-date information on the molecular pathology of single gene disorders is through one of the Web sites on the Internet that have been developed and maintained as part of the Human Genome Project (see appendix).

Animal models of inherited disease

Animal models of human inherited diseases are essential to understand the molecular basis at the DNA, biochemical and cellular levels as well as to provide a test system for new treatments before clinical trials can be considered in humans (p. 323). Spontaneously occurring animal mutants for human inherited disease are limited in number. Exposure to chemical mutagens, such as ethyl nitrosourea (ENU) produces mutations in DNA (p. 27) which occur on a random basis. Identification of mutants in particular genes requires a systematic research screening programme to identify and characterize induced mutants. A number of such programmes are under way at present and hold great promise for identifying large numbers of new mouse mutants which will serve as powerful tools for the analysis of inherited diseases in humans.

The development of *gene targeting* which allows the introduction of specific mutations into genes by homologous recombination (p. 64) in mouse embryonic stem cells, along with the ability to produce *knock-out* mutations which result in the complete loss of function of the gene, allow modelling of the functional effects of various mutations including complete loss of function. This involves the targeted introduction of a mutation into a specific gene in a mouse *embryonic stem (ES) cell*. The modified ES cell is injected into a blastocyst which is then allowed to continue to develop in a foster mother. The subsequent offspring, which are mosaics for the introduced mutation, are interbred and their offspring are then screened for the presence/absence of the mutation (Fig. 4.23). In some instances, the targeted or knock-out mutation is found to be prenatally lethal. In this instance it is possible to engineer a mutation that is only expressed under certain conditions, e.g. raised temperature, or what is known as a *conditional knock-out*.

The targeted introduction of mutations, along with the study of spontaneous and induced mutants in model organisms such as the mouse promises to greatly facilitate our understanding of the developmental basis of a large number of inherited disorders in humans, as well as enhancing the possibility of therapeutic intervention, e.g. the CF mouse (p. 19).

DIAGNOSIS IN NON-GENETIC DISEASE

DNA technology, especially PCR, has found application

Table 4.3   Single gene diseases in humans with their molecular basis

Disorder	Nature of molecular defect
Autosomal dominant	
Antithrombin III deficiency	Deletions, point mutations, insertions
Familial hypercholesterolaemia	Deletions, point mutations, duplications, insertions (Alu repeat)
Huntington's disease	CAG triplet repeat expansion
Myotonic dystrophy	CTG triplet repeat expansion
Neurofibromatosis type I (von Recklinghausen's disease)	Deletions (Alu repeat), point mutations, insertions, splice site mutations
Osteogenesis imperfecta	Deletions, point mutations
Autosomal recessive	
α_1-antitrypsin deficiency	Point mutations, deletions, insertions, duplications
Congenital adrenal hyperplasia (21-hydroxylase deficiency)	Point mutations, deletions
Cystic fibrosis	Deletions, point mutations, insertions
Growth hormone deficiency (rare familial form)	Deletions
Phenylketonuria	Point mutations, deletions, insertions
Tay–Sachs disease	Deletions, point mutations
X-linked	
Chronic granulomatous disease	Deletions, point mutations
Duchenne/Becker muscular dystrophy	Deletions, duplications, point mutations
Fragile X mental retardation	CGG triplet repeat expansion
Haemophilia A (factor VIII deficiency)	Point mutations, deletions, insertions, duplications, inversions
Haemophilia B (factor IX deficiency)	Point mutations, deletions, insertions
Lesch–Nyhan syndrome (HGPRT deficiency)	Deletions, point mutations, insertions, duplications
Ornithine transcarbamylase deficiency	Deletions, point mutations
Emery–Dreifuss muscular dystrophy	Deletion, insertion, point mutations

HGPRT = hypoxanthine-guanine phosphoribosyl transferase.

in the diagnosis and management of both infective and malignant disease.

Infective disease

The polymerase chain reaction can be used to detect the presence of DNA sequences specific to a particular infectious organism before conventional evidence such as an antibody response or the results of cultures are available. An example is the screening of blood products for the presence of DNA sequences from the human immunodeficiency virus (HIV) to ensure the safety of their use, e.g. screening pooled factor VIII concentrate for use in males with haemophilia A. Another example is the identification of DNA sequences specific to bacterial or viral organisms responsible for acute overwhelming infections, where early diagnosis allows prompt institution of the correct antibiotic or antiviral agent with the prospect of reducing morbidity and mortality.

Malignant disease

The extreme sensitivity of PCR means it has potential applications in malignancy for detecting residual disease or recurrence after treatment for disorders such as leukaemia. This can be vital to the choice of timing, continuation, duration and reinstitution of chemotherapy with relapse of the malignant disease.

MAPPING, IDENTIFICATION AND CLONING OF GENES IN HUMANS

The identification of the gene responsible for an inherited single gene disorder, as well as having immediate clinical diagnostic application, will enable an understanding of the developmental basis of the pathology (p. 81) with the prospect of possible therapeutic interventions (p. 325). The physical mapping of a gene is an essential first step in its identification and cloning.

Gene mapping

Gene mapping can be divided into two main types. The first involves techniques used to assign a gene or DNA fragment to a specific chromosome or a particular region of a chromosome, or what can be called *chromosome* or *low resolution mapping*. The second, finer level of analysis provides detailed mapping information which includes the physical relationship to flanking DNA sequence polymorphisms or what is called *high resolution DNA mapping*.

Chromosome/low resolution mapping techniques

Chromosome mapping techniques include gene dosage, somatic cell hybridization, chromosome-specific DNA libraries and in situ hybridization studies.

Gene dosage

The study of persons with chromosome abnormalities looking for increased amounts of a particular protein in trisomic individuals (p. 44), and decreased amounts in individuals with deletions (p. 49), can allow assignment of structural genes to a particular chromosome. Although the genes for the enzymes superoxide dismutase and red cell acid phosphatase were provisionally assigned to chromosomes 21 and 2 respectively by this means, gene dosage studies have found limited use in mapping studies, being superseded by somatic cell hybridization and in situ hybridization techniques.

Somatic cell hybridization

Somatic cell hybridization involves taking cells from two different species and fusing them, a process facilitated by the presence of the Sendai virus or by the use of the chemical polyethyleneglycol. The chromosome constitution of the resulting somatic cell hybrid shows a preferential loss of the human chromosomes from the cells (Fig. 4.24). It is possible to determine which human chromosomes have been retained and select interspecific hybrids which contain different human chromosome(s). A panel of somatic cell hybrid clones which retain different human chromosomes can be selected which will enable assignment of any DNA sequence or expressed enzyme or protein to a particular human chromosome. Cells from individuals with chromosome rearrangments, e.g. deletions or translocations, can be used to more precisely map a gene to a particular region of a chromosome. As a further refinement of this approach, cells exposed to radiation which fragments their chromosomes, allow the establishment of so-called *radiation hybrids*. These contain subchromosomal fragments enabling assignment of a

Fig. 4.23
Gene targeting by homologous recombination to create a transgenic 'knock-out' mouse for cystic fibrosis.

Fig. 4.24
The hybridization of human and mouse cells and subsequent selective loss of chromosomes from the hybrid cells.

particular gene or DNA sequence to a specific region of a chromosome.

Chromosome specific DNA libraries

Chromosomes can be sorted through the technique of *fluorescent activated chromosome sorting*, or FACS. FACS utilizes the differential fluoresence of the various chromosomes with DNA-binding dyes on exposure to laser light of a particular wavelength which arises through their variation in size, DNA content and composition (p. 37). This allows the creation of chromosome-specific DNA libraries which can be screened to assign DNA sequences or genes to specific chromosomes.

In situ hybridization

Single stranded radiolabelled DNA sequences incubated under special conditions with standard chromosome preparations will hybridize with homologous DNA sequence(s) in the genome. This allows mapping of single copy genes or DNA sequences on the chromosomes by exposure of the preparation to an X-ray film, or what is known as *in situ hybridization*. The availability of non-radioactive labelling techniques has allowed development of fluorescent in situ hybridization (p. 34) which has found widespread use in mapping of genes and DNA fragments.

DNA/high resolution mapping techniques

In single gene disorders which have been mapped by linkage studies (p. 121) to a particular region of a chromosome, even with closely adjacent markers, the gene of interest can still only be located within a region of several million base pairs. Sequencing of DNA fragments of this size to identify a gene of interest is possible but can still be technically difficult, labour intensive and expensive. The techniques of pulsed field gel electrophoresis, high resolution FISH and yeast artificial chromosome clone contig analysis can be used to give mapping information at this intermediate level of analysis.

Pulsed field gel electrophoresis

Conventional agarose gel electrophoresis can resolve DNA fragments up to approximately 20 000 base pairs in size. Use of *pulsed field gel electrophoresis*, or *PFGE*, in which DNA fragments are subjected alternately to two approximately perpendicular fields in the electrophoretic gel, enables separation of DNA fragments of up to 2 000 000 base pairs in size. Digestion of DNA with restriction enzymes such as *Not*I and *Pvu*I, which have 6–8 base pair nucleotide recognition sequences which occur less frequently at random in DNA, results in relatively larger DNA fragments. Analysis of restriction digests of genomic DNA using these infrequently cutting restriction enzymes allows construction of physical maps of relatively large

stretches of DNA not amenable to resolution by conventional restriction mapping studies. DNA for PFGE analysis must be extracted in situ in the gel since genomic DNA extracted by conventional methods results in physical fragmentation of the DNA.

High resolution FISH

Fluorescent in situ hybridization of metaphase chromosomes (p. 34) has a limit of resolution in mapping of at least one or more megabases. FISH utilizing preparations of cells in which the chromosomes are in interphase (p. 38) allows mapping of DNA sequences which are 50–500 kb apart. Use of chromatin or DNA fibres which have been artificially extended, or what is known as *chromatin fibre FISH*, enables mapping of DNA fragments which are separated by 2–3 and up to 700 kb (Fig. 4.25).

Yeast artificial chromosome clone contigs

The development of cloning vectors such as yeast artificial chromosomes (p. 57) allows cloning of large segments of genomic DNA. YACs are commonly used in long-range physical mapping by the production of overlapping YAC clones. A number of means of sequence tagging and repetitive DNA fingerprinting of the YAC clones allows an ordered assembly of clones extending in both directions from a start point, or what is known as

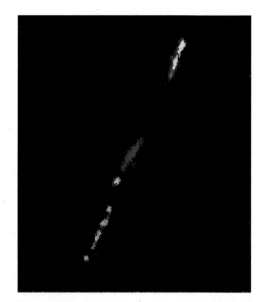

Fig. 4.25
Simultaneous use of three different fluorescently labelled cosmid clones, 203H12 (green), ABO.17 (red) and 255A6 (yellow), hybridized to single stranded genomic DNA fibres in the region of the tuberous sclerosis locus (TSC1) on the long arm of chromosome 9 allowing their physical order in relation to each other to be determined. (From Hornigold N, van Slegtenhorst M, Nahmias J et al 1997 A 1.7 megabase sequence-ready cosmid contig covering the TSC1 candidate region in 9q34. Genomics 41: 385–390, with permission.)

chromosome walking, to establish a *YAC contig*. Use of standardized gridded arrays of YAC libraries along with automation of certain techniques greatly reduces the effort involved.

Identification of genes

There are a number of techniques which can be used to identify coding sequences or genes with DNA fragments or clones. This includes the identification of HTF/CpG islands, zoo blotting, exon trapping, expressed sequence tags, homology to genes in model organisms and analysis of databases from the Human Genome Project (see appendix).

HTF/CpG islands

A number of the infrequently cutting restriction enzymes, such as *Hpa*II, contain one or more CpG dinucleotides (cytosine-guanine dinucleotide with the intervening phosphate molecule) within the nucleotide recognition sequence necessary for DNA cleavage. Methylation of the cytosine residue of this dinucleotide pair prevents cleavage of the DNA by these restriction enzymes. It has been found that CpG dinucleotides occur with one-quarter of the frequency which would be predicted from the base composition of genomic DNA and that they are non-randomly distributed within the genome. Clusters of undermethylated CpG dinucleotides have been found near transcription initiation sites at the 5' end of many genes and are called methylation-free *Hpa*II tiny fragments, *HTF* or *CpG islands*. Cleavage at one of these sites which identifies a methylation-free region can be used to determine the likely location of genes within a stretch of DNA. Just over one-half of genes, however, are associated with HTF/CpG islands while only approximately 40% of genes which show tissue-specific expression are associated with an HTF/CpG island. Conversely not all HTF/CpG islands are found in association with genes.

Zoo blots

The structure and relative position of many genes have been highly conserved during evolution so that in closely related species the same DNA sequences or genes, or what are known as *homologues*, often occur in the same relative position to each other. Southern blots of DNA from a number of different species comprise what is known as a *zoo blot*. If a DNA fragment is found to be present in a number of different species then it is thought likely to contain coding sequences of an important functional gene which has been conserved by being highly selected for during evolution.

Exon trapping

Exon trapping involves the use of expression cloning vectors containing DNA sequences, which, when used to transfect a suitably modified eukaryotic cell line, result in transcription of the inserted target DNA into RNA which undergoes splicing. The production of an abnormally sized splice product after insertion of a target DNA fragment indicates the presence of an exon in the cloned DNA fragment which is likely to contain the coding sequence of a gene.

Expressed sequence tags

Sequence-specific primers from cDNA clones can be designed to identify sequences of expressed genes constituting what are known as *expressed sequence tags* or *ESTs*. ESTs can be assigned to a specific chromosomal location by a variety of methods which include chromosomal and radiation hybrids (p. 71), fluorescent in situ hybridization (p. 34) and PCR analysis of gridded arrays of yeast artificial chromosomes (p. 72). By virtue of their mapping location and the cell or tissue origin of the mRNA from which the cDNA is derived, ESTs provide a rich source of partial sequences of a large number of positional candidate genes for inherited diseases in humans.

Analysis of Human Genome Project databases

A number of computer programs have been developed which can search genomic DNA sequence databases for sequence homology to known genes, as well as DNA sequences specific to all genes such as the conserved intron–exon splice junctions, promoter sequences, poly-adenylation sites and stretches of open reading frames (ORFs). The use of this approach offers the prospect of what is known as *cloning in silico*!

Homology to genes in model organisms

The recognition of phenotypic features in a model organism, such as the mouse, which are similar to those seen in persons affected with an inherited disorder, allows the possibility that the cloning of the gene in the model organism, can lead to more rapid identification of the gene responsible in humans. An example of this approach was the mapping of the gene responsible for the inherited disorder of pigmentation and deafness known as Waardenburg's syndrome which was mapped to the long arm of human chromosome 2. This region of chromosome 2 shows extensive homology, or what is known as *synteny*, to the region of mouse chromosome 1 to which the gene for the murine pigmentary mutant known as *Splotch* had been assigned. The mapping of the murine

Pax3 gene, which codes for a transcription factor expressed in the developing nervous system, to this region suggested it as a positional candidate gene for the disorder. It was suggested that the pigmentary abnormalities could arise on the basis that melanocytes, in which melanin synthesis takes place, are derived from the neural crest. Identification of mutations in *PAX3*, the human homologue, confirmed it as the gene responsible for Waardenburg's syndrome.

Cloning of genes

Although a single gene disorder can be physically mapped to a specific region of a chromosome, there are usually a large number of genes, often several hundred or thousand within that interval, which could potentially be the particular gene reponsible for the inherited disorder. Three main ways have been used to clone genes.

Functional cloning

If the protein product of a gene can be isolated by biochemical or immunological methods then its amino acid sequence can be determined. Knowledge of the genetic code allows synthesis of oligonucleotide sequences which can then be used to screen appropriate cDNA libraries. cDNA clones so identified are used to screen a genomic DNA library for genomic DNA clones which will enable identification and characterization of the gene. This process, called *functional cloning*, has been of limited use because in only a minority of single gene disorders has the gene product been identified.

Positional cloning

Once a gene has been assigned to a particular region of a chromosome, despite lack of information about the gene product and its function, it is possible to identify the gene responsible, by what was originally incorrectly called *reverse genetics* and what is more correctly called *positional cloning*. Identification of some of the first genes by positional cloning often involved important clinical observations.

Individuals with single gene disorders and chromosomal abnormalities

Occasionally individuals are recognized with single gene disorders who are also found to have structural chromosomal abnormalities. The first clue that the gene responsible for Duchenne muscular dystrophy, DMD (p. 280), was located on the short arm of the X chromosome was the identification of a number of females with DMD who were also found to have a chromosomal rearrange-

ment between an autosome and a specific region of the short arm of one of their X chromosomes. Isolation of DNA clones spanning the region of the X chromosome involved in the rearrangement led in one such female to more detailed gene mapping information as well as to the eventual cloning of the DMD or dystrophin gene (p. 281).

At the same time as these observations, a male was reported with three X-linked disorders: Duchenne muscular dystrophy, chronic granulomatous disease and retinitis pigmentosa. He also had an unusual X-linked red cell group known as the McLeod phenotype. It was suggested that he could have a deletion of a number of genes of the short arm of his X chromosome including the Duchenne muscular dystrophy gene, or what is now termed a *contiguous gene syndrome*. Detailed prometaphase chromosome analysis revealed this to be the case. DNA from this individual was used in vast excess to hybridize in competitive reassociation, under special conditions, with DNA from persons with multiple X chromosomes to enrich for DNA sequences which he lacked, the so-called *p*henol *e*nhanced *r*eassociation *t*echnique, or *pERT*, which allowed isolation of DNA clones containing portions of the DMD gene.

The occurrence of individuals with a chromosome abnormality and a single gene disorder is rare, but identification of such individuals is important since they have led to the cloning of several other important disease genes in humans, e.g. tuberous sclerosis (p. 99) and familial adenomatous polyposis (p. 200).

Positional candidate genes

Searching databases for cloned genes with a function likely to be involved in the pathogenesis of the inherited disorder can also suggest what are known as *candidate genes*. If a disease has been mapped to a particular chromosomal region, any gene mapping to that region is a *positionial candidate gene*. Data on the pattern of expression, the timing and the distribution of tissue and cells types, may suggest that a certain positional candidate gene or genes are more likely to be responsible for the phenotypic features seen in persons affected with a particular single gene disorder. The observation of a similar disease phenotype in another species, such as the mouse, may suggest obvious candidate genes based on the conservation of homologous, or what more correctly are called *orthologous* regions of chromosomes between species.

Identification of a gene with homology to a known gene causing a recognized inherited disorder can suggest it as a possible candidate gene for other inherited disorders with a similar phenotype. For example, the identification of mutations in the connexin 26 gene which codes for one of the proteins which constitute the gap-junctions between cells causing sensorineural hearing impairment/

deafness has led to the identification of other connexins being responsible for inherited hearing impairment/deafness.

Confirmatory testing that a candidate gene is a disease gene

Confirmation that a candidate gene is responsible for a single gene disorder requires the following criteria to be fulfilled. Mutations in candidate genes can be screened for by a variety of methods (p. 63) and confirmed by DNA sequencing (p. 61). Sequence changes in the gene such as substitution of a polar for a hydrophobic amino acid in an important functional domain of the protein, or a nonsense mutation leading to premature termination of translation through generation of a stop codon (p. 19), are likely to have significant functional effects. These provide particularly convincing evidence that a potential candidate gene is responsible for a single gene disorder.

Further support is provided by the observation that the candidate gene is expressed in the appropriate tissues and at the relevant stages of development. The production of a transgenic animal model by the targeted introduction of the mutation into the homologous gene in another species (p. 69), which is shown to exhibit similar phenotypic features to those seen in persons affected with the disorder, and restoration of the normal phenotype by transfection of the normal gene into a cell line, provides final proof that the candidate gene and the disease gene are one and the same.

THE HUMAN GENE MAP

The rate at which single gene disorders and their genes are being mapped in humans is increasing exponentially (see Fig. 1.4, p. 6). Many of the more common and clinically important single gene disorders have been mapped to produce the 'morbid anatomy of the human genome' (Fig. 4.26).

POSSIBLE BIOLOGICAL HAZARDS OF DNA TECHNOLOGY

DNA technology has a very great deal to offer to medicine but there is genuine concern, amongst the public in particular, that potentially serious hazards of DNA technology should not be ignored. Recombinant DNA technology is being used to improve animal and plant stocks for food production, and recombinant microbial strains are being engineered to deal with environmental waste products. Some factions suggest that insufficient consideration is being given to the serious potential consequences which could follow introduction of the use of these techniques. For example, it is claimed that the engineered microbial strains, if released into the environment, could cause far more problems than they solve. These concerns, in many instances, are likely to be more theoretical than practical.

The main concern surrounding DNA technology is the danger of producing transgenic organisms which could contain genes for cancer susceptibility or be resistant to all known antibiotics. After all, one of the host organisms which is commonly used in such experiments is *E. coli*, which is ubiquitous being a normal bowel commensal. These are matters which have been of considerable public concern and were the subject of the famous Asilomar Conferences in California in the mid-1970s. The consensus of scientific opinion now, however, seems to be that these dangers have been very much exaggerated. Various authorities, such as the Genetic Manipulation Advisory Group (GMAG) in Britain and the National Institutes of Health in the United States, have laid down very careful guidelines for the use of recombinant DNA techniques.

TECHNIQUES TO MINIMIZE BIOHAZARDS

There have been two main approaches to limiting potential hazards of DNA technology. These can be separated into physical and biological containment methods.

Physical containment

Here the object is to make sure that any microorganisms of potential danger are contained by use of specially designed laboratories having special ventilator systems. Laboratories are graded, according to the type of experiments being conducted, from C I (minimum containment), which involves little more than the use of careful techniques, to C IV (maximum containment), where containment is of an exceptionally high order. This high level of containment is used in laboratories involved in biological warfare such as Porton Down in Britain and Camp Detrick in the United States.

Biological containment

Host organisms used in recombinant DNA work have been attenuated, or 'crippled', so that they cannot survive outside the confines of specialized laboratory culture conditions. This is achieved by careful selection of particular mutants which led, for example, to the production of the *E. coli* K12 strain 1776 (after the year of American independence!) which requires many complex growth factors if it is to survive outside the laboratory. At the same time, complementary work has produced

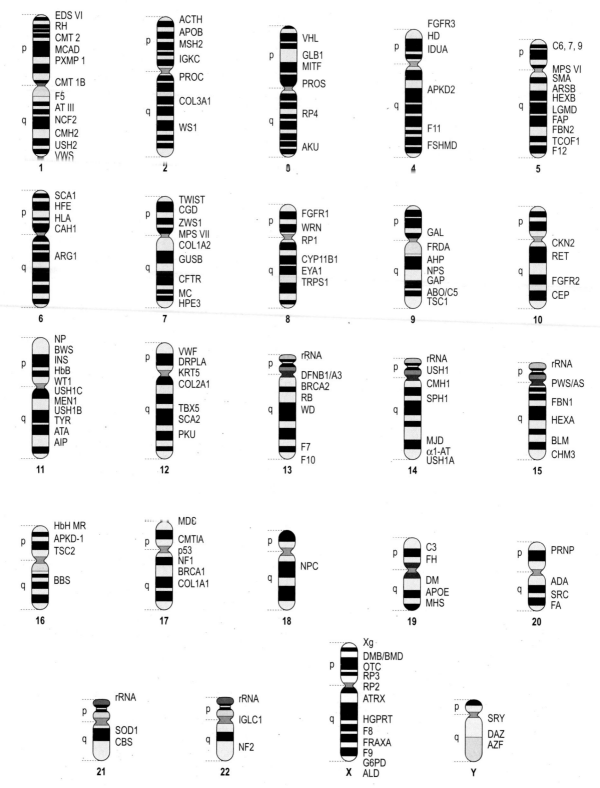

Fig. 4.26

A gene map of the human genome with examples of some of the more common or important single genes and disorders.

α1-AT – 14q32 – α₁-antitrypsin deficiency
ABO – 9q34 – ABO blood group
ACTH – 2p25 – Adrenocorticotrophic hormone deficiency
ADA – 20q13.11 – Severe combined immunodeficiency, ADA deficiency

AHP – 9q34 – Acute hepatic porphyria
AIP – 11q23.3 – Acute intermittent porphyria
AKU – 3q2 – Alkaptonuria
ALD – Xq28 – Adrenoleukodystrophy

APKD1 — 16p13 — Adult polycystic kidney disease, locus 1
APKD2 — 4q21-23 — Adult polycystic kidney disease, locus 2
APOB — 2p24 — Apolipoprotein B
APOE — 19q.13.2 — Apolipoprotein E
ARG1 — 6q23 — Arginase deficiency, argininaemia
ARSB — 5q11-13 — Mucopolysaccharidosis type VI, Maroteaux–Lamy syndrome
AS — 15q11-13 — Angelman syndrome
ATA — 11q22.3 — Ataxia telangiectasia
AT III — 1q23-25 — Antithrombin III
ATRX — Xq13 — α thalassaemia mental retardation
AZF — Yq11 — Azoospermia factor
BBS2 — 16q21 — Bardet–Biedl syndrome
BLM — 15q26.1 — Bloom's syndrome
BRCA1 — 17q21 — Familial breast/ovarian cancer, locus 1
BRCA2 — 13q12.3 — Familial breast/ovarian cancer, locus 2
BWS — 11p15.4 — Beckwith-Wiedemann syndrome
C3 — 19p13.2-13.3 — Complement factor 3
C5 — 9q34.1 — Complement factor 5
C6 — 5p13 — Complement factor 6
C7 — 5p13 — Complement factor 7
C9 — 5p13 — Complement factor 9
CAH1 — 6p21.3 — Congenital adrenal hyperplasia, 21-hydroxylase
CBS — 21q22.3 — Homocystinuria
CEP — 10q25.2-26.3 — Congenital erythropoietic porphyria
CFTR — 7q31.2 — Cystic fibrosis transmembrane conductance regulator
CKN2 — 10q11 — Cockayne syndrome 2, late onset
CMH1 — 14q12 — Hypertrophic obstructive cardiomyopathy type 1
CMH2 — 1q3 — Hypertrophic obstructive cardiomyopathy type 2
CMH3 - 15q22 — Hypertrophic obstructive cardiomyopathy type 3
CMT1A — 17p11.2 — Charcot-Marie-Tooth disease type 1A
CMT1B — 1q22 — Charcot-Marie-Tooth disease type 1B
CMT2 — 1p35-36 — Charcot-Marie-Tooth disease type 2
COL1A1 — 17q21.31-22 — Collagen type I, α_1 chain, osteogenesis imperfecta
COL1A2 — 7q22.1 — Collagen type I, α_2 chain, osteogenesis imperfecta
COL2A1 — 12q13.11-13.2 — Collagen type II, Stickler syndrome
COL3A1 — 2q31 — Collagen type III, α_1 chain, Ehlers–Danlos syndrome type IV
CYP11B1 — 8q21 — Congenital adrenal hyperplasia, 11β-hydroxylase
DAZ — Yq11 — Deleted in azoospermia
DFNB1/A3 — 13q12 — Non-syndromic sensorineural deafness, 1st recessive, 3rd dominant locus
DM — 19q13.2-13.3 — Myotonic dystrophy
DMD/BMD — Xp21.2 — Dystrophin, Duchenne and Becker muscular dystrophy
DRPLA — 12p13.1-12.3 — Dentatorubropallidoluysian disease
EDS VI — 1p36.2-36.3 — Ehlers–Danlos syndrome type VI
EYA1 — 8q13.3 — Brachio-oto-renal syndrome
F5 — 1q23 — Coagulation protein V
F7 — 13q34 — Coagulation protein VII
F8 — Xq28 — Coagulation protein VIII, haemophilia A
F9 — Xq27.1-27.2 — Coagulation protein IX, Christmas disease, haemophilia B
F10 — 13q34 — Coagulation protein X
F11 — Xq27.1-27.2 — Coagulation factor XI
F12 — 5q33-qter — Coagulation factor XII
FAP — 5q21-22 — Familial adenomatous polyposis, Gardner's syndrome

FBN1 — 15q21.1 — Fibrillin-1, Marfan syndrome
FBN2 — 5q23-31 — Fibrillin-2, contractural arachnodactyly
FGFR1 — 8p11.1-11.2 — Fibroblast growth factor receptor 1, Pfeiffer's syndrome
FGFR2 — 10q26 — Fibroblast growth factor receptor 2, Crouzon's, Pfeiffer's, Apert's syndrome
FGFR3 — 4p16.3 — Fibroblast growth factor receptor 3, achondroplasia, thanatophoric dysplasia
FH — 19p13.1-13.2 — Familial hypercholesterolaemia
FRAXA (FMR1) — Xq27.3 — Fragile X mental retardation
FRDA — 9q13-21.1 — Friedreich's ataxia
FSHMD — 4q35 — Facio-scapulo-humeral muscular dystrophy
GAL — 9p13 — Galactosaemia
GAP — 9q31 — Basal cell naevus syndrome, Gorlin's syndrome
GLB1 — 3p21.33 — GM$_1$ gangliosidosis
G6PD — Xq28 — Glucose-6-phosphate dehydrogenase
GUSB — 7q21.11 — Mucopolysaccharidosis type VII, Sly syndrome
HbB — 11p15.5 — β-globin gene
HD — 4p16.3 — Huntington's disease
HEXA — 15q23-24 — Hexosaminidase A, Tay–Sachs disease
HEXB — 5q13 — Hexosaminidase B, Sandhoff disease
HFE — 6p21.3 — Haemochromatosis
HGPRT — Xq26-27.2 — Hypoxanthine guanine phosphoribosyl transferase, Lesch–Nyhan syndrome
HLA — 6p21.3 — Major histocompatibility locus
HPE3 — 7q36 — Holoprosencephaly
IDUA — 4p16.3 — Mucopolysaccharidosis type I, Hurler's syndrome
IGKC — 2p12 — Immunoglobulin κ light chain
IGLC1 — 22q11 — Immunoglobulin λ light chains
INS — 11p15.5 — Insulin-dependent diabetes mellitus type 2
KRT5 — 12q11-13 — Epidermolysis bullosa simplex, Koebner type
LGMD7 — 5q31 — Limb-girdle muscular dystrophy
MCAD — 1p31 — Acyl Co-A dehydrogenase, medium chain
MDS — 17p13.3 — Miller–Dieker lissencephaly syndrome
MEN1 — 11q13 — Multiple endocrine neoplasia syndrome type 2
MHS — 19q13.1 — Malignant hyperpyrexia susceptibility, locus 1
MITF — 3p14.1 — Waardenburg's syndrome type 2
MJD — 14q24.3-31 — Machado-Joseph disease, spinocerebellar ataxia type 3
MPS VI — 5q11-13 — Maroteaux–Lamy syndrome
MSH2 — 2p15-16 — Hereditary non-polyposis colorectal cancer type 1
NCF2 — 1q25 — Chronic granulomatous disease, NCF2 deficiency
NF1 — 17q11.2 — Neurofibromatosis type I, von Recklinghausen's disease
NF2 — 22q12.2 — Neurofibromatosis type II, bilateral acoustic neuroma
NP — 11p15.1-15.4 — Niemann–Pick disease type A and B
NPC — 18q11-12 — Niemann–Pick disease type C
NPS — 9q43 — Nail-patella syndrome
OTC — Xp21.1 — Ornithine transcarbamylase
p53 — 17p13.1 — p53 protein, Li-Fraumeni syndrome
PKU — 12q24.1 — Phenylketonuria
PROC — 2q13-14 — Protein C, coagulopathy disorder
PROS — 3p11.1-q11.2 — Protein S, coagulopathy disorder
PRNP — 20p12-pter — Prion disease protein
PWS — 15q11 — Prader–Willi syndrome
PXMP1 — 1p21-22 — Zellweger's syndrome, type 2
RB — 13q14.1-14.2 — Retinoblastoma
RET — 10q11.2-Familial medullary thyroid carcinoma, MEN IIA and IIB, familial Hirschsprung's disease

RH — 1p34–36.2 — Rhesus null disease, Rhesus blood group
RP1 — 8p11–q21 — Retinitis pigmentosa, locus 1
RP2 — Xp11.3 — Retinitis pigmentosa, locus 2
RP3 — Xp21.1 — Retinitis pigmentosa, locus 3
rRNA — Ribosomal RNA
SCA1 — 6p23 — Spinocerebellar ataxia, locus 1
SCA2 — 12q24 — Spinocerebellar ataxia, locus 2
SPH1 — 14q22–23.2 — Spherocytosis type I
SMA — 5q12.2-13.3 — Spinal muscular atrophy
SOD1 — 21q22.1 — Superoxide dismutase, familial motor neurone disease
SRY — Yp11.3 — Sex-determining region Y, testis-determining factor
TBX5 — 12q21.3–22 — Holt–Oram syndrome
TCOF1 — 5q32–33.1 — Treacher–Collins syndrome
TRPS1 — 8q24.12 — Tricho-rhino-phalangeal syndrome

TSC1 — 9q34 — Tuberous sclerosis, locus 1
TSC2 — 16p13.3 — Tuberous sclerosis, locus 2
TYR — 11q14–21 — Oculocutaneous albinism
USH1A — 14q32 — Usher's syndrome type IA
USH1B — 11q13.5 — Usher's syndrome type IB
USH1C — 11p15.1 — Usher's syndrome type IC
USH2 — 1q41 — Usher's syndrome type II
VWS — 1q32 — van der Woude syndrome
VHL — 3p25–26 — von Hippel–Lindau syndrome
VWF — 12p13.3 — von Willebrand disease
WD — 13q14.3–21.1 — Wilson's disease
WRN — 8p11.2–12 — Werner's syndrome
WS1 — 2q35 — Waardenburg's syndrome type 1
WT1 — 11p13 — Wilms' tumour 1 gene
ZWS1 — 7q11.23 — Zellweger's syndrome type 1

safer vectors. The combination of physical containment and the use of attenuated organisms should reduce the risk of any possible hazard.

From the evidence available to date, it seems that the hazards of genetic engineering have, perhaps, been over-emphasized in the past and that the risks are more imaginary than real. Accordingly, the guidelines set out by the GMAG on which types of procedure can be carried out at the various levels of containment have been relaxed. Nevertheless, great care will continue to have to be exercised in this field, if for no other reason than to allay the fears of the general public as exemplified by recent adverse publicity surrounding genetically modified foods.

ELEMENTS

1 Restriction enzymes allow DNA from any source to be cleaved into reproducible fragments based on the presence of specific nucleotide recognition sequences. These fragments can be made to recombine enabling their incorporation into a suitable vector, with subsequent transformation of a host organism by the vector leading to the production of clones containing a particular DNA sequence.

2 Low resolution mapping techniques, which include gene dosage, somatic cell hybridization, chromosome-specific libraries and in situ hybridization enable assignment of a gene to a chromosome or a region of a chromosome. Pulsed field gel electrophoresis, chromatin fibre FISH and analysis of yeast artificial chromosome contigs allow high level resolution mapping.

3 Identification of DNA fragments containing genes is facilitated by identification of HTF/CpG islands, demonstration of their presence in zoo blots, exon trapping, expressed sequence tags, homology to genes in model organisms and analysis of Human Genome Project databases.

4 The approaches of functional and positional candidate cloning allow the identification of genes on the basis of knowledge of their function or position. Confirmation that a specific gene is responsible for a particular inherited disorder can be obtained by tissue and developmental expression studies, in vitro cell culture studies or the introduction and analysis of mutations in a homologous gene in another species. As a consequence the 'anatomy of the human genome' is beginning to be revealed.

5 Techniques including Southern and Northern blotting, DNA sequencing and mutation screening can be used to identify or analyse specific DNA sequences of interest. These techniques can be used for analysing normal gene structure and function as well as revealing the molecular pathology of inherited disease. This provides a means for presymptomatic diagnosis, carrier detection and prenatal diagnosis either by direct mutational analysis or indirectly using polymorphic markers in family studies.

6 Recombinant DNA technology is potentially biologically hazardous but these risks can be minimized by physical and biological containment methods.

FURTHER READING

Botstein D, White R L, Skolnick M, Davis R W 1980 Construction of a genetic linkage map in man using restriction fragment length polymorphisms. Am J Hum Genet 32: 314–331
One of the original papers describing the concept of linked RFLPs.
Emery A E H, Malcolm S 1995 An introduction to recombinant DNA medicine, 2nd edn. John Wiley, London
The second edition of this text which covers the techniques and applications of DNA technology in clinical medicine.
McKusick V A 1998 Mendelian inheritance in man, 12th edn. Johns Hopkins University Press, London
A computerized catalogue of the dominant, recessive and X-linked Mendelian traits and disorders in humans with a brief clinical commentary and details of the mutational basis if known. Also available online, updated regularly.
Strachan T, Read A P 1999 Human molecular genetics, 2nd edn. βios Scientific, Oxford
An up-to-date, comprehensive textbook of all aspects of molecular and cellular biology as it relates to inherited disease in humans.
Weatherall D J 1991 The new genetics and clinical practice, 3rd edn. Oxford Medical, Oxford
One of the original texts which provided a lucid overview of the application of DNA techniques in clinical medicine.

Developmental genetics

The formation and subsequent development of a human being are extremely complex processes which are still only poorly understood. Both genetic and environmental factors play important roles. Given a suitable environment, genes inherited from both parents determine how a small cluster of undifferentiated cells derived from the fertilized egg or zygote develops over a period of approximately 12 weeks into a recognizably human fetus. The developmental processes which take place within these first 12 weeks following conception fall within the realm of embryology. In this chapter we are not concerned so much with the mechanics of these structural changes as with the way these processes are under genetic control. It is this aspect of biology which constitutes the field of developmental genetics.

Prenatal life can be divided into three main stages — pre-embryonic, embryonic and fetal (Table 5.1). During the pre-embryonic stage a small collection of cells becomes distinguishable, firstly as a double layered or bilaminar disc, and then as a triple layered or trilaminar disc which is destined to develop into the human infant. During the embryonic stage, cranio-caudal and dorso-ventral axes are established, as cellular aggregation and differentiation lead to tissue and organ formation. The final fetal stage is characterized by rapid growth and development as the embryo, now known as a fetus, matures into a viable human infant.

On average this extraordinary process takes approximately 38 weeks. By convention pregnancy is usually dated from the first day of the last menstrual period (LMP) which usually precedes conception by around 2 weeks so that the normal period of gestation is often stated incorrectly as lasting for 40 weeks.

FERTILIZATION AND GASTRULATION

Fertilization, the process by which the male and female gametes fuse, occurs in the Fallopian tube. Of the 100–200 million spermatozoa deposited in the female genital tract only a few hundred reach the site of

Table 5.1 Main events in the development of a human infant

Stage	Time from conception	Length of embryo/fetus
Pre-embryonic		
First cell division	30 hours	
Zygote reaches uterine cavity	4 days	
Implantation	5–6 days	
Formation of bilaminar disc	12 days	0.2 mm
Lyonization in female	16 days	
Formation of trilaminar disc and primitive streak	19 days	1 mm
Embryonic stage		
Organogenesis	4–8 weeks	
Brain and spinal cord are forming	4 weeks	4 mm
First signs of heart and limb buds		
Brain, eyes, heart and limbs developing rapidly	6 weeks	17 mm
Bowel and lungs beginning to develop		
Digits have appeared. Ears, kidneys, liver and muscle are developing	8 weeks	4 cm
Palate closes and joints form	10 weeks	6 cm
Sexual differentiation almost complete	12 weeks	9 cm
Fetal stage		
Fetal movements felt	16–18 weeks	20 cm
Eyelids open. Fetus is now viable with specialized care	24–26 weeks	35 cm
Rapid weight gain due to growth and accumulation of fat as lungs mature	28–38 weeks	40–50 cm

fertilization. Of these only a single spermatozoon succeeds in penetrating first the corona radiata, then the zona pellucida and finally the oocyte cell membrane, whereupon the oocyte completes its second meiotic division (Fig. 3.19, p. 41).

After the sperm has penetrated the oocyte and the meiotic process has been completed, the two nuclei, now known as pronuclei, fuse, thereby restoring the diploid number of 46 chromosomes. The fertilized ovum or zygote then undergoes a series of mitotic divisions to consist of two cells by 30 hours, four cells by 40 hours and 12–16 cells by 3 days when it is known as a *morula*.

Further cell division leads to formation of a *blastocyst* which consists of an inner cell mass or *embryoblast*, destined to form the embryo, and an outer cell mass or *trophoblast*, which gives rise to the placenta. The process of converting the inner cell mass into firstly a bilaminar and then a trilaminar disc is known as *gastrulation*, and takes place between the beginning of the second and the end of the third weeks.

Between 4 and 8 weeks the body form is established beginning with the formation of the primitive streak at the caudal end of the embryo. The germinal layers of the trilaminar disc give rise to ectodermal, mesodermal and endodermal structures (Table 5.2). The neural tube is formed and neural crest cells migrate to form sensory ganglia, the sympathetic nervous system, pigment cells, and both bone and cartilage in parts of the face and branchial arches.

Disorders involving cells of neural crest origin, such as neurofibromatosis (p. 272), are sometimes referred to as neurocristopathies. This period between 4 and 8 weeks is referred to as the period of organogenesis as it is during this interval that all of the major organs are formed as regional specialization proceeds in a cranio-caudal direction down the axis of the embryo.

DEVELOPMENTAL GENE FAMILIES

Information about the genetic factors which initiate, maintain and direct embryogenesis is limited. However, genetic studies of the fruit fly, *Drosophila melanogaster*, have identified several genes and gene families which play important roles in the early developmental processes. Most of these genes produce proteins called transcription factors (p. 20). These control RNA transcription from the DNA template by binding to specific regulatory DNA sequences forming complexes which initiate transcription by RNA polymerase.

Transcription factors can switch genes on and off by activating or repressing gene expression. It is likely that important transcription factors control many other genes in a coordinated sequential cascade involving the regulation of fundamental embryological processes such as segmentation, induction, migration, differentiation and programmed cell death or what is known as *apoptosis*. It is believed that these processes are mediated by growth factors, cell receptors and chemicals known as *morphogens*.

Several gene families have been identified in vertebrates, most commonly mice, which show strong sequence homology with developmental regulatory genes in *Drosophila*. Recent studies in humans have revealed

Table 5.2 Organ and tissue origins

Ectodermal
Central nervous system
Peripheral nervous system
Epidermis including hair and nails
Subcutaneous glands
Dental enamel

Mesodermal
Connective tissue
Cartilage and bone
Smooth and striated muscle
Cardiovascular system
Urogenital system

Endodermal
Thymus and thyroid
Gastro-intestinal system
Liver and pancreas

that mutations in various members of these gene families can result in either isolated malformations or multiple congenital anomaly syndromes (p. 229).

SEGMENTATION GENES

Insect bodies consist of series of repeated body segments which differentiate into particular structures according to their position. Three main groups of segmentation determining genes have been classified on the basis of their mutant phenotypes. These are *gap mutants*, which delete groups of adjacent segments, *pair-rule mutants*, which delete alternate segments, and *segment polarity mutants*, which cause portions of each segment to be deleted and duplicated on the wrong side.

The segment polarity genes produce two main morphogens known as *hedgehog* and *wingless*, which have been conserved throughout evolution. Three mammalian hedgehog homologues, known as *Sonic Hedgehog*, *Desert Hedgehog* and *Indian Hedgehog*, have been identified. These are involved in the control of left–right asymmetry, the determination of polarity in the central nervous system, somites and limbs, and in both organogenesis and the formation of the skeleton. Sonic hedgehog (*SHH*) plays a major role in development of the ventral neural tube with loss-of-function mutations resulting in a serious and often lethal malformation known as holoprosencephaly (Fig. 5.1). The primary underlying defect in holoprosencephaly lies in incomplete cleavage of the developing forebrain into separate hemispheres and ventricles.

HOMEOBOX (HOX) GENES

In *Drosophila* a class of genes known as the *homeotic* genes have been shown to determine segment identity.

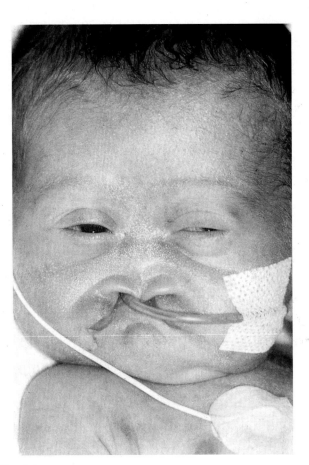

Fig. 5.1
The facial features in holoprosencephaly. The eyes are close together and there is a midline cleft lip due to failure of normal prolabia development.

Table 5.3   Homeobox gene clusters in humans

Cluster	Number of genes	Chromosome location
HOXA (= HOX1)	11 (1–7, 9–11, 13)	7p
HOXB (= HOX2)	10 (1–9, 13)	17q
HOXC (= HOX3)	9 (4–6, 8–13)	12q
HOXD (= HOX4)	9 (1, 3, 4, 8–13)	2q

Note that *HOX* genes bearing the same number are paralogous, e.g. *HOXD13* shows greater homology with *HOXA13* and *HOXC13* than with other members of the *HOXD* group.

Mutations in these genes result in major structural abnormalities such as the development of a leg instead of an antenna. Homeotic genes contain a conserved 180 bp sequence known as the *homeobox* which is believed to be characteristic of genes involved in spatial pattern control and development. This encodes a 60 amino acid domain which binds to DNA. Proteins from homeobox containing, or what are known as *HOX*, genes are therefore important transcription factors which specify cell fate and establish a regional anterior/posterior axis.

Four homeobox gene clusters have been identified in humans (Table 5.3). Each cluster contains a series of closely linked genes. In vertebrates such as mice it has been shown that these genes are expressed in segmental units in the hindbrain and in the somites formed from axial mesoderm. In each *HOX* cluster there is a direct linear correlation between the position of the gene and its temporal and spatial expression. These observations indicate that these genes play a crucial role in early morphogenesis. Thus in the developing limb bud (p. 87) *HOXA9* is expressed both anteriorly to and before *HOX10*, etc.

Mutations in *HOXA13* cause a rare condition known as the hand–foot–genital syndrome. This shows autosomal dominant inheritance and is characterized by shortening of the first and fifth digits with hypospadias in males and bicornuate uterus in females. Mutations in *HOXD13* result in an equally rare limb developmental abnormality known as synpolydactyly. This also shows autosomal dominant inheritance and is characterized by insertion of an additional digit between the third and fourth digits which are webbed (Fig. 5.2). The phenotype in homozygotes is more severe with the metacarpals and metatarsals being converted into short carpal and tarsal-like bones respectively. Reported mutations take the form of an increase in the number of residues in a polyalanine tract. This triplet repeat expansion probably alters the structure and function of the protein thereby constituting a gain-of-function mutation (p. 24).

Given that there are 39 *HOX* genes in mammals it is surprising that no other recognized syndromes or malformations have been attributed to *HOX* gene mutations. One possible explanation is that most *HOX* mutations are so devastating that the embryo cannot survive. Alternatively the high degree of homology between *HOX* genes in the different clusters could lead to functional redundancy so that one *HOX* gene could compensate for a loss-of-function mutation in another. In this context *HOX* genes are said to be *paralogous* because family members from different clusters, such as *HOXA13* and *HOXD13*, are more similar than adjacent genes in the same cluster.

Several other developmental genes also contain a homeobox-like domain. These include *MSX2* and *EMX2*. Mutations in *MSX2* can cause craniosynostosis, i.e. premature fusion of the cranial sutures. Mutations in *EMX2* cause a severe cerebral malformation known as schizencephaly in which there is a large full thickness cleft in one or both cerebral hemispheres.

Fig. 5.2
(A) Clinical and (B) X-ray views of the hands in synpolydactyly.

Table 5.4 Developmental abnormalities associated with *PAX* gene mutations

Gene	Chromosome location	Developmental abnormality
PAX2	10q24	Renal-coloboma syndrome
PAX3	2q35	Waardenburg's syndrome type 1
PAX6	11p13	Aniridia
PAX8	2q12	Absent or ectopic thyroid gland

Fig. 5.3
Iris heterochromia in a person with Waardenburg's syndrome.
(Courtesy of Dr C P Bennett, St James's Hospital, Leeds.)

PAIRED–BOX (*PAX*) GENES

The paired-box is a highly conserved DNA sequence which encodes a 130 amino acid DNA-binding transcription regulator domain. Nine *PAX* genes have been identified in mice and humans. In mice these have been shown to play important roles in the developing nervous system and vertebral column. In humans loss-of-function mutations in four *PAX* genes have been identified in association with developmental abnormalities (Table 5.4). Waardenburg's syndrome type 1 is caused by mutations in *PAX3*. It shows autosomal dominant inheritance and is characterized by sensorineural hearing loss, areas of depigmentation in hair and skin, and abnormal patterns of pigmentation in the iris (Fig. 5.3). Waardenburg's syndrome shows genetic heterogeneity with the more common type 2 form, in which the inner canthi are not widely separated, being caused by mutations in the human microphthalmia (*MITF*) gene on chromosome 3.

The importance of expression of the *PAX* gene family in eye development is illustrated by the effects of mutations in *PAX2* and *PAX6*. Mutations in *PAX2* cause the renal-coloboma syndrome in which renal malformations occur in association with structural defects in various parts of the eye including the retina and optic nerve. Mutations in *PAX6* lead to absence of the iris, which is known as aniridia (Fig. 5.4). This is a key feature of the WAGR syndrome (p. 254) which results from a contiguous gene deletion involving the *PAX6* locus on chromosome 11.

SRY–TYPE HMG BOX (*SOX*) GENES

SRY is the Y-linked gene which plays a major role in male sex determination (p. 90). A series of genes known as the *SOX* genes show homology with *SRY* by sharing a 79 amino acid domain known as the HMG (high mobility group) box. This HMG domain activates transcription by bending DNA in such a way that other regulatory factors can bind with the promoter regions of genes which encode for important structural proteins. These *SOX* genes are thus transcription regulators and are expressed in specific tissues during embryogenesis. For example *SOX1*, *SOX2* and *SOX3* are expressed in the developing mouse nervous system.

In humans it has been shown that loss-of-function mutations in *SOX9* on chromosome 17 cause campomelic dysplasia. This very rare disorder is characterized by

Fig. 5.4
An eye showing absence of the iris (aniridia). The cornea shows abnormal vascularization. (Courtesy of Mr R Gregson, Queen's Medical Centre, Nottingham.)

bowing of the long bones, sex reversal in chromosomal males and very poor long term survival. In situ hybridization studies in mice have shown that *SOX9* is expressed in the developing embryo in skeletal primordial tissue, where it regulates type II collagen expression, as well as in the genital ridges and early gonads. *SOX9* is now thought to be one of several genes which are expressed downstream of *SRY* in the process of male sex determination (p. 90). Mutations in *SOX10* on chromosome 22 cause a rare form of Waardenburg's syndrome in which affected individuals have a high incidence of Hirschsprung's disease.

T–BOX (*TBX*) GENES

The *T* gene in mice plays an important role in mesoderm formation and notochord differentiation. Heterozygotes for loss-of-function mutations have a short tail and mal-formed sacral vertebrae. This gene, which is also known as *Brachyury*, encodes a transcription factor which contains both activator and repressor domains. It shows homology with a series of genes through the shared possession of the T domain which is also referred to as the T-box. These T-box or *TBX* genes are dispersed throughout the human genome with some family members existing in

small clusters. One of these clusters on chromosome 12 contains *TBX3* and *TBX5*. Loss-of-function mutations in *TBX3* cause the ulnar-mammary syndrome in which ulnar ray developmental abnormalities in the upper limbs are associated with hypoplasia of the mammary glands. Loss-of-function mutations in *TBX5* cause the Holt–Oram syndrome. This autosomal dominant disorder is characterized by congenital heart abnormalities, most notably atrial septal defects, and upper limb reduction defects which can vary from mild hypoplasia of the thumbs to almost complete absence of the forearms.

ZINC FINGER GENES

The term *zinc finger* refers to a finger-like loop projection which is formed by a series of four amino acids which form a complex with a zinc ion. Genes which contain a zinc finger motif act as transcription factors through binding of the zinc finger to DNA. Consequently they are good candidates for single gene developmental disorders (Table 5.5).

For example a zinc finger motif containing gene known as *GLI3* on chromosome 7 has been implicated as the cause of two developmental disorders. Large deletions or translocations involving *GLI3* cause Greig cephalopolysyndactyly which is characterized by head, hand and foot abnormalities such as polydactyly and syndactyly (Fig. 5.5). In contrast, frameshift mutations in *GLI3* have been reported in the Pallister–Hall syndrome in which the key features are polydactyly, hypothalamic hamartomata and imperforate anus.

Mutations in another zinc finger motif containing a gene known as *WT1* on chromosome 11 can cause both Wilms' tumour and a rare developmental disorder, the Denys–Drash syndrome, in which the external genitalia are ambiguous and there is progressive renal failure as a result of nephritis. Finally mutations in two other zinc finger motif containing genes, *ZIC2* and *ZIC3*, have recently been shown to cause holoprosencephaly and laterality defects respectively. Laterality defects are characterized by abnormal development and positioning of unpaired organs such as the heart, liver and spleen.

Table 5.5 Developmental abnormalities associated with genes containing a zinc finger motif

Gene	Chromosome location	Developmental abnormality
GLI3	7p13	Greig's syndrome and Pallister–Hall syndrome
WT1	11p13	Denys–Drash syndrome
ZIC2	13q32	Holoprosencephaly
ZIC3	Xq26	Laterality defects

Fig. 5.5
The feet of a child with Greig cephalopolysyndactyly. Note that they show both polydactyly (extra digits) and syndactyly (fused digits).

SIGNAL TRANSDUCTION ('SIGNALLING') GENES

Signal transduction is the process whereby extracellular growth factors regulate cell division and differentiation by a complex pathway of genetically determined intermediate steps. Mutations in many of the genes involved in signal transduction play a role in causing cancer (p. 194). In some cases they can also cause development abnormalities.

The *RET* proto-oncogene

The proto-oncogene *RET* on chromosome 10q11.2 encodes a cell surface tyrosine kinase. Gain-of-function mutations, whether inherited or acquired, are found in a high proportion of thyroid cancers. Loss-of-function mutations in *RET* have been identified in approximately 50% of familial cases of Hirschsprung's disease, in which there is failure of migration of ganglionic cells to the submucosal and myenteric plexuses of the large bowel. The clinical consequences are usually apparent shortly after birth when the child presents with abdominal distension and intestinal obstruction.

Fibroblast growth factor receptors (FGFRs)

Fibroblast growth factors play key roles in embryogenesis including cell division, migration and differentiation. The transduction of extracellular *FGF* signals is mediated by a family of four transmembrane tyrosine kinase receptors. These are the fibroblast growth factor receptors, each of which contains three main components — an extracellular region with three immunoglobulin-like domains, a transmembrane segment and two intracellular tyrosine kinase domains (Fig. 5.6).

Mutations in the genes which code for FGFRs have been identified in two groups of developmental disorders (Table 5.6). These are the craniosynostosis syndromes and the achondroplasia family of skeletal dysplasias. The craniosynostosis syndromes, of which Apert's syndrome

Fig. 5.6
Fibroblast growth factor receptor (*FGFR*) structure. Arrows indicate the location of mutations in the craniosynostosis syndromes and achondroplasia group of skeletal dysplasias. Ig = immunoglobulin-like domain; TM = transmembrane domain; TK = tyrosine kinase domain; P = Pfeiffer's syndrome; A = Apert's syndrome; C = Crouzon's syndrome; J = Jackson–Weiss syndrome; TD = thanatophoric dysplasia; ACH = achondroplasia, HCH = hypochondroplasia.

Table 5.6   Developmental disorders caused by mutations in fibroblast growth factor receptors

Gene	Chromosome	Syndrome
Craniosynostosis syndromes		
FGFR1	8p11	Pfeiffer
FGFR2	10q25	Apert
		Crouzon
		Jackson–Weiss
		Pfeiffer
FGFR3	4p16	Crouzon (with acanthosis nigricans)
Skeletal dysplasias		
FGFR3	4p16	Achondroplasia
		Hypochondroplasia
		Thanatophoric dysplasia

(Fig. 5.7) is the best known, are characterized by premature fusion of the cranial sutures often in association with hand and foot abnormalities such as syndactyly (fusion of the digits). Apert's syndrome is caused by a mutation in one of the adjacent *FGFR2* residues in the peptides which link the second and third immunoglobulin loops (Fig. 5.6). In contrast mutations in the third immunoglobulin loop can cause either Crouzon's syndrome, in which the limbs are normal, or Pfeiffer's syndrome in which usually only the thumbs and big toes are abnormal. At present the relationship between genotype and phenotype in this group of disorders is not well understood.

Achondroplasia is the most commonly encountered form of genetic short stature (Fig. 5.8). The limbs show proximal ('rhizomelic') shortening and the head is enlarged with frontal bossing. Intelligence and life expectancy are entirely normal. Achondroplasia is almost always caused by a mutation in or close to the transmembrane domain

Fig. 5.7
Views of (A) the face, (B) the hand and (C) the foot of a child with Apert's syndrome.

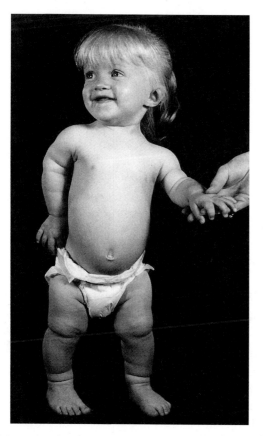

Fig. 5.8
A young child with achondroplasia.

of *FGFR3*. Hypochondroplasia, a milder form of skeletal dysplasia with similar trunk and limb changes but normal head shape and size, is caused by mutations in the proximal tyrosine kinase domain of *FGFR3*. Finally thanatophoric dysplasia, a much more severe and invariably lethal form of skeletal dysplasia, is caused by mutations in either the peptides linking the second and third immunoglobulin domain of *FGFR3*, or the distal *FGFR3* tyrosine kinase domain.

The mechanism by which these mutations cause skeletal shortening is not understood at present. The mutations cannot have loss-of-function effects as children with the Wolf–Hirschhorn syndrome (p. 253) due to chromosome microdeletions which include *FGFR3* do not show similar skeletal abnormalities. Instead the mutations probably involve a gain-of-function mediated by increased ligand binding or receptor activation.

THE LIMB AS A DEVELOPMENTAL MODEL

Four main phases are recognized in limb development. These are (1) initiation, (2) specification, (3) tissue differentiation and (4) growth. Although none of these stages is fully understood, insight into the probable underlying mechanisms has been gleaned from the study of limb development in chicks and mice in particular.

INITIATION AND SPECIFICATION

Limb bud formation is thought to be initiated at around 28 days by a member of the *FGF* family as illustrated by the development of an extra limb if *FGF1, -2* or *-4* is applied to the side of a developing chick embryo. During normal limb initiation *FGF8* transcripts have been identified in mesenchyme near the initiation site. *FGF8* expression is probably controlled by *HOX* genes which determine limb type (i.e. forelimb or hindlimb) and number.

TISSUE DIFFERENTIATION AND GROWTH

Once limb formation has been initiated a localized area of thickened ectoderm at the limb tip, known as the *apical ectodermal ridge* (AER), produces growth signals such as *FGF4* and *FGF8* which maintain further growth and establish the proximo-distal axis (Fig. 5.9). Similar signals from another localized area on the posterior margin of the developing bud, known as the *zone of polarizing activity* (ZPA), determine the antero-posterior axis. One of these signals is Sonic Hedghog (*SHH*) (p. 82) which acts in concert with other *FGF* genes, *GLI3* and another gene family which produces bone morphogenetic proteins (BMPs). Another morphogen, retinoic acid, is believed to play a major role at this stage in determining development at the anterior margin of the limb bud.

Subsequent development involves the activation of genes from the *HOXA* and *HOXD* clusters in the un-differentiated proliferating mesenchymal cells beneath the AER. This area is known as the *progress zone*. Cells in different regions express different combinations of *HOX* genes which determine local cell proliferation, adhesion and differentiation. Downstream targets of the *HOX* gene clusters remain to be identified.

Fibroblast growth factors continue to be important during the later stages of limb development. In this context it becomes easy to understand why limb abnormalities are a feature of disorders such as Apert's syndrome (see Fig. 5.7) in which mutations have been identified in the extracellular domains of *FGFR2*.

DEVELOPMENTAL GENES AND CANCER

Several genes which play important roles in embryo-genesis have also been shown to play a role in causing cancer (Table 5.7). This is not surprising given that many developmental genes are expressed throughout life in processes such as signal transduction and signal tran-scription (p. 193). It has been shown that several different mechanisms can account for the phenotypic diversity demonstrated by these so-called *teratogenes*.

Limb bud

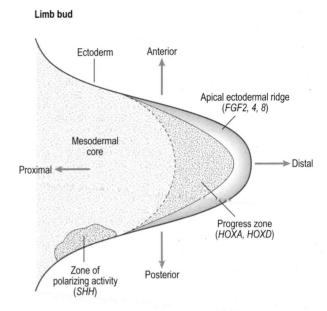

Fig. 5.9
Simplified representation of vertebrate limb development.

Table 5.7	Genes which can cause both developmental anomalies and cancer		
Gene	**Chromosome**	**Developmental anomaly**	**Cancer**
PAX3	2q35	Waardenburg's syndrome type 1	Alveolar rhabdomyosarcoma
KIT	4q12	Piebaldism	Mast cell leukaemia
PTC (Patched)	9q22	Gorlin's syndrome	Basal cell carcinoma
RET	10q11	Hirschsprung's disease	MEN2A, MEN2B, thyroid carcinoma
WT1	11p13	Denys–Drash syndrome	Wilms' tumour

GAIN-OF-FUNCTION VS LOSS-OF-FUNCTION MUTATIONS

Mention has already been made of the causal role of the *RET* proto-oncogene in familial Hirschsprung's disease as well as in both inherited and sporadic thyroid cancer (pp. 24, 86). The protein product encoded by *RET* consists of three main domains: an extracellular domain which binds to a glial cell line-derived neurotrophil factor, a transmembrane domain, and an intracellular tyrosine kinase domain which activates signal transduction (Fig. 5.10). Mutations which cause loss-of-function result in Hirschsprung's disease. These include whole gene deletions, small intragenic deletions, nonsense mutations

Fig. 5.10
The *RET* proto-oncogene. The most common mutation sites in the different clinical entities associated with *RET* are indicated. Numbers refer to amino acid residues. SP = signal peptide; ECD = extracellular domain; TMD = transmembrane domain; TKD = tyrosine kinase domain; MEN = multiple endocrine adenomatosis; FMTC = familial medullary thyroid carcinoma. The arrow above PTC (= papillary thyroid carcinoma) indicates the somatic rearrangement site for the formation of new hybrid forms of *RET*. (Adapted from Pasini B, Ceccherini I, Romeo G 1996 *RET* mutations in human disease. Trends in Genetics 12: 138–144.)

Table 5.8 Developmental genes which show a position effect

Gene	Chromosome	Developmental anomaly
GLI3	7p13	Greig's cephalopolysyndactyly
SHH	7q36	Holoprosencephaly
PAX6	11p13	Aniridia
SOX9	17q24	Campomelic dysplasia

and splicing mutations leading to synthesis of a truncated protein.

In contrast mutations which cause a gain-of-function effect result in either type 2A or type 2B multiple endocrine adenomatosis (MEN) (p. 203). These disorders are characterized by a high incidence of medullary thyroid carcinoma and phaeochromocytoma. The activating mutations which cause MEN 2A are clustered in five cysteine residues in the extracellular domain. MEN 2B, which differs from MEN 2A in that affected individuals are tall and thin, is caused by a unique mutation in a methionine residue in the tyrosine kinase domain.

SOMATIC REARRANGEMENTS

Activation of the *RET* proto-oncogene can occur by a different mechanism whereby the genomic region encoding the intracellular domain is juxtaposed to one of several activating genes which are normally preferentially expressed in the thyroid gland. The newly formed hybrid *RET* gene produces a novel protein whose activity is not ligand dependent. These somatic rearrangements are found in a high proportion of papillary thyroid carcinomas, which show a particularly high incidence in children who were exposed to radiation following the Chernobyl accident in 1986.

PAX3 provides another example of a developmental gene which can cause cancer if it is fused to new DNA sequences. A specific translocation between chromosomes 2 and 13 which results in a new chimeric transcript leads to the development in children of a rare lung tumour called alveolar rhabdomyosarcoma.

MUTATIONS IN DEVELOPMENT CONTROL GENES

The *hedgehog* gene family are segment polarity genes which induce cell differentiation and cell to cell communication. Their action is antagonized by a gene called *PTC* or *patched* which is able to shut down the *hedgehog* signalling pathway. Loss-of-function in *PTC* is believed to lead to ectopic expression of *hedgehog* genes, which clinically results in a condition called Gorlin's syndrome, also known as the basal cell naevus syndrome. Characteristic features of Gorlin's syndrome include multiple basal cell carcinomas, mandibular cysts and ovarian fibromata.

POSITION EFFECTS AND DEVELOPMENTAL GENES

The discovery of a chromosomal abnormality, such as a translocation or inversion, in a person with a single gene developmental syndrome provides a strong indication of the probable position of the disease locus as it is likely that one of the break-points involved in the rearrangement will have disrupted the relevant gene. However in a few instances it has emerged that the chromosome break-point actually lies approximately 10–1000 kb upstream or downstream of the gene which is subsequently shown to be mutated in other affected individuals (Table 5.8). The probable explanation is that the break-point has separated the coding part of the gene from contiguous regulatory elements (p. 20). These observations have created obvious difficulties for those carrying out the original research when the putative disease gene in translocation families has been found not to contain an intragenic mutation.

HYDATIDIFORM MOLES

Occasionally conception results in an abnormal pregnancy in which the placenta consists of a proliferating disorganized mass known as a hydatidiform mole. These changes can be either partial or complete (Table 5.9).

Table 5.9   Characteristics of partial and complete hydatidiform moles

	Partial	Complete
Number of chromosomes	69	46
Parental origin of chromosomes	23 — maternal 46 — paternal	All 46 paternal
Fetus present	Yes — but not viable	No
Malignant potential	Very low	High

PARTIAL HYDATIDIFORM MOLE

Chromosome analysis of tissue from partial moles reveals the presence of 69 chromosomes, i.e. triploidy (p. 256). Using DNA polymorphisms it has been shown that 46 of these chromosomes are always derived from the father with the remaining 23 being maternal in origin. This doubling of the normal haploid paternal contribution of 23 chromosomes can be due to either fertilization by two sperm, which is known as *dispermy*, or to duplication of a haploid sperm chromosome set by a process known as *endoreduplication*.

In these pregnancies the fetus rarely if ever survives to term. Triploid conceptions only survive to term if the additional chromosome complement is maternally derived, in which cases partial hydatidiform changes do not occur. Even in these situations it is extremely uncommon for a triploid infant to survive for more than a few hours or days after birth.

COMPLETE HYDATIDIFORM MOLE

Complete moles have only 46 chromosomes, but these are exclusively paternal in origin. A complete mole is caused by fertilization of an empty ovum by either two sperm or by a single sperm which undergoes endoreduplication. The opposite situation of an egg undergoing development without being fertilized by a sperm, a process known as parthenogenesis, occurs in lower animals such as arthropods but has been reported in a human on only one occasion, this being in the form of chimeric fusion with another cell line which had a normal male-derived complement.

The main importance of complete moles lies in their potential to undergo malignant change into invasive choriocarcinoma. This can usually be treated very successfully by chemotherapy, but if untreated the outcome can be fatal. Malignant change is seen only very rarely with partial moles.

DIFFERENT PARENTAL EXPRESSION IN TROPHOBLAST AND EMBRYOBLAST

Studies in mice have shown that when all nuclear genes

in a zygote are derived from the father, the embryo fails to develop, whereas trophoblast development proceeds relatively unimpaired. In contrast, if all of the nuclear genes are maternal in origin, the embryo develops normally but extra-embryonic development is very poor. The observations outlined above on partial and complete moles indicate that a comparable situation exists in humans with paternally derived genes being essential for trophoblast development and maternally derived genes being necessary for early embryonic development. These phenomena are relevant to the concept of genomic imprinting (p. 109).

SEXUAL DIFFERENTIATION AND DETERMINATION

The sex of an individual is determined by the X and Y chromosomes (p. 30). The presence of a Y chromosome leads to maleness regardless of the number of X chromosomes present. Absence of a Y chromosome results in female development.

Although the sex chromosomes are present from conception, differentiation into a phenotypic male or female does not commence until approximately 6 weeks. Up to this point both the Müllerian and Wolffian duct systems are present and the embryonic gonads, although consisting of cortex and medulla, are still undifferentiated. From 6 weeks onwards the embryo develops into a female unless the testis-determining factor initiates a sequence of events which prompt the undifferentiated gonads to develop into testes.

THE TESTIS-DETERMINING FACTOR — *SRY*

In 1990 it was shown that the testis-determining factor or gene is located on the short arm of the Y chromosome close to the pseudoautosomal region (p. 105). This gene is now referred to as being located in the sex-determining region of the Y chromosome (*SRY*). It consists of a single exon which encodes a protein of 204 amino acids which include a 79 amino acid HMG box (p. 84), indicating that it is likely to be a transcription regulator.

Evidence that the *SRY* gene is the primary factor which determines maleness comes from several observations:

1. *SRY* sequences are present in XX males. These are infertile phenotypic males who appear to have a normal 46,XX karyotype.

2. Mutations or deletions in the *SRY* sequences are found in many XY females. These are infertile phenotypic females who are found to have a 46,XY karyotype.

3. In mice the *SRY* gene is expressed only in the male gonadal ridge as the testes are developing in the embryo.

4. Transgenic XX mice which have a tiny portion of the Y chromosome containing the *SRY* region develop into males with testes.

Considered from the evolutionary point of view and for the maintenance of the species, it would clearly be impossible for the *SRY* gene to be involved in crossing over with the X chromosome during meiosis I. Hence *SRY* has to lie outside the pseudoautosomal region.

However there has to be pairing of the X and Y chromosomes, as otherwise they would segregate together into the same gamete during on average 50% of meioses. Nature's compromise has been to ensure that only a small portion of the X and Y chromosomes are homologous and therefore pair during meiosis I. Unfortunately the close proximity of *SRY* to the pseudoautosomal region means that, occasionally, it can get caught up in a recombinational event. This almost certainly accounts for the majority of XX males, in whom molecular and FISH studies show evidence of Y chromosome sequences at the distal end of one X chromosome short arm (Fig. 17.20, p. 261).

Expression of *SRY* triggers off a series of events, which involves other genes such as *SOX9*, leading to the medulla of the undifferentiated gonad developing into a testis, in which the Leydig cells begin to produce testosterone (Fig. 5.11). This leads to stimulation of the Wolffian ducts, which form the male internal genitalia, and also to masculinization of the external genitalia. This latter step is mediated by dihydrotestosterone which is produced from testosterone by the action of 5α-reductase (p. 261). The Sertoli cells in the testes produce a hormone known as Müllerian inhibitory factor which causes the Müllerian duct system to regress.

In the absence of normal *SRY* expression, the cortex of the undifferentiated gonad develops into an ovary. The Müllerian duct forms the internal genitalia. The external genitalia fail to fuse and grow as in the male and instead evolve into normal female external genitalia. This normal process of female development is sometimes referred to rather chauvinistically as the 'default' pathway. Without the stimulating effects of testosterone, the Wolffian duct system regresses.

Normally sexual differentiation is complete by 12–14 weeks gestation, although the testes do not migrate into the scrotum until late pregnancy. Abnormalities of sexual differentiation are uncommon but they are important causes of infertility and sexual ambiguity and are considered further in Chapter 17.

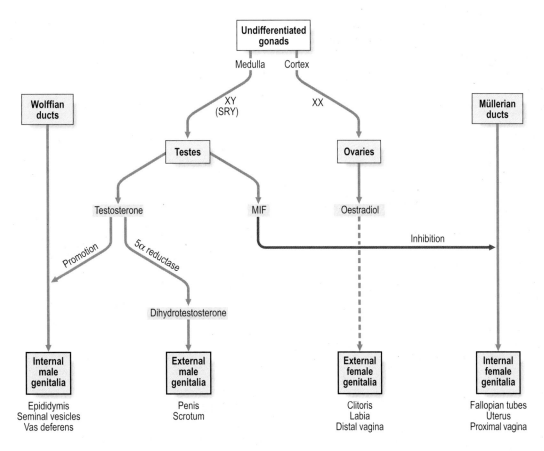

Fig. 5.11
Summary of the main events involved in sex determination. SRY = sex determining region of the Y chromosome; MIF = Müllerian inhibitory factor.

X CHROMOSOME INACTIVATION

As techniques were developed for studying chromosomes it was noted that in female mice one of the X chromosomes often differed from all other chromosomes in the extent to which it was condensed. In 1961 Dr Mary Lyon proposed that this *heteropyknotic X* chromosome was inactivated, citing as evidence her observations on the mosaic pattern of skin coloration seen in mice known to be heterozygous for X-linked genes which influence coat colour. Subsequent events have confirmed the validity of Dr Lyon's hypothesis, and in recognition of her foresight the process of X-inactivation is often referred to as *Lyonization*.

The process of X-inactivation occurs early in development at around 15–16 days gestation when the embryo consists of approximately 5000 cells. Normally either of the two X chromosomes can be inactivated in any particular cell. Thereafter the same X chromosome is inactivated in all daughter cells (Fig. 5.12). This differs from marsupials in which the paternally derived X chromosome is consistently inactivated.

The inactive X chromosome exists in a condensed form during interphase when it appears as a darkly staining mass of chromatin known as the *sex-chromatin* or *Barr body*. During mitosis the inactive X chromosome is late replicating. Laboratory techniques have been developed for distinguishing which X chromosome is late replicating in each cell. This can be useful for confirming that one of the X chromosomes is structurally abnormal, as usually an abnormal X chromosome will be preferentially inactivated, or more correctly only those haematopoietic stem cells in which the normal X

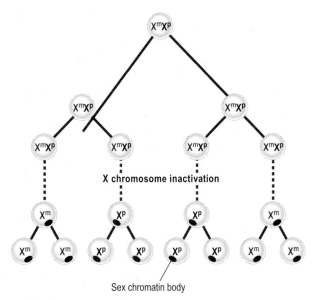

X chromosome inactivation

Sex chromatin body

Fig. 5.12
X chromosome inactivation during development. The maternally and paternally derived X chromosomes are represented as Xm and Xp respectively.

chromosome is active will have survived. Apparent non-random inactivation also occurs if one of the X chromosomes is involved in a translocation with an autosome (p. 104).

The process of X-inactivation is achieved by differential methylation and is initiated by a gene, *XIST* ('X inactivation specific transcript'), which maps within the *X-inactivation centre* at Xq13.3. *XIST* is expressed only from the inactive X chromosome and produces RNA which spreads an inactivation methylation signal up and down the X chromosome on which it is located. This differential methylation of the X chromosomes has been utilized in carrier detection studies for X-linked immuno-deficiency diseases using methylation-sensitive restriction enzymes (p. 185). Not all of the X chromosome is inactivated. Genes in the pseudoautosomal region at the tip of the short arm remain active as do other loci elsewhere on the short and long arms such as *XIST*. If all loci on the X chromosome were inactivated then all women would have the clinical features of Turner's syndrome and the presence of more than one X chromosome in a male, e.g. 47,XXY or two in a female, e.g. 47,XXX, would have no phenotypic effects. There are, in fact, quite characteristic clinical features in these disorders (p. 256).

X chromosome inactivation provides a satisfactory explanation for several observations:

1. Barr bodies — In men and women with more than one X chromosome, the number of Barr bodies (p. 40) visible at interphase is always one less than the total number of X chromosomes. For example men with a 47,XXY karyotype have a single Barr body, whereas women with a 47,XXX karyotype have two Barr bodies.

2. Dosage compensation — Women with two normal X chromosomes have the same blood levels of X chromosome protein products, such as factor VIII, as normal men who of course have only one X chromosome. An exception to this phenomenon of dosage compensation is the level of steroid sulphatase in blood which is increased in women as compared with men. Not surprisingly it has been shown that the locus for steroid sulphatase, deficiency of which causes a skin disorder known as ichthyosis, is in the pseudoautosomal region.

3. Mosaicism — Mice which are heterozygous for X-linked genes affecting coat colour show mosaicism with alternating patches of different colour rather than a homogeneous pattern. This is consistent with patches of skin being clonal in origin in that they are derived from a single stem cell in which one or other of the X chromosomes is expressed but not both. Thus, each patch reflects which of the X chromosomes was active in the original stem cell. Similar effects are seen in tissues of clonal origin in women who are heterozygous for X-linked mutations such as ocular albinism (Fig. 5.13).

Other evidence confirming that X-inactivation leads to mosaicism in females comes from studies of the expression of the enzyme glucose-6-phosphate dehydrogenase (p. 171) in clones of cultured fibroblasts from women heterozygous for variants of this gene. Each clone is derived from a single cell and expresses one of the variants but never both. The clonal origin of tumours can be confirmed in women who are heterozygous for such variants by demonstration of expression of only one of the variants in the tumour.

4. Problems of carrier detection — Carrier detection for X-linked recessive disorders based only on examination of clinical features or on indirect assay of gene function is notoriously difficult and unreliable. Cells in which the X chromosome with the normal gene is active can have a selective advantage, or they can correct the defect in closely adjacent cells in which the X chromosome with the mutant gene is active. For example, only a proportion of carriers of Duchenne muscular dystrophy show evidence of muscle damage as indicated by measurement of creatine kinase in serum (p. 288). Fortunately the development of molecular methods for carrier detection in X-linked disorders can bypass these problems as techniques such as Southern blotting are not influenced by methylation unless methylation-sensitive restriction enzymes are used. When methylation-sensitive enzymes are used this can in fact provide a means of carrier detection if there has been strong selection against the cell line in which the mutant-bearing X chromosome is active (Fig. 5.14).

5. Manifesting heterozygotes — Occasionally a woman is encountered who shows mild or even full expression of an X-linked recessive disorder. One possible explanation is that she is a manifesting heterozygote in whom, by chance, the X chromosome bearing the normal gene has been inactivated in significantly more than 50% of relevant cells. This is referred to as skewed X-inactivation (p. 103). There is some evidence that X chromosome inactivation can itself be under genetic control as families with several manifesting carriers of disorders such as Duchenne muscular dystrophy and Fabry's disease have been reported. In a few families marked skewing of X inactivation in several females has been shown to be associated with an underlying mutation in *XIST*.

6. The 46,Xr(X) phenotype — A 46,Xr(X) karyotype is found in some women with typical Turner's syndrome features. This is consistent with the ring lacking X sequences which are normally not inactivated and which are needed for a normal phenotype. Curiously a few 46,Xr(X) women have congenital abnormalities and show mental retardation. In these women it has been shown that *XIST* is not expressed on the ring X, so that it is likely that their relatively severe phenotype is caused by functional disomy for those genes present on their ring X chromosome.

Fig. 5.13
The fundus of a carrier of X-linked ocular albinism showing a mosaic pattern of retinal pigmentation. (Courtesy of Mr S J Charles, The Royal Eye Hospital, Manchester.)

TWINNING

Twinning occurs frequently in humans although the incidence in early pregnancy as diagnosed by ultrasonography is greater than at delivery, presumably as a result of death and subsequent resorption of one of the twins in a proportion of twin pregnancies. The overall incidence of twinning in the United Kingdom is approximately 1 in 80 of all pregnancies, so that approximately 1 in 40 (i.e. 2 out of 80) of all individuals is a twin.

Twins can be identical or non-identical — *monozygotic* (MZ) or *dizygotic* (DZ) — depending on whether they originate from a single conception or from two separate conceptions (Table 5.10). Comparison of the incidence of disease in identical and non-identical twins reared apart and together can provide information about the relative contributions of genetics and environment to the cause of many of the common diseases of adult life, as discussed in Chapter 14.

MONOZYGOTIC TWINS

Monozygotic twinning occurs in about 1 in 300 births in all populations which have been studied. MZ twins originate from a single egg which has been fertilized by a single sperm. A very early division, occurring in the zygote before separation of the cells which make the

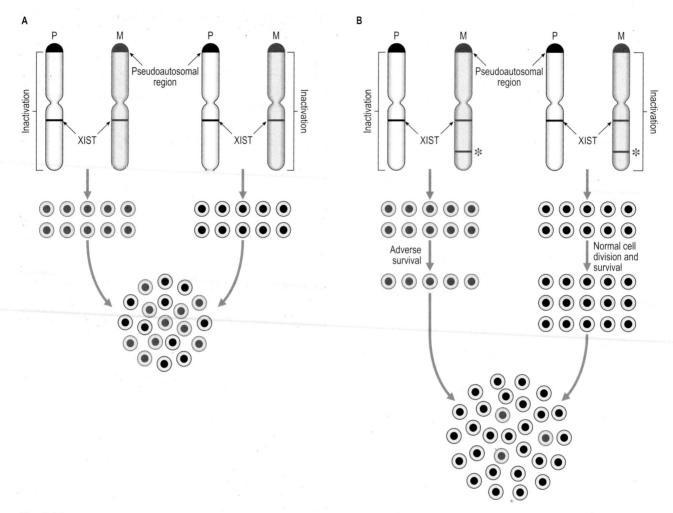

Fig. 5.14
(A) Normal X chromosome inactivation resulting in survival of roughly equal numbers of cells with the paternally (P) and maternally (M) derived X chromosome active. (B) In this situation the maternally derived X chromosome has a mutation* which results in selection against those cells in which it is active. Thus surviving cells show preferential expression of the paternally derived X chromosome.

Table 5.10 Summary of differences between monozygotic and dizygotic twins		
	Monozygotic	**Dizygotic**
Origin	Single egg fertilized	Two eggs each fertilized by a single sperm
Incidence	1 in 300 pregnancies	Varies from 1 in 100 to 1 in 500 pregnancies
Proportion of genes in common	100%	50%
Fetal membranes	70% monochorionic and diamniotic 30% dichorionic and diamniotic, rarely monochorionic and monoamniotic	Always dichorionic and diamniotic

chorion, results in dichorionic twins. Division during the blastocyst stage from days 3 to 7 results in monochorionic diamniotic twins. Division after the first week leads to monoamniotic twins.

MZ twins are genetically identical although rarely they can be discordant for a single gene trait or chromosome abnormality because of a post-zygotic somatic mutation or non-disjunction respectively. Curiously, MZ female twins can show quite striking discrepancy in X chromosome inactivation. There are several reports of female MZ twin pairs only one of whom is affected with an X-linked recessive condition such as Duchenne muscular dystrophy or haemophilia. In these rare examples both twins have the mutation and both show non-random X-inactivation but in opposite directions.

Very late division occurring more than 2 weeks after conception can result in conjoined twins. This occurs in less than 1 in 50 000 pregnancies. Conjoined twins are sometimes referred to as Siamese, in memory of Chang and Eng who were born in 1811 in Thailand, then Siam, joined at the upper abdomen. Chang and Eng made a successful living out of showing themselves at travelling shows in the United States, where they settled and married. Somehow they both managed to have large numbers of children despite remaining conjoined until they died within a few hours of each other at the age of 61 years.

DIZYGOTIC TWINS

The incidence of DZ twinning varies from approximately 1 in 100 deliveries in Afro-Caribbean populations to 1 in 500 deliveries in Asia and Japan. In Western European Caucasians the incidence is approximately 1 in 120 deliveries. Factors which convey an increased risk for DZ twinning are increased maternal age, a positive family history and the use of ovulation-inducing drugs such as clomiphene.

DZ twins result from the fertilization of two ova by two sperm and are no more closely related genetically than brothers and sisters. Hence they are sometimes referred to as *fraternal* twins. DZ twins are dichorionic and diamniotic although they can have a single fused placenta if implantation occurs at closely adjacent sites.

DETERMINATION OF ZYGOSITY

This used to be established by study of the placenta and membranes and also by analysis of polymorphic systems such as the blood groups, the HLA antigens and other biochemical markers. Now zygosity is most reliably determined using highly polymorphic molecular markers such as those identified by DNA fingerprinting (Fig. 16.4, pp. 67, 247).

FURTHER READING

Dreyer S D, Zhou G, Lee B 1998 The long and the short of it: developmental genetics of the skeletal dysplasias. Clin Genet 54: 464–473
A short review of developmental genes known to cause abnormal skeletal development.

Hammerschmidt M, Brook A, McMahon A P 1997 The world according to hedgehog. Trends Genet 13: 14–20
A comprehensive account of the role of the hedgehog gene family in early vertebrate development.

Kleinjan D J, van Heyningen V 1998 Position effect in human genetic disease. Hum Mol Genet 7: 1611–1618
An outline of the various theories and mechanisms which have been proposed to account for observed positional effects in developmental gene expression.

Lacombe D 1999 Transcription factors in dysmorphology. Clin Genet 55: 137–143
As the title indicates a description of the role of transcription regulatory genes in causing multiple congenital abnormality syndromes.

Lindor N M, Ney J A, Gaffey T A et al 1992 A genetic review of complete and partial hydatidiform moles and nonmolar triploidy. Mayo Clin Proc 67: 791–799
A detailed review of the mechanisms which can lead to the formation of hydatidiform moles.

Lyon M F 1961 Gene action in the X chromosome of the mouse (*Mus musculus* L). Nature 190: 372–373
The original proposal of X-inactivation. Very short and easily understood.

Manouvrier-Hanu S, Holder-Espinasse M, Lyonnet S 1999 Genetics of limb anomalies in humans. Trend Genet 15: 409–417
A detailed and well illustrated account of vertebrate limb development.

Muenke M, Schell U 1995 Fibroblast-growth-factor receptor mutations in human skeletal disorders. Trend Genet 11: 308–313
A concise review of the functions of the fibroblast growth factors and their receptors.

Muragaki Y, Mundlos S, Upton J, Olsen B R 1996 Altered growth and branching patterns in synpolydactyly caused by mutations in HOXD13. Science 272: 548–551
The long-awaited first report of a human malformation caused by a mutation in a HOX gene.

ELEMENTS

❶ Several developmental gene families first identified in *Drosophila* and mice also play important roles in human morphogenesis. These include segment polarity genes, homeobox containing genes (*HOX*), and paired-box containing genes (*PAX*). Many of these genes act as transcription factors which regulate sequential developmental processes. Others are important in cell signalling. It has recently been shown that several human malformations and multiple malformation syndromes are caused by mutations in these genes.

❷ For normal development a haploid chromosome set must be inherited from each parent. A paternal diploid complement results in a complete hydatidiform mole if there is no maternal contribution and in triploidy with a partial hydatidiform mole if there is a haploid maternal contribution.

❸ A testis-determining factor on the Y chromosome, known as *SRY*, stimulates the undifferentiated gonads to develop into testes. This, in turn, sets off a series of events leading to male development. In the absence of *SRY* expression the human embryo develops into a female.

4 In females one of the X chromosomes is inactivated in each cell in early embryogenesis. This can be either the maternally derived or the paternally derived X chromosome. Thereafter in all daughter cells the same X chromosome is inactivated. This process, known as Lyonization, explains the presence of the Barr body in female nuclei and achieves dosage compensation of X chromosome gene products in males and females.

5 Twins can be monozygotic (identical) or dizygotic (fraternal). Monozygotic twins originate from a single zygote which divides into two during the first 2 weeks after conception. Monozygotic twins are genetically identical. Dizygotic twins originate from two separate zygotes and are no more genetically alike than brothers and sisters.

Patterns of inheritance

FAMILY STUDIES

If we wish to investigate the genetics of a particular trait or disorder in humans, we usually have to rely either on observation of the way in which it is transmitted from one generation to another, or on study of its frequency among relatives.

An important reason for studying the pattern of inheritance of disorders within families is to enable advice to be given to members of a family regarding the likelihood of their developing it or passing it on to their children, i.e. *genetic counselling* (p. 241). Taking a family history can, in itself, provide a diagnosis. For example, a child could come to the attention of a doctor having a fracture after a seemingly trivial injury. A family history of relatives with a similar tendency to fracture and blue sclerae would suggest the diagnosis of osteogenesis imperfecta (p. 70). In the absence of a positive family history other diagnoses would have to be considered.

PEDIGREE DRAWING AND TERMINOLOGY

A family tree is a shorthand system of recording the pertinent information about a family. It usually begins with the person through whom the family came to the attention of the investigator. This person is referred to as the *index case*, *proband* or *propositus*, or if female, the *proposita*. The position of the proband in the family tree is indicated by an arrow. Information about the health of the rest of the family is obtained by asking about brothers, sisters, parents and maternal and paternal relatives with the relevant information about the sex of the individual, affection status and relationship to other individuals being carefully recorded in the pedigree chart (Fig. 6.1).

MENDELIAN INHERITANCE

Over 11 000 traits or disorders in humans exhibit single gene *unifactorial* or *Mendelian inheritance*. However, charac-

teristics such as height, and many common familial disorders, such as diabetes, hypertension, etc., do not usually follow a simple pattern of inheritance (p. 127).

A trait or disorder which is determined by a gene on an autosome is said to show *autosomal inheritance*, whereas a trait or disorder determined by a gene on one of the sex chromosomes is said to show *sex-linked inheritance*.

AUTOSOMAL DOMINANT INHERITANCE

An *autosomal dominant* trait is one which manifests in the heterozygous state, i.e. in a person possessing both an abnormal or mutant allele and the normal allele. It is often possible to trace a dominantly inherited trait or disorder through many generations of a family (Fig. 6.2). In South Africa the vast majority of cases of porphyria variegata can be traced back to one couple in the late seventeenth century. This is a metabolic disorder characterized by skin blistering through increased sensitivity to sunlight and the excretion of urine which becomes 'port wine' coloured on standing as a result of the presence of porphyrins (p. 166) (Fig. 6.3). This pattern of inheritance is sometimes referred to as 'vertical' transmission.

Genetic risks

Each gamete from an individual with a dominant trait or disorder will contain either the normal allele or the mutant allele. If we represent the dominant mutant allele as 'A' and the recessive normal allele as 'a', then the various possible combinations of the gametes can be represented in a Punnett's square (Fig. 6.4). Any child born to a person affected with a dominant trait or disorder has a 1 in 2 (50%) chance of inheriting it and being similarly affected.

Pleiotropy

Autosomal dominant traits can involve only one organ or part of the body. A common example is having an extra finger, or what is known as polydactyly. However,

Individuals

Relationships

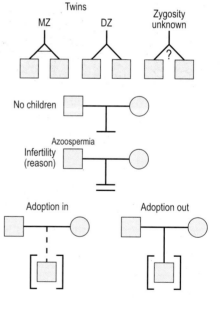

Fig. 6.1
Symbols used to represent individuals and relationships in family trees.

many autosomal dominant disorders in humans can manifest in a number of different systems of the body in a variety of ways, so-called *pleiotropy*. An example is tuberous sclerosis (p. 290), in which affected individuals can present with learning difficulties, epilepsy and a facial rash known as adenoma sebaceum which, although it can be confused with acne, is histologically composed of

blood vessels and fibrous tissue or what is known as an angiokeratoma(ta) (Fig. 6.5).

Variable expressivity

The clinical features in autosomal dominant disorders can show striking variation from person to person. This

Fig. 6.2
Family tree of an autosomal dominant trait.

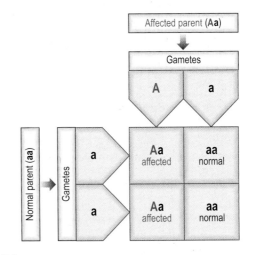

Fig. 6.4
Punnett's square showing possible gamete combinations for an autosomal dominant allele.

Fig. 6.3
Blistering skin lesions on the hand in porphyria variegata.

Fig. 6.5
Facial rash of angiokeratoma in a male with tuberous sclerosis.

difference in involvement between individuals is referred to as *variable expressivity*, e.g. in the autosomal dominant disorder neurofibromatosis Type I (p. 272) individuals vary enormously in the number of cutaneous neurofibromata which they have, varying from none to several hundred.

Reduced penetrance

In some individuals heterozygous for certain autosomal disorders, the presence of the mutation can be undetected clinically, representing so-called *reduced penetrance* or what is known in lay terms as the disorder 'skipping a generation'. Reduced penetrance is thought to be the result of the modifying effects of other genes, as well as being due to interaction of the gene with environmental factors. An individual who is heterozygous for a dominant mutation but has no features of the disorder is said to represent *non-penetrance*.

Reduced penetrance, variable expressivity along with the pleiotropic effects of a mutant allele all need to be taken into account when providing genetic counselling to individuals at risk for autosomal dominantly inherited disorders (p. 290).

New mutations

In autosomal dominant disorders an affected person will usually have an affected parent. Sometimes, however, a trait can appear in an individual in one generation when no one else in previous generations has been affected. An example is achondroplasia, a form of short-limbed dwarfism (p. 86), in which the parents are usually of normal stature. The sudden unexpected appearance of a condition arising as a result of a mistake occurring in the transmission of a gene is called a *new mutation*. The dominant mode of inheritance of achondroplasia could only be confirmed by the offspring of persons with achondroplasia having an equal chance of having achondroplasia or being of normal stature.

There are other possible explanations for a disorder appearing to arise as a new dominant mutation. One possibility is that one of the parents can, in fact, be heterozygous for the mutant allele but be so mildly affected that it has not previously been detected, i.e. non-penetrance. The variable expressivity of a mutant allele also needs to be considered as a second possible explanation. Another possibility for the appearance of an apparent new mutation is that the stated father is not the child's biological father, i.e. *non-paternity* (p. 247).

New dominant mutations, in certain instances, have been associated with an increased age of the father. It is believed that this is because of the large number of mitotic divisions which male gamete stem cells undergo during a man's reproductive lifetime (p. 43).

Codominance

Codominance is the term used for two allelic traits which are both expressed in the heterozygous state. In persons with blood group AB it is possible to demonstrate both A and B blood group substances on the red blood cells so that the A and B blood groups are therefore codominant (p. 186).

Homozygosity for autosomal dominant traits

The rarity of most autosomal dominant disorders and diseases means that they usually only occur in the heterozygous state. There are, however, a few reports of children born to couples where both parents are heterozygous for a dominantly inherited disorder. Offspring of such couples are, therefore, at risk of being homozygous. In some instances affected individuals appear to be either more severely affected, as has been reported with achondroplasia, or have an earlier age of onset, as in familial hypercholesterolaemia (p. 160). The heterozygote having a phenotype intermediate between the homozygotes for the normal and mutant alleles is

consistent with a haploinsufficiency loss-of-function mutation (p. 23).

Conversely, with other dominantly inherited disorders, homozygous affected individuals seem to have the same age of onset and severity as heterozygotes, e.g. Huntington's disease (p. 267). There is also an intriguing report of individuals who have been shown by DNA analysis to be homozygous for expansions in the triplet repeat in the myotonic dystrophy gene (p. 269) but who are clinically unaffected, as if the two different mutations have cancelled each other out!

AUTOSOMAL RECESSIVE INHERITANCE

Recessive traits and disorders are only manifest when the mutant allele is present in a double dose, i.e. homozygosity. Individuals heterozygous for a recessive mutant allele show no features of the disorder and are perfectly healthy, i.e. they are *carriers*. The family tree for recessive traits differs considerably from that found in autosomal dominant traits (Fig. 6.6). It is not possible to trace an autosomal recessive trait or disorder through the family, i.e. all the affected individuals in a family are usually in a single *sibship*, that is, they are brothers and sisters. This is sometimes referred to as 'horizontal' transmission.

Consanguinity

Enquiry into the family history of individuals affected with rare recessive traits or disorders can reveal that their parents are related, i.e. *consanguineous*. The rarer a recessive trait or disorder, the greater the frequency of consanguinity among the parents of affected individuals. In cystic fibrosis, the commonest autosomal recessive disorder in persons of Western European origin (p. 276), the frequency of parental consanguinity is only slightly greater than that seen in the general population. By contrast, in alkaptonuria, one of the original inborn errors of metabolism (pp. 61, 155) which is an exceedingly rare recessive disorder, Bateson and Garrod, in their original

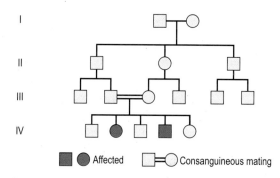

Fig. 6.6
Family tree of an autosomal recessive trait.

description of the disorder, observed that a quarter or more of the parents were first cousins. They reasoned that rare alleles for disorders such as alkaptonuria are more likely to 'meet up' in the offspring of cousins than in the offspring of parents who are unrelated.

Genetic risks

If we represent the normal dominant allele as 'A' and the recessive mutant allele as 'a', then each parental gamete carries either the mutant or the normal allele (Fig. 6.7). The various possible combinations of gametes mean that the offspring of two heterozygotes have a 1 in 4 (25%) chance of being homozygous affected, a 1 in 2 (50%) chance of being heterozygous unaffected and a 1 in 4 (25%) chance of being homozygous unaffected.

Pseudodominance

If an individual who is homozygous for an autosomal recessive disorder marries a carrier of the same disorder, their children have a 1 in 2 (50%) chance of being affected. Such a pedigree is said to exhibit *pseudo-dominance* (Fig. 6.8).

Locus heterogeneity

A disorder inherited in the same manner can be due to mutations in more than one gene, or what is known as *locus heterogeneity*. For example, it is recognized that sensorineural hearing impairment/deafness most commonly shows autosomal recessive inheritance. Deaf persons, by virtue of their schooling and involvement in the deaf community, often choose to have children with another deaf person. It would be expected that if two deaf persons were homozygous for the same recessive gene, all of their children would be similarly affected. Families have been described in which all the children born to parents deaf due to autosomal recessive genes have had perfectly normal hearing and are what is known as *double heterozygotes*. The explanation for this must be that the parents were homozygous for mutant alleles at different loci, i.e. that a number of different genes can cause autosomal recessive sensorineural deafness. In fact, over the past 10 years, six genes and a further 28 loci have been shown to be involved!

Disorders with the same phenotype due to different genetic loci are known as *genocopies*, while the same phenotype being the result of environmental causes is known as a *phenocopy*.

Mutational heterogeneity

Heterogeneity can also occur at the allelic level. In the majority of single gene disorders, e.g. β thalassaemia, a

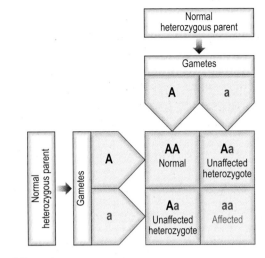

Fig. 6.7
Punnett's square showing possible gametic combinations for heterozygous carrier parents of an autosomal recessive allele.

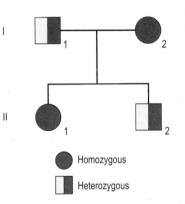

Fig. 6.8
A pedigree with a woman (I₂) homozygous for an autosomal recessive disorder whose husband is heterozygous for the same disorder. They have a homozygous affected daughter so that the pedigree shows pseudodominant inheritance.

large number of different mutations have been identified as being responsible (p. 146). Individuals have been identified who have two different mutations at the same locus and are known as *compound heterozygotes*, constituting what is known as allelic or *mutational heterogeneity*. Most individuals affected with an autosomal recessive disorder are probably, in fact, compound heterozygotes rather than true homozygotes, unless their parents are related when they are likely to be homozygous for the same mutation by descent, having inherited the same mutation from a common ancestor.

SEX-LINKED INHERITANCE

Sex-linked inheritance refers to the pattern of inheritance shown by genes which are located on either of the sex chromosomes. Genes carried on the X chromosome are referred to as being *X-linked* while genes carried on the Y chromosome are referred to as exhibiting *Y-linked* or *holandric inheritance*.

X-linked recessive inheritance

An X-linked recessive trait is one determined by a gene carried on the X chromosome and usually only manifests in males. A male with a mutant allele on his single X chromosome is said to be *hemizygous* for that allele. Diseases inherited in an X-linked manner are transmitted by healthy heterozygous female carriers to affected males, as well as by affected males to their obligate carrier daughters with a consequent risk to male grandchildren through these daughters (Fig. 6.9). This type of pedigree is sometimes said to show 'diagonal' or a 'knight's move' pattern of transmission.

The mode of inheritance whereby only males are affected by a disease which is transmitted by normal females was appreciated by the Jews nearly 2000 years ago. They excused from circumcision the sons of all the sisters of a mother who had sons with the 'bleeding disease', in other words, haemophilia (p. 282). The sons of the father's sibs were not excused. Queen Victoria was a carrier of haemophilia and her carrier daughters, who were perfectly healthy, introduced the gene into the Russian and Spanish royal families. Fortunately for the British royal family, Queen Victoria's son, Edward VII, did not inherit the gene, and so could not transmit it to his descendants.

Genetic risks

A male transmits his X chromosome to each of his daughters and his Y chromosome to each of his sons. If a male affected with haemophilia has children with a normal female, then all his daughters will be *obligate carriers* but none of his sons will be affected (Fig. 6.10). A male cannot transmit an X-linked trait to his son, with

the very rare exception of uniparental heterodisomy (p. 109).

For a carrier female of an X-linked recessive disorder having children with a normal male, each son has a 1 in 2 (50%) chance of being affected and each daughter has a 1 in 2 (50%) chance of being a carrier (Fig. 6.11).

Some X-linked disorders are not compatible with survival to the reproductive age and are not, therefore, transmitted by affected males. Duchenne muscular dystrophy is the commonest form of muscular dystrophy and is a severe disease (p. 280). The first signs in an affected male are a waddling gait, difficulty in climbing stairs unaided and a tendency to fall over easily. By about the age of ten affected boys usually can no longer

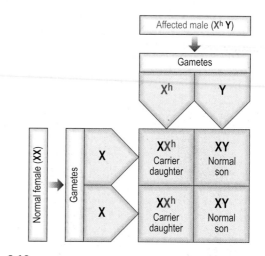

Fig. 6.10
Punnett's square showing possible gamete combinations for the offspring of a male affected by an X-linked recessive disorder (X^h represents a mutation for an X-linked gene).

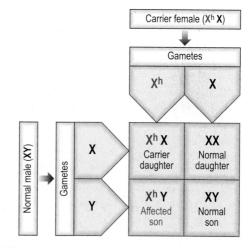

Fig. 6.11
A Punnett's square showing possible gamete combinations for the offspring of a female carrier of an X-linked recessive disorder (X^h represents a mutation for an X-linked gene).

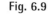

Fig. 6.9
Family tree of an X-linked recessive trait in which affected males reproduce.

walk and have to use a wheelchair. The muscle weakness gradually progresses and affected males ultimately become confined to bed and will often die before reaching the age of 20 years (Fig. 6.12). Since affected boys do not usually survive to reproduce, the disease is transmitted almost entirely by healthy female carriers (Fig. 6.13).

Variable expression in heterozygous females

In humans, several X-linked disorders are known in which heterozygous females have a mosaic phenotype with a mixture of features of the normal and mutant alleles. In X-linked ocular albinism the iris and ocular fundus of affected males are completely lacking in pigment. Careful examination of the ocular fundus in females heterozygous for ocular albinism reveals a mosaic pattern of pigmentation (Fig. 5.13, p. 93). This mosaic pattern of involvement can be explained through the random process of X-inactivation (p. 92). In the pigmented areas the normal gene is on the active X

chromosome while in the depigmented areas the mutant allele is on the active X chromosome.

Females affected with X-linked recessive disorders

Very rarely a woman can exhibit an X-linked recessive trait. There are several explanations for how this can happen.

Homozygosity for X-linked recessive disorders

Another example of an X-linked recessive trait is red–green colour blindness, the inability to distinguish between the colours red and green. About 8% of males are red–green colour blind and, although it is unusual, because of the high frequency of this allele in the population, about 1 in 150 women are red–green colour blind. Therefore a female can be affected with an X-linked recessive disorder as a result of homozygosity for an X-linked allele, although this is uncommon because of the rarity of most X-linked conditions. A female could be a homozygote because her mother was a carrier and her father was affected. Much less likely is that a female could be homozygous if her father was affected and her mother was normal but a new mutation occurred on the X chromosome transmitted to the daughter. Alternatively, again very rarely a female could be homozygous if her mother was a carrier and her father was normal but a new mutation occurred on the X chromosome he transmitted to his daughter.

Skewed X-inactivation

The process of X-inactivation usually occurs randomly, there being an equal chance of either of the two X chromosomes in a heterozygous female being inactivated in any one cell. By chance, however, in an occasional heterozygous carrier female, the active X chromosome in most of her cells could be the one bearing the mutant allele. If this happens, a carrier female would exhibit some of the symptoms and signs of the disease and be a so-called *manifesting heterozygote* or *carrier*. This has been

Fig. 6.12
Boy with Duchenne muscular dystrophy; note the enlarged calves and wasting of the thigh muscles.

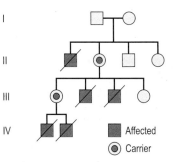

Fig. 6.13
Family tree of Duchenne muscular dystrophy with the disorder being transmitted by carrier females and affecting males who do not survive to transmit the disorder.

reported in a number of X-linked disorders including Duchenne muscular dystrophy and haemophilia A (p. 93). In addition, there are reports of several X-linked disorders in which there are several manifesting carriers in the same family, consistent with the coincidental inheritance of an abnormality of X-inactivation (p. 93).

Numerical X chromosome abnormalities

A female could manifest an X-linked recessive disorder through being a carrier of an X-linked recesssive mutation and having only a single X chromosome, i.e. Turner's syndrome (p. 257). Women with Turner's syndrome and haemophilia or Duchenne muscular dystrophy have been reported.

X-autosome translocations

Females with a translocation involving one of the X chromosomes and an autosome can be affected with an X-linked recessive disorder. If the break-point of the translocation disrupts a gene on the X chromosome, then a female can be affected with an X-linked recessive disorder. This is because the X chromosome involved in the translocation survives preferentially so as to maintain functional disomy of the autosomal genes (Fig. 6.14). The observation of females affected with Duchenne muscular dystrophy with X-autosome translocations involving the same region of the short arm of the X chromosome helped to map the Duchenne muscular dystrophy gene (p. 281). This type of observation has been vital in the positional cloning of a number of genes in humans (p. 74).

X-linked dominant inheritance

Although uncommon, there are disorders which are manifest in the heterozygous female as well as in the male who has the mutant allele on his single X chromosome. This is known as X-linked dominant inheritance (Fig. 6.15). X-linked dominant inheritance superficially resembles that of an autosomal dominant trait because both daughters and sons of an affected female have a 1 in 2 (50%) chance of being affected. There is, however, an important difference. With an X-linked dominant trait an affected male transmits the trait to all his daughters but to none of his sons. Therefore in families with an X-linked dominant disorder there is an excess of affected females and direct male to male transmission cannot occur.

An example of an X-linked dominant trait is vitamin D-resistant rickets. Rickets can be due to a dietary deficiency of vitamin D, but in vitamin D-resistant rickets the disorder occurs even when there is an adequate dietary intake of vitamin D. In the X-linked dominant form of vitamin D-resistant rickets both males and females are affected, though the females usually have less severe skeletal changes than the males.

Fig. 6.14
Shows the generation of an X-autosome translocation with break point in a female and how this results in the development of Duchenne muscular dystrophy.

A mosaic pattern of involvement can be demonstrated in females heterozygous for some X-linked dominant disorders. An example is the mosaic pattern of abnormal pigmentation of the skin which follows developmental lines (p. 256) seen in females heterozygous for the X-linked dominant disorder incontinentia pigmenti.

Y-linked inheritance

Y-linked or *holandric inheritance* implies that only males are affected. An affected male transmits Y-linked traits to

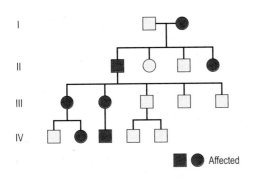

Fig. 6.15
Family tree of an X-linked dominant trait.

all his sons but to none of his daughters. In the past it has been suggested that bizarre sounding conditions such as porcupine skin, hairy ears and webbed toes are Y-linked traits. With the possible exception of hairy ears, these claims of holandric inheritance have not stood up to more careful study. Recent evidence clearly indicates, however, that the H–Y histocompatibility antigen (p. 182) and genes involved in spermatogenesis are carried on the Y chromosome and therefore manifest holandric inheritance. The latter, if deleted, lead to infertility due to azoospermia (absence of the sperm in semen) in males. The recent advent of techniques of assisted reproduction, particularly the technique of intracytoplasmic sperm injection (ICSI), means that if a pregnancy with a male conceptus results after the use of this technique, the child will also necessarily be infertile!

Partial sex-linkage

Partial sex-linkage has been used in the past for certain disorders which appear to exhibit autosomal dominant inheritance in some families and X-linked inheritance in others. This is now known to be likely to be because of genes carried on the portion of the X chromosome which shows homology with the Y chromosome and escapes X-inactivation. During meiosis pairing occurs between the homologous distal parts of the short arms of the X and Y chromosomes, the so-called *pseudoautosomal region*. As a result of a cross-over, a gene could be transferred from the X to the Y chromosome or vice versa allowing the possibility of male to male transmission. The latter instances would be consistent with autosomal dominant inheritance. A rare skeletal dysplasia Leri–Weil dyschondrosteosis, in which affected individuals have short stature and a characteristic wrist deformity (Madelung's deformity), has been reported to show both autosomal dominant and X-linked inheritance. The disorder has been shown to be due to deletions of or mutations in the short stature homeobox (SHOX) gene (p. 257) which is in the pseudoautosomal region.

Sex influence

Some autosomal traits are expressed more frequently in one sex than another, so-called *sex influence*. Gout and presenile baldness are examples of sex-influenced autosomal dominant traits, males being predominantly affected in both cases. The influence of sex in these two examples is probably through the effect of male hormones. Gout, for example, is very rare in women before the menopause but the frequency increases in later life. Baldness does not occur in males who have been castrated.

Sex limitation

Sex limitation refers to the appearance of certain features in individuals of only one sex. Examples include virilization of female infants affected with the autosomal recessive endocrine disorder, congenital adrenal hyperplasia (p. 158).

ESTABLISHING THE MODE OF INHERITANCE OF A GENETIC DISORDER

In experimental animals it is possible to arrange specific types of mating to establish the mode of inheritance of a trait or disorder. In humans when a disorder is newly recognized, the geneticist approaches the problem indirectly by fitting likely models of inheritance to the observed outcome in the offspring. Certain features are necessary to support a particular mode of inheritance. Formally establishing the mode of inheritance is not usually possible with a single family and normally requires study of a number of families (Table 6.1).

Autosomal dominant inheritance

In order to determine whether a trait or disorder is inherited in an autosomal dominant manner, there are three specific features which need to be observed. The first is that it affects both males and females in equal proportions. The second is that it is transmitted from one generation to the next. The third is that all forms of transmission between the sexes are observed, i.e. male to male, female to female, male to female and the converse. The first two types of transmission exclude the possibility of the gene being on one of the sex chromosomes. In the case of sporadically occurring disorders, increased paternal age is suggestive of a new autosomal dominant mutation.

Autosomal recessive inheritance

There are three features which suggest the possibility of autosomal recessive inheritance. The first is that the

Table 6.1 Features which support the single gene or Mendelian patterns of inheritance

Autosomal dominant
— Males and females affected in equal proportions
— Affected individuals in multiple generations
— Transmission by individuals of both sexes, i.e. male to male, female to female, male to female and female to male

Autosomal recessive
— Males and females affected in equal proportions
— Affected individuals usually only in a single generation
— Parents can be related, i.e. consanguineous

X-linked recessive
— Males usually only affected
— Transmitted through unaffected females
— Males cannot transmit the disorder to their sons, i.e. no male to male transmission

X-linked dominant
— Males and females affected but often with an excess of females
— Females less severely affected than males
— Affected males can transmit the disorder to their daughters but not sons

Y-linked inheritance
— Affected males only
— Affected males must transmit it to their sons

Y-linked inheritance

There are two features necessary to establish a Y-linked pattern of inheritance. The first is that it affects males only. The second is that affected males must transmit the disorder to their sons, e.g. male infertility by ICSI (p. 105).

MULTIPLE ALLELES

So far, each of the traits we have considered has involved only two alleles, the normal and the mutant. Some genes have more than two allelic forms, i.e. multiple alleles. Multiple alleles are the result of a normal gene having mutated to produce various different alleles, some of which can be dominant and others recessive to the normal allele. In the case of the ABO blood group system (p. 186), there are at least four alleles (A_1, A_2, B and O). An individual can possess any two of these alleles which can be the same or different (AO, A_2B, OO, and so on). Alleles are carried on homologous chromosomes and therefore a person transmits only one allele for a certain trait to any particular offspring. For example, if a person has the genotype AB, he will transmit to any particular offspring either the A allele or the B allele but never both or neither (Table 6.2).

The preceding remarks concerning the inheritance of multiple alleles relate only to genes located on the autosomes. If a series of alleles are carried on the X chromosome then a woman would have two, either of which she could transmit to a particular offspring, whereas a man would only have one allele to transmit.

disorder affects males and females in equal proportions. The second is that it usually only affects individuals in one generation in a single sibship, i.e. brothers and sisters, and does not occur in previous and subsequent generations. Lastly, consanguinity in the parents provides further support for autosomal recessive inheritance.

X-linked recessive inheritance

There are three main features necessary to establish X-linked recessive inheritance. The first is that the trait or disorder should affect males almost exclusively. The second is that X-linked recessive disorders are transmitted through unaffected carrier females to their sons. Affected males, if they survive to reproduce, can have affected grandsons through their daughters who are obligate carriers. The third is that male to male transmission is not observed, i.e. affected males cannot transmit the disorder to their sons.

X-linked dominant inheritance

There are three features necessary to establish X-linked dominant inheritance. The first is that males and females are affected but affected females are more frequent than affected males. Secondly, females are usually less severely affected than males. Thirdly, while affected females can transmit the disorder to both male and female offspring, affected males can only transmit the disorder to their daughters, all of whom will be affected.

NON-MENDELIAN INHERITANCE

A number of disorders are known which do not follow classical patterns of Mendelian inheritance. In recent

Table 6.2 Possible genotypes, phenotypes and gametes formed from the four alleles A_1, A_2, B and O at the ABO locus

Genotype	Phenotype	Gametes
A_1A_1	A_1	A_1
A_2A_2	A_2	A_2
BB	B	B
OO	O	O
A_1A_2	A_1	A_1 or A_2
A_1B	A_1B	A_1 or B
A_1O	A_1	A_1 or O
A_2B	A_2B	A_2 or B
A_2O	A_2	A_2 or O
BO	B	B or O

Fig. 6.16
Newborn baby with severe hypotonia requiring ventilation as a result of having inherited myotonic dystrophy from his mother.

Fig. 6.17
Silver staining of a 5% denaturing gel of the PCR products of the CAG triplet in the 5' untranslated end of the Huntington's disease gene from an affected male and his wife showing her to have two similar size repeats in the normal range (20 and 24 copies) and him to have one normal sized triplet repeat (18 copies) and an expanded triplet repeat (44 copies). The bands in the left lane are standard markers to allow sizing of the CAG repeat. (Courtesy of Alan Dodge, Regional DNA Laboratory, St Mary's Hospital, Manchester.)

years several different novel mechanisms have been recognized which account for this.

ANTICIPATION

In some autosomal dominant traits or disorders, such as myotonic dystrophy, the onset of the disease occurs at an earlier age in the offspring than in the parents, or the disease occurs with increasing severity in subsequent generations. This phenomenon is called *anticipation*. It used to be believed that this effect was the result of a bias of ascertainment, because of the way in which the families were collected. It was argued that this arose because persons in whom the disease begins earlier or is more severe are more likely to be ascertained and only those individuals who are less severely affected tend to have children. In addition, it was felt that because the observer is in the same generation as the affected presenting probands, many individuals who at present are unaffected would, by necessity, develop the disease later in life.

Recent studies, however, have shown that in a number of disorders, including Huntington's disease and myotonic dystrophy, anticipation is, in fact, a real biological phenomenon occurring as a result of the expansion of unstable triplet repeat sequences (p. 22). An expansion of the CTG triplet repeat in the 3' untranslated end of the myotonic dystrophy gene occurring predominantly in maternal meiosis appears to be the explanation for the severe neonatal form of myotonic dystrophy which usually only occurs when the gene is transmitted by the mother (Fig. 6.16). A similar expansion in the CAG expansion in the 5' end of the Huntington's disease gene (Fig. 6.17) in paternal meiosis appears to account for the increased risk of juvenile Huntington's disease when the gene is transmitted by the father.

MOSAICISM

An individual, or a particular tissue of the body, can consist of more than one cell type or line, through an error occurring during mitosis at any stage after conception, or what is known as *mosaicism* (p. 52). Mosaicism of either somatic or germ cells can account for some instances of unusual patterns of inheritance or phenotypic features in an affected individual.

Somatic mosaicism

The possibility of *somatic mosaicism* is suggested by the features of a single gene disorder being less severe in an individual than usual or by being confined to a particular part of the body in a segmental distribution, e.g. as occasionally occurs in neurofibromatosis type I (p. 272). Depending on when a mutation arises in development, it may or may not be transmitted to the next generation with full expression depending on whether the mutation is also present in all or some of the germ line cells.

Gonadal mosaicism

There have been many reports of families with autosomal dominant disorders, such as achondroplasia and osteogenesis imperfecta, and X-linked recessive disorders, such as Duchenne muscular dystrophy and haemophilia, in which the parents are phenotypically normal and the results of investigations or genetic tests have also all been normal, but in which more than one of their children has been affected. The most favoured

explanation for these observations is *gonadal* or *germ line mosaicism* in one of the parents, i.e. the mutation being present in a proportion of the gonadal cells. An elegant example of this was provided by the demonstration of a mutation in the collagen gene responsible for osteogenesis imperfecta in a proportion of individual sperm from a clinically normal father who had two affected infants with different partners. Germ line mosaicism is an important possibility to keep in mind when providing recurrence risks in genetic counselling for apparently new autosomal dominant and X-linked recessive mutations (p. 298).

UNIPARENTAL DISOMY

An individual normally inherits one of a pair of homologous chromosomes from each parent (p. 40). Over the last decade, with the advent of DNA technology, individuals have been identified who have been shown to have inherited both homologues of a chromosome pair from only one of their parents, so-

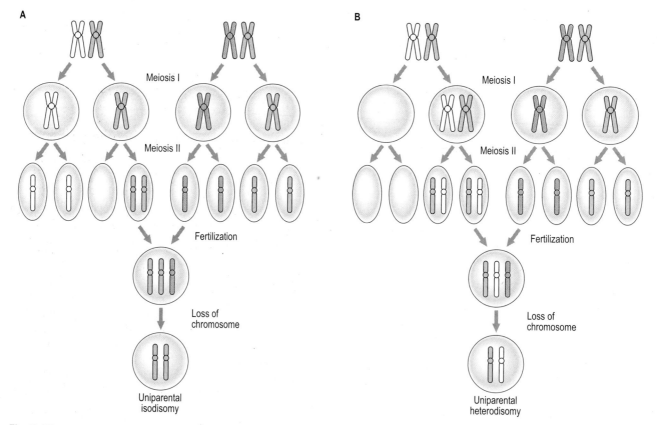

Fig. 6.18
Mechanism of origin of uniparental disomy. (A) Uniparental isodisomy occurring through a disomic gamete arising from non-disjunction in meiosis II fertilizing a monosomic gamete with loss of the chromosome from the parent contributing the single homologue. (B) Uniparental heterodisomy occurring through a disomic gamete arising from non-disjunction in meiosis I fertilizing a monosomic gamete with loss of the chromosome from the parent contributing the single homologue.

called *uniparental disomy*. If an individual inherits two copies of the same homologue from one parent, through an error in meiosis II (p. 42), this is called *uniparental isodisomy* (Fig. 6.18). If, however, the individual inherits the two different homologues from one parent through an error in meiosis I (p. 40), this is termed *uniparental heterodisomy*. In either instance, it is presumed that the conceptus would originally be trisomic with loss of a chromosome leading to the 'normal' disomic state. One-third of such chromosome losses, if they occurred with equal frequency, would result in uniparental disomy. Alternatively, it is postulated that uniparental disomy could arise as a result of a gamete from one parent which does not contain a particular chromosome homologue, or what is termed *nullisomic*, being 'rescued' by fertilization with a gamete which, through a second separate chance error in meiosis, is disomic.

Using DNA techniques, uniparental disomy has been shown to be the cause of a father with haemophilia having an affected son and of a child with cystic fibrosis being born to a couple in which only the mother was a carrier (with proven paternity!). Uniparental paternal disomy for chromosome II has also been shown in some cases of the rare overgrowth syndrome known as the Beckwith–Wiedemann syndrome.

GENOMIC IMPRINTING

Although it was originally believed that genes on homologous chromosomes were expressed equally, it is now recognized that different clinical features can result, depending on whether a gene is inherited from the father or from the mother. This 'parent of origin' effect is referred to as *genomic imprinting*. Although the mechanism by which differential expression of the maternally and paternally derived alleles in early development occurs was thought to involve differential methylation, at present there is no clear methylation pattern observed when the active and inactive alleles of the imprinted genes are compared in all instances. Only a small proportion of the human genome is imprinted.

Evidence of genomic imprinting has been observed in two dysmorphic syndromes associated with learning difficulties known as the Prader–Willi and Angelman syndromes.

The Prader–Willi syndrome

The Prader–Willi syndrome is characterized by short stature, obesity, hypogonadism and learning difficulty (Fig. 6.19). Approximately 50–60% of individuals with the Prader–Willi syndrome can be shown to have an interstitial deletion of the proximal portion of the long arm of chromosome 15 visible by conventional cyto-

genetic means and in a further 15% a submicroscopic deletion can be demonstrated by FISH (p. 34) or molecular means. DNA analysis has revealed that the chromosome deleted is almost always the paternally derived homologue. Most of the remaining 25% of individuals with the Prader–Willi syndrome found not to have a chromosome deletion, have been shown to have maternal uniparental disomy. This is functionally the equivalent of a deletion in the paternally derived chromosome 15.

Recent findings have shown that only the paternally inherited allele of a critical region of the proximal portion of chromosome 15, which includes the gene for the small nuclear ribonucleoprotein polypeptide N (SNRPN), is expressed, i.e. the SNRPN gene and adjacent genes are maternally imprinted. These findings are consistent with the hypothesis that expression of a functional SNRPN gene product or closely adjacent genes is lacking in the Prader–Willi syndrome and its deficiency could lead, in part, to the features of the disorder.

The Angelman syndrome

The Angelman syndrome (p. 254) is characterized by epilepsy, severe learning difficulties, an unsteady or ataxic gait and a happy affect (Fig. 6.20). Interestingly

Fig. 6.19
Male child with the Prader–Willi syndrome.

Fig. 6.20
Female child with the Angelman syndrome.

preferentially or exclusively expressed from the maternally derived chromosome 15 in brain. How mutations in UBE3A lead to the features seen in persons with the Angelman syndrome is not clear but it is thought that it could involve ubiquitin-mediated destruction of proteins in the central nervous system in development.

A small proportion of individuals with the Prader–Willi syndrome, around 2%, and in the region of 5% of individuals with the Angelman syndrome have abnormalities of the imprinting process itself. This last group, unlike the other three, is associated with a risk of recurrence which presumably occurs due to gonadal mosaicism for the mutation in the mother.

Families have been reported in which a translocation of the proximal portion of the long arm of chromosome 15 involved in these two syndromes is segregating. Depending on whether the translocation is transmitted by the father or mother, the affected offspring within the family have had either the Prader–Willi syndrome or the Angelman syndrome!

75% of individuals with the Angelman syndrome have been shown to have an interstitial deletion of the same region of chromosome 15 as is involved in the Prader–Willi syndrome, but on the maternally derived homologue. In approximately a further 2–3% of individuals with the Angelman syndrome, it can be shown to have arisen through paternal uniparental disomy. In approximately 15% of individuals with the Angelman syndrome, mutations have been identified in a gene, UBE3A which is one of the ubiquitin genes, which appears to be

MITOCHONDRIAL INHERITANCE

Each cell contains many thousands of copies of mitochondrial DNA with more being found in cells which have high energy requirements such as brain and muscle. Mitochondria and therefore their DNA are almost exclusively inherited from the mother through the oocyte (p. 17). Mitochondrial DNA has a higher rate of spontaneous mutation than nuclear DNA and the accumulation of mutations in mitochondrial DNA has been proposed as being responsible for some of the somatic effects seen with ageing.

Table 6.3 Some of the more common mitochondrially inherited disorders, features, gene and mutation usually involved

Disorder	Features	Mitochondrial gene	Mutation
Leber's hereditary optic neuropathy	Visual loss, neurodegenerative features	ND1, ND4, ND6	3460A, 11778A, 14459A, 14484C
MELAS	Encephalopathy, lactic acidosis, stroke-like episodes	tRNA$^{Leu(UUR)}$	3243G
MERRF	Myoclonic epilepsy, mitochondrial myopathy with ragged-red fibres	tRNA^{Lys}	8344G, 8356C
Chronic progressive external ophthalmoplegia	Ptosis, ophthalmoplegia	tRNA^{Asn}	5692G, 5703G
Hypertrophic cardiomyopathy with myopathy	HOCM, muscle weakness	tRNA^{Ile} tRNA$^{Leu(UUR)}$	4317G, 4269G, 4300G, 3303T, 3260G
Diabetes with deafness	Diabetes mellitus, sensorineural deafness	tRNA$^{Leu(CUIN)}$	3243G
Aminoglycoside-induced deafness	Deafness induced by use of aminoglycoside antibiotics	12S RNA, tRNA^{SER}	1555G, 7445G, 7472Cins

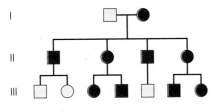

Fig. 6.21
Family tree consistent with mitochondrial inheritance.

In humans, *cytoplasmic* or *mitochondrial inheritance* has been proposed as a possible explanation for the pattern of inheritance observed in some rare disorders which affect both males and females but are transmitted only through females, so-called *maternal* or *matrilineal inheritance* (Fig. 6.21).

A number of rare disorders with unusual combinations of muscle and neurological features, sometimes occurring in association with other conditions such as diabetes or deafness, have been characterized as being due to mutations in mitochondrial genes (Table 6.3). As mitochondria have an important role in cellular metabolism, it is not surprising that the organs most susceptible to mitochondrial mutations are the central nervous system, skeletal muscle and heart.

In most persons the mitochondrial DNA from different mitochondria is identical, or shows what is termed *homoplasmy*. If a mutation occurs in the mitochondrial DNA of an individual, initially there will be two populations of mitochondrial DNA, so-called *heteroplasmy*. The proportion of mitochondria with a mutation in their DNA and mutational heterogeneity are possible explanations for the range of phenotypic severity seen in persons affected with mitochondrially inherited disorders.

FURTHER READING

Bateson W, Saunders E R 1902 Experimental studies in the physiology of heredity. Royal Society Reports to the Evolution Committee, pp. 132–134
Early observations on Mendelian inheritance.

Hall J G 1988 Somatic mosaicism: observations related to clinical genetics. Am J Hum Genet 43: 355–363
Good review of findings arising from somatic mosaicism in clinical genetics.

Hall J G 1990 Genomic imprinting: review and relevance to human diseases. Am J Hum Genet 46: 857–873
Extensive review of examples of imprinting in inherited diseases in humans.

Heinig R M 2000 The monk in the garden: The lost and found genius of Gregor Mendel. Houghton Mifflin, London
The life and work of Gregor Mendel as the history of the birth of genetics.

Kingston H M 1994 An ABC of clinical genetics, 2nd edn. British Medical Association, London
A simple outline primer of the basic principles of clinical genetics.

Reik W, Surami A (eds) 1997 Genomic imprinting (Frontiers in Molecular Biology), IRL Press, London
Detailed discussion of examples and mechanisms of genomic imprinting.

Vogel F, Motulsky A G 1996 Human genetics, 3nd edn. Springer-Verlag, Berlin
This text has detailed explanations of many of the concepts in human genetics outlined in this chapter.

ELEMENTS

❶ Family studies are often necessary to determine the mode of inheritance of a trait or disorder and to give appropriate genetic counselling. A standard shorthand convention exists for pedigree documentation of the family history.

❷ Mendelian, or single gene, disorders can be inherited in five ways: autosomal dominant, autosomal recessive, X-linked dominant, X-linked recessive and Y-linked inheritance.

❸ Autosomal dominant alleles are manifest in the heterozygous state and are usually transmitted from one generation to the next but can occasionally arise as a new mutation. They usually affect both males and females equally. Each offspring of a parent with an autosomal dominant gene has a 1 in 2 chance of inheriting it from the affected parent. Autosomal dominant alleles can exhibit reduced penetrance, variable expressivity and sex limitation.

❹ Autosomal recessive disorders are only manifest in the homozygous state and normally only affect individuals in one generation, usually in one sibship in a family. They affect both males and females equally. Offspring of parents who are heterozygous for the same autosomal recessive allele have a 1 in 4 chance of being homozygous for that allele. The less common an autosomal recessive allele, the greater the likelihood that the parents of a homozygote are consanguineous.

5 X-linked recessive alleles are normally only manifest in males. Offspring of females heterozygous for an X-linked recessive allele have a 1 in 2 chance of inheriting the allele from their mother. Daughters of males with an X-linked recessive allele are obligate heterozygotes while sons cannot inherit the allele. Rarely, females manifest an X-linked recessive trait because they are homozygous for the allele, have a single X chromosome, have a structural rearrangement of one of their X chromosomes, or are heterozygous but show skewed or non-random X-inactivation.

6 There are only a few disorders known to be inherited in an X-linked dominant manner. In X-linked dominant disorders hemizygous males are more severely affected than heterozygous females.

7 Unusual features in single gene patterns of inheritance can be explained by phenomena such as genetic heterogeneity, mosaicism, anticipation, imprinting, uniparental disomy and mitochondrial inheritance.

Mathematical and population genetics

In this chapter some of the more mathematical aspects of the ways in which genes are inherited shall be considered together with how genes are distributed and maintained at particular frequencies in populations. This subject constitutes what is known as *population genetics*. By its very nature genetics lends itself to a numerical approach with many of the most influential pioneering figures in human genetics having come from a mathematical background. They were particularly attracted by the challenges of trying to determine the frequencies of genes in populations and the rates at which they mutate. Much of this early work impinges on the specialty of medical genetics, and in particular on genetic counselling, and by the completion of this chapter it is hoped that the reader will have gained an understanding of the following.

1. Why a dominant trait does not increase in a population at the expense of a recessive one.
2. How the carrier frequency and mutation rate can be determined knowing the disease incidence.
3. Why a particular genetic disorder can be more common in one population or community than in another.
4. How it can be confirmed that a genetic disorder shows a particular pattern of inheritance.
5. The concept of genetic linkage and how this differs from linkage disequilibrium.
6. The effects of medical intervention.

ALLELE FREQUENCIES IN POPULATIONS

On first reflection it would be reasonable to predict that dominant genes and traits in a population would tend to increase at the expense of recessive ones. After all, on average three-quarters of the offspring of two heterozygotes will manifest the dominant trait, but only one-quarter will have the recessive trait. It might be concluded therefore that eventually almost everyone in the population would have the dominant trait. However, it can be shown that in a large randomly mating population, in which there is no disturbance by outside influences, dominant traits do not increase at the expense of recessive ones. In fact, in such a population, the relative proportions of the different genotypes (and phenotypes) remain constant from one generation to another. This is known as the *Hardy–Weinberg principle* as it was proposed, independently, by an English mathematician, G. H. Hardy, and a German physician, W. Weinberg, in 1908. This is one of the most important fundamental principles in human genetics.

THE HARDY–WEINBERG PRINCIPLE

Consider an 'ideal' population in which there is an autosomal locus with two alleles A and a, which have frequencies of p and q respectively. These are the only alleles found at this locus so that p + q = 100% or 1. The frequency of each genotype in the population can be determined by construction of a Punnett's square which shows how the different genes can combine (Fig. 7.1).

From Figure 7.1 it can be seen that the frequencies of the different genotypes are:

Genotype	Phenotype	Frequency
AA	A	p^2
Aa	A	$2pq$
aa	a	q^2

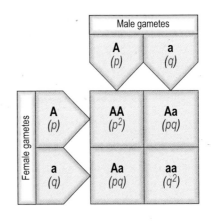

Fig. 7.1
Punnett's square showing the allele frequencies and resulting genotype frequencies for a two allele system in the first generation.

We have now established that if there is random mating of sperm and ova the frequencies of the different genotypes in the first generation will be as shown above. Next consider that these individuals mate with each other to produce a second generation. Once again a Punnett's square is used to show the different matings and their frequencies (Fig. 7.2).

From Figure 7.2 a table can be drawn up to calculate the total frequency for each genotype in the second generation (Table 7.1). This reveals that the relative frequency or proportion of each genotype is the same in the second generation as in the first. In fact it can be shown that no matter how many generations are studied the relative frequencies will remain constant. The actual numbers of individuals with each genotype will change as the population size increases or decreases, but their relative frequencies or proportions remain constant. This is the fundamental tenet of the Hardy–Weinberg principle. When studies confirm that the relative proportions of each genotype are indeed remaining constant with frequencies of p^2, $2pq$ and q^2, then that population is said to be in a state of *Hardy–Weinberg equilibrium* for that particular genotype.

FACTORS WHICH CAN DISTURB HARDY–WEINBERG EQUILIBRIUM

The discussion above relates to an 'ideal' population. By definition such a population is large and shows random mating with no new mutations and no selection for or against any particular genotype. For some human characteristics, such as neutral genes for blood groups or enzyme variants, these criteria can be fulfilled. However, in genetic disorders, several factors can disturb the Hardy–Weinberg equilibrium by influencing either the distribution of genes in the population or by altering the gene frequencies. These factors include:

1. Non-random mating
2. Mutation
3. Selection
4. Small population size
5. Gene flow (migration).

Non-random mating

Random mating, or *panmixis*, refers to the selection of a partner regardless of that partner's genotype. *Non-random mating* can lead to an increase in the frequency of affected homozygotes by two mechanisms, either assortative mating or consanguinity.

Assortative mating

Assortative mating is the tendency for human beings to chose partners who share characteristics such as height, intelligence and racial origin. If assortative mating extends to conditions such as autosomal recessive deafness, which accounts for a large proportion of all congenital

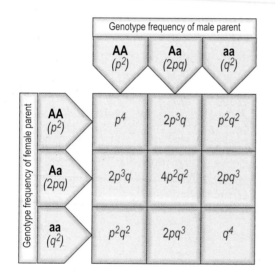

Fig. 7.2
Punnett's square showing the frequencies of the different matings in the second generation.

Table 7.1   Shows the frequency of the various types of offspring from the matings shown in Figure 7.2

Mating type	Frequency	Frequency of offspring		
		AA	Aa	aa
AA × AA	p^4	p^4	—	—
AA × Aa	$4p^3q$	$2p^3q$	$2p^3q$	—
Aa × Aa	$4p^2q^2$	p^2q^2	$2p^2q^2$	p^2q^2
AA × aa	$2p^2q^2$	—	$2p^2q^2$	—
Aa × aa	$4pq^3$	—	$2pq^3$	$2pq^3$
aa × aa	q^4	—	—	q^4
Total		$p^2(p^2+2pq+q^2)$	$2pq(p^2+2pq+q^2)$	$q^2(p^2+2pq+q^2)$
Relative frequency		p^2	$2pq$	q^2

hearing loss, then this will lead to a small increase in the relative frequency of affected homozygotes.

Consanguinity

Consanguinity is the term used to describe marriage between blood relatives who have at least one common ancestor no more remote than a great-great grandparent. Widespread consanguinity in a community will lead to a relative increase in the frequency of affected homozygotes with a relative decrease in the frequency of heterozygotes.

Mutation

The validity of the Hardy–Weinberg principle is based on the assumption that no new mutations occur. If a particular locus shows a high mutation rate then there will be a steady increase in the proportion of mutant alleles in a population. In practice mutations do occur at almost all loci, albeit at different rates, but the effect of their introduction is usually balanced by the loss of mutant alleles due to reduced fitness of affected individuals. If a population is found to be in Hardy–Weinberg equilibrium, it is generally assumed that these two opposing factors have roughly equal effects. This is discussed further in the section which follows on the estimation of mutation rates.

Selection

In the 'ideal' population there is no selection for or against any particular genotype. In reality for deleterious characteristics there is likely to be negative selection with affected individuals having reduced reproductive (= biological = 'genetic') fitness. This infers that they do not have as many offspring as unaffected control members of the same population. In the absence of new mutations this reduction in fitness will lead to a gradual reduction in the frequency of the mutant gene and disturbance of Hardy–Weinberg equilibrium.

Selection can act in the opposite direction by increasing fitness. For some autosomal recessive disorders there is evidence that heterozygotes show a slight increase in biological fitness as compared with unaffected homozygotes. This is referred to as *heterozygote advantage*. The best understood example is sickle-cell disease in which affected homozygotes have severe anaemia and often show persistent ill-health (p. 144). However, heterozygotes are relatively immune to infection with *Plasmodium falciparum* malaria because if their red blood cells are invaded by the parasite they undergo sickling and are rapidly destroyed. In areas in which this form of malaria is endemic, carriers of sickle-cell anaemia, who are described as having sickle-cell trait, are at a biological advantage as compared with unaffected homozygotes.

Therefore, in these communities, there will be a tendency for the proportion of heterozygotes to increase relative to the proportions of normal and affected homozygotes. Once again this will result in a disturbance of Hardy–Weinberg equilibrium.

Small population size

In a large population the numbers of children produced by individuals with different genotypes, assuming no alteration in fitness for any particular genotype, will tend to balance out, so that gene frequencies will remain stable. However, in a small population it is possible that by random statistical fluctuation one allele could be transmitted to a high proportion of offspring by chance, resulting in marked changes in allele frequency from one generation to the next, so that Hardy–Weinberg equilibrium is disturbed. This phenomenon is referred to as *random genetic drift*. If one allele is lost altogether then it is said to be extinguished and the other allele is described as having become fixed (Fig. 7.3).

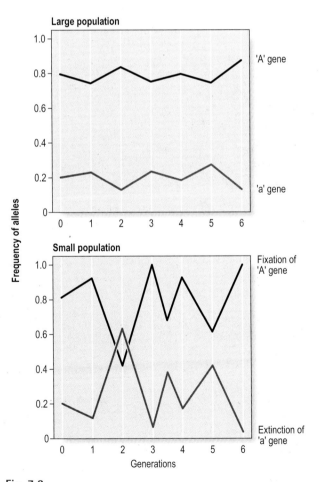

Fig. 7.3
The possible effects of random genetic drift in large and small populations.

Gene flow (migration)

If new alleles are introduced into a population as a consequence of migration with subsequent intermarriage, this will lead to a change in the relevant allele frequencies. This slow diffusion of alleles across a racial or geographical boundary is known as *gene flow*. The most widely quoted example is the gradient shown by the incidence of the B blood group allele throughout the world (Fig. 7.4). This allele is thought to have originated in Asia and spread slowly westward as a result of admixture through invasion.

VALIDITY OF HARDY–WEINBERG EQUILIBRIUM

It is relatively simple to establish whether a population is in Hardy–Weinberg equilibrium for a particular trait if all possible genotypes can be identified. Consider a system with two alleles A and a, with three resulting genotypes AA, Aa/aA and aa. Amongst 1000 individuals selected at random, the following genotype distributions are observed:

AA	800
Aa/aA	185
aa	15

From these figures the incidence of the A allele (p) equals $[(2 \times 800) + 185]/2000 = 0.8925$ and the incidence of the a allele (q) equals $[185 + (2 \times 15)]/2000 = 0.1075$.

Now consider what the expected genotype frequencies would be if the population is in Hardy–Weinberg equilibrium and compare these with the observed values.

Genotype	Observed	Expected
AA	800	796.5 ($p^2 \times 1000$)
Aa/aA	185	192 ($2pq \times 1000$)
aa	15	11.5 ($q^2 \times 1000$).

These observed and expected values correspond closely and formal statistical analysis with a χ^2 test would confirm that the observed values do not differ significantly from those expected if the population is in equilibrium.

Next consider a different system with two alleles B and b. Amongst 1000 randomly selected individuals the observed genotype distributions are:

BB	430
Bb/bB	540
bb	30

From these figures the incidence of the B allele (p) equals $[(2 \times 430) + 540]/2000 = 0.7$ and the incidence of the b allele (q) equals $[540 + (2 \times 30)]/2000 = 0.3$.

Using these values for p and q the observed and expected genotype distributions can be compared.

Genotype	Observed	Expected
BB	430	490 ($p^2 \times 1000$)
Bb/bB	540	420 ($2pq \times 1000$)
bb	30	90 ($q^2 \times 1000$)

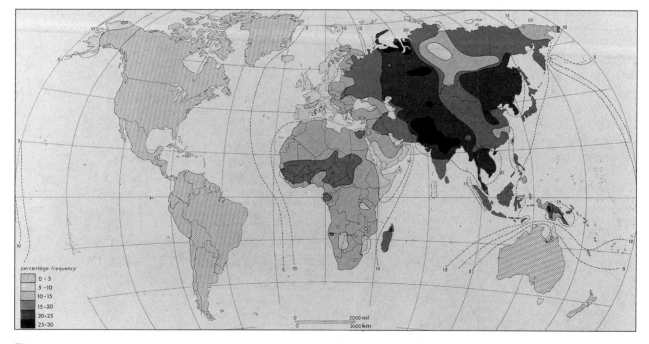

Fig. 7.4
Distribution of blood group B throughout the world. (From Mourant, Kopéc and Domianiewska-Sobczaz 1976 The distribution of the human blood groups and other polymorphisms, 2nd edn. Oxford University Press, with permission.)

percentage frequency
0 - 5
5 - 10
10 - 15
15 - 20
20 - 25
25 - 30

These values differ considerably with an increased number of heterozygotes at the expense of homozygotes. Deviation such as this from Hardy–Weinberg equilibrium should prompt a search for factors which could result in increased numbers of heterozygotes such as heterozygote advantage or negative assortative mating, i.e. the attraction of opposites!

Unless there is strong evidence to the contrary it is usually assumed that most populations are in equilibrium for most genetic traits, despite the number of factors which can disturb this equilibrium, as it is very unusual to find a population in which genotype frequencies show significant deviation from those which would be expected.

APPLICATIONS OF HARDY–WEINBERG EQUILIBRIUM

Estimation of carrier frequencies

If the incidence of an autosomal recessive disorder is known then it is possible to calculate the carrier frequency using some relatively simple algebra. If, for example, the disease incidence equals 1 in 10 000, then $q^2 = \frac{1}{10\,000}$ and $q = \frac{1}{100}$. As $p + q = 1$, therefore $p = \frac{99}{100}$. The carrier frequency can then be calculated as $2 \times \frac{99}{100} \times \frac{1}{100}$, i.e. 2pq, which approximates to 1 in 50. Thus a rough approximation of the carrier frequency can be obtained by doubling the square root of the disease incidence. Approximate values for gene frequency and carrier frequency derived from the disease incidence can be extremely useful when calculating risks for genetic counselling (p. 297) (Table 7.2). Note that if the disease incidence includes cases resulting from consanguineous relationships, then it is not valid to use the Hardy–Weinberg principle to calculate heterozygote frequences as a relatively high incidence of consanguinity disturbs the equilibrium by leading to a relative increase in the proportion of affected homozygotes.

For an X-linked disorder the frequency of affected males equals the frequency of the mutant allele, q. Thus for a trait such as red–green colour blindness, which affects approximately 1 in 12 male Western European caucasians, q equals $\frac{1}{12}$ and p equals $\frac{11}{12}$. This means that the frequency of affected females (q^2) and carrier females (2pq) equals $\frac{1}{144}$ and $\frac{22}{144}$ respectively.

Estimation of mutation rates

Direct method

If an autosomal dominant disorder shows full penetrance and is therefore always expressed in heterozygotes, an estimate of its mutation rate can be made relatively easily by counting the number of new cases in a defined

Table 7.2 Approximate values for gene frequency and carrier frequency calculated from the disease incidence assuming Hardy–Weinberg equilibrium

Disease incidence (q2)	Gene frequency (q)	Carrier frequency (2pq)
$\frac{1}{1000}$	$\frac{1}{32}$	$\frac{1}{16}$
$\frac{1}{2000}$	$\frac{1}{45}$	$\frac{1}{23}$
$\frac{1}{5000}$	$\frac{1}{71}$	$\frac{1}{36}$
$\frac{1}{10\,000}$	$\frac{1}{100}$	$\frac{1}{50}$
$\frac{1}{50\,000}$	$\frac{1}{224}$	$\frac{1}{112}$
$\frac{1}{100\,000}$	$\frac{1}{316}$	$\frac{1}{158}$

number of births. Consider a sample of 100 000 children, 12 of whom have a particular autosomal dominant disorder such as achondroplasia (p. 86). Only two of these children have an affected parent so that the remaining 10 must have acquired their disorder as a result of new mutations. Therefore 10 new mutations have occurred among the 200 000 genes inherited by these children (each child inherits two genes) giving a mutation rate of 1 per 20 000 gametes per generation.

Indirect method

For an autosomal dominant disorder with reproductive fitness (f) equal to zero, all cases must result from new mutations. If the incidence of a disorder is denoted as I and the mutation rate as μ, then as each child inherits two alleles, either of which can mutate to cause the disorder, the incidence equals twice the mutation rate, i.e. I = 2μ.

If fitness is greater than zero, and the disorder is in Hardy–Weinberg equilibrium, then genes lost through reduced fitness must be counterbalanced by new mutations. Therefore, 2μ = I (1–f) or μ = [I (1–f)]/2.

Thus if an estimate of genetic fitness can be made by comparing the average number of offspring born to affected parents as compared with controls such as their unaffected siblings, it will be possible to calculate the mutation rate.

A similar approach can be used to estimate mutation rates for autosomal recessive and sex-linked recessive disorders. With an autosomal recessive condition, two genes will be lost for each homozygote who fails to reproduce. These will be balanced by new mutations. Therefore, 2μ = I(1–f) × 2 or μ = I(1–f).

For a sex-linked recessive condition with incidence in males equal to I^M, three X chromosomes are transmitted per couple per generation. Therefore, 3μ = I^M (1–f) or μ = [I^M (1–f)]/3.

Why is it helpful to know mutation rates?

At first sight it might seem that knowledge of these formulae linking mutation rates with disease incidence and fitness is of little practical value. However, there are several ways in which this information can be useful.

Estimation of gene size

If a disorder has a high mutation rate this could yield information about the structure of the gene which would help expedite its isolation and characterization. For example, the gene could contain a high proportion of GC residues which are thought to be particularly prone to copy error (p. 21), or it could contain a high proportion of repeat sequences (p. 16) which could predispose to misalignment in meiosis resulting in deletion and duplication, or it could simply be that the gene is very large.

Determination of mutagenic potential

If valuable information is to be gained about the potential mutagenic effects of nuclear accidents such as Chernobyl, it will be necessary to have accurate methods for determining mutation rates and how these are related to observed changes in disease incidence (p. 25).

Consequences of treatment of genetic disease

Knowledge of the relationship between disease incidence, fitness and mutation rate is necessary to determine the possible effects of improved treatment for serious genetic disorders. This is discussed further towards the end of this chapter.

WHY ARE SOME GENETIC DISORDERS MORE COMMON THAN OTHERS?

It is axiomatic that if a gene shows a high mutation rate, then this will usually result in a high incidence of the relevant disease. However, factors other than the mutation rate and the fitness of affected individuals can also be involved. Mention has already been made of some of the mechanisms which can account for a high gene frequency of a particular disorder in a specific population. These will now be considered in the context of population size.

Small populations

Several rare autosomal recessive disorders show a relatively high incidence in certain populations and communities (Table 7.3). The most likely explanation for most of these observations is that the high allele frequency has resulted from a combination of a *founder effect* coupled with social, religious or geographical isolation of the relevant group. Such groups are referred to as *genetic isolates*. In some of the smaller populations genetic drift could also have played a role.

For example, several otherwise very rare autosomal recessive disorders have been found to occur at a relatively high frequency in the Old Order Amish, a religious isolate of European origin now living in Pennsylvania. Presumably, by chance, one or two original founders of the group carried these alleles which became established

Table 7.3   Rare recessive disorders which are relatively common in certain groups of people

Group	Disorder	Clinical features
Finns	Congenital nephrotic syndrome	Oedema, proteinuria, susceptibility to infection
	Aspartylglycosaminuria	Progressive mental and motor deterioration, coarse features
	MULIBREY–nanism	MUscle, LIver, BRain and EYe involvement
	Congenital chloride diarrhoea	Reduced Cl⁻ absorption, diarrhoea
Amish	Cartilage–hair hypoplasia	Dwarfism, fine, light-coloured and sparse hair
	Ellis–van Creveld syndrome	Dwarfism, polydactyly, congenital heart disease
Hopi and San Blas Indians	Albinism	Lack of pigmentation
Ashkenazi Jews	Tay–Sachs disease	Progressive mental and motor deterioration, blindness
	Gaucher's disease	Hepatosplenomegaly, bone lesions, skin pigmentation
	Dysautonomia	Indifference to pain, emotional lability, lack of tears, hyperhidrosis
Karaite Jews	Werdnig–Hoffmann disease	Infantile spinal muscular atrophy
Afrikaners	Sclerosteosis	Increased stature, syndactyly, cranial nerve palsies
	Lipoid proteinosis	Thickening of skin and mucous membranes
Ryukyan islands (off Japan)	'Ryukyan' spinal muscular atrophy	Muscle weakness, club foot, scoliosis

at relatively high frequency because of the restricted number of partners available to members of the religious sect.

A founder effect can also be observed for autosomal dominant disorders. Variegate porphyria, which is characterized by photosensitivity and drug-induced neurovisceral disturbance, has a much higher incidence in the Afrikaner population of South Africa than in any other country or race. This is thought to be due to one of the early Dutch settlers having the condition and transmitting it to a large number of his or her descendants (p. 97).

One particularly novel explanation for a high gene frequency in a small population is provided by the Hopi Indians of Arizona, who show a high incidence of albinism. Affected males were protected from outdoor farming activity because of their susceptibility to bright sunlight and it seems that this provided them with opportunity for reproductive activity in the absence of their unaffected peers. It is worth noting that several famous historical figures were affected with albinism: these include Noah and the Reverend William Spooner who was famous for transposing the initial letters of words — hence 'Spoonerism'.

Large populations

When a serious autosomal recessive disorder, which results in reduced fitness in affected homozygotes, has a high incidence in a large population, the explanation must lie in either a very high mutation rate or in heterozygote advantage. The latter explanation is the more probable for most autosomal recessive disorders (Table 7.4).

Heterozygote advantage

For sickle-cell anaemia (p. 144) and thalassaemia (p. 145) there is good evidence that heterozygote advantage results from reduced susceptibility to *Plasmodium falciparum* malaria. The mechanism by which this is thought to occur is that the red cells of heterozygotes for sickle-cell can more effectively express malarial or altered self antigens which will result in more rapid removal of parasitized cells from the circulation. Americans of Afro-Caribbean origin are no longer exposed to malaria so it would be expected that the frequency of the sickle-cell allele amongst these individuals would gradually decline. However, the predicted rate of decline is so slow that it will be many generations before it is detectable.

For several autosomal recessive disorders the mechanisms proposed for heterozygote advantage are largely speculative (Table 7.4). The recent discovery of the cystic fibrosis gene, with the subsequent elucidation of the role of its protein product in membrane permeability (p. 277), supports the hypothesis of selective advantage through increased resistance to the effects of gastro-intestinal infections such as cholera and dysentery in the heterozygote. This relative resistance could result from reduced loss of fluid and electrolytes. It is likely that this selective advantage was of greatest value several hundred years ago when these infections were endemic in Western Europe. If this is so then a gradual decline in the incidence of cystic fibrosis would be expected.

An alternative and entirely speculative mechanism for the high incidence of a condition such as cystic fibrosis is that the mutant allele is preferentially transmitted at meiosis. This type of segregation distortion whereby an allele at a particular locus is transmitted more often than would be expected by chance, i.e. in more than 50% of

Table 7.4   Presumed increased resistance in heterozygotes which could account for the maintenance of various genetic disorders in certain populations

Disorder	Genetics	Region/population	Resistance or advantage
Sickle-cell disease	AR	Tropical Africa	*Falciparum* malaria
α and β thalassaemia	AR	South-east Asia and Mediterranean	*Falciparum* malaria
G6PD deficiency	XR	Mediterranean	*Falciparum* malaria
Cystic fibrosis	AR	Western Europe	Tuberculosis? The plague? Cholera?
Tay–Sachs disease	AR	Eastern European Jews	Tuberculosis?
Congenital adrenal hyperplasia	AR	Yupik Eskimos	Influenza B
Non-insulin dependent diabetes	AD	Pima Indians and others	Periodic starvation
Phenylketonuria	AR	Western Europe	Spontaneous abortion rate lower?

AR = autosomal recessive; XR = X-linked recessive; AD = autosomal dominant.

gametes, is referred to as *meiotic drive*. Firm evidence for this phenomenon in cystic fibrosis is lacking although it has been demonstrated in the autosomal dominant disorder myotonic dystrophy (p. 269).

A major practical problem when studying heterozygote advantage is that even a tiny increase in heterozygote fitness as compared with the fitness of unaffected homozygotes can be sufficient to sustain a high allele frequency. For example in cystic fibrosis, with an allele frequency of approximately 1 in 44, a heterozygote advantage of between 2% and 3% would be sufficient to account for this high allele frequency.

GENETIC POLYMORPHISM

A *polymorphism* is defined as the occurrence in a population of two or more genetically determined forms in such frequencies that the rarest of them could not be maintained by mutation alone. By convention, a polymorphic locus is one at which there are at least two alleles each with frequencies greater than 1%. Alleles with frequencies of less than 1% are referred to as rare variants.

Studies of enzyme and protein variability have shown that in humans at least 30% of structural gene loci are polymorphic, with each individual being heterozygous at between 10% and 20% of all structural loci. Known polymorphic protein systems include the ABO blood groups (p. 186) and many serum proteins. A large number of enzymes exhibit polymorphic electrophoretic differences or what are known as *isozymes*.

Polymorphism at the DNA level has proved particularly valuable in the positional cloning studies which have led to the isolation of many disease genes (p. 74). Polymorphic DNA markers are also of use in gene tracking (p. 68), which can be used in presymptomatic diagnosis, prenatal diagnosis and carrier detection for a large number of single gene disorders. The value of a particular polymorphic system is assessed by determining its *polymorphic information content* (PIC). The higher the PIC value, the more likely it is that a polymorphic marker will be of value in linkage analysis and gene tracking.

Finally, mention should be made of the distinction between *balanced* and *transient polymorphisms*. In a balanced polymorphism, two or more different forms are maintained by a balance between the selective advantage of the heterozygote and the reduced fitness of the affected homozygote. Thus the high incidence of the sickle-cell allele in areas where malaria is endemic is an example of a balanced polymorphism. However, as has already been discussed, the incidence of the sickle-cell allele is likely to decline in populations which are no longer exposed to malaria, so that in these situations the polymorphism can be considered as transient.

SEGREGATION ANALYSIS

Segregation analysis refers to the study of the way in which a disorder is transmitted in families so as to establish the underlying mode of inheritance. The mathematical aspects of segregation analysis are extremely complex and fall far beyond the scope of this book and most doctors! However, it is important that those who encounter families with genetic disease have some understanding of the principles involved in segregation analysis as well as an awareness of some of the pitfalls and problems.

AUTOSOMAL DOMINANT INHERITANCE

For an autosomal dominant disorder the simplest approach is to compare the observed numbers of affected offspring born to affected parents with what would be expected based on the disease penetrance, i.e. 50% if penetrance is complete. A χ^2 test can be used to see if the observed and expected numbers differ significantly. Care must be taken to ensure that a bias is not introduced by excluding parents who were ascertained through an affected child.

AUTOSOMAL RECESSIVE INHERITANCE

For disorders believed to show autosomal recessive inheritance, formal segregation analysis is much more difficult. This is because some couples who are both carriers will by chance not have any affected children. Usually such couples and their healthy offspring will not be ascertained. To illustrate this consider 64 possible sibships of size 3 in which both parents are carriers, drawn from a large hypothetical population (Table 7.5). The sibship structure shown in Table 7.5 is that which would be expected on average, assuming that the birth of an affected child does not deter the parents from having further children.

In this population, on average, 27 of the 64 sibships will not contain any affected individuals. This can be calculated simply by cubing $\frac{3}{4}$, i.e. $\frac{3}{4} \times \frac{3}{4} \times \frac{3}{4} = \frac{27}{64}$. Therefore when the families are analysed these 27 sibships containing only healthy individuals will not be ascertained. This is referred to as *truncate* or *incomplete ascertainment*. If this is not taken into account, a falsely high segregation ratio of 0.43 will be obtained instead of the correct figure of 0.25.

Mathematical methods have been devised to cater for truncate ascertainment, but analysis is usually further complicated by the problems associated with achieving full or complete ascertainment. In practice it can actually be very difficult to 'prove' that a disorder shows autosomal recessive inheritance unless accurate molecular or bio-

Table 7.5 Shows the expected sibship structure in a hypothetical population which contains 64 sibships each of size 3, in which both parents are carriers of an autosomal recessive disorder. If no allowance is made for truncate ascertainment, in that the 27 sibships with no affected cases will not be ascertained, then a falsely high segregation ratio of 48/111 (= 0.43) will be obtained

No. of affected in sibship	Structure of sibship	No. of sibships	No. of affected	Total no. of sibs
3	■ ■ ■	1	3	3
2	■ ■ □	3	6	9
	□ ■ ■	3	6	9
	■ □ ■	3	6	9
1	■ □ □	9	9	27
	□ ■ □	9	9	27
	□ □ ■	9	9	27
0	□ □ □	27	0	81
Total		64	48	192

chemical methods are available for carrier detection. A high incidence of parental consanguinity provides strong supportive evidence for autosomal recessive inheritance, a point first noted by Bateson and Garrod as long ago as 1902 (p. 100).

GENETIC LINKAGE

Mendel's third law, the principle of independent assortment, states that members of different gene pairs assort to gametes independently of one another (p. 4). Stated more simply, the alleles of genes at different loci segregate independently. While this is true of genes on different chromosomes, it is not always true for genes which are located on the same chromosome, i.e. *syntenic*.

If two loci are positioned close together on the same chromosome, so that alleles at these loci are inherited together more often than not, then these loci are said to be *linked*. In effect the two loci are sufficiently close together for it to be unlikely that they will be separated by a cross-over or recombination in meiosis I (Fig. 7.5).

Alleles at linked loci on the same chromosome are said to be in *coupling*, whereas those on opposite homologous chromosomes are described as being in *repulsion*. This is

known as the linkage *phase*. Thus in Fig 7.5C, in the parental chromosomes A and B are in coupling whereas A and b are in repulsion.

RECOMBINATION FRACTION

The *recombination fraction*, which is usually designated as θ (Greek theta), is a measure of the distance separating two loci, or more precisely an indication of the likelihood that a cross-over will occur between them. If two loci are not linked then θ equals 0.5, as on average genes at unlinked loci will segregate together during 50% of all meioses. If θ equals 0.05, this means that on average the syntenic alleles will segregate together 19 times out of 20, i.e. a cross-over will occur between them during on average only 1 in 20 meioses.

CENTIMORGANS

The unit of measurement for genetic linkage is known as a *map unit* or *centiMorgan* (cM). If two loci are 1 cM apart, then a cross-over occurs between them during on average only 1 in every 100 meioses, i.e. $\theta = 0.01$. CentiMorgans are a measure of the genetic or linkage distance between two loci. This is not the same as physical distance which is measured in base pairs.

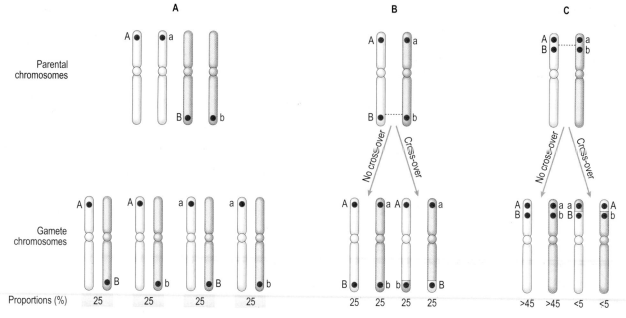

Fig. 7.5

Segregation at meiosis of alleles at two loci. In (A) the loci are on different chromosomes and in (B) they are on the same chromosome but widely separated. Hence these loci are not linked and there is independent assortment. In (C) the loci are closely adjacent so that separation by a cross-over is unlikely, i.e. the loci are linked.

The human genome has been estimated by recombination studies to be about 3000 cM in length in males. As the physical length of the haploid human genome is approximately 3×10^9 bp, 1 cM corresponds to approximately 10^6 bp (or 1000 kb). However, the relationship between linkage map units and physical length is not linear. Some chromosome regions appear to be particularly prone to recombination, so-called 'hot spots', and for reasons which are not understood, recombination tends to occur less often during meiosis in males than in females in whom the genome 'linkage' length has been estimated to be 4200 cM. Generally in humans there are one or two recombination events between each pair of homologous chromosomes in meiosis I with a total of around 40 across the entire genome. Recombination events are rare close to the centromeres and relatively common in telomeric regions.

LINKAGE ANALYSIS

Linkage analysis has proved to be an extremely valuable tool for mapping genes (p. 70). The basic methodology involves study of the segregation of the disease in large families with polymorphic markers from each chromosome. Eventually a marker will be identified which cosegregates with the disease more often than would be expected by chance, i.e. the marker and disease loci are linked. The mathematical analysis tends to be very complex, particularly if lots of closely adjacent markers are being used

as in *multipoint linkage analysis*. However, the underlying principle is relatively straightforward and involves the use of likelihood ratios, the logarithms of which are known as *LOD scores*.

LOD SCORES

When studying the segregation of alleles at two loci which could be linked, a series of likelihood ratios is calculated for different values of the recombination fraction (θ), ranging from $\theta = 0$ to $\theta = 0.5$. The likelihood ratio at a given value of θ equals the likelihood of the observed data if the loci are linked at recombination value of θ divided by the likelihood of the observed data if the loci are not linked ($\theta = 0.5$). The logarithm to the base 10 of this ratio is known as the LOD score (Z), i.e. LOD (θ) = $\log_{10} [L\theta / L(0.5)]$. Logarithms are used because they allow results from different families to be added together.

For example, when a research paper reports that linkage of a disease with a DNA marker has been identified with a LOD score (Z) of 4 at recombination fraction (θ) 0.05, this means that in the families which have been studied the results indicate that it is 10 000 (10^4) times more likely that the disease and marker loci are closely linked (i.e. 5 cM apart) than that they are not linked. It is generally agreed that a LOD score of +3 or greater is confirmation of linkage. This would yield a ratio of 1000 to 1 in favour of linkage, but because there is a prior probability of only 1 in 50 that any two given loci are linked, a LOD score of +3 means that the overall probability that the loci are linked is approximately 20 to 1, i.e. $[1000 \times \frac{1}{50}]$:1. The importance of taking prior probabilities into account in probability theory is discussed in the section on Bayes' theorem (p. 293).

A 'simple' example

Consider a three-generation family in which several members have an autosomal dominant disorder (Fig. 7.6). A and B are alleles at a locus which is being tested for linkage to the disease locus.

To establish whether it is likely that these two loci are linked, the LOD score is calculated for various values of θ. The value of θ which gives the highest LOD score is taken as the best estimate of the recombination fraction. This is known as a *maximum likelihood method*.

To demonstrate the underlying principle, the LOD score will be calculated for a value of θ equal to 0.05. If θ equals 0.05 then the loci are linked, in which case the disease gene and the B marker must be on the same chromosome in II_2, as both of these characteristics have been inherited from her mother. Thus in II_2 the linkage phase is known — the disease allele and the B allele are in coupling. Therefore the probability that III_1 would be affected and would also inherit the B marker equals 0.95, i.e. 1–θ. A similar result is obtained for the remaining three members of the sibship in generation III, giving a value for the numerator of $(0.95)^4$. If the loci are not linked, then the likelihood of observing both the disease and marker B in III_1 equals 0.5. A similar result is obtained for his three siblings, giving a value for the denominator of $(0.5)^4$.

Therefore the LOD score for this family given a value of θ = 0.05 equals $\log_{10} 0.95^4/0.5^4 = \log_{10} 13.032 = 1.12$. For a value of θ = 0 the LOD score equals $\log_{10} 1^4/0.5^4 = \log_{10} 16 = 1.20$. For a value of θ = 0.1 the LOD score equals $\log_{10} 0.9^4/0.5^4 = \log_{10} 10.498 = 1.02$. The highest LOD score is obtained for a value of θ equals 0, which is consistent with the fact that if the disease and marker loci are linked then there have been no recombinations between the two loci in members of generation III.

To confirm linkage other families would have to be studied by pooling all the results until a LOD score of +3 or greater is obtained. A LOD score of –2 or less is taken as proof that the loci are not linked. This less stringent requirement for proof of non-linkage, i.e. a LOD score of –2 as compared with +3 for proof of linkage, is due to the high prior probability of $\frac{49}{50}$ that any two loci are not linked.

MULTIPOINT LINKAGE ANALYSIS

Two-point linkage analysis is often used to map a disease locus to a specific chromosome region. This gives

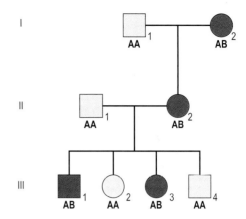

Fig. 7.6

A three-generation pedigree showing segregation of an autosomal dominant disorder and alleles (A and B) at a locus which may or may not be linked to the disease locus.

a rather rough or 'coarse' indication of the location of the disease locus. The next step often involves multipoint linkage analysis using a series of polymorphic markers which are known to map to the disease region. This process allows 'fine' tuning of the probable position of the disease locus within the narrow interval defined by the small number of previously ordered polymorphic marker loci.

Using this approach the results of linkage studies with the various markers are analysed using a computer program which calculates the overall likelihood of the position of the disease locus in relation to the marker loci. The results are presented in the form of a likelihood ratio known as a *location score*. This is calculated for different positions of the disease locus and a graph is drawn up of location score against map distance (Fig. 7.7). On this graph the peaks represent possible positions of the disease locus with the tallest peak being the most probable location. The troughs represent the positions of the polymorphic marker loci.

Multipoint linkage analysis is used to define the smallest possible interval in which a disease locus is located, so that physical mapping methods can then be applied to isolate the disease gene (p. 73).

AUTOZYGOSITY MAPPING

This is an ingenious form of linkage analysis which has been used to map several rare autosomal recessive disorders. *Autozygosity* occurs when individuals are homozygous at particular loci through identity by descent from a common ancestor. In an inbred pedigree containing two or more children with a rare autosomal recessive disorder it is very likely that the children will be homozygous not only at the disease locus but at closely linked loci also. In other words all affected relatives in an

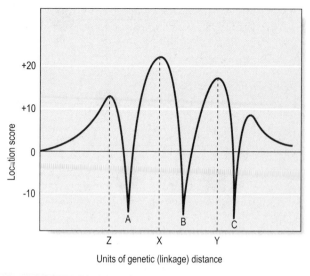

Fig. 7.7
Multipoint linkage analysis. A, B and C represent the known linkage relationships of three polymorphic marker loci. X, Y and Z represent in descending order of likelihood the probable position of the disease locus.

inbred family will be homozygous at the region surrounding the disease locus. Thus a search can be made for shared areas of homozygosity in affected relatives using highly polymorphic markers such as microsatellites (p. 16). In a pedigree with a relatively large number of affected individuals only a small number of shared homozygous regions will be identified; one of these will harbour the relevant disease locus which can then be isolated using physical mapping strategies.

Autozygosity mapping can be applied in both small inbred families and in genetic isolates (p. 118) with a shared common genetic ancestry. This technique has met with particular success in locating several of the genes which cause autosomal recessive sensorineural hearing loss.

LINKAGE DISEQUILIBRIUM

Linkage disequilibrium is defined formally as the association of two alleles at linked loci more frequently than would be expected by chance. In the pedigree shown in Figure 7.6 support was obtained for linkage of the disease gene with the B marker allele. Assume that further studies confirm linkage of these loci and that the A and B alleles have an equal frequency of 0.5. It would be reasonable to expect that the disease gene would be in coupling with allele A in approximately 50% of families and with allele B in the remaining 50%. If, however, the disease allele was found to be in coupling almost exclusively with one particular marker allele this would be an example of linkage disequilibrium.

The demonstration of linkage disequilibrium in a particular disease suggests that the mutation which has caused the disease has occurred relatively recently and that the marker locus being studied is very closely linked to the disease locus. For example, one of the very small number of the original mutations for sickle-cell disease occurred in a β-globin gene which was closely adjacent to a very rare syntenic RFLP (Fig. 4.21, p. 68). Selection for this sickle-cell mutation, with only very rare recombination having occurred between it and the adjacent tightly linked locus, has resulted in a very high proportion of present day sickle-cell alleles being in coupling with this otherwise rare RFLP.

MEDICAL AND SOCIETAL INTERVENTION

Recent developments in molecular biology, such as the human genome project (p. 321) and pilot studies using gene therapy (p. 327), have reawakened concern that future generations could have to cope with an ever increasing burden of genetic disease. The term *eugenics* was first used by Charles Darwin's cousin, Francis Galton, to refer to the improvement of a population by selective breeding. The notion that this should be applied to human populations became popular during the early years of the twentieth century, culminating in the horrifying and totally unacceptable practices of Nazi Germany. Ensuing revulsion led to the total abandonment of eugenic programmes in humans with universal condemnation and agreement that these have no place in modern medical practice.

Nevertheless, doctors who care for patients and families with hereditary disease are faced with a dilemma. On the one hand, by helping patients with serious genetic disease to survive and reproduce they are indeed increasing the numbers of 'bad genes' in society, thereby potentially adding to humanity's future genetic load. Such behaviour could be interpreted as dysgenic. On the other hand, most medical practitioners would argue that their responsibility to an individual patient far outweighs their obligation to either contemporary society or to future generations.

Before returning to this ethical debate it is worth considering the possible long-term effects of artificial selection for or against genetic disorders.

AUTOSOMAL DOMINANT DISORDERS

If everyone with an autosomal dominant disorder was successfully encouraged not to reproduce, then the incidence of that disorder would decline rapidly with all future cases only being the result of new mutations. This would have a particularly striking effect on the incidence of relatively mild conditions such as familial hypercholesterolaemia in which genetic fitness is close to 1.

Alternatively, if successful treatment became available for all patients with a serious autosomal dominant disorder which at present is associated with a marked reduction in genetic fitness, then there would be an immediate increase in the frequency of the disease gene followed by a more gradual levelling off at a new equilibrium level. If, at one time, all those with a serious autosomal dominant disorder died in childhood (f = 0) then the incidence of affected individuals would be 2μ. If treatment raised the fitness from 0 to 0.9, then the incidence of affected children in the next generation would rise to 2μ due to new mutations plus 1.8μ inherited which equals 3.8μ. Eventually a new equilibrium would be reached by which time the disease incidence would have risen tenfold to 20μ. This can be calculated relatively easily using the formula $\mu = [I(1-f)]/2$ (p. 117), which can be expressed alternatively as $I = 2\mu/(1-f)$. The net result would be that the proportion of affected children who die would be less (100% down to 10%), but the total number affected would be much greater, although the actual number who die from the disease would remain unchanged at 2μ.

AUTOSOMAL RECESSIVE DISORDERS

In contrast to an autosomal dominant disorder, artificial selection against an autosomal recessive condition will have only a very slow effect.

The reason for this difference is that in autosomal recessive conditions most of the genes in a population are present in healthy heterozygotes who would not be affected by eugenic measures. It can be shown that if there is complete selection against an autosomal recessive disorder so that no homozygotes reproduce, then the number of generations (n) required to change the allele frequency from q_o to q_n equals $1/q_n - 1/q_o$. Therefore, for a condition with an incidence of approximately 1 in 2000 and an allele frequency of roughly 1 in 45, if all affected patients refrained from reproduction then it would take over 500 years (18 generations) to reduce the disease incidence by half and over 1200 years (45 generations) to reduce the gene frequency by half, assuming an average generation time of 27 years.

Now consider the opposite situation where selection operating against a serious autosomal recessive disorder is relaxed because of improvement in medical treatment. More affected individuals will reach adult life and transmit the mutant allele to their offspring. The result will be that the frequency of the mutant allele will increase until a new equilibrium is reached. Using the

formula $\mu = I(1-f)$ (p. 117), it can be shown that when the new equilibrium is eventually reached, an increase in fitness from 0 to 0.9 will have resulted in a tenfold increase in the disease incidence.

SEX-LINKED RECESSIVE DISORDERS

When considering the effects of selection against these disorders, it is necessary to take into account the fact that a large proportion of the relevant genes are present in entirely healthy female carriers, who are often unaware of their carrier status. For a very serious condition, such as Duchenne muscular dystrophy (p. 280), with fitness equal to 0 in affected males, selection will have no effect unless female carriers choose to limit their families. If all female carriers opted not to have any children, then the incidence would be reduced by two-thirds, i.e. from 3μ to μ.

A much more plausible possibility is that effective treatment will be forthcoming for these disorders. This will result in a steady increase in the disease incidence. For example, an increase in fitness from 0 to 0.5 will lead to a doubling of the disease incidence by the time a new equilibrium has been established. This can be calculated using the formula $\mu = [I^M (1-f)]/3$ (p. 117).

CONCLUSION

In reality it is extremely difficult to predict the long term impact of medical intervention on the incidence and burden of genetic disease. Non-directive genetic counselling could lead to a reduction in the number of affected children being born, but it is quite likely that many of these children will be 'replaced' by carrier siblings, either by such couples compensating by having large families, or through the use of prenatal diagnosis, so that the overall effects on gene frequency are almost impossible to determine. While it is true that improvements in medical treatment could result in an increase in genetic load in future generations, it is equally possible that successful gene therapy will have eased the overall burden of these disorders in terms of human suffering. Some of these arguments could have been made many years ago for other major medical developments such as the discovery of insulin and antibiotics which have had overwhelming financial implications in terms of burgeoning pharmaceutical costs and an increasingly ageing population. Ultimately it can reasonably be argued that it is how a society copes with these challenges that gives a true measure of the validity of its claim to be civilized.

ELEMENTS

1 According to the Hardy–Weinberg principle the relative proportions of the possible genotypes at a particular locus remain constant from one generation to the next.

2 Factors which may disturb Hardy–Weinberg equilibrium are non-random mating, mutation, selection for or against a particular genotype, small population size, and migration.

3 If an autosomal recessive disorder is in Hardy–Weinberg equilibrium the carrier frequency can be estimated by doubling the square root of the disease incidence.

4 The mutation rate for an autosomal dominant disorder can be measured directly by estimating the proportion of new mutations among all members of one generation. Indirect estimates of mutation rates can be made using the formulae:

$\mu = [I(1-f)]/2$ for autosomal dominant inheritance
$\mu = I(1-f)$ for autosomal recessive inheritance
$\mu = [I^M(1-f)]/3$ for sex-linked recessive inheritance.

5 Otherwise rare single gene disorders can show a high incidence in a small population because of a founder effect coupled with genetic isolation.

6 When a serious autosomal recessive disorder has a relatively high incidence in a large population this is likely to be due to heterozygote advantage.

7 Closely adjacent loci on the same chromosome are said to be linked if genes at these loci segregate together during more than 50% of meioses. The recombination fraction (θ) indicates how often two such genes will be separated (recombine) at meiosis.

8 The LOD score is a mathematical indication of the relative likelihood that two loci are linked. A LOD score of +3 or greater is taken as confirmation of linkage. Two-point linkage analysis is used to map a disease locus to a chromosome region. Then multipoint linkage analysis can be used to determine the probable order of polymorphic loci within that region and to narrow down the size of the interval to be studied by physical mapping.

FURTHER READING

Allison A C 1954 Protection afforded by sickle-cell trait against subtertian malarial infection. BMJ i: 290–294
A landmark paper providing clear evidence that the sickle-cell trait provides protection against parasitaemia by falciparum malaria.
Emery A E H 1986 Methodology in medical genetics, 2nd edn. Churchill Livingstone, Edinburgh
A useful handbook of basic population genetics and mathematical methods for analysing the results of genetic studies.
Haldane J B S 1935 The rate of spontaneous mutation of a human gene. J Genet 31: 317–326
The first estimate of the mutation rate for haemophilia using an indirect method.

Hardy G H 1908 Mendelian proportions in a mixed population. Science 28: 49–50
A short letter in which Hardy pointed out that in a large randomly mating population dominant 'characters' would not increase at the expense of recessives.
Khoury M J, Beaty T H, Cohen B H 1993 Fundamentals of genetic epidemiology. Oxford University Press, New York
A comprehensive textbook of population genetics and its areas of overlap with epidemiology.
Ott J 1991 Analysis of human genetic linkage. Johns Hopkins University Press, Baltimore
A detailed mathematical explanation of linkage analysis.
Vogel F, Motulsky A G 1997 Human genetics, problems and approaches, 3rd edn. Springer-Verlag, Berlin
The definitive textbook of human genetics with extensive coverage of mathematical aspects.

Polygenic and multifactorial inheritance

CHAPTER

8

Many disorders demonstrate familial clustering which does not conform to any recognized pattern of Mendelian inheritance. Examples include several of the most common congenital malformations and many of the common acquired diseases of childhood and adult life (Table 8.1). These conditions show a definite familial tendency but the incidence in close relatives of affected individuals is usually around 2–4%, instead of the much higher figures which would be seen if these conditions were caused by mutations in single genes.

As it is likely that many factors, both genetic and environmental, are involved in causing these disorders, they are generally referred to as showing *multifactorial* inheritance. This does not mean that the underlying genetic mechanisms are well understood — in fact they are not! The prevailing view until recently has been that in multifactorial inheritance environmental factors interact with many genes to generate a normally distributed susceptibility. According to this theory individuals are affected if they lie at the wrong end of the distribution curve. This concept of a normal distribution generated by many genes, known as *polygenes*, each acting in an additive fashion is plausible for physiological characteristics such as height and possibly blood pressure. However, for disease states such as insulin-dependent diabetes mellitus (IDDM) recent research has shown that the genetic contribution is not straightforward and probably involves many loci, some of which play a much more important role than others.

POLYGENIC INHERITANCE AND THE NORMAL DISTRIBUTION

Before considering the impact of recent research in detail, it is necessary to outline briefly the scientific basis of what is known as *polygenic* or *quantitative* inheritance. This involves the inheritance and expression of a phenotype being determined by many genes at different loci, with each gene exerting a small additive effect. Additive implies that the effects of the genes are cumulative, i.e. no one gene is dominant or recessive to another.

Several human characteristics (Table 8.2) show a continuous distribution in the general population, which closely resembles a normal distribution. This takes the form of a symmetrical bell-shaped curve distributed evenly about a mean (Fig. 8.1). The spread of the distribution about the mean is determined by the standard deviation. Approximately 68%, 95% and 99.7% of observations fall within the mean plus or minus one, two or three standard deviations respectively.

It is possible to show that a phenotype with a normal distribution in the general population can be generated

---

Table 8.1 Disorders which show multifactorial inheritance

Congenital malformations
  Cleft lip/palate
  Congenital dislocation of the hip
  Congenital heart defects
  Neural tube defects
  Pyloric stenosis
  Talipes
Acquired diseases of childhood and adult life
  Asthma
  Autism
  Diabetes mellitus
  Epilepsy
  Glaucoma
  Hypertension
  Ischaemic heart disease
  Manic depression
  Schizophrenia

Table 8.2 Human characteristics which show a continuous normal distribution

Blood pressure
Dermatoglyphics (ridge count)
Head circumference
Height
Intelligence
Skin colour

Fig. 8.1
The normal (Gaussian) distribution.

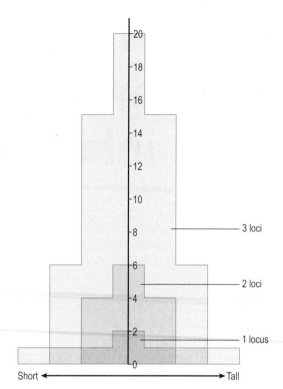

Fig. 8.2
Shows the distribution of genotypes for a characteristic such as height with 1, 2 and 3 loci each with two alleles of equal frequency. The values for each genotype can be obtained from the binomial expansion $(p+q)^{2n}$ where $p = q = 1/2$ and n equals the number of loci.

Table 8.3   Degrees of relationship

Relationship	Proportion of genes shared
First degree	$\frac{1}{2}$
Parents	
Siblings	
Children	
Second degree	$\frac{1}{4}$
Uncles and aunts	
Nephews and nieces	
Grandparents	
Grandchildren	
Half-siblings	
Third degree	$\frac{1}{8}$
First cousins	
Great-grandparents	
Great-grandchildren	

by polygenic inheritance involving the action of many genes at different loci, each of which exerts an equal additive effect. This can be illustrated by considering a trait such as height. If height were to be determined by two equally frequent alleles, a (tall) and b (short), at a single locus, then this would result in a discontinuous phenotype with three groups in a ratio of 1 (tall–aa) to 2 (average–ab/ba) to 1 (short–bb). If the same trait were to be determined by two alleles at each of two loci interacting in a simple additive way, then this would lead to a phenotypic distribution of five groups in a ratio of 1 (4 tall genes) to 4 (3 tall + 1 short) to 6 (2 tall + 2 short) to 4 (1 tall + 3 short) to 1 (4 short). For a system with three loci each with two alleles the phenotypic ratio would be 1-6-15-20-15-6-1 (Fig. 8.2).

It can be seen that as the number of loci increases, the distribution increasingly comes to resemble a normal curve, thereby lending support to the concept that characteristics such as height are determined by the additive effects of many genes at different loci. Further support for this concept comes from the study of familial correlations for characteristics such as height and, to a lesser extent, intelligence. *Correlation* is a statistical measure of the degree of association of variable phenomena, or in more simple terms a measure of the degree of resemblance or relationship between two parameters. As first-degree relatives share on average 50% of their genes (Table 8.3), it would be reasonable to predict that, if a parameter such as height is polygenic, then the correlation between first-degree relatives such as siblings should be 0.5. Several studies have shown that the sib–sib correlation for height is indeed close to 0.5.

In reality, human characteristics such as height and intelligence are also influenced by environment and possibly also by genes which are not additive in that they exert a dominant effect. These factors probably account for the observed tendency of offspring to show what is known as 'regression to the mean'. This is demonstrated by tall or intelligent parents (the two are not mutually exclusive!) having children whose average height or intelligence is slightly lower than the average or mid-parental value.

Similarly, parents who are very short or of low intelligence tend to have children whose average height or intelligence is lower than the general population average, but higher than the average value of the parents. If a trait was to show true polygenic inheritance with no external influences then the measurements in offspring would be distributed evenly around the mean of their parents' values.

MULTIFACTORIAL INHERITANCE — THE LIABILITY/THRESHOLD MODEL

Efforts have been made to extend the polygenic theory for the inheritance of quantitative or continuous traits to try to account for *discontinuous* multifactorial disorders. According to the *liability/threshold* model, as originally proposed by Falconer, all of the factors which influence the development of a multifactorial disorder, whether genetic or environmental, can be considered as a single entity known as liability. The liabilities of all individuals in a population form a continuous variable, which has a normal distribution in both the general population and in relatives of affected individuals. However, the curves for these relatives will be shifted to the right, with the extent to which they are shifted being directly related to the closeness of their relationship to the affected index case (Fig. 8.3).

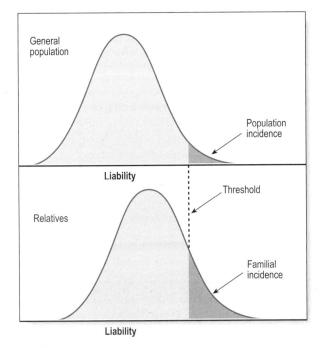

Fig. 8.3
Hypothetical liability curves in the general population and in relatives for a hereditary disorder in which the genetic predisposition is multifactorial.

To account for a discontinuous phenotype (i.e. affected or not affected) with an underlying continuous distribution, it is proposed that a threshold exists above which the abnormal phenotype is expressed. In the general population the proportion beyond the threshold is the population incidence and among relatives the proportion beyond the threshold is the familial incidence.

It is important to emphasize once again that liability includes all factors which contribute to the cause of the condition. Looked at very simply a deleterious liability can be viewed as consisting of a combination of several 'bad' genes and adverse environmental factors. Liability cannot be measured but the mean liability of a group can be determined from the incidence of the disease in that group using statistics of the normal distribution. The units of measurement are standard deviations and these can be used to estimate the correlation between relatives.

CONSEQUENCES OF THE LIABILITY/ THRESHOLD MODEL

Part of the attraction of this model, and it should be emphasized once again that this is a hypothesis rather than proven fact, is that it provides a simple explanation for the observed patterns of familial risks in conditions such as cleft lip/palate, pyloric stenosis and spina bifida. For example:

1. The incidence of the condition is greatest among relatives of the most severely affected patients, presumably because they are the most extreme deviants along the liability curve. For example, in cleft lip/palate the proportion of affected first-degree relatives (parents, siblings and offspring) is 6% if the index patient has bilateral cleft lip and palate, but only 2% if the index patient has a unilateral cleft lip (Fig. 8.4).

2. The risk is greatest among close relatives of the index case and decreases rapidly in more distant relatives. For example, in spina bifida the risks to first-, second- and third- degree relatives of the index case are approximately 4%, 1% and less than 0.5% respectively.

3. If there is more than one affected close relative then the risks for other relatives are increased. In spina bifida, if two siblings are affected, the risk to a subsequent sibling is approximately 10%.

4. If the condition is more common in individuals of one particular sex, then relatives of an affected individual of the less frequently affected sex will be at higher risk than relatives of an affected individual of the more frequently affected sex. This is illustrated by the condition pyloric stenosis. Pyloric stenosis shows a male to female ratio of 5 to 1. The proportions of affected offspring of male index patients are 5.5% for sons and 2.4% for daughters, whereas the risks to the offspring of female

A

B

Fig. 8.4
(A) Severe and (B) mild forms of cleft lip/palate.

index patients are 19.4% for sons and 7.3% for daughters. The probable explanation for these different risks is that in order for a female to be affected she has to lie at the extreme of the liability curve, so that her close relatives will also have a very high liability for developing the condition. As males are more susceptible to developing the disorder, risks in male offspring are higher than in female offspring regardless of the sex of the affected parent.

5. The risk of recurrence for first-degree relatives, i.e. siblings and offspring, approximates to the square root of the general population incidence. Thus if the incidence is 1 in 1000, the sibling and offspring risk will equal approximately 1 in 32 or 3%.

Table 8.4   Estimates of heritability of various disorders

Disorder	Frequency (%)	Heritability
Schizophrenia	1	85
Asthma	4	80
Cleft lip ± cleft palate	0.1	76
Pyloric stenosis	0.3	75
Ankylosing spondylitis	0.2	70
Club foot	0.1	68
Coronary artery disease	3	65
Hypertension (essential)	5	62
Congenital dislocation of the hip	0.1	60
Anencephaly and spina bifida	0.3	60
Peptic ulcer	4	37
Congenital heart disease	0.5	35

HERITABILITY

Though it is not possible to assess an individual's liability for a particular disorder, it is possible to estimate what proportion of the aetiology can be ascribed to genetic factors as opposed to environmental factors. This is referred to as *heritability*, which can be defined as the proportion of the total phenotypic variance of a condition which is caused by additive genetic variance. In statistical terms, variance equals the square of the standard deviation. Heritability is often depicted using the symbol h^2 and is expressed either as a proportion of 1 or as a percentage.

Estimates of the heritability of a condition or trait provide an indication of the relative importance of genetic factors in its causation, so that the greater the value for the heritability the greater the role of genetic factors.

Heritability is estimated from the degree of resemblance between relatives expressed in the form of a correlation coefficient which is calculated using statistics of the normal distribution. Alternatively, heritability can be calculated using data on the concordance rates in monozygotic and dizygotic twins. In practice it is desirable to try to derive heritability estimates using different types of relatives and to measure the disease incidence in relatives reared together and living apart so as to try to disentangle the possible effects of common environmental factors. Estimates of heritability for some common diseases are given in Table 8.4.

IDENTIFYING GENES WHICH CAUSE MULTIFACTORIAL DISORDERS

Multifactorial disorders are common and make a major contribution to human morbidity and mortality (p. 7). It is therefore not surprising that vigorous efforts are being made to try to identify and isolate genes which contribute to their aetiology. Towards this end several strategies can be employed.

DISEASE ASSOCIATIONS

The study of disease associations is undertaken by comparing the incidence of a particular polymorphism in affected patients with the incidence in a carefully matched control group. If the incidences in the two groups differ significantly, this provides evidence for a positive or negative association.

The polymorphic system which has been studied most often is the HLA histocompatibility complex on chromosome 6 (p. 181). One of the strongest known HLA associations is that between ankylosing spondylitis and the B27 allele. This is present in approximately 90% of all patients and in only 5% of controls. The strength of an HLA association is indicated by the ratio of the risk of developing the disease in those with the antigen to the risk of developing the disease in those without the antigen (Table 8.5). This is known as the relative risk and it gives an indication of how much more frequently the disease occurs in individuals with a specific marker than in those without that marker.

Progress in molecular biology has led to a huge increase in the number of polymorphic systems which can be studied in a search for disease associations. The many alleles at the HLA complex can now be studied at the molecular level using the polymerase chain reaction (p. 58). This has resulted in many more HLA associations being identified than was possible previously.

One of the major difficulties with disease associations is to establish how they should best be interpreted. In particular it is important to try to rule out a chance or spurious observation by ensuring as far as possible that the proposed association is biologically plausible and that the patient and control groups are closely matched. If evidence for a strong association is forthcoming this suggests that the allele encoded by the marker locus is directly involved in causing the disease (i.e. a susceptibility locus) or that the marker locus is in linkage disequilibrium (p. 124) with a closely linked susceptibility locus. When considering disease associations it is important to remember that the identification of a susceptibility locus does not mean that *the* definitive disease gene has been identified. This is illustrated by the association of HLA B27 with ankylosing spondylitis. Although this is one of the strongest disease associations known, only 1% of all HLA B27 individuals develop ankylosing spondylitis so that many other factors, genetic and environmental, must be involved in causing this condition.

LINKAGE ANALYSIS

Linkage analysis has proved extremely valuable in mapping single gene disorders by studying the cosegregation of polymorphisms with the disease until a linked marker has been identified (p. 122). However, this type of approach is much more difficult in multifactorial disorders for the following reasons:

1. If a multifactorial disorder has a true polygenic underlying genetic susceptibility, then in theory it is unlikely that alleles at a single locus will make a major contribution. It is extremely difficult mathematically to develop strategies for detecting linkage of additive 'polygenes' each of which makes only a small contribution to the phenotype.

2. Many multifactorial diseases show a variable age of onset so that the genetic status of unaffected family members cannot be known with certainty.

3. Most families in which a multifactorial disease is, or has been, present have only one or two living affected members so that the number of 'informative meioses' available for study is usually very small.

4. Some apparent multifactorial disorders, such as coronary artery disease and schizophrenia, are probably aetiologically heterogeneous, with different genetic and environmental mechanisms involved in different subtypes which cannot be easily distinguished at the phenotypic level. This makes analysis of linkage results very difficult.

Despite these limitations progress is being made towards identifying susceptibility loci using modifications of the approaches utilized for mapping single gene loci. Some of this progress is discussed in the following sections on autism and diabetes and further examples are given in Chapter 14 on the 'common diseases'. It has been recognized for some time that one of the best approaches would be to undertake disease association studies and linkage analysis utilizing a so-called 'ideal' population. Such a population would be relatively large yet historically isolated and therefore genetically homogeneous, with extensive medical records dating back many generations, a large tissue bank, good medical services and a co-operative willing citizenship. The 270 000 citizens of

---

Table 8.5   Calculation of relative risk for a disease association

	Marker positive	Marker negative
Patients	a	b
Controls	c	d
Relative risk	$= \dfrac{a}{c} \div \dfrac{b}{d}$	
	$= \dfrac{ad}{bc}$	

Iceland have been deemed to represent such an ideal population and a genomics company, known as DeCODE Genetics, has been granted a licence to set up a national medical database and undertake genetic research. While on the one hand this initiative has raised serious concern about the issue of informed consent (p. 341), on the other hand it could lead to the relatively rapid isolation of genes which make a significant contribution to human morbidity and mortality.

Sib-pair analysis

If affected siblings inherit a particular allele more or less often than would be expected by chance, this indicates that that allele or its locus is involved in some way in causing the disease.

Consider a set of parents with alleles AB (father) and CD (mother) at a particular locus. The probability that any two of their children will have both alleles in common is 1 in 4 (Fig. 8.5). The probability that they will have one allele in common is 1 in 2 and the probability that they will have no alleles in common equals 1 in 4. If siblings who are affected with a particular disease show deviation from this 1:2:1 ratio for a particular polymorphism, this implies that there is a causal relationship between the locus and the disease.

The strength of this relationship can be quantified by determining the ratio of the expected to observed proportions of affected sib-pairs which share zero alleles at the relevant locus. This risk ratio is known as λ. For example, sib-pair analysis might indicate that at a particular locus only 15% of affected siblings share zero alleles, in contrast to the expected proportion of 25%. This would yield a sib risk ratio for that locus of $\frac{25}{15} = 1.67$.

Degree of familial clustering

The degree of familial clustering shown by a multifactorial disorder can be estimated by measuring the ratio of the risk to siblings of affected individuals to the general population incidence. For example, for a disease with a population incidence of 1 in 1000 and a sibling recurrence risk of 1 in 40 the sib risk to population incidence ratio would be 25 (i.e. $\frac{1}{40} : \frac{1}{1000}$).

This ratio of sib risk to population incidence is known as λ_s. It can be shown that for a multifactorial disorder with an underlying polygenic susceptibility the sib risk to population incidence ratio (λ_s) equals the product of the individual λ values contributed by each susceptibility locus, i.e. $\lambda_s = \lambda_1 \times \lambda_2 \times \lambda_3 \ldots \times \lambda_n$. This assumes that the various susceptibility loci interact in a multiplicative manner, perhaps by exerting their effects at different points on a common underlying biochemical or immunological pathway.

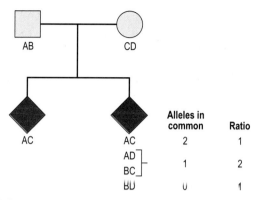

Fig. 8.5
The probability that siblings will have 2, 1 or 0 parental alleles in common. Significant deviation from the 1:2:1 ratio indicates that the locus is causally related to the disease.

Multilocus sib-pair analysis

This is essentially an extension of single locus sib-pair analysis, in which a total genome screen is carried out on a large number of sib-pairs looking for regions of the genome which are 'identical by descent' (IBD). A panel of highly polymorphic markers, such as microsatellites (p. 16) or single nucleotide polymorphisms (p. 67), can be used for each chromosome to facilitate what is sometimes referred to as 'saturation genomic linkage analysis'. The power of multilocus sib-pair analysis can be enhanced by:

1. Including only sib-pairs both of whom are severely affected and who are therefore likely to share several susceptibility loci.

2. Including only sibships with more than two affected members. This increases the mathematical power of the analysis but in practice such sibships are rare.

3. Looking for linkage disequilibrium (p. 124) in identified susceptibility regions. This is particularly applicable when studying multifactorial disorders in relatively isolated populations (e.g. Iceland, p. 131) in which the disorders in question are likely to be homogeneous.

Once a chromosome region which appears to confer susceptibility is identified a search for the relevant locus can be made using positional cloning strategies (p. 74). Known candidate genes in the relevant region can be analysed for mutations. Alternatively reference can be made to internationally accessible databases of partial gene sequences and expressed sequence tags (p. 73) to enable genes in the relevant region to be scrutinized for mutations.

Linkage analysis in animal models

An alternative approach to identifying susceptibility loci involves the use of a suitable animal model in which breeding experiments can be undertaken. These usually take the form of mating inbred highly susceptible strains of mice with other inbred strains which have very low susceptibility. The F1 offspring are then 'backcross' mated with the high risk parental strain. By studying the cosegregation of polymorphic markers at multiple loci with the disease and then analysing the results with an appropriate computer-based linkage program, susceptibility regions can be identified. Subsequently mapping studies can be undertaken in humans by focusing in on areas of human–mouse chromosome homology.

DISEASE MODELS FOR MULTIFACTORIAL INHERITANCE

The search for susceptibility loci and polygenes, sometimes also referred to as *quantitative trait loci*, in human multifactorial disorders has met with only limited success, although it is hoped that knowledge gained from the Human Genome Project (p. 321), together with research in Iceland and elsewhere, will help accelerate the rate of progress. Recent research in two conditions will be considered to illustrate the extent of the challenges which lie ahead.

AUTISM

Autism is a severe neurodevelopmental disorder which affects approximately 1 in 2500 children, with onset during the first three years of life. The characteristic features are an absence of verbal communication, lack of social responsivenesss and ritualistic behaviour. Many affected children show significant developmental delay and, conversely, many children with developmental delay can show autistic features. For example, autistic behaviour is well recognized in children with tuberous sclerosis and various forms of chromosome imbalance, as well as in boys with the Fragile X syndrome (p. 258).

The cause of autism in isolation (non-syndromal) is not clear, but there is increasing evidence that genetic factors play an important role. This is based on the results of twin studies, which yield concordance rates of 80% and 3% in monozygotic and dizygotic twins respectively, and on evidence of familial aggregation with the empiric recurrence risk for siblings being between 2 and 6% in many different studies.

In an attempt to clarify the genetic contribution to autism, a large study has been undertaken in the United States based on genome screening of 139 affected sib-pairs. Using complex computer based statistical analysis it was concluded that non-syndromal autism is associated with 15 or more susceptibility loci, each of which makes

only a modest additive contribution to the overall disease phenotype. The authors in this study concluded that positional cloning of susceptibility loci using linkage analysis will be a 'formidable task' and that other approaches such as genome-wide association and linkage disequilibrium studies will be required. These conclusions indicate that full understanding of the genetic contribution to autism and genetically based therapeutic strategies are a long way off.

INSULIN–DEPENDENT DIABETES MELLITUS

There are two main forms of diabetes mellitus (p. 212). Type 1 is the rarer juvenile onset insulin-dependent form (IDDM) which affects 0.4% of the population and shows a high incidence of potentially serious renal, retinal and vascular complications. Type 2 is the maturity onset non-insulin-dependent form which affects 5–6% of the population and is relatively benign. Both type 1 and type 2 show complex patterns of familial clustering which led to diabetes being labelled as the 'geneticist's nightmare'.

Because of its severity and associated complications research has tended to focus on type 1 diabetes mellitus. The concordance rates in monozygotic and dizygotic twins are around 50% and 12% respectively. The sibling recurrence risk is 6%. These observations point to a multifactorial aetiology with both environmental and genetic contributions. Known environmental factors include diet, viral exposure in early childhood and certain drugs. The disease process involves irreversible destruction of insulin-producing islet β-cells in the pancreas by the body's own immune system, probably as a result of an interaction between infection and an abnormal genetically programmed immune response.

IDDM1

Over the last 20 years the genetic contribution to IDDM has become much better understood. The first major breakthrough came with the recognition of strong associations with the HLA region on chromosome 6p21. The original associations were with the HLA B8 and B15 antigens which are in linkage disequilibrium with the DR3 and DR4 alleles (p. 182). It is with these that the IDDM association is strongest with 95% of affected individuals having DR3 and/or DR4 compared with 50% of the general population. Following the development of PCR analysis for the HLA region, it was shown that the HLA contribution to IDDM susceptibility is determined by the 57th amino acid residue at the DQ locus where aspartic acid conveys protection, in contrast to other alleles which increase susceptibility. As this was the first susceptibility locus identified for type 1 diabetes it was labelled *IDDM1*.

IDDM2

The next locus to be identified was that of the insulin gene on chromosome 11p15 where it was shown that variation in the number of tandem repeats of a 14 bp sequence upstream to the gene influences disease susceptibility. Long repeats convey protection by increasing expression of the insulin gene in the fetal thymus gland thereby reducing the likelihood that insulin producing β-cells will be viewed as foreign by the mature immune system.

Other IDDM loci

IDDM1 and *IDDM2* contribute λ values of approximately 3 and 1.3 respectively. However, the total risk ratio for IDDM is around 15 (i.e. the sibling risk of 6% divided by the population incidence of 0.4%). Confirmation that other loci are involved came first of all from linkage analysis using breeding experiments with the non-obese diabetic (NOD) strain of mice. These mice show a very high incidence of IDDM with immunopathological features similar to those seen in IDDM in humans. These linkage data pointed to the existence of nine or ten different susceptibility loci in mice. Shortly afterwards, in 1994, the results of multilocus sib-pair analysis based on the segregation of 289 genome-wide polymorphic markers in three large sets of around 100 affected British sib-pairs provided evidence for the existence of between 12 and 20 susceptibility loci in humans.

However this relatively simplistic view of IDDM as being caused by a small number of polygenes, more correctly described as *oligogenes*, has been challenged by two subsequent studies. An extension of the original British study confirmed and developed its initial findings, whereas analysis of a very large sample of 679 affected sib-pairs in the United States yielded conflicting results with little if any support for several of the loci identified in the British study. The most probable explanation for these discrepancies is that of causal heterogeneity as it is perfectly plausible that different susceptibility loci and environmental factors interact in different populations. This emphasizes once again the potential value of studying a homogeneous group such as the Icelandic population (p. 131).

Summary

The currrent understanding is that IDDM is indeed a multifactorial disorder with an underlying oligogenic or polygenic susceptibility consisting of one major locus (*IDDM1* = HLA) and up to 20 minor loci. The products of these loci are believed to interact in a complex and poorly understood way to confer susceptibility to environmental triggers of autoimmune pancreatic β-cell destruction. This phenomenon of gene interaction is referred to as *epistasis*. The long term research goals are firstly to map all the IDDM loci, then identify the relevant genes and finally devise new strategies for prevention and possibly treatment based on a full understanding of the underlying aetiology and pathogenesis. These objectives are ambitious but if successfully achieved the rewards in terms of preventing the health burden posed by IDDM will be huge.

CONCLUSION

The term multifactorial has been coined to describe the pattern of inheritance displayed by a large number of common disorders which show familial clustering and which are probably caused by the interaction of genetic with environmental factors. The genetic mechanisms underlying these disorders are not well understood. The liability/threshold model should be viewed as an attractive hypothesis rather than as proven scientific fact. Research in molecular biology is beginning to unravel some of the mysteries of multifactorial inheritance and in particular some progress has been achieved in elucidating the genetic contribution to type 1 diabetes mellitus. However, for many other conditions, such as autism, schizophrenia and the affective disorders, progress has been disappointingly slow and probably awaits the development of more sophisticated methods for simultaneous multilocus linkage analysis.

This emphasis on the underlying genetic contribution to multifactorial disorders should not in any way detract from the importance of trying to identify major environmental causal factors. This is amply demonstrated by the beneficial effect of folic acid supplementation in preventing neural tube defects (p. 232).

FURTHER READING

Davies J L, Kawaguchi Y, Bennett S T et al 1994 A genome-wide search for human type 1 diabetes susceptibility genes. Nature 371: 130–136
The results of a major study to identify polygenic IDDM susceptibility loci.

Falconer D S 1965 The inheritance of liability to certain diseases estimated from the incidence among relatives. Ann Hum Genet 29: 51–76
The original exposition of the liability/threshold model and how correlations between relatives can be used to calculate heritability.

Fraser F C 1980 Evolution of a palatable multifactorial threshold model. Am J Hum Genet 32: 796–813
An amusing and 'reader-friendly' account of models proposed to explain multifactorial inheritance.

King R A, Rotter J I, Motulsky A G (eds) 1992 The genetic basis of common diseases. Oxford University Press, Oxford
A lengthy and detailed review of the genetic aspects of common adult onset disorders.
Lernmark A, Ott J 1998 Sometimes it's hot, sometimes it's not. Nature Genet 19: 213–214

A brief account of possible explanations for the conflicting results obtained in studies to identify susceptibility loci in IDDM.
Risch N, Spiker D, Lotspeich L et al 1999 A genomic screen of autism: evidence for a multilocus etiology. Am J Hum Genet 65: 493–507
The results of multilocus sib-pair analysis in 139 sibships with autism.

ELEMENTS

1 The concept of multifactorial inheritance has been proposed to account for the common congenital malformations and acquired disorders which show non-Mendelian familial aggregation. These disorders are thought to result from the interaction of genetic and environmental factors.

2 Human characteristics such as height and intelligence, which show a normally distributed continuous distribution in the general population, are probably caused by the additive effects of many genes, i.e. polygenic inheritance.

3 According to the liability/threshold model for multifactorial inheritance the population's genetic and environmental susceptibility, which is known as liability, is normally distributed. Individuals are affected if their liability exceeds a threshold superimposed on the liability curve.

4 Recurrence risks to relatives for multifactorial disorders are influenced by the disease severity, the degree of relationship to the index case, the number of affected close relatives and, if there is a higher incidence in one particular sex, the sex of the index case.

5 Heritability is a measure of the proportion of the total variance of a character or disease which is due to the genetic variance.

6 Loci which contribute to susceptibility for multifactorial disorders can be identified by (a) a search for disease associations and (b) linkage analysis looking for example for chromosomal regions which are identical by descent in affected sib-pairs. Strategies for multilocus sib-pair analysis have been devised. These approaches have led to the identification of one major and 10–20 minor susceptibility loci for type 1 diabetes mellitus.

GENETICS IN MEDICINE

Haemoglobin and the haemoglobinopathies

It has been estimated that more than a quarter of a million people are born in the world each year with one of the disorders of the structure or synthesis of haemoglobin (Hb), the so-called *haemoglobinopathies*. As a consequence the haemoglobinopathies have the greatest impact on morbidity and mortality of any single group of inherited disorders. The mobility of modern society means that appreciable numbers of individuals from areas of high prevalence often constitute significant minority populations with a high risk of the haemoglobinopathies in countries where they are uncommon in the endemic population. This means that it is incumbent for all clinicians to be familiar with this group of disorders. In addition, during the course of the last 40 years, the haemoglobinopathies have also served as a paradigm for our understanding of the pathology of inherited disease in humans at the clinical, protein and DNA level.

In order to better understand the various types of haemoglobinopathies and their clinical consequences, it is first necessary to consider the structure, function and synthesis of Hb.

STRUCTURE OF HAEMOGLOBIN

Hb is the protein present in red blood cells responsible for oxygen transport. There are large quantities of Hb in blood making it amenable to analysis.

PROTEIN ANALYSIS

By fractionating the peptide products of digestion of human Hb with the proteolytic enzyme, trypsin, Ingram, in 1956, found 30 discrete peptide fragments. Trypsin cuts polypeptide chains at the amino acids arginine and lysine. Analysis of the 580 amino acids of human Hb had previously shown there to be a total of 60 arginine and lysine residues, suggesting that Hb was made up of two identical peptide chains with 30 arginine and lysine residues on each chain.

About the same time a family was reported in which two haemoglobin variants, Hb S and Hb Hopkins II, were both present in some family members. Several members of the family who possessed both variants had children with normal Hb, offspring who were heterozygous for only one Hb variant, as well as offspring who like their parents were doubly heterozygous for the two Hb variants. These observations provided further support for the suggestion that there were at least two different genes involved in the production of human Hb.

Shortly thereafter, the amino–terminal amino acid sequence of human Hb was determined and showed valine–leucine and valine–histidine sequences in equimolar proportions, with two moles of each of these sequences per mole of Hb. This was consistent with human Hb being made up of a tetramer consisting of two pairs of different polypeptides referred to as the α- and β-globin chains.

Analysis of the iron content of human Hb revealed it to constitute 0.35% of its weight, from which it was calculated that human Hb should have a minimum molecular weight of 16 000. In contrast, determination of the molecular weight of human Hb by physical methods gave values of the order of 64 000, consistent with the suggested tetrameric structure, $\alpha_2\beta_2$, with each of the globin chains having its own iron containing group, *haem* (Fig. 9.1).

Subsequent investigators demonstrated that Hb from normal adult individuals also contained a minor fraction, constituting 2–3% of the total Hb, with an electrophoretic mobility different from the majority of human Hb. The main component was called Hb A, while the minority component was called Hb A_2. Subsequent studies revealed Hb A_2 to be a tetramer of two normal α-globin chains and two other polypeptide chains whose amino acid sequence resembled most closely the β-globin chain and was designated delta (δ).

DEVELOPMENTAL EXPRESSION OF HAEMOGLOBIN

Analysis of Hb from a human fetus revealed it to consist primarily of a Hb with a different electrophoretic mobility than normal Hb A, which was called fetal Hb or Hb F. Subsequent analysis showed Hb F to be a tetramer of two α-globin chains and two polypeptide chains whose sequence resembled the β-globin chain and which were designated gamma (γ). Hb F makes up somewhere in the region of 0.5% of haemoglobin in the blood of normal adults.

Analysis of Hb from embryos earlier in gestation reveals there to be a developmental or ontological succession of different embryonic Hbs. Hb Gower I and II, and Hb Portland, which are produced in varying amounts at different times of gestation. Subsequent analysis has revealed that these various Hbs, which are transiently expressed in development, are in fact tetramers of various combinations of α or α-like zeta (ζ) chains with β or β-like γ- and epsilon (ε)-globin chains (Table 9.1). Apart from the transient expression of the ζ chain early in embryonic life, the α-globin chain gene is expressed throughout development. Similarly, ε-globin chain expression occurs early in embryonic life with γ chain expression occurring throughout fetal life followed by increasing levels of expression of the β-globin chain towards the end of fetal life. The ordered expression of these chains results in the various Hb tetramers seen during development (Fig. 9.2).

GLOBIN CHAIN STRUCTURE

The analysis of the structure of the individual globin chains was initially carried out at the protein level.

PROTEIN STUDIES

Amino acid sequencing of the various globin polypeptides, carried out in the 1960s by a number of different investigators, showed that the α-globin chain was 141 amino acids long while the β chain contained 146 amino acids. The α and β chains were found to have a similar sequence of amino acids but were by no means identical. Analysis of the amino acid sequence of the δ chain showed it to differ from the β-globin chain by 10 amino acids. Similar analysis of the γ-globin chain showed that it also most closely resembled the β-globin chain, differing by 39 amino acids. In addition, it was found that there were two types of fetal Hb in which the γ chain contained either the amino acid glycine or alanine at position 136, which were consequently named $^G\gamma$ and $^A\gamma$ respectively. More recently, partial sequence analyses of the ζ and ε chains of embryonic Hb suggest the former to be similar in amino acid sequence to the α chain, while the latter resembles the β chain.

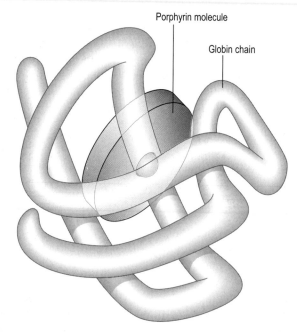

Fig. 9.1
Diagrammatic representation of one of the globin chains and associated porphyrin molecule of human haemoglobin.

Table 9.1 Human haemoglobins

Stage in development	Haemoglobin	Structure	Proportion in normal adult (%)
Embryonic	Gower I	$\zeta_2\varepsilon_2$	—
	Gower II	$\alpha_2\varepsilon_2$	—
	Portland I	$\zeta_2\gamma_2$	—
Fetal	F	$\alpha_2\gamma_2$	<1
Adult	A	$\alpha_2\beta_2$	97–98
	A₂	$\alpha_2\delta_2$	2–3

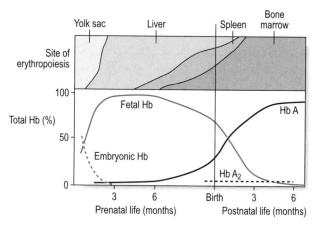

Fig. 9.2
Haemoglobin synthesis during prenatal and postnatal development. There are several embryonic haemoglobins. (After Huehns E R, Shooter E M 1965 Human haemoglobins. J Med Genet 2: 48–90, with permission.)

Thus, it appeared that there are two groups of globin chains, the α-like and β-like, all of which seem to be derived from an ancestral primordial Hb gene, which has undergone a number of gene duplications, and diverged during the course of evolution.

GLOBIN GENE MAPPING

The first evidence for the arrangement of the various globin structural genes on the human chromosomes was provided by analysis of the Hb electrophoretic variant, Hb Lepore. Comparison of trypsin digests of Hb Lepore with Hb from normal persons revealed that the α chains were normal, whereas the non-α chains appeared to consist of an amino-terminal δ-globin-like sequence and a carboxy-terminal β-globin-like sequence.

It was therefore proposed that Hb Lepore could represent a 'fusion' globin chain which had arisen as a result of a cross-over coincidental with mispairing of the δ- and β-globin genes during meiosis as a result of the sequence similarity of the two genes and the close proximity of the δ- and β-globin genes on the same chromosome (Fig. 9.3). If this hypothesis was correct, it was argued that there should also be an 'anti-Lepore' Hb, i.e. a β-δ-globin fusion product in which the non-α-globin chains contained β chain residues at the amino-terminal end and δ chain residues at the carboxy-terminal end. In the late 1960s, a new Hb electrophoretic variant, Hb Miyada, was identified by investigators in Japan in which analysis of trypsin digests did, indeed, show it to contain β-globin sequence at the amino-terminal end and δ-globin sequence at the carboxy-terminal end, as predicted.

Further evidence at the protein level for the physical mapping of the human globin genes was provided by the report of another Hb electrophoretic variant, Hb Kenya. Amino acid sequence analysis of this variant suggested that it was a γ-β fusion product with a cross-over having occurred somewhere between amino acids 81 and 86 in the two globin chains. It was suggested that, in order for this fusion polypeptide to have occurred, the γ-globin structural gene must also be in close physical proximity to the β-globin gene.

Little evidence was forthcoming from protein studies about the mapping of the α-globin genes. The presence of normal Hb A in individuals who, by family studies, should have been homozygous for a particular α-globin chain variant or obligate compound heterozygotes (p. 101) suggested that there could be more than one α-globin gene. In addition, the proportion of the total Hb made up by the α-globin chain variant, in persons heterozygous for those variants, was consistently lower (less than 20%) than that seen with the β-globin chain variants (usually more than 30%), suggesting that there could be more than one α-globin structural gene.

GLOBIN GENE STRUCTURE

Detailed information on the structure of the globin genes has been made possible by DNA techniques (p. 55). Immature red blood cells, reticulocytes, provide a rich source of globin mRNA for the synthesis of cDNA because they synthesize little else! Use of β-globin cDNA for restriction mapping studies of DNA from normal persons revealed that the non-α or β-like globin genes are located in a 50 kb stretch on the short arm of chromosome 11 (Fig. 9.4). The whole of this 50 kb stretch has been cloned and the nucleotide sequence of each of the various globin structural genes is known. Of particular interest are regions with sequences similar to the globin structural genes but which are non-functional and do not produce an identifiable message or protein product, that is pseudogenes (p. 15).

Similar studies of the α-globin structural genes have shown that there are, in fact, two α-globin structural genes, α1 and α2, located on the short arm of chromosome 16 (Fig. 9.4). DNA sequence analysis has revealed nucleotide sequence differences between these two structural genes even though the α-globin chains produced have an identical amino acid sequence, evidence of the 'degeneracy' of the genetic code. In addition, there are pseudo-α, pseudo-ζ and ζ genes to the 5' side of the α-globin genes as well as a recently discovered theta (θ)-globin gene to the 3' side of the α1-globin gene. This latter gene, whose function is unknown, is of interest because, unlike the globin pseudogenes, which are not

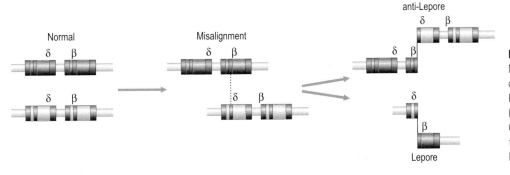

Fig. 9.3
Mechanism of unequal crossing over which generates Hb Lepore and anti-Lepore. (Adapted from Weatherall D J, Clegg J B 1981 The thalassaemia syndromes. Blackwell, Oxford.)

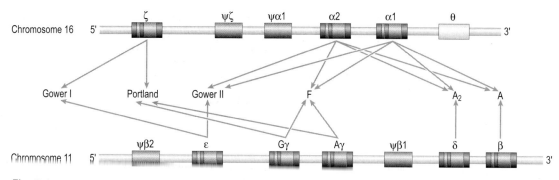

Fig. 9.4
The α- and β-globin regions on chromosomes 16 and 11 showing the structural genes and pseudogenes (ψ) and the various haemoglobins produced. (Adapted from Carrell R W, Lehman H 1985 The haemoglobinopathies. In: Dawson A M, Besser G, Compston N (eds) Recent advances in medicine 19. Churchill Livingstone, Edinburgh, pp. 223–225.)

expressed, its structure is compatible with expression. It has been suggested that it could be expressed in very early erythroid tissue such as the fetal liver and yolk sac.

SYNTHESIS AND CONTROL OF HAEMOGLOBIN EXPRESSION

From in vitro translation studies with reticulocyte mRNA from normal persons it is known that α- and β-globin chains are synthesized in roughly equal proportions. In vitro studies of globin chain synthesis have shown, however, that β-globin mRNA is slightly more efficient in protein synthesis than α-globin mRNA and that this difference is compensated for in the red blood cell precursors by a relative excess of α-globin mRNA. It seems that the most important level of regulation of expression of the globin genes, like other eukaryotic genes, is likely to occur at the level of transcription (p. 19).

DNA studies of the β-globin genes and flanking regions have revealed that, in addition to promoter sequences in the 5' flanking regions of the various globin genes, there are sequences 6–20 kb 5' to the ε-globin gene necessary for the expression of the various β-like globin genes. This region has been called the *locus control region* or *lcr*, and is involved in the timing and tissue specificity of expression or *switching* of the β-like globin genes in development. There is a similar region 5' to the α-globin genes involved in the control of their expression. Both are involved in the binding of proteins and transcription factors involved in the control of expression of the globin genes.

DISORDERS OF HAEMOGLOBIN

The disorders of human Hb can be divided into two main groups, structural globin chain variants such as sickle-cell disease and disorders of synthesis of the globin chains, the thalassaemias.

STRUCTURAL VARIANTS/DISORDERS

In 1975, Ingram demonstrated that the difference between Hb A and Hb S lay in the substitution of valine for glutamic acid in the β-globin chain. Since then more than 300 Hb electrophoretic variants have been described due to a variety of types of mutation (Table 9.2). Some 200 of these electrophoretic variants are single amino acid substitutions resulting from a point mutation. The majority of these are rare and not associated with clinical disease. A few are associated with disease and relatively prevalent in certain populations.

Types of mutation

Point mutation

A point mutation which results in substitution of one amino acid for another can lead to an altered haemoglobin, such as Hb S, C or E, which are missense mutations (p. 21).

Deletion

There are a number of Hb variants in which one or more amino acids of one of the globin chains is missing or deleted, e.g. Hb Freiburg.

Insertion

Conversely, there are variants in which the globin chains are longer than normal because of insertions, such as Hb Grady.

Table 9.2   Structural variants of haemoglobin

Type of mutation	Examples	Chain/residue(s)/alteration
Point (over 200 variants)	Hb S Hb C Hb E	β, 6 glu to val β, 6 glu to lys β, 26 glu to lys
Deletion (shortened chain)	Hb Freiburg Hb Lyon Hb Leiden Hb Gun Hill	β, 23 to 0 β, 17–18 to 0 β, 6 or 7 to 0 β, 92–96 or 93–97 to 0
Insertion (elongated chain)	Hb Grady	α, 116–118 (glu, phe, thr) duplicated
Frameshift (insertion/deletion of other than multiples of three base pairs)	Hb Tak, Hb Cranston Hb Wayne Hb McKees Rock	*β, + 11 residues, loss of termination codon, insertion of 2 base pairs in codon 146/147 *α, + 5 residues, due to loss of termination codon by single base pair deletion in codon 138/139 *β, –2 residues, point mutation in 145, generating premature termination codon
Chain termination	Hb Constant Spring	*α, + 31 residues, point mutation in termination codon
Fusion chain (unequal crossing over)	Hb Lepore/anti-Lepore Hb Kenya/anti-Kenya	non-α, δ-like residues at N-terminal end and β-like residues at C-terminal end and vice versa, respectively non-α, γ-like residues at N-terminal end and β-like residues at C-terminal end and vice versa, respectively

*Residues are either added (+) or lost (–).

Frameshift mutation

Frameshift mutations involve disruption of the normal triplet reading frame, i.e. addition or removal of a number of bases which are not a multiple of three (p. 21). In this instance, translation of the mRNA continues until a termination codon is read 'in frame'. These variants can result in either an elongated or shortened globin chain.

Chain termination

A mutation in the termination codon itself can lead to an elongated globin chain, e.g. Hb Constant Spring.

Fusion polypeptides

The last type of structural variants are the fusion *polypeptides*, Hbs Lepore and Kenya, which result from unequal cross-over events in meiosis, as previously detailed (p. 141).

Clinical aspects

Some of the haemoglobin variants are associated with disease but many are harmless and do not interfere with normal function, having been identified only in the course of population surveys of Hb electrophoretic variants. A number, however, do interfere in a variety of ways with the normal function of Hb (Table 9.3).

Table 9.3   Functional abnormalities of structural variants of haemoglobin

Clinical features	Examples
Haemolytic anaemia	
Sickling disorders	Hb S Hb C Hb E
Unstable haemoglobin	Hb Köln Hb Gun Hill Hb Bristol
Cyanosis	
Haemoglobin M (methaemoglobinaemia)	Hb M (Boston) Hb M (Hyde Park)
Low O$_2$ affinity	Hb Kansas
Polycythaemia	
High O$_2$ affinity	Hb Chesapeake Hb Heathrow

If the mutation is on the inside of the globin subunits, in close proximity to the haem pockets or at the interchain contact areas, this can produce an unstable Hb molecule which precipitates in the red blood cell, damaging the membrane and resulting in haemolysis of the red blood cell. Alternatively, mutations can interfere with the normal oxygen transport function of Hb leading either to an enhanced or reduced oxygen affinity or to a Hb which is stable in its reduced form, so-called *methaemoglobin*.

The structural variants of Hb identified by electrophoretic techniques probably represent a minority of the

Fig. 9.5
Haemoglobin electrophoresis showing haemoglobin A, C and S.
(Courtesy of Dr D Norfolk, General Infirmary, Leeds.)

Fig. 9.6
Blood film showing sickling of red cells in sickle-cell disease. Sickled cells are arrowed. (Courtesy of Dr D Norfolk, General Infirmary, Leeds.)

total number of variants that exist since it is predicted that only one-third of the possible Hb mutations which could occur will produce an altered charge in the Hb molecule and thereby be detectable by electrophoresis (Fig. 9.5).

SICKLE–CELL DISEASE

Although the severe hereditary haemolytic anaemia, *sickle-cell disease*, was first recognized early in the twentieth century, it was only in 1940 that the red blood cells from persons with sickle-cell disease were noted to appear birefringent when viewed in polarized light under the microscope, reflecting polymerization of the sickle haemoglobin, leading to distortion in the shape of the red blood cells under deoxygenated conditions, so-called *sickling* (Fig. 9.6). Pauling, in 1949, analysing Hb from patients with sickle-cell disease by electrophoresis, demonstrated that it had a different mobility when compared to Hb A, and called it Hb S for sickle.

Clinical aspects of sickle-cell disease

Sickle-cell disease is the most common haemoglobinopathy and the clinical manifestations are multifold including cerebral symptoms, kidney failure, 'pneumonia', heart failure, weakness and lassitude. All of these are a manifestation of the mutant allele. Hb S is less soluble than normal haemoglobin and tends to polymerize, causing the sickle-shaped deformation of the red cells. A proportion of sickle cells become irreversibly sickled because of damage to the red cell membrane and are taken up by the reticuloendothelial system. The shorter red cell survival time leads to a more rapid red cell turnover with consequent anaemia. In addition the sickle cells have a reduced deformability tending to obstruct small arteries, resulting in an inadequate oxygen supply to the tissues (Fig. 9.7).

Persons with sickle-cell disease can present acutely unwell with a sudden onset of chest, back, or limb pain, fever and dark urine, the latter due to the presence of free haemoglobin in the urine, a so-called *sickle-cell crisis*.

When compared to the general population, persons with sickle-cell disease have an increased risk of early death; earlier recognition and treatment of the known complications of sickle-cell disease have resulted in improved life expectancy. Some simple measures, such as prophylactic penicillin to prevent the risk of overwhelming sepsis due to splenic infarction, have met with limited success in treating specific complications. It is fair to state that although there has been an understanding of the molecular basis of sickle-cell disease for over 30 years, the therapeutic approaches available to date to prevent the sickling process have had limited benefit.

Sickle-cell trait

The heterozygous or carrier state for the sickle-cell allele is known as *sickle-cell trait* and is not thought, in general, to be associated with any significant risk to health. There are, however, reports suggesting a small increased risk of sudden death associated with strenuous exercise. In addition, there is continuing controversy about whether there are risks from hypoxia in persons with sickle-cell trait on airplane flights.

Mutational basis of sickle-cell disease

In sickle-cell disease, knowledge of the genetic code (p. 18) suggested that the substitution of valine at the

Fig. 9.7

The pleiotropic effects of the gene for sickle-cell disease.

sixth position of the β-globin chain was due to an alteration in the second base of the triplet coding for glutamic acid, i.e. GAG to GTG. Using the restriction enzyme, *Mst* II, the nucleotide recognition sequence of which is abolished by the point mutation in Hb S, it is possible to demonstrate a difference between persons with sickle-cell disease and normal persons in the restriction fragments when hybridized with a radioactively labelled β-globin probe (p. 65).

Use of a mutation-specific RFLP is possible with Hb E using the restriction enzymes *Hph*I or *Mn*II. Family studies using linked polymorphic DNA sequence variants are needed for carrier testing and prenatal diagnosis for the other haemoglobinopathies (p. 68).

DISORDERS OF HAEMOGLOBIN SYNTHESIS

The *thalassaemias* are the commonest single group of inherited disorders in humans occurring in persons from the Mediterranean area, the Middle East, the Indian subcontinent and South-East Asia. They are a heterogeneous group of disorders and are classified according to the particular globin chain or chains synthesized in reduced amounts, e.g. α, β, δβ thalassaemia.

The pathophysiology is similar in all forms of thalassaemia. An imbalance of globin chain production results in the accumulation of free globin chains in the red blood cell precursors, which, being insoluble, precipitate, resulting in haemolysis of the red blood cells, i.e. a haemolytic anaemia, with consequent compensatory hyperplasia of the bone marrow.

α thalassaemia

α *thalassaemia* results from an underproduction of the α-globin chains. It occurs most commonly in persons from

Fig. 9.8

Longitudinal ultrasound scan of a coronal section of the head (to the right) and thorax of a fetus with hydrops fetalis due to the severe form of a thalassaemia, Hb Barts, showing a large pleural effusion (arrowed). (Courtesy Mr J Campbell, St James's Hospital, Leeds.)

South-East Asia. There are two main types of α thalassaemia which differ in their severity: the severe form, in which no α-globin chains are produced, is associated with death of the fetus in utero, as a result of massive oedema because of heart failure from the severe in utero anaemia, so-called *hydrops fetalis* (Fig. 9.8).

Analysis of the Hb present in fetuses with hydrops fetalis reveals it to be a tetramer of γ-globin chains, which used to be called Hb Barts. In the milder forms of α thalassaemia compatible with survival, although some α-globin chains are produced, there is still a relative excess of β-globin chains which results in the production of the β-globin tetramer, Hb H, or what is known as Hb H disease. Both the Hb Barts and Hb H globin tetramers have an oxygen affinity similar to that of myoglobin and do not release oxygen normally in the peripheral tissues. In addition, Hb H is unstable and precipitates, resulting in haemolysis of the red blood cells.

Mutational basis of α thalassaemia

In vitro translation studies using mRNA from reticulocytes from fetuses with hydrops fetalis show no synthesis of α-globin. However, when mRNA from reticulocytes of persons with the milder form of α thalassaemia, Hb H disease, is used, α-globin is produced but in reduced amounts when compared to mRNA from reticulocytes from normal persons. Studies comparing the quantitative hybridization of radioactively labelled α-globin cDNA to DNA from fetuses with hydrops fetalis, persons with Hb H disease and normal persons are consistent with α thalassaemia being due to deletions of the α-globin genes.

Restriction mapping studies of the α-globin region of chromosome 16 reveal that there are two α-globin structural genes on the short arm of chromosome 16. The various forms of α thalassaemia have been shown to be mostly due to deletions of one or more of these structural genes (Fig. 9.9).

Deletions of the α-globin genes in α thalassaemia are believed to have arisen as a result of unequal cross-over events in meiosis which are thought to be more likely to occur where genes with homologous sequences are in close proximity. Support for this hypothesis comes from the finding of the other product of such an event, i.e. persons with three α-globin structural genes located on one chromosome.

These observations resulted in the recognition of two other milder forms of α thalassaemia which are not associated with anaemia and can only be detected by the transient presence in the immediate newborn period of Hb Barts. The results of the DNA mapping studies of the α-globin genes have shown that these milder forms of α thalassaemia are due to the deletion of one or two of the α-globin genes. Less commonly, non-deletion mutations which include point mutations in the α-globin genes and mutations in the 5' region involved in the control of their transcription have been found to cause α thalassaemia.

An exception to this classification of the α thalassaemias is the Hb variant Constant Spring, named after the town in the USA where the original patient came from. This was detected as an electrophoretic variant in a person with Hb H disease, i.e. α thalassaemia. Hb Constant Spring is due to an abnormally long α chain which is the result of a mutation in the normal termination codon at position 142 in the α-globin gene. Translation of this α-globin mRNA continues until the occurrence of another termination codon, resulting in an abnormally long α-globin chain variant. In addition, this abnormal α-globin mRNA molecule is unstable with a consequent relative deficiency of α-globin chains, resulting in the presence of the α-globin tetramer, Hb H.

β thalassaemia

β thalassaemia is caused by underproduction of the β-globin chain of haemoglobin. In vitro translation studies using mRNA from persons with β thalassaemia due to these different types of mutation show either reduced or absent production of β-globin chains, β^+ and β^0 respectively. Persons homozygous for β^0 thalassaemia mutations have a severe transfusion dependent anaemia.

Mutational basis of β thalassaemia

Restriction mapping studies have shown that β thalassaemia is rarely due to a deletion and DNA sequencing has often been necessary to reveal the molecular pathology. In excess of 100 different mutations have been shown to cause β thalassaemia. These involve a wide variety of different types of mutation including point mutations, insertions and deletions of one or more bases. These occur at a number of places, both within the coding and non-coding portions of the β-globin genes as well as in the 5' flanking promoter region, the 5' capping sequences (p. 18) and the 3' polyadenylation sequences (p. 18) (Fig. 9.10).

αα / αα   αα / α−   αα / − −   α− / α−   α− / − −   − − / − −

Normal   Alpha heterozygote   Alpha heterozygote   Alpha heterozygote   Hb H disease   Hydrops fetalis

Fig. 9.9
The structure of the normal and deleted α-globin structural genes in the various forms of α thalassaemia. (Adapted from Emery A E H 1984 An introduction to recombinant DNA. John Wiley, Chichester.)

The various types of mutation causing β thalassaemia are often unique to certain population groups and can be considered to fall into six main functional types.

Transcription mutations
Mutations in the 5′ flanking TATA box or the promoter region of the β-globin gene can result in reduced transcription levels of the β-globin mRNA.

mRNA splicing mutations
Mutations involving the invariant 5′ GT or 3′ AG dinucleotides of the introns in the β-globin gene or the consensus donor or acceptor sequences (p. 17) result in abnormal splicing with consequent reduced levels of β-globin mRNA. In the most common β thalassaemia mutation in persons from the Mediterranean region, the mutation leads to the creation of a new acceptor AG dinucleotide splice site sequence in the first intron of the β-globin gene creating a so-called cryptic splice site (p. 23). The cryptic splice site competes with the normal splice site leading to reduced levels of the normal β-globin mRNA. Mutations in the coding regions of the β-globin region can also lead to cryptic splice sites.

Polyadenylation signal mutations
Mutations in the 3′ end of the untranslated region of the β-globin gene can lead to loss of the signal for cleavage and polyadenylation of the β-globin gene transcript.

RNA modification mutations
Mutations in the 5′ and 3′ DNA sequences, involved respectively in the capping (p. 18) and polyadenylation (p. 18) of the mRNA, can result in abnormal processing and transportation of the β-globin mRNA to the cytoplasm with consequent reduced levels of translation.

Chain termination mutations
Insertions, deletions and point mutations can all generate a nonsense or chain termination codon, resulting in the premature termination of translation of the β-globin mRNA. This will result in the majority of instances in a shortened β-globin mRNA which is often unstable and more rapidly degraded with consequent reduced levels of translation of an abnormal β-globin.

Missense mutations
Missense mutations which lead to a β-globin which is highly unstable can rarely result in β thalassaemia. An example is Hb Indianapolis.

Clinical aspects of β thalassaemia

Children affected with thalassaemia major, or Cooley's anaemia as it was originally known, usually present in the first year of life with a severe transfusion-dependent anaemia. Unless the child is adequately transfused compensatory expansion of the bone marrow results in an unusually shaped face and skull (Fig. 9.11). Although persons with thalassaemia major used to die in their late teens or early twenties as a result of complications due to iron overload from repeated transfusions, the regular daily use of iron-chelating drugs, such as desferrioxamine, has improved their long-term survival.

Individuals heterozygous for β thalassaemia, *thalassaemia trait* or *thalassaemia minor*, usually have no symptoms

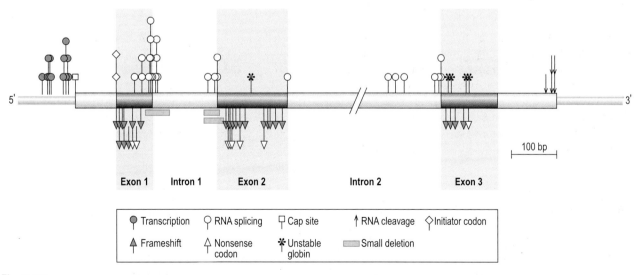

Fig. 9.10
Location and some of the types of mutation in the β-globin gene and flanking region which result in β thalassaemia. (Adapted from Orkin S H, Kazazian H H 1984 The mutation and polymorphism of the human β-globin gene and its surrounding DNA. In: Roman H L, Campbell A, Sandler L M (eds) Annu Rev Genet 18: 131–171.)

Fig. 9.11
Facies of a child with β thalassaemia showing prominence of the forehead through changes in skull shape as a result of bone marrow hypertrophy. (Courtesy of Dr D Norfolk, General Infirmary, Leeds.)

aemia produce no δ- or β-globin chains. Although one would expect such persons to have a fairly profound illness, they are only mildly anaemic, because of increased production of γ-globin chains, with Hb F levels being much higher than the mild compensatory increase seen in homozygotes for β thalassaemia.

Mutational basis of δβ thalassaemia

δβ thalassaemia has been shown to be caused by extensive deletions in the β globin region involving the δ- and β-globin structural genes (Fig. 9.12). Some deletions extend to include the ^{A}γ-globin gene so that only the ^{G}γ-globin chain is synthesized.

Hereditary persistence of fetal haemoglobin

Hereditary persistence of fetal Hb, or HPFH, in which there is persistence of the production of fetal Hb into childhood and adult life is included in the thalassaemias. Most forms of HPFH are, in fact, a form of δβ thalassaemia in which continued γ chain synthesis compensates for the lack of production of δ- and β-globin chains. Persons with hereditary persistence of fetal Hb continue to produce significant amounts of fetal Hb after birth accounting for 20–30% of total Hb in heterozygotes and 100% in homozygotes. This is not associated with any symptoms and was originally considered more of a scientific curiosity than a medical problem.

Mutational basis of HPFH

Some forms of HPFH have been shown to be due to deletions of the δ- and β-globin genes. Analysis of the non-deletion forms of HPFH has shown point mutations in the 5' flanking promoter region of either the ^{G}γ or ^{A}γ

or signs. They do have, however, a mild hypochromic, microcytic anaemia, which can often mistakenly be confused with iron deficiency anaemia.

δβ thalassaemia

In *δβ thalassaemia* there is underproduction of both the δ- and β-globin chains. Persons homozygous for δβ thalass-

Fig. 9.12
Some of the deletions in the β-globin region which result in some forms of thalassaemia and hereditary persistence of fetal haemoglobin.

globin genes near the CAAT box sequences (p. 20) involved in the control of expression of the haemoglobin genes.

CLINICAL VARIATION OF THE HAEMOGLOBINOPATHIES

The marked mutational heterogeneity of β thalassaemia means that affected individuals are often compound heterozygotes (p. 101), i.e. they have different mutations in their β-globin genes, leading to a broad spectrum of severity in the disorder. One form of β thalassaemia of intermediate severity, known as *thalassaemia intermedia*, requires less frequent transfusions.

In certain populations many of the haemoglobinopathies are relatively 'common' and, not unexpectedly, persons are reported who have two different disorders of Hb. Understandably, in the past, recognition of such individuals was often quite difficult. Because of the high prevalence in certain populations of some of the structural variants of haemoglobin, such as Hb S, individuals can present with severe anaemia who are found to be heterozygous for both Hb S and β thalassaemia, i.e. are compound heterozygotes (p. 101).

Finally, certain combinations of haemoglobinopathies can also result in a previously unexplained mild form of what is normally thought to be an invariably severe haemoglobinopathy. For example, deletion of one or two of the α-globin genes in a person homozygous for β+ thalassaemia results in a milder illness because there is less of an imbalance in globin chain production. Similarly, the presence of one of the forms of HPFH in a person homozygous for β thalassaemia or sickle-cell disease can contribute to amelioration of the disease as the increased production of γ-globin chains compensates for the deficient β-globin chain production. This finding has been exploited therapeutically by the use of drugs, such as hydroxyurea and butyrate, which have been found to be associated with increased Hb F levels. Recent developments in gene therapy for the haemoglobinopathies in a mouse model for sickle-cell disease (p. 327), in which the introduction of the fetal Hb gene resulted in increased Hb F levels, led to a reduction in the sickling phenomenon. This approach holds great promise for a reduction in the morbidity and mortality associated with this disorder.

FURTHER READING

Cay J C, Phillips J A, Kazazian H H 1996 Haemoglobinopathies and thalassemias. In: Rimoin D L, Connor J M, Pyeritz R E (eds) Principles and practice of medical genetics, 3rd edn. Churchill Livingstone, Edinburgh, pp. 1599–1626
A useful up-to-date concise summary of the haemoglobinopathies.
Cooley T B, Lee P 1925 A series of cases of splenomegaly in children with anemia and peculiar bone changes. Trans Am Pediat Soc 37: 29–40
The original description of β thalassaemia.
Pauling L, Itano H A, Singer S J, Wells I C 1949 Sickle-cell anaemia, a molecular disease. Science 110: 543–548
The first genetic disease in which a molecular basis was described, leading to a Nobel Prize.
Serjeant G R 1992 Sickle cell disease, 2nd edn. Oxford University Press, Oxford
Excellent comprehensive text covering all aspects of this important disorder.
Weatherall D J, Clegg J B, Higgs D R, Woods W G 1995 The hemoglobinopathis. In: Scriver C R, Beaudet A L, Sly W S, Valle D (eds) The metabolic and molecular basis of inherited disease, 7th edn. McGraw Hill, New York, pp. 3417–3484
A very comprehensive detailed account of haemoglobin and the haemoglobinopathies.

ELEMENTS

1 Hb, the protein present in red blood cells responsible for oxygen transport, is a tetramer made up of two dissimilar pairs of polypeptide chains and the iron-containing molecule, haem.

2 Human Hb is heterogeneous. During development it comprises a succession of different globin chains which are differentially expressed during embryonic, fetal and adult life, i.e. $\alpha_2\varepsilon_2$, $\alpha_2\gamma_2$, $\alpha_2\delta_2$, $\alpha_2\beta_2$, etc.

3 The disorders of Hb — the haemoglobinopathies — can be divided into two main groups: the structural disorders, e.g. sickle-cell Hb or Hb S, and disorders of synthesis, the thalassaemias. The former can be subdivided by the way in which they interfere with the normal function of Hb and/or the red blood cell, e.g. abnormal oxygen affinity or haemolytic anaemia. The latter can be subdivided according to which globin chain is synthesized abnormally, i.e. α, β or δβ thalassaemia.

4 Family studies of the various disorders of human Hb and analysis of the mutations responsible for these at the protein and DNA level have led to an understanding of the normal structure, function and synthesis of Hb. This has allowed demonstration of the molecular pathology of these disorders and prenatal diagnosis of a number of the inherited disorders of human Hb is possible.

Biochemical genetics

In this chapter we shall consider single gene biochemical or metabolic disorders. Garrod at the beginning of the twentieth century introduced the concept of 'chemical individuality', leading to the concept of the *inborn error of metabolism*. Beadle and Tatum later developed the idea that metabolic processes, whether in humans or any other organism, proceed by steps. They proposed that each step was controlled by a particular enzyme and that this, in turn, was the product of a particular gene. This was referred to as the 'one gene–one enzyme concept'.

THE INBORN ERRORS OF METABOLISM

In excess of 200 inborn errors of metabolism are known which can be grouped either by the metabolite, metabolic pathway, function of the enzyme or cellular organelle involved (Table 10.1). Most inborn errors of metabolism are inherited in an autosomal recessive or X-linked manner with only a few being inherited in an autosomal dominant manner. This is because the defective protein in most inborn errors is an enzyme which is diffusible and there is usually sufficient residual activity in the heterozygous state (i.e. loss-of-function mutation, p. 23) for the enzyme to function normally in most situations. If, however, the reaction catalysed by an enzyme is rate-limiting (i.e. haploinsufficiency mutation, p. 23) or the gene product is part of a multimeric complex (i.e. dominant-negative mutation, p. 24), the disorder can manifest in the heterozygous state, i.e. be dominantly inherited (p. 97).

DISORDERS OF AMINO ACID METABOLISM

There are a number of disorders of amino acid metabolism, the best known of which is phenylketonuria.

PHENYLKETONURIA

Children with phenylketonuria (PKU), if untreated, are severely mentally retarded and often have convulsions. In PKU, the particular enzyme necessary for the conversion of phenylalanine to tyrosine, phenylalanine hydroxylase (PAH), is deficient. In other words there is a 'genetic block' in the metabolic pathway (Fig. 10.1).

PKU was, in fact, the first genetic disorder in humans shown to be caused by a specific enzyme deficiency by Jervis in 1953. As a result of the enzyme defect, phenylalanine accumulates and is converted into phenylpyruvic acid and other metabolites which are excreted in the urine. The enzyme block leads to a deficiency of tyrosine with a consequent reduction in melanin formation. Affected children therefore often have blond hair and blue eyes (Fig. 10.2). In addition, areas of the brain which are usually pigmented, e.g. the substantia nigra, can also lack pigment.

Treatment of PKU

An obvious method of treating children with PKU would be to replace the missing enzyme but this cannot be done simply by any conventional means of treatment (p. 325). Bickel, only a year after the enzyme deficiency had been identified, suggested that PKU could be treated by removal of phenylalanine from the diet. This has proved to be an effective treatment. If PKU is detected early enough in infancy, mental retardation can be prevented by giving a diet containing a restricted amount of phenylalanine. Phenylalanine is an essential amino acid and therefore cannot be entirely removed from the diet. By monitoring the level of phenylalanine in the blood, it is possible to supply sufficient amounts to meet normal requirements and avoid levels which would result in mental retardation.

The mental retardation seen in children with phenylketonuria is most likely the result of an elevation of phenylalanine and/or its metabolites rather than a deficiency of tyrosine, since an adequate amount of the latter amino acid is usually available in a normal diet. It

Table 10.1   Characteristics of some inborn errors of metabolism

Type of defect	Genetics	Deficient enzyme	Main clinical features
Amino acid metabolism			
Phenylketonuria	AR	Phenylalanine hydroxylase	Mental retardation, fair skin, eczema, epilepsy
Alkaptonuria	AR	Homogentisic acid oxidase	Arthritis
Oculocutaneous albinism	AR	Tyrosinase	Lack of skin and hair pigment, eye defects
Homocystinuria	AR	Cystathione β-synthetase	Mental retardation, dislocation of lens, thrombosis, skeletal abnormalities
Maple syrup urine disease	AR	Branched chain α-ketoacid decarboxylase	Mental retardation
Urea cycle disorders			
Carbamyl synthetase deficiency	AR	Carbamyl synthetase	Hyperammonaemia, coma, death
Ornithine carbamyl transferase deficiency	XD	Ornithine carbamyl transferase	Hyperammonaemia, death in early infancy
Citrullinaemia	AR	Argininosuccinic acid synthetase	Variable clinical course
Argininosuccinic aciduria	AR	Argininosuccinic acid lyase	Hyperammonaemia, mild mental retardation, protein intolerance
Hyperargininaemia	AR	Arginase	Hyperammonaemia, progressive spasticity, intellectual deterioration
Carbohydrate metabolism			
Monosaccharide metabolism			
Galactosaemia	AR	Galactose-1-phosphate uridyl transferase	Cataracts, mental retardation, cirrhosis
Hereditary fructose intolerance	AR	Fructose-1-phosphate aldolase	Failure to thrive, vomiting, jaundice, convulsions
Glycogen storage diseases			
Primarily affecting liver			
von Gierke's disease (GSD I)	AR	Glucose-6-phosphatase	Hepatomegaly, hypoglycaemia
Cori disease (GSD III)	AR	Amylo-1,6-glucosidase	Hepatomegaly, hypoglycaemia
Anderson's disease (GSD IV)	AR	Glycogen brancher enzyme	Abnormal liver function/failure
Hepatic phosphorylase deficiency (GSD VI)	AR/X-linked	Hepatic phosphorylase	Hepatomegaly, hypoglycaemia, failure to thrive
Primarily affecting muscle			
McArdle's disease (GSD V)	AR	Muscle phosphorylase	Muscle cramps
Pompe's disease (GSD II)	AR	Lysosomal α-1,4-glucosidase	Heart failure, muscle weakness
Steroid metabolism			
Congenital adrenal hyperplasia	AR	21-hydroxylase, 11β-hydroxylase, 3β-dehydrogenase	Virilization, salt-losing
Androgen insensitivity	XR	Androgen receptor	Female external genitalia, testes, male chromosomes
Lipid metabolism			
Familial hypercholesterolaemia	AD	Low density lipoprotein receptor	Early coronary artery disease
Lysosomal storage diseases			
Mucopolysaccharidoses			
Hurler's syndrome (MPS I)	AR	α-L-iduronidase	Mental retardation, skeletal abnormalities, hepatosplenomegaly, corneal clouding
Hunter's syndrome (MPS II)	XR	Iduronate sulphate sulphatase	Mental retardation, skeletal abnormalities, hepatosplenomegaly

Table 10.1   Continued

Type of defect	Genetics	Deficient enzyme	Main clinical features
Sanfilippo syndrome (MPS III)	AR	Heparan-S-sulphaminidase (MPS III A), N-ac-α-D-glucosaminidase (MPS III B), Ac-CoA-α-glucosaminidase, N-acetyltransferase (MPS III C), N-ac-glucosaminine-6-sulphate sulphatase (MPS III D)	Behavioural problems, dementia, fits
Morquio syndrome (MPS IV)	AR	Galactosamine-6-sulphatase (MPS IV A), β-galactosidase (MPS IV B)	Corneal opacities, short stature, skeletal abnormalities
MPS V (formerly Scheie — now known to be a mild allelic form of MPS I)			
Maroteaux–Lamy syndrome (MPS VI)	AR	Arylsulphatase B, N-acetyl-galactosamine, α-4-sulphate sulphatase	Corneal clouding, skeletal abnormalities, cardiac abnormalities
Sly syndrome (MPS VII)	AR	β-glucuronidase	Variable presentation, skeletal and cardiac abnormalities, hepatosplenomegaly, corneal clouding, mental retardation
Sphingolipidoses			
Tay–Sachs disease	AR	Hexosaminidase-A	Developmental regression, blindness, cherry-red spot, deafness
Gaucher's disease	AR	Glucosylceramide β-glucosidase	Type I — joint and limb pains, splenomegaly Type II — spasticity, fits, death
Niemann–Pick disease	AR	Sphingomyelinase	Failure to thrive, hepatomegaly, cherry red spot, developmental regression
Purine/pyrimidine metabolism			
Lesch–Nyhan disease	XR	Hypoxanthine guanine phosphoribosyltransferase	Mental retardation, uncontrolled movements, self-mutilation
Adenosine deaminase deficiency	AR	Adenosine deaminase	Severe combined immunodeficiency
Purine nucleoside phosphorylase	AR	Purine nucleoside phosphorylase	Severe viral infections due to impaired T cell function
Hereditary orotic aciduria	AR	Orotate phosphoribosyltransferase, orotidine 5'-phosphate decarboxylase	Megaloblastic anaemia, failure to thrive, developmental delay
Porphyrin metabolism			
Hepatic porphyrias			
Acute intermittent porphyria (AIP)	AD	Uroporphyrinogen I synthetase	Abdominal pain, CNS effects
Hereditary coproporphyria	AD	Coproporphyrinogen oxidase	As for AIP, photosensitivity
Porphyria variegata	AD	Protoporphyrinogen oxidase	Photosensitivity, as for AIP
Erythropoietic porphyrias			
Congenital erythropoietic porphyria	AR	Uroporphyrinogen III synthase	Haemolytic anaemia, photosensitivity
Erythropoietic protoporphyria	AD	Ferrochelatase	Photosensitivity, liver disease
Organic acid disorders			
Methylmalonic acidaemia	AR	Methylmalonyl-CoA mutase	Hypotonia, poor feeding, acidosis, developmental delay
Propionic acidaemia	AR	Propionyl-CoA carboxylase	Poor feeding, failure to thrive, vomiting, acidosis, hypoglycaemia

Table 10.1 Continued

Type of defect	Genetics	Deficient enzyme	Main clinical features
Copper metabolism			
Wilson's disease	AR	ATPase membrane copper transport protein	Spasticity, rigidity, dysphagia, cirrhosis
Menkes' disease	XR	ATPase membrane copper transport protein	Failure to thrive, neurological deterioration
Peroxisomal disorders			
Peroxisomal biogenesis disorders			
Zellweger's syndrome	AR	All peroxisomal enzymes	Dysmorphic features, hypotonia, large liver, renal cysts
Isolated peroxisomal enzyme deficiency			
Adrenoleukodystrophy	XR	Very long chain fatty acid-CoA synthetase	Mental deterioration, fits, behavioural changes, adrenal failure

AR = autosomal recessive; AD = autosomal dominant; XR = X-linked recessive; XD = X-linked dominant.

Fig. 10.1

Sites of 'biochemical block' in phenylketonuria, alkaptonuria, congenital hypothyroidism and oculocutaneous albinism.

could well be that there are both prenatal as well as postnatal factors responsible for the mental retardation in persons with untreated PKU.

Diagnosis of PKU

Although PKU only affects approximately 1 in 10 000 persons of Western European origin, PKU was the first inborn error routinely screened for in newborns. This can be done by tests which detect the presence of the metabolite of phenylalanine, phenylpyruvic acid, in the urine by its reaction with ferric chloride or through elevated levels of phenylalanine in the blood. The latter test, known as the Guthrie test, involves taking blood samples from children in the first week of life and comparing the amount of growth induced by the sample with standards in a strain of the bacterium *Bacillus subtilis* which requires phenylalanine for growth. This technique has been replaced by the use of a variety of biochemical assays of phenylalanine levels.

Fig. 10.2
Facies of a male with phenylketonuria; note the fair complexion.

Heterogeneity of hyperphenylalaninaemia

Elevated phenylalanine levels in the newborn period can be the result of causes other than PKU. A small proportion of newborn infants have a condition called benign hyperphenylalaninaemia caused by a transient immaturity of liver cells to metabolize phenylalanine; they do not require treatment as they are not at risk of developing mental retardation. There are, however, two other rare causes of hyperphenylalanaemia with serious consequences: in these two disorders the enzyme phenylalanine hydroxylase is normal but there is a deficiency of either dihydropteridine reductase or dihydrobiopterin synthetase. These two enzymes are involved in the synthesis of tetrahydrobiopterin, a cofactor necessary for normal activity of phenylalanine hydroxylase. Both disorders are more serious than classical PKU because there is a high likelihood of mental handicap despite satisfactory management of phenylalanine levels.

Mutational basis of PKU

Although all cases of classical PKU arise from a deficiency of phenylalanine hydroxylase, more than 70 different mutations in the PAH gene have now been identified (p. 70). Certain mutations are more common in persons with PKU from specific population groups. In

addition, in persons of Western European origin with PKU, the mutations occur on a limited number of DNA haplotypes (p. 68). Interestingly, however, a variety of different individual mutations have been found in association with some of these haplotypes.

Maternal phenylketonuria

Children born to mothers with phenylketonuria have an increased risk of mental retardation even when their mothers are on closely controlled dietary restriction (p. 151). It has been suggested that the reduced ability of the mother with PKU to deliver an appropriate amount of tyrosine to her fetus in utero could result in reduced fetal brain growth.

ALKAPTONURIA

Alkaptonuria was the original autosomal recessive inborn error of metabolism described by Garrod. In alkaptonuria there is a block in the breakdown of homogentisic acid, a metabolite of tyrosine, through a deficiency of the enzyme homogentisic acid oxidase (Fig. 10.1). As a consequence, homogentisic acid accumulates and is excreted in the urine, to which it imparts a dark colour on exposure to air. Dark pigment is also deposited in certain tissues such as the ear wax, cartilage and joints, where it is known as ochronosis, which in the latter location can lead to arthritis later in life.

OCULOCUTANEOUS ALBINISM

Oculocutaneous albinism (OCA) is an autosomal recessive disorder due to deficiency of the enzyme tyrosinase, which is necessary for the formation of melanin pigment from tyrosine (see Fig. 10.1). In persons with OCA there is a lack of pigment in the skin, hair, iris and ocular fundus (Fig. 10.3). The lack of pigment in the eye results in poor visual acuity and typical uncontrolled pendular eye movement (nystagmus). The reduced pigmentation appears to lead to underdevelopment of the part of retina for fine vision, the fovea, and abnormal projection of the visual pathways to the optic cortex.

Heterogeneity of oculocutaneous albinism

Oculocutaneous albinism is genetically and biochemically heterogeneous. Cells from persons with classical albinism have no measurable tyrosinase activity, the so-called *tyrosinase-negative* form. However, cells from some persons with albinism show reduced but residual tyrosinase activity and are termed *tyrosinase-positive*. This is usually reflected clinically by variable development of pigmentation of their hair and skin with age. Both types

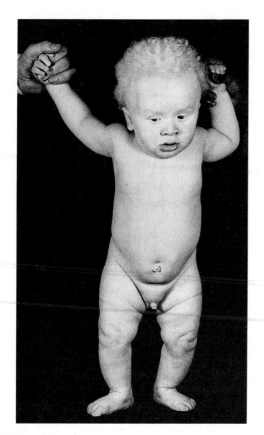

Fig. 10.3
Oculocutaneous albinism in a child of Afro-Caribbean origin.
(Courtesy of Dr V A McKusick.)

are known as tyrosinase gene-related oculocutaneous albininism type 1, or OCA 1.

DNA studies have revealed classical tyrosinase-negative and some tyrosinase-positive families with oculocutaneous albinism to be due to mutations in the tyrosinase gene on the long arm of chromosome 11. Linkage studies in some of the families with tyrosinase-positive oculocutaneous albinism, however, have excluded the tyrosinase gene as being responsible. A number of these families, interestingly, have a mutation in the P gene, the human homologue of a gene in the mouse called *pink-eyed dilution*, or pink-eye for short, located on the long arm of chromosome 15. This has been termed oculocutaneous albinism type 2, or OCA 2. In addition, in a proportion of families with oculocutaneous albinism linkage to both of these two loci has been excluded, consistent with the existence of a third locus responsible for OCA.

HOMOCYSTINURIA

Homocystinuria is a recessively inherited inborn error of sulphur amino acid metabolism characterized by mental retardation, fits, thromboembolic episodes, osteoporosis and a tendency to dislocation of the lenses. This last feature along with a tendency to develop a curvature of the spine (scoliosis), together with a pectus excavatum, and long fingers and toes (arachnodactyly) can lead to confusion with the autosomal dominant disorder, the Marfan syndrome (p. 292).

Homocystinuria is caused by a deficiency of the enzyme cystathionine β-synthetase and can be screened for by means of a positive cyanide nitroprusside test which detects the presence of increased levels of homocystine in the urine. The diagnosis is confirmed by elevated plasma homocystine levels. Treatment involves a low methionine diet with cystine supplementation. A proportion of individuals with homocystinuria are responsive to the enzyme cofactor, pyridoxine, or what is known as the pyridoxine responsive form. A small proportion of affected individuals have mutations in genes leading to deficiencies of enzymes involved in the synthesis of cofactors for cystathionine β-synthetase.

DISORDERS OF BRANCHED CHAIN AMINO ACID METABOLISM

The essential branched chain amino acids, leucine, isoleucine and valine, have a part of their metabolic pathways in common. Deficiency of the enzyme involved results in maple syrup urine disease.

MAPLE SYRUP URINE DISEASE

Newborn infants with this autosomal recessive disorder present in the first week of life with vomiting, then alternating decreased and increased tone proceeding on to death within a few weeks if left untreated. There is a characteristic odour of the urine likened to that of maple syrup. The disorder is caused by a deficiency of the branched chain ketoacid decarboxylase producing increased excretion of the branched chain amino acids valine, leucine and isoleucine in the urine, the presence of which suggest the diagnosis which is confirmed by the presence of the three essential branched chain amino acids in blood. Treatment involves a diet limiting the intake of the three branched chain amino acids to the amount necessary for growth. Affected individuals are particularly susceptible to deterioration in association with intercurrent illnesses resulting from the catabolic degradation of proteins.

UREA CYCLE DISORDERS

The urea cycle is a five-step metabolic pathway which takes place primarily in liver cells for the removal of waste nitrogen from the amino groups of amino acids arising from the normal turnover of protein. It converts two molecules of ammonia and one of bicarbonate into urea (Fig. 10.4). Deficiencies of enzymes in the urea cycle result in intolerance to protein due to the accumulation of ammonia in the body, or what is known as hyper-ammonaemia. Elevated ammonia levels are toxic to the central nervous system and can lead to coma and, with some of the urea cycle disorders if left untreated, death. The various disorders of the urea cycle are collectively rare and individually very rare. They are all inherited as autosomal recessive disorders except ornithine trans-carbamylase deficiency which is X-linked.

DISORDERS OF CARBOHYDRATE METABOLISM

The inborn errors of carbohydrate metabolism can be considered in two main groups, disorders of mono-saccharide metabolism and the glycogen storage disorders.

DISORDERS OF MONOSACCHARIDE METABOLISM

Two examples of disorders of monosaccharide metabolism are galactosaemia and hereditary fructose intolerance.

Galactosaemia

Galactosaemia is an autosomal recessive disorder due to deficiency of the enzyme galactose-1-phosphate uridyl transferase, which is necessary for the metabolism of the dietary sugar galactose. Newborn infants with

galactosaemia present with vomiting, letharg[y, failure to] thrive and jaundice in the second week [of life. If] untreated, they go on to develop complica[tions which] include mental retardation, cataracts and cir[rhosis of the] liver. Galactosaemia can be screened for by the presence of reducing substances in the urine with specific testing for galactose. The complications of galactosaemia can be prevented by early diagnosis and feeding of affected infants with milk substitutes which do not contain galactose or lactose, the sugar found in milk, which is broken down into galactose. Early diagnosis and treatment are essential if the severe complications are to be prevented.

Hereditary fructose intolerance

Hereditary fructose intolerance is an autosomal recessive disorder due to deficiency of the enzyme fructose-1-phosphate aldolase. Dietary fructose is present in honey, fruit and certain vegetables and in combination with glucose in the disaccharide sucrose in cane sugar. Individuals with hereditary fructose intolerance present at different ages, depending on when fructose is introduced into the diet. Symptoms can be minimal but can be as severe as those seen in galactosaemia which include failure to thrive, vomiting, jaundice and convulsions. The diagnosis is confirmed by the presence of fructose in the urine and enzyme assay on an intestinal mucosal or a liver biopsy sample. Dietary restriction of fructose is associated with a good long term prognosis.

GLYCOGEN STORAGE DISEASES

Glycogen is the form in which the sugar glucose is stored in muscle and liver as a polymer, acting as a reserve

Fig. 10.4
Diagram indicating the position of the various inborn errors of the urea cycle.

energy source. In the glycogen storage diseases (GSDs) glycogen accumulates in excessive amounts in skeletal muscle, cardiac muscle and/or liver due a variety of inborn errors of the enzymes involved in synthesis and degradation of glycogen. In addition, because of the metabolic block, glycogen is unavailable as a normal glucose source. This can result in hypoglycaemia, impairment of liver function and neurological abnormalities.

In each of the six major types of GSD there is a specific enzyme defect involving one of the steps in the metabolic pathways of glycogen synthesis or degradation. The various types can be grouped according to whether they affect primarily the liver or muscle. All six types are inherited as autosomal recessive disorders, although there are variants of the hepatic phosphorylase which are X-linked.

Glycogen storage diseases which primarily affect liver

von Gierke's disease (GSD I)

Von Gierke's disease was the first described disorder of glycogen metabolism and is due to deficiency of the enzyme glucose-6-phosphatase which is responsible for degradation of liver glycogen to release glucose. Affected infants present with an enlarged liver (hepatomegaly) and/or sweating and a fast heart rate due to hypoglycaemia which can occur after fasting of only 3–4 hours' duration. Treatment is simple: frequent feeding and the avoidance of fasting to maintain the blood sugar.

Cori disease (GSD III)

Cori disease is caused by deficiency of the enzyme amylo-1,6-glucosidase, which is also known as the debrancher enzyme. Deficiency of the enzyme results in glycogen accumulation in the liver and other tissues resulting from the inability to cleave the 'branching' links of the glycogen polymer. Affected infants can present with hepatomegaly because of glycogen accumulation and/or muscle weakness. Treatment involves avoiding hypoglycaemia by frequent feeding and avoiding prolonged periods of fasting.

Anderson's disease (GSD IV)

Anderson's disease results from deficiency of glycogen brancher enzyme which leads to formation of abnormal glycogen consisting of long chains with few branches which cannot be broken down by the enzymes normally responsible for glycogen degradation. Affected infants present with hypotonia and abnormal liver function in the first year of life, the latter progressing rapidly to liver failure. No effective treatment is available apart from the possibility of a liver transplant.

Hepatic phosphorylase deficiency (GSD VI)

Hepatic phosphorylase is a multimeric enzyme complex with subunits coded for by both autosomal and X-linked genes. Deficiency of hepatic phosphorylase obstructs glycogen degradation which results in children presenting in the first 2 years of life with hepatomegaly, hypoglycaemia and failure to thrive. Treatment is with carbohydrate supplements which improve growth.

Glycogen storage diseases which primarily affect muscle

Pompe's disease (GSD II)

Infants with Pompe's disease usually present in the first few months of life with floppiness (hypotonia) and delay in the gross motor milestones because of muscle weakness. They then develop an enlarged heart and die of cardiac failure in the first or second year. Voluntary and cardiac muscle accumulates glycogen due to the deficiency of the lysosomal enzyme α-1,4-glucosidase which is needed to break down glycogen. The diagnosis can be confirmed by enzyme assay on white blood cells or fibroblasts. Early reports of enzyme replacement therapy appear promising.

McArdle's disease (GSD V)

Persons with McArdle's disease present with muscle cramps on exercise in the teenage years. It is caused by a deficiency of muscle phosphorylase, which is necessary for degradation of muscle glycogen. There is no effective form of treatment, although in some affected individuals the muscle cramps tend to decline if exercise is continued, probably as a result of other energy sources becoming available from alternative metabolic pathways.

DISORDERS OF STEROID METABOLISM

The disorders of steroid metabolism include a number of autosomal recessive inborn errors of the biosynthetic pathways of cortisol. These can result in the virilization of a female fetus along with an associated salt loss in both affected male and female infants due to deficiency of the hormone aldosterone. In addition, defects of the androgen receptor result in lack of virilization of chromosomally male individuals (Fig. 10.5).

CONGENITAL ADRENAL HYPERPLASIA (ADRENOGENITAL SYNDROME)

The diagnosis of congenital adrenal hyperplasia (CAH) should be considered in any newborn female infant

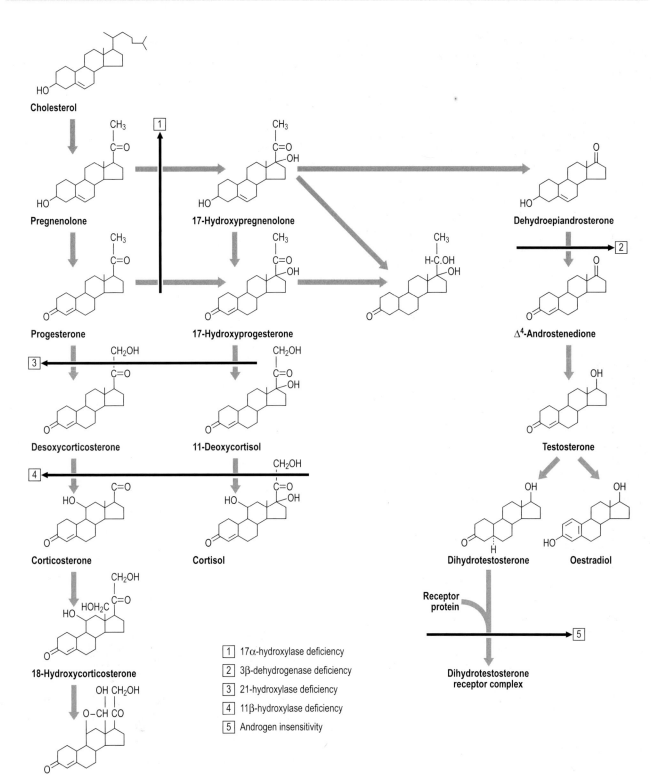

Fig. 10.5
Steroid biosynthesis indicating the site of the common inborn errors of steroid biosynthesis.

1 17α-hydroxylase deficiency
2 3β-dehydrogenase deficiency
3 21-hydroxylase deficiency
4 11β-hydroxylase deficiency
5 Androgen insensitivity

Fig. 10.6
Virilized external genitalia in a female with congenital adrenal hyperplasia.

presenting with virilization of the external genitalia as this is the commonest cause of ambiguous genitalia in female newborns (p. 260) (Fig. 10.6). 21-hydroxylase deficiency accounts for over 90% of cases. About one-quarter of affected infants will have the salt-losing form, presenting in the second week of life with circulatory collapse. Less commonly CAH is due to deficiency of the enzymes 11β-hydroxylase or 3β-dehydrogenase and very rarely occurs as a result of deficiencies of enzymes 17α-hydroxylase and 17,20-lyase.

Affected females have normal Müllerian-derived internal genitalia, the virilization of the external genitalia being caused by an accumulation of the adrenocortical steroids proximal to the enzyme block in the steroid biosynthetic pathway, many of which have testosterone-like activity (Fig. 10.5). The possibility of CAH should not be forgotten in male infants presenting with circulatory collapse in the first few weeks of life.

Affected infants, in addition to requiring urgent correct assignment of gender, are treated with replacement cortisol, along with fludrocortisone if they have the salt-losing form. Virilized females may require plastic surgery in due course. Steroid replacement is lifelong and needs to be increased during intercurrent illness or times of stress, e.g. surgery.

ANDROGEN INSENSITIVITY SYNDROME

Individuals with the androgen insensitivity syndrome (AIS) have female external genitalia, and undergo breast development in puberty (p. 261). They classically present either with primary amenorrhoea, which is the lack of onset of menstrual periods, or with an inguinal hernia containing a gonad which turns out to be a testis. There is often scanty secondary sexual hair and investigation of the internal genitalia reveals an absent uterus and Fallopian tubes with a blind-ending vagina. Chromosome analysis reveals a normal male karyotype, 46,XY.

Androgen production by the testes is normal in affected individuals but they do not bind androgen normally because of abnormal androgen receptors. This can be functionally assayed in skin fibroblasts (see Fig. 10.5). Some individuals have incomplete or partial androgen insensitivity and undergo variable virilization. Affected individuals usually have a female sexual orientation but obviously will be sterile. They require removal of their testes because of an increased risk of developing a testicular malignancy and should be placed on oestrogen for secondary sexual development and to prevent osteoporosis in the longer term.

DISORDERS OF LIPID METABOLISM

Familial hypercholesterolaemia is the commonest autosomal dominant single gene disorder in Western society and is associated with a high morbidity and mortality through premature coronary artery disease (p. 217).

FAMILIAL HYPERCHOLESTEROLAEMIA

Persons with familial hypercholesterolaemia (FH) have elevated cholesterol levels with a significant risk of developing early coronary artery disease (p. 217). They can present in childhood or adolescence with sub-cutaneous deposition of lipid, known as xanthomata (Fig. 10.7). Starting with families who presented with

Fig. 10.7
Legs of a person homozygous for familial hypercholesterolaemia, showing multiple xanthomata. (Courtesy of Dr E Wraith, Royal Manchester Children's Hospital, Manchester.)

early coronary artery disease, Brown and Goldstein unraveled the biology of the low density lipoprotein (LDL) receptor (p. 218) and the pathological basis of FH.

Cells normally derive their cholesterol from either endogenous cholesterol synthesis or by uptake of dietary cholesterol from LDL receptors on the cell surface. Intracellular cholesterol levels are maintained by a feedback system with free cholesterol inhibiting LDL receptor synthesis as well as reducing the level of de novo endogenous cholesterol synthesis.

The high cholesterol levels in persons with FH are due to deficient or defective function of the LDL receptors which leads to increased levels of endogenous cholesterol synthesis. Four main functional types or classes of mutation in the LDL receptor have been identified: reduced or defective biosynthesis of the receptor; reduced or defective transport of the receptor from the endoplasmic reticulum to the Golgi apparatus; abnormal binding of the LDL by the receptor; and abnormal internalization of the LDL by the receptor (Fig. 10.8). Specific mutations are found more commonly in persons with FH from certain ethnic groups, as a result of founder effects (p. 118).

Dietary restriction of cholesterol intake and drug treatment with agents such as cholestyramine, which sequesters cholesterol from the enterohepatic circulation, can lower cholesterol levels and, in part, reduce the risk of coronary artery disease. The recent detailed elucidation of the metabolic and biosynthetic pathways of cholesterol has enabled further therapeutic measures through the development of drugs which inhibit the endogenous synthesis of cholesterol by inhibiting the enzyme HMG CoA reductase. These are proving to be more effective in preventing long-term complications.

LYSOSOMAL STORAGE DISORDERS

In addition to the inborn errors of metabolism, in which an enzyme defect leads to deficiency of an essential metabolite and accumulation of intermediate metabolic precursors, there are a number of disorders in which a deficiency of a lysosomal enzyme involved in the degradation of complex macromolecules leads to their accumulation. This accumulation occurs because macromolecules are normally in a constant state of flux with a delicate balance between their rates of synthesis and breakdown. Children born with lysosomal storage diseases are usually normal at birth but with the passage of time commence a downhill course of differing duration due to accumulation of one or more of a variety or type of macromolecules.

MUCOPOLYSACCHARIDOSES

Children with one of the mucopolysaccharidoses (MPSs) present with skeletal, vascular or central nervous system findings along with coarsening of the facial features. These features are due to progressive accumulation of sulphated polysaccharides (also known as glycosaminoglycans) caused by defective degradation of the carbohydrate side-chain of acid mucopolysaccharide.

Six different MPSs are recognized, based on clinical and genetic differences. Each specific MPS type has a characteristic pattern of excretion in the urine of the glycosaminoglycans, dermatan, heparan, keratan and chondroitin sulphate. Subsequent biochemical investigation has revealed the various types to be due to deficiency of different individual enzymes. All but

Fig. 10.8
Stages in cholesterol biosynthesis and in the metabolism of low density lipoprotein receptors indicating the types of mutation in familial hypercholesterolaemia. (Adapted from Brown M S, Goldstein J L 1986 A receptor-mediated pathway for cholesterol homeostasis. Science 232: 34–47.)

Hunter's syndrome, which is X-linked, are inherited as autosomal recessive disorders.

Hurler's syndrome (MPS I)

Hurler's syndrome is the most severe of the muco-polysaccharidoses. Affected infants present in the first year with corneal clouding, a characteristic curvature of the lower spine and subsequent poor growth. They develop hearing loss, coarse facial features, an enlarged liver and spleen, joint stiffness and vertebral changes in the second year. There is progression of these features along with mental deterioration and eventually death by the mid-teens from a combination of cardiac failure and respiratory infections.

The diagnosis of the Hurler syndrome was initially made by demonstration of the presence of meta-chromatic granules in the cells, i.e. lysosomes distended by the storage material which is primarily dermatan sulphate. Increased urinary excretion of dermatan and heparan sulphate is commonly used as a screening test but confirmation of the diagnosis involves demonstration of reduced activity of the lysosomal hydrolase, α-L-iduronidase. Less severe allelic forms of Hurler's syndrome, caused by varying levels of residual α-L-

iduronidase activity, were previously classified separately as Scheie's disease (MPS I S) and Hurler/Scheie disease (MPS I H/S).

Hunter's syndrome (MPS II)

Males with Hunter's syndrome usually present between the ages of 2 and 5 years with hearing loss, a history of recurrent infection, diarrhoea and poor growth. Examination reveals a characteristic coarsening of their facial features (Fig. 10.9), along with enlargement of their liver and spleen and stiffness of their joints. X-rays of the spine reveal abnormalities in the shape of the vertebrae. There is progressive physical and mental deterioration with death usually in the teenage years.

The diagnosis is confirmed by the presence of excess amounts of dermatan and heparan sulphate in the urine and deficient or decreased activity of the enzyme iduronate sulphate sulphatase in serum or white blood cells.

Sanfilippo syndrome (MPS III)

Sanfilippo syndrome is the most common MPS. Affected individuals present in their second year with mild coarsening of features, skeletal changes and progressive intellectual loss with behavioural problems, proceeding to convulsions and death in early adult life. The diagnosis is confirmed by the presence of increased urinary heparan and chondroitin sulphate excretion and deficiency of one of four enzymes involved in degradation of heparan sulphate; sulphaminidase (MPS III A), N-acetyl-α-D-glucosaminidase (MPS III B), acetyl-CoA-α-glucosaminidase-N-acetyltransferase (MPS III C) or N-acetyl-glucosamine-6-sulphate sulphatase (MPS III D). Individuals with these different enzyme deficiencies cannot be distinguished clinically.

Morquio syndrome (MPS IV)

Children with Morquio's syndrome present in the second or third year of life with skeletal abnormalities which include short stature, thoracic deformity and curvature of the spine (kyphoscoliosis). Intelligence is normal and survival is long term although there is a risk of spinal cord compression due to progression of skeletal involvement. The diagnosis is confirmed by the presence of keratan sulphate in the urine and deficiency of either galactosamine-6-sulphatase (MPS IV A) or β-galactosidase (MPS IV B).

Maroteaux–Lamy syndrome (MPS VI)

Individuals affected with the Maroteaux–Lamy syndrome present with Hurler-like features in early childhood. These include coarse facial featues, short stature with thoracic deformity, kyphosis and restriction of joint mobility. In addition they develop corneal clouding and cardiac valve abnormalities but retain normal intelligence. A less severe form presents later with survival into late adulthood, in contrast to the more severe form in which survival is usually only until the third decade. The diagnosis is confirmed by the presence of increased urinary dermatan sulphate excretion and arylsulphatase B deficiency in white blood cells or fibroblasts.

Sly syndrome (MPS VII)

Sly syndrome shows marked variability in the severity of presentation. This ranges from skeletal features which include mild kyphoscoliosis and hip dysplasia to coarse facial features, hepatosplenomegaly, corneal clouding, cardiac abnormalities and mental retardation with death in childhood or adolescence. Increased urinary glycosaminoglycans excretion and β-glucuronidase deficiency in serum, white blood cells or fibroblasts confirm the diagnosis.

Fig. 10.9
Facies of a male with the mucopolysaccharidosis, Hunter's syndrome. (Courtesy of Dr E Wraith, Royal Manchester Children's Hospital, Manchester.)

Treatment of the mucopolysaccharidoses

Treatment of the mucopolysaccharidoses has been attempted by enzyme replacement but there are a number of practical difficulties which have been responsible for its lack of success (p. 326). More recently, however, treatment by bone marrow transplantation has been attempted with varying reports of success biochemically and clinically in the skeletal and cerebral features (p. 327).

SPHINGOLIPIDOSES (LIPID STORAGE DISEASES)

In the sphingolipidoses there is an inability to degrade sphingolipid, resulting in the progressive deposition of lipid or glycolipid primarily in the brain, liver and spleen. Central nervous system involvement results in progressive mental deterioration, often with fits, usually resulting in death in childhood. There are at least 10 different types with specific enzyme deficiencies: Tay–Sachs, Gaucher's and Niemann–Pick disease are the most common.

Tay–Sachs disease

This is the best known sphingolipidosis and affects approximately 1 in 3600 persons of Ashkenazi-Jewish ancestry (p. 118). Affected infants usually present by 6 months of age with poor feeding, lethargy and floppiness. Loss of developmental milestones or developmental regression will usually become apparent in the second half of the first year. Feeding becomes increasingly difficult and the infant progressively deteriorates with deafness, visual impairment and spasticity which progresses to rigidity. Death usually occurs by the age of 3 years as a result of respiratory infection. Less severe juvenile, adult and chronic forms are also reported.

The diagnosis of Tay–Sachs disease is further supported clinically by the presence of a 'cherry-red' spot in the centre of the macula of the fundus. Biochemical confirmation of Tay–Sachs disease is by demonstration of reduced hexosaminidase A levels in serum, white blood cells or cultured fibroblasts. Reduced hexosaminidase A activity is due to deficiency of the α subunit of the enzyme β-hexosaminidase which leads to accumulation of the sphingolipid, GM_2 ganglioside. Deficiency of the β subunit of β-hexosaminidase leads to reduced activity of the isozyme, hexosaminidase B, causing the other GM_2 gangliosidosis, Sandhoff disease in which affected individuals present with similar clinical features.

Gaucher's disease

This is the commonest sphingolipidosis, and like Tay–Sachs disease, it occurs with an increased frequency among persons of Ashkenazi-Jewish ancestry. There are two main types based on the age of onset. In type I, or the adult type which is the most common form of Gaucher's disease, affected persons present with febrile episodes and limb, joint or trunk pain and a tendency to pathologic fractures. Clinical examination usually reveals an enlarged spleen and liver. Affected persons often show mild anaemia and X-ray changes in the vertebral bodies and proximal femora. The central nervous system is spared.

In type II, or infantile Gaucher's disease, central nervous involvement is a major feature. Affected infants usually present between 3–6 months of age with failure to thrive and hepatosplenomegaly. By 6 months of age they begin to show developmental regression and neurological deterioration with spasticity and fits leading on to recurrent pulmonary infection and death in the second year.

The diagnosis of Gaucher's disease is confirmed by reduced activity of the enzyme glucosylceramide β-glucosidase in white blood cells or cultured fibroblasts.

Treatment of individuals with the adult type of Gaucher's disease involves symptomatic relief of pain. In addition, it is often necessary to remove the enlarged spleen because it causes a secondary anaemia due to premature sequestering of red blood cells, a condition known as hypersplenism.

The lack of central nervous system involvement in type I Gaucher's disease meant that it was an obvious candidate for enzyme replacement therapy since it was not necessary for the enzyme to cross the blood-brain barrier (p. 326). Initial attempts to treat adults with Gaucher's disease by enzyme replacement therapy met with little success because of difficulty in obtaining sufficient quantities of enzyme and targeting the appropriate sites. However, modification of β-glucosidase by the addition of mannose-6-phosphate which targets the enzyme to macrophage lysosomes has led to dramatic alleviation of symptoms and regression of the organomegaly in affected persons. The treatment is, however, expensive and treatment regimens using lower doses and alternative methods to target the enzyme more efficiently are being assessed.

Niemann–Pick disease

Infants with Niemann–Pick disease present in infancy with failure to thrive and hepatomegaly and can be found to have a cherry-red spot on their macula. Developmental regression rapidly progresses by the end of the first year, with death by the age of four. A characteristic finding is the presence of what are called foam cells in the bone marrow due to sphingomyelin accumulation. Confirmation of the diagnosis is by demonstration of deficiency of the enzyme sphingomyelinase. A less severe form without neurological involvement has been reported. Niemann–Pick disease, like Tay–Sachs and Gaucher's disease, occurs more commonly in Jews of Ashkenazi Eastern European ancestry.

DISORDERS OF PURINE/PYRIMIDINE METABOLISM

Gout is the disorder in humans which is classically associated with abnormalities of purine metabolism. Joint pain, swelling and tenderness are a result of the inflammatory response of the body to deposits of crystals of a salt of uric acid. In fact, only a minority of persons who present with gout are found to have an inborn error of metabolism. The cause in most instances results from a combination of genetic and environmental factors; it is, however, always important to consider disorders which can result in an increased turnover of purines (e.g. a malignancy such as leukaemia) or reduced secretion of the metabolites (e.g. renal impairment) as a possible underlying precipitating cause.

LESCH–NYHAN SYNDROME

A particularly disabling disorder of purine metabolism is the Lesch–Nyhan syndrome. This X-linked disorder is due to the deficiency of the enzyme hypoxanthine guanine phosphoribosyltransferase which results in increased levels of phosphoribosylpyrophosphate. The latter is normally a rate-limiting chemical in the synthesis of purines. Its excess leads to an increased rate of purine synthesis which results in an accumulation of excessive amounts of uric acid and some of its metabolic precursors. The main effect is on the central nervous system, resulting in uncontrolled movements, spasticity, mental retardation and compulsive self-mutilation. Although drugs such as allopurinol, which inhibit uric acid formation, can lower uric acid levels, none yet offers any satisfactory treatment for the debilitating central nervous system effects.

IMMUNODEFICIENCY DISEASES CAUSED BY DEFECTS IN PURINE METABOLISM

Two inherited immunodeficiency disorders (p. 183), somewhat surprisingly, are inborn errors of purine metabolism.

Adenosine deaminase deficiency

About a half of all children with the autosomal recessive form of severe combined immunodeficiency with impaired B and T cell function (p. 184) have deficiency of the enzyme adenosine deaminase. Affected children present in the first year of life with recurrent viral and bacterial infections and, if untreated, will die of overwhelming infection in the first year. The diagnosis is confirmed by deficient red blood cell adenosine deaminase activity. Correction of the immunodeficiency by transfusion of irradiated red blood cells has been reported. More recently bone marrow transplantation has been successfully carried out, even antenatally in utero!

Purine nucleoside phosphorylase deficiency

A proportion of children susceptible to severe, recurrent and potentially lethal viral infections with isolated impaired T cell function have been shown to have a deficiency of the enzyme purine nucleoside phosphorylase. Treatment with irradiated red blood cells has been reported to result in a temporary improvement in immune function.

HEREDITARY OROTIC ACIDURIA

Children with hereditary orotic aciduria present in the first year of life with a megaloblastic anaemia, failure to thrive and developmental delay. They have deficiency of one of two enzymes, orotate phosphoribosyltransferase or orotidine-5'-phosphate decarboxylase, both of which are necessary for the synthesis of pyrimidines, resulting in excretion of large quantities of orotic acid in the urine. Treatment with the pyrimidine, uridine, has been reported to reduce urinary orotic acid excretion, correct the anaemia and restore growth.

DISORDERS OF PORPHYRIN METABOLISM

There are several different disorders of porphyrin metabolism which are due to deficiency of enzymes in the biosynthetic pathway of the iron containing group in haemoglobin, haem (p. 139). They are all inherited as autosomal dominant disorders, except for congenital erythropoietic porphyria which is an autosomal recessive disorder. This is because the enzymes are rate limiting (p. 23), so that haploinsufficiency results in clinical disease.

The different types of porphyria are variably associated with neurological or visceral involvement and cutaneous photosensitivity due to accumulation of the different porphyrin precursors in those organs. The porphyrias are divided into two types depending on whether the excess production of porphyrins occurs predominantly in the liver or in the erythropoietic system.

HEPATIC PORPHYRIAS

These include acute intermittent porphyria, hereditary coproporphyria and porphyria variegata.

Acute intermittent porphyria

Acute intermittent porphyria (AIP) is characterized by attacks of abdominal pain, vomiting and mental disturbance in the form of confusion, emotional upset or hallucinations. Attacks can be precipitated by the administration of certain drugs, such as exogenous steroids, anticonvulsants and barbiturates. It is caused by a partial deficiency of the enzyme uroporphyrinogen I synthetase leading to increased excretion of the porphyrin precursors porphobilinogen and δ-aminolevulinic acid in urine.

Hereditary coproporphyria

In hereditary coproporphyria, a related condition, also inherited as a dominant trait, there is partial deficiency of the enzyme coproporphyrinogen oxidase. The disorder is clinically indistinguishable from acute intermittent porphyria although approximately one-third of affected persons also have photosensitivity of their skin.

Porphyria variegata

Persons with this form of porphyria, which is particularly prevalent in those of Afrikaner origin in South Africa (p. 97), have variable skin photosensitivity with neurological and visceral findings which can also be triggered by drugs. Increased faecal excretion of the porphyrin precursors protoporphyrin and coproporphyrin can be demonstrated and the disorder has been shown to be due to deficiency of the enzyme protoporphyrinogen oxidase.

ERYTHROPOIETIC PORPHYRIAS

The erythropoietic porphyrias include congential erythropoietic porphyria and erythropoietic protoporphyria.

Congenital erythropoietic porphyria

The main feature of congenital erythropoietic porphyria (CEP) is an extreme photosensitivity with blistering of the skin leading to extensive scarring, to the extent that most affected persons are unable to go out in normal daylight. In addition, many have a haemolytic anaemia requiring regular blood transfusion and frequently splenectomy. Affected individuals have red-brown discolouration of their teeth, which show red fluorescence under ultraviolet light. Congential erythropoietic porphyria is due to deficiency of the enzyme uroporphyrinogen III synthase.

Erythropoietic protoporphyria

Erythropoietic protoporphyria (EPP) is due to deficiency of the enzyme ferrochelatase which is responsible for the insertion of ferrous iron into the porphyrin precursor to form haem. Affected persons have photosensitivity and can sometimes develop chronic liver disease. Successful treatment of the photosensitivity has been reported with β-carotene.

ORGANIC ACID DISORDERS

Children affected with one of the organic acid disorders present with periodic episodes of poor feeding, vomiting and lethargy in association with a severe metabolic acidosis, low white cell (neutropenia) and platelet (thrombocytopenia) counts, low blood sugar (hypoglycaemia) and high blood ammonia levels (hyperammonaemia). These episodes are often precipitated by intercurrent illness or increased protein intake and, after such an episode, affected children can lose developmental skills. Analysis of blood from children at the time of these episodes reveals high levels of glycine, i.e. hyperglycinaemia. It was subsequently found that the acidosis in these episodes was due to increased levels of the organic acids, either propionic or methylmalonic acid.

The two autosomal recessive organic acid disorders methylmalonic acidaemia (MMA) and propionic acidaemia (PPA) are caused by deficiency of the enzymes methylmalonyl-CoA mutase and proprionyl-CoA carboxylase respectively. The enzyme deficiency results in accumulation of the toxic organic acid metabolites derived from deamination of certain amino acids, specific long chain fatty acids and cholesterol sidechains. Therapy of the acute episode involves treatment of any infection, fluid replacement, correction of the metabolic acidosis and cessation of protein intake. Long-term prophylactic treatment involves restriction of protein intake and rapid recognition and management of any intercurrent illness. A proportion of individuals affected with propionic acidaemia are responsive to biotin while some persons with methylmalonic acidaemia are sensitive to vitamin B_{12}.

DISORDERS OF COPPER METABOLISM

There are two inborn errors of copper metabolism, Menkes' disease and Wilson's disease.

MENKES' DISEASE

Menkes' disease is an X-linked disorder with affected males presenting in the first few months of life with feeding difficulties, vomiting and poor weight gain. Subsequently floppinesss (hypotonia), fits and progressive neurological deterioration ensue with death due to recurrent respiratory infection usually occurring by the age of three years. A characteristic feature is the hair, which lacks pigment and is kinky and brittle and breaks easily. This was noted to resemble the wool of sheep suffering from copper deficiency. Serum copper and caeruloplasmin levels are very low. Cloning of the gene for Menkes' disease was facilitated through an affected female with an X;autosome translocation (p. 74) and revealed it to code for an ATPase cation transport protein for copper. Treatment regimens with different exogenous copper sources have had limited benefit to date.

WILSON'S DISEASE

Persons affected with the autosomal recessive disorder Wilson's disease commonly present in childhood or the early teenage years with fits and abnormal neurological findings. These can include deterioration of coordination, involuntary movements, abnormal tone, dysarthria (difficulty in speaking), dysphagia (difficulty with swallowing) and changes in behaviour or frank pyschiatric disturbance. Clinical examination can reveal the presence of what is called a Kayser–Fleischer ring, which is a golden brown or greenish collarette at the corneal margin. Investigation can reveal the presence of abnormal liver function, which can progress on to cirrhosis.

High copper levels in the liver, decreased serum concentrations of the copper transport protein, caeruloplasmin, and abnormal copper loading tests are suggestive of the diagnosis. The gene for Wilson's disease was cloned on the basis of anticipated homology to the Menkes' gene and the gene product has been shown to be an ATPase cation transport protein involved in copper transfer from the hepatocytes to the biliary collecting system.

There are dramatic reports of striking improvement of the neurological features in persons with Wilson's disease using the chelating agents D-penicillamine and trientine, although these can cause side-effects (p. 326).

PEROXISOMAL DISORDERS

The peroxisomes are subcellular organelles bound by a single trilayer lipid membrane present in all cells; they are especially abundant in liver and renal parenchymal cells. The organelle matrix contains more than 40 enzymes which carry out a number of reactions involved in fatty acid oxidation and cholesterol biosynthesis interacting with metabolic pathways outside the peroxisomes. The enzymes of the peroxisomal matrix are synthesized on the polyribosomes, enter the cytosol and are transferred into the peroxisomes.

There are two main categories of peroxisomal disorders, disorders of peroxisome biogenesis, such as the Zellweger's syndrome, in which there are severely reduced numbers of peroxisomes in all cells and single isolated peroxisomal enzyme deficiencies, such as X-linked adrenoleukodystrophy.

ZELLWEGER'S SYNDROME

Newborn infants with Zellweger's syndrome present with hypotonia and weakness and have mildly dysmorphic facial features (Fig. 10.10) consisting of a prominent forehead and a large anterior fontanelle ('soft spot'). They may also have cataracts and an enlarged liver. They generally go on to have fits with developmental regression and usually die by 1 year of age. Investigations can reveal renal cysts and abnormal

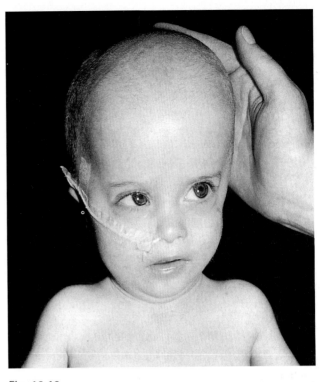

Fig. 10.10
Facies of an infant with Zellweger's syndrome showing a prominent forehead.

Fig. 10.11
Radiograph of the knee of a newborn infant with Zellweger's syndrome showing abnormal punctate calcification of the distal femoral epiphyses.

calcification in the cartilaginous growing ends of the long bones (Fig. 10.11). There is a range of severity of this disorder with different clinical diagnoses being given to the less severe types. The diagnosis can be confirmed by elevated levels of plasma long chain fatty acids. The gene for the Zellweger syndrome encodes a protein involved in the peroxisome assembly.

It is unusual for inborn errors of metabolism to be associated with a dysmorphic syndrome (p. 229). In addition to the Zellweger syndrome, the Smith–Lemli–

Opitz syndrome has recently been found to be caused by an inborn error of cholesterol biosynthesis.

ADRENOLEUKODYSTROPHY

Males with the X-linked disorder adrenoleukodystrophy (ALD) classically present in late childhood with deteriorating school performance, although affected males can present at any age and even, on occasion, be asymptomatic. A proportion of affected males can also present in adult life with less severe neurological features and adrenal insufficiency, or what is termed adrenomyeloneuropathy. ALD has been shown to be associated with a deficiency of the enzyme very long chain fatty acid (VLCFA) CoA synthetase but is secondary to deficiency of a peroxisomal membrane protein.

Treatment of ALD is being undertaken with a diet which uses an oil as a source of fat which has low levels of the very long chain fatty acids. This has been popularly called 'Lorenzo's oil' after a film of that name made about a child with adrenoleukodystrophy. The efficacy of this diet has, however, been disappointing.

PRENATAL DIAGNOSIS OF THE INBORN ERRORS OF METABOLISM

In the majority of the inborn errors of metabolism in which an abnormal or deficient gene product can be identified, prenatal diagnosis is possible. Until recently this has been by biochemical analysis of cultured amniocytes obtained at mid-trimester amniocentesis. Techniques are now available for detection of many of the inborn errors of metabolism using direct or cultured chorionic villi, allowing first-trimester diagnosis (p. 303). In addition, in many instances, biochemical assays are being replaced by the use of linked DNA sequence variants or identification of specific mutations (p. 68). This latter approach is of particular value for the inborn errors of metabolism in which the biochemical basis has not yet been identified or the enzyme is not expressed in amniocytes or chorionic villi.

FURTHER READING

Benson P F, Fensom A H 1985 Genetic biochemical disorders. Oxford University Press, Oxford
A good reference source for detailed basic further information on the inborn errors of metabolism.
Cohn R M, Roth K S 1983 Metabolic disease: a guide to early recognition. Saunders, Philadelphia
Useful text as it considers the inborn errors from their mode of presentation rather than starting from the diagnosis.
Garrod A E 1908 Inborn errors of metabolism. Lancet ii: 1–7, 73–79, 142–148, 214–220
Reports of the first inborn errors of metabolism.
Rimoin D L, Connor J M, Pyeritz R E, Korf B R (eds) 2001 Principles and practice of medical genetics, 4th edn. Churchill Livingstone, Edinburgh
The section on metabolic disorders includes 13 chapters covering in succinct detail the various groups of metabolic disorders.
Scriver C R, Beaudet A L, Sly W S, Valle D (eds) 2000 The metabolic basis of inherited disease, 8th edn. McGraw Hill, New York
A huge multiauthor three volume comprehensive detailed text on biochemical genetics with an exhaustive reference list and, with this edition, a CD-ROM.

ELEMENTS

① Metabolic processes in all species occur in steps, each being controlled by a particular enzyme which is the product of a specific gene, leading to the one gene–one enzyme concept.

② A block in a metabolic pathway results in the accumulation of metabolic intermediates and/or a deficiency of the end-product of the particular metabolic pathway concerned, a so-called inborn error of metabolism.

③ The majority of the inborn errors of metabolism are inherited as autosomal recessive or X-linked recessive traits. A few are inherited as autosomal dominant disorders involving rate-limiting enzymes, cell surface receptors or multimeric enzymes, through haploinsufficiency or dominant negative mutations.

④ A number of the inborn errors of metabolism can be screened for in the newborn period and successfully treated by dietary restriction or supplementation.

⑤ Prenatal diagnosis of many of the inborn errors of metabolism is possible either by conventional biochemical methods, the use of linked DNA markers or by direct mutation detection.

Pharmacogenetics

DEFINITION

Some individuals can be especially sensitive to the effects of a particular drug, whereas others can be quite resistant. Such individual variation can be the result of factors which are not genetic. For example, both the young and the elderly are very sensitive to morphine and its derivatives, as are persons with liver disease. Individual differences in response to drugs in humans are, however, often genetically determined.

The term *pharmacogenetics* was introduced by Vogel in 1959 for the study of genetically determined variations that are revealed solely by the effects of drugs. Such a definition would strictly exclude those hereditary disorders in which symptoms are usually only precipitated or aggravated by drugs. Many investigators, however, also include these latter disorders within the sphere of pharmacogenetics.

Pharmacogenetics is an important branch of genetics because adverse drug reactions are a major cause of morbidity and mortality. It is also likely to be of increasing importance in the future, particularly as a result of the development of new drugs from information which becomes available from the Human Genome Project, or what has been termed *pharmacogenomics*. In addition, these developments will extend our understanding of the inherited differences which lead to susceptibility for the common diseases which are the consequence of interaction with environmental or occupational exposures, or what is termed *ecogenetics*.

DRUG METABOLISM

The metabolism of a drug usually follows a common sequence of events (Fig. 11.1). A drug is first absorbed from the gut, passes into the bloodstream, and so becomes distributed and partitioned in the various tissues and tissue fluids. Only a small proportion of the total dose of a drug will be responsible for producing a specific

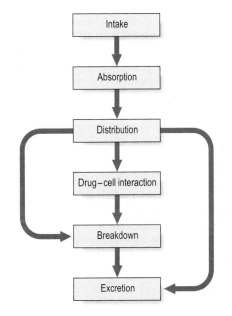

Fig. 11.1
Stages of metabolism of a drug.

pharmacological effect, most of it being broken down or excreted unchanged.

BIOCHEMICAL MODIFICATION

The actual breakdown process, which usually takes place in the liver, varies with different drugs. Some are completely oxidized to carbon dioxide which is exhaled through the lungs. Others are excreted in modified forms either via the kidneys into the urine, or by the liver into the bile and thence the faeces. Many drugs undergo biochemical modifications which increase their solubility resulting in them being more readily excreted.

One important biochemical modification of many drugs is conjugation, which involves union with the carbohydrate glucuronic acid. Glucuronide conjugation occurs primarily in the liver. The elimination of morphine and its derivatives, such as codeine, is almost entirely dependent on this process. Isoniazid, used in the treatment of tuberculosis, and a number of other drugs, including the sulphonamides, are modified by the introduction of an acetyl group into the molecule, a process known as acetylation (Fig. 11.2).

KINETICS OF DRUG METABOLISM

The study of the metabolism and effects of a particular drug usually involves giving a standard dose of the drug and then after a suitable time interval determining the response, measuring the amount of the drug circulating in the blood or determining the rate at which it is metabolized. Such studies show that there is considerable variation in the way different individuals respond to certain drugs. This variability in response can be continuous or discontinuous.

If a dose–response test is carried out on a large number of subjects, their results can be plotted. A number of different possible responses can be seen (Fig. 11.3). In continuous variation the results form a bell-shaped or unimodal distribution. With discontinuous variation the curve is bimodal or sometimes even trimodal. A discontinuous response suggests that the metabolism of the drug is under monogenic control. For example, if the normal metabolism of a drug is controlled by a dominant gene, R, and if some people are unable to metabolize the drug because they are homozygous for a recessive gene, r, there will be three classes of individuals: RR, Rr and rr. If the responses of RR and Rr are indistinguishable, then a bimodal distribution will result. If RR and Rr are distinguishable, then a trimodal distribution will result, each peak or mode representing a different genotype. A unimodal distribution implies that the metabolism of the drug in question is under the control of many genes, i.e. is polygenic (p. 127).

GENETIC VARIATIONS REVEALED SOLELY BY THE EFFECTS OF DRUGS

Among the best known examples of drugs which have been responsible for revealing genetic variation in response are isoniazid, succinylcholine, primaquine, coumarin anticoagulants, certain anaesthetic agents, the thiopurines, phenylbutazone, debrisoquine and alcohol.

N-ACETYLTRANSFERASE ACTIVITY

Isoniazid is one of the drugs used in the treatment of tuberculosis. It has been shown that it is rapidly absorbed from the gut, resulting in an initial high blood level which is slowly reduced as the drug is inactivated and excreted. The metabolism of isoniazid allows two groups to be distinguished: rapid and slow inactivators. In the former, blood levels of the drug fall rapidly after an oral

Fig. 11.2
Acetylation of the antituberculosis drug isoniazid.

Fig. 11.3
Various types of response to different drugs consistent with polygenic and monogenic control of drug metabolism. (A) Continuous variation, multifactorial control of drug metabolism, (B) discontinous bimodal variation, (C) discontinuous trimodal variation.

dose; in the latter, blood levels remain high for some time. Family studies have shown that slow inactivators of isoniazid are homozygous for an autosomal recessive allele of the liver enzyme N-acetyltransferase with lower activity levels. N-acetyltransferase activity varies in different populations. In the United States and Western Europe about 50% of the population are slow inactivators, in contrast to the Japanese who are predominately rapid inactivators.

In some individuals, isoniazid can cause side-effects such as polyneuritis, a systemic lupus erythematosus-like disorder, or liver damage. Blood levels of isoniazid remain higher for longer periods in slow inactivators than in rapid inactivators on equivalent doses. Slow inactivators have a significantly greater risk of developing side-effects on doses which rapid inactivators require to ensure adequate blood levels for successful treatment of tuberculosis. Conversely, rapid inactivators have an increased risk of liver damage due to isoniazid. A number of other drugs are also metabolized by *N*-acetyltransferase and therefore slow inactivators of isoniazid are also more likely to exhibit side-effects. These drugs include hydralazine which is an antihypertensive and sulphasalazine which is a sulphonamide derivative used to treat Crohn's disease.

DNA studies

Studies in other animal species led to the cloning of the genes responsible for *N*-acetyltransferase activity in humans. This has revealed that there are three genes, one of which is not expressed and represents a pseudogene (NATP), one which does not exhibit differences in activity between individuals (NAT1), and a third (NAT2), mutations in which are responsible for the inherited polymorphic variation. These inherited variations in NAT2 have been reported to modify the risk of developing a number of cancers which include bladder, colorectal, breast and lung cancer. This is thought to be through differences in acetylation of aromatic and heterocyclic amine carcinogens.

SUCCINYLCHOLINE SENSITIVITY

Curare is a plant extract used in hunting by certain South American Indian tribes, which produces profound muscular paralysis. Medically, curare is used in surgical operations because of the muscular relaxation it produces. Succinylcholine, also known as suxamethonium, is another drug which produces muscular relaxation, though by a different mechanism from curare. Suxamethonium has the advantage over curare that the relaxation of skeletal and respiratory muscles and the consequent apnoea (cessation of breathing) it induces is only short-lived. Therefore it is most often used in the induction phase of an anaesthetic for intubation. The anaesthetist, therefore, needs to maintain respiration by artificial means for only 2–3 minutes before it returns spontaneously. However, about one patient in every 2000 has a period of apnoea which can last an hour or more after the use of suxamethonium. It was found that the apnoea in such instances can be corrected by transfusion of blood or plasma from a normal person. The anaesthetist, if a suxamethonium induced apnea occurs, has to maintain respiration until the effects of the drug have worn off.

Succinylcholine is normally destroyed in the body by the plasma enzyme pseudocholinesterase. In patients who are highly sensitive to succinylcholine, the plasma pseudocholinesterase in their blood destroys the drug at a markedly slower rate than normal or in some very rare cases is entirely deficient. Family studies have shown that succinylcholine sensitivity is inherited as an autosomal recessive trait.

A refined method of studying plasma pseudocholinesterase activity in the blood involves determining the percentage inhibition of the enzyme by the local anaesthetic dibucaine (syn: cinchocaine). The result is termed the dibucaine number. The frequency distribution of dibucaine number values in families with succinylcholine-sensitive individuals gives a trimodal curve. The three modes represent the normal homozygotes, the heterozygotes and the affected homozygotes.

GLUCOSE-6-PHOSPHATE DEHYDROGENASE VARIANTS

For many years, quinine was the drug of choice in the treatment of malaria. Although it has been very effective in acute attacks, it is not very effective in preventing relapses. In 1926 primaquine was introduced and proved to be much better than quinine in preventing relapses. However, it was not long after primaquine was introduced that some people were found to be sensitive to the drug. The drug could be taken for a few days with no apparent ill effects, and then suddenly some individuals would begin to pass very dark, often black, urine. Jaundice developed and the red cell count and haemoglobin concentration gradually fell as a consequence of haemolysis of the red blood cells. Affected individuals usually recovered from such a haemolytic episode but occasionally the destruction of the red cells was extensive enough to be fatal. The cause of such cases of primaquine sensitivity was subsequently shown to be a deficiency in the red cell enzyme glucose-6-phosphate dehydrogenase (G6PD).

Family studies have shown that G6PD deficiency is inherited as an X-linked recessive trait (p. 102). G6PD deficiency is rare in most Caucasians but affects about 10% of Afro-Caribbean males and is also relatively common in males of Mediterranean origin. G6PD deficiency is thought to be relatively common in these populations as a result of conferring increased resistance to the malarial parasite. The red cell G6PD levels in persons of Mediterranean extraction with G6PD deficiency are very much lower than in persons of Afro-Caribbean origin with G6PD deficiency.

Persons with G6PD deficiency are sensitive not only to primaquine but also to many other compounds which include phenacetin, nitrofurantoin and certain sulphonamides. These drugs should be used with caution in males of Afro-Caribbean and Mediterranean origin if their G6PD status is unknown, and in a person known to be G6PD-deficient such drugs are absolutely contra-indicated. Drug-induced haemolysis is uncommon and, in fact, the main risk of G6PD deficiency is favism, in which a haemolytic crisis occurs after eating fava beans. This is thought to be the first recognized pharmacogenetic disorder, having been described by Pythagoras around 500 BC!

COUMARIN METABOLISM

Coumarin anticoagulant drugs, such as warfarin, are used in the treatment of a number of different disorders to prevent the blood from clotting, e.g. after a deep venous thrombosis. There is discontinuous variation in the response of some patients taking these drugs, which involves an increased resistance to the effects of the anti-coagulant and is transmitted as an autosomal dominant trait.

MALIGNANT HYPERTHERMIA

Malignant hyperthermia (MH) is a rare complication of anaesthesia. Susceptible individuals develop muscle rigidity as well as an increased temperature (hyper-thermia), often as high as 42.3°C (108°F) during anaes-thesia. This usually occurs when halothane is used as the anaesthetic agent, particularly when succinylcholine is used as the muscle relaxant for intubation. If it is not recognized rapidly and treated with vigorous cooling, the affected individual will die.

MH susceptibility is inherited as an autosomal dominant trait affecting approximately 1 in 10 000 persons. Susceptible individuals occasionally have a raised serum creatine kinase level but this cannnot be used as a reliable screening test for at risk family members. The most reliable prediction of an individual's susceptibility status requires a muscle biopsy with in vitro muscle contracture testing in response to exposure to halothane and caffeine.

A person known or suspected of being susceptible to MH can undergo a general anaesthetic provided that recognized precipitating anaesthetic agents are avoided. Should hyperthermia develop during surgery, it is treated by cooling and intravenous procaine or procainamide but most effectively with dantrolene.

Malignant hyperthermia is genetically heterogeneous with a number of different genes having been identified as being responsible. Only a minority of families show linkage to or mutations in the ryanodine receptor gene on the long arm of chromosome 19.

THIOPURINE METHYLTRANSFERASE

A group of potentially toxic substances known as the thiopurines, which include 6-mercaptopurine, 6-thioguanine and azathioprine, are used extensively in the treatment of leukaemia, to suppress the immune response in patients with autoimmune disorders such as systemic lupus erythematosus and to prevent rejection of organ transplants. They are very effective drugs clinically but have serious side-effects such as leucopenia and severe liver damage. The response to these drugs varies widely and it has not been possible to predict either those who are likely to develop such side-effects or the possible therapeutic response in the individual patient. An important step in the metabolism of these compounds is methylation catalysed by the enzyme thiopurine methyltransferase (TPMT). It appears that erythrocyte TPMT activity is polymorphic, with roughly 0.3% of the population having undetectable activity. Individuals with these low levels are likely to respond less well to these drugs but could also be in danger of developing serious side-effects. Those with high TPMT activity levels could be treated more aggressively with these drugs, resulting in a better therapeutic response, which has been suggested to be the case in childhood leukaemia.

PHENYLBUTAZONE METABOLISM

Phenylbutazone is used in the treatment of the more severe forms of arthritis. The metabolism of this drug differs from the examples discussed so far in that it appears to be under polygenic control. Individuals who are relatively slow in metabolizing phenylbutazone are more likely to develop drug-associated side-effects such as hypoplastic anaemia.

DEBRISOQUINE METABOLISM

Debrisoquine is a drug which was frequently used in the past for the treatment of hypertension. There is a bimodal distribution in the response to the drug in the general population. Approximately 5–10% of persons of European origin are poor metabolizers, being homozygotes for an autosomal recessive gene with reduced hydroxylation activity. Such individuals are more prone to overreact to the drug and develop hypotension with treatment. They are also more susceptible to adverse reactions to several other drugs such as the β-blockers propranolol and metoprolol, the antidepressants amitryptiline and imipramine and the antipsychotics thioridazine and haloperidol.

DNA studies

Molecular studies have revealed that the gene involved in debrisoquine metabolism is one of the P450 family of genes on chromosome 22, known as CYP2D6. The mutations responsible for the poor metabolizer phenotype are heterogeneous, either a splice site mutation (p. 23) resulting in a truncated gene product or a deletion of the gene. It is postulated that these enzymes could have evolved in the past to metabolize dietary toxic plant alkaloids.

ALCOHOL METABOLISM

Under the heading of pharmacogenetics we can also include alcoholism and alcoholic cirrhosis, which in terms of its frequency and social implications dwarf all others, although some persons would debate whether alcohol should really be considered a drug. Alcoholism is clearly related to the amount consumed as well as to dietary and various social and economic factors. Nevertheless, evidence is gradually emerging which clearly indicates that genetic factors can also be involved. Some of this evidence is based on twin studies, which have shown high concordance rates (p. 210), and family studies, which have shown a high prevalence of alcohol-related problems among relatives of alcoholics. Clearly, however, behaviour patterns within families could artificially inflate what would appear to be genetic factors. Similarly, apparent racial or ethnic differences in the incidence of alcoholism, such as the high incidence among certain American Indians and Eskimos, could well be affected by social factors.

Perhaps the most convincing evidence for the possible role of genetic factors in alcoholism comes from the study of the enzymes involved in alcohol metabolism. Alcohol is metabolized in the liver by alcohol dehydrogenase (ADH) to acetaldehyde, and then further degraded by acetaldehyde dehydrogenase (ALDH). Human ADH consists of dimers of various combinations of subunits of three different polypeptide units coded for by three loci, ADH1 coding for the α subunit, ADH2 for the β subunit and ADH3 for the γ subunit. ADH1 is primarily expressed in early fetal life, while ADH2 is expressed in adult life.

Persons of Far East Asian origin tolerate alcohol less well than persons of Caucasian origin and often exhibit an acute flushing reaction to it (p. 213). This sensitivity is due to differences in the rate of metabolism of acetaldehyde. There are two major acetaldehyde dehydrogenase variants or isozymes, ALDH1 which is present in the cytosol and ALDH2 which is present in the mitochondria. The acute flushing reaction to alcohol in Far East Asians has been shown, in fact, to be due to absent ALDH2 activity. It has been suggested that this unpleasant reaction could account for the reported lower incidence of alcoholism and alcohol-related liver disease in that population.

HEREDITARY DISORDERS WITH ALTERED DRUG RESPONSE

Not all investigators include hereditary disorders with altered drug response within the sphere of pharmacogenetics. However, this is of immense importance in medical practice.

PORPHYRIA VARIEGATA

Porphyria variegata, one of the types of porphyria (p. 166), is inherited as an autosomal dominant trait. Some affected individuals develop skin lesions particularly on sun-exposed surfaces. Others have attacks of severe abdominal pain, muscular paralysis or mental disturbance. During an acute attack the patient can die. An acute attack can be precipitated by barbiturates and a number of other medications.

HAEMOGLOBINOPATHIES

Sulphonamides can cause severe haemolysis in individuals with certain haemoglobinopathies. Examples include haemoglobin H, a haemoglobin which consists entirely of β-globin chains, and haemoglobin Zurich which was first described in members of a Swiss family in 1962. These haemoglobinopathies are, however, very rare.

GOUT AND CHLOROTHIAZIDE

The treatment of congestive heart failure often involves the use of diuretics. These drugs increase the excretion of water and consequently reduce the amount of oedema. One of the most widely used diuretics is chlorothiazide. Not long after it was first used, it was realized that chlorothiazide diuretics could cause problems in persons who suffer from gout. In genetically predisposed individuals attacks often follow dietary excesses which lead to an elevation in serum uric acid. Chlorothiazide has a similar effect by raising the serum level of uric acid in genetically predisposed individuals.

CRIGLER–NAJJAR SYNDROME

The Crigler–Najjar syndrome is characterized by a severe non-haemolytic jaundice, appearing on the first or second day after birth, and can result in deposition of unconjugated bilirubin in the central nervous system leading to neurological sequelae. Affected children often die in infancy. The condition is inherited as an autosomal recessive trait, heterozygotes being perfectly healthy. The basic defect is an inability of the liver to conjugate bilirubin with glucuronides due to a deficiency of the enzyme glucuronyl transferase. Affected individuals are unable to conjugate certain drugs such as salicylates.

NON–INSULIN DEPENDENT DIABETES

In the form of non-insulin-dependent diabetes inherited as an autosomal dominant trait, maturity onset diabetes of the young (p. 213), it has been suggested that those at risk of developing the disease develop facial flushing after alcohol if they are first given the oral hypoglycaemic drug chlorpropamide. Although it was hoped that this could prove a useful test for familial susceptibility to diabetes and more recently to identify those at risk of developing complications of diabetes, there have been no consistent findings.

EVOLUTIONARY ORIGIN OF VARIATION IN DRUG RESPONSES

What is the evolutionary significance of genetic variations in response to certain drugs in particular ethnic groups (Table 11.1)? Man has been exposed to these drugs for no more than a few decades yet there is no doubt that mutations in genes conferring abnormal responses to these drugs arose, in many instances, many thousands of years ago. There is evidence in the case of G6PD deficiency that it can confer some protection against malaria. With most hereditary variation in response to drugs we have very little idea of how or why it arose. A mutation could have conferred selective advantage under certain past dietary or environmental conditions or have conferred resistance to particular infections.

PHARMACOGENOMICS

Pharmacogenomics is defined as the development of new drugs from the discovery of new genes and DNA sequence information from the Human Genome Project (p. 322). The premise is that inherited variation at the DNA level results in functional variation in the gene products which will play an essential role in determining the variability in responses, both therapeutic and adverse, to a drug. If polymorphic DNA sequence variation occurs in the coding portion or regulatory regions of genes, it is likely to result in variation in the gene product through alteration of function, activity or level of expression. Automated analysis of SNPs (p. 67) allows the possibility of identifying genes involved in drug metabolism, transport and receptors, which are likely to play a role in determining the variability in efficacy, side effects and toxicity of a drug.

ECOGENETICS

An extension of pharmacogenetics is the study of genetically determined differences in susceptibility to the action of physical, chemical and infectious agents in the environment. This has been referred to as *ecogenetics*, a term first coined by Brewer in 1971. Such differences in susceptibility can be either unifactorial or multifactorial in causation (Table 11.2).

ORGANOPHOSPHATE METABOLISM

Paraoxonase is an enzyme which catalyses the breakdown of organophosphates which are widely used as insecticides in agriculture. Individuals can have different enzyme activity levels which result from a two allele

Table 11.1   Ethnic variations in some pharmacogenetic disorders

Disorder	Ethnic group	Frequency (%)
Slow acetylation	Europeans	50
	Orientals	10
Pseudocholinesterase variants	Europeans	<1
	Eskimos	1–2
G6PD deficiency	N. Europeans	<1
	S. Europeans	up to 25
	Afro-Caribbeans	10
Atypical ADH	Europeans	5
	Orientals	85

Table 11.2   Ecogenetics: genetic variation in susceptibility to environmental agents

Environment agent	Genetic susceptibility	Disease
UV light	Fair complexion	Skin cancer
Drugs (see text)		
Foods		
Fats	Hypercholesterolaemia	Atherosclerosis
Fava beans	G6PD deficiency	Favism
Gluten	Gluten sensitivity	Coeliac disease
Salt	Na–K pump defective	Hypertension
Milk	Lactase deficiency	Lactose intolerance
Alcohol	Atypical ADH	Alcoholism
Oxalates	Hyperoxaluria	Renal stones
Fortified flour	Haemochromatosis	Iron overload
Inhalants		
Dust	α_1-antitrypsin deficiency	Emphysema
Allergens	Atopy	Asthma
Infections	Defective immunity	Diabetes mellitus? Spondylitis?

polymorphic system. Those who are homozygous for the low activity allele are likely to be particularly sensitive to accidental or occupational exposure to organophosphates. Reports of individuals experiencing either acute or chronic neurological or psychiatric symptoms through exposure to organophosphates could be the result of these inherited differences in paraoxonase activity.

DISEASE SUSCEPTIBILITY

An extension of ecogenetics which will be particularly important is the identification of individuals at high risk of developing diseases after environmental exposures, e.g. particular cancers after exposure to mutagens or carcinogens (p. 24).

There are reports of an increased risk of bladder cancer in persons who are slow acetylators and who have had occupational exposure to aromatic amines which are used as industrial dyes. There is also the possibility of an increased risk of bladder cancer for slow acetylators in the general population in which no specific hazardous exposure has been recognized. Conversely, there are recent reports suggesting the possibility of an increased risk of colorectal cancer in rapid acetylators.

Recent studies have suggested that poor debrisoquine metabolizer status is less common than would be expected in persons with cancer of the lung. This is in contrast to another recently discovered activity level polymorphism for the enzyme glutathione S-transferase (GSTM1), which shows an increase in the incidence of the null phenotype, i.e. no activity, in persons with adenocarcinoma of the lung when compared to the general population. This enzyme is involved in the conjugation of glutathione with electrophilic compounds, including carcinogens such as benzpyrene, and could have a protective role against the development of cancer.

This susceptibility to disease is not just limited to cancer. Many of the common diseases in humans could be due to genetically determined differences in response to environmental agents or susceptibilities (p. 209). There are reports of a possible increased risk of developing Parkinson's disease because of differences in the detoxification of potential neurotoxins in association with a poor metabolizer phenotype in the hepatic cytochrome P450 CYP2D6 gene.

The ability to screen large numbers of persons for SNPs (p. 67) should allow identification of genes involved in determining the inherited contribution for many of the common diseases. As well as identifying individuals at high risk of developing a common disease, this will allow a better understanding of the disease pathways involved, which holds the promise of directly linking possible therapeutic interventions for those individuals. The major international/multinational pharmaceutical and biotechnology companies, not surprisingly, are investing heavily in these developments. While there is the prospect of reducing the likelihood of individuals developing many of the common diseases, this raises however, many social and ethical problems when the knowledge of genetic variation and susceptibility is translated into public policy with vested commercial interests (p. 343).

FURTHER READING

Beutler E 1991 Glucose-6-phosphate dehydrogenase deficiency. N Engl J Med 324: 169–174
  Recent review of an important ethnic pharmacogenetic polymorphism.
Nebert D W 1999 Pharmacogenetics and pharmacogenomics: why is this relevant to the clinical geneticist? Clin Genet 56: 247–258
  A good summary of the two areas.
Neumann D A, Kimmel C A 1998 Human variability in response in chemical exposures: measures, modelling, and risk assessment. CRC Press, London
  A detailed discussion of the inherited human variability to exposure to the toxic effects of environmental chemicals.
Vogel F, Buselmaier W, Reichert W, Kellerman G, Berg P (eds) 1978 Human genetic variation in response to medical and environmental agents: pharmacogenetics and ecogenetics. Springer-Verlag, Berlin
  One of the early definitive outlines of the field of pharmacogenetics.
Wendell W 1997 Pharmacogenetics (Oxford Monographs on Medical Genetics, 32). Oxford University Press, Oxford
  A detailed comprehensive text on pharmacogenetics.

ELEMENTS

1 Pharmacogenetics is defined as the study of genetically determined variations revealed solely by the effects of drugs. Hereditary disorders in which symptoms can occur spontaneously or can be exacerbated or precipitated by drugs are often also included.

2 The metabolism of many drugs involves biochemical modification, often by conjugation with another molecule, which usually takes place in the liver. This biochemical transformation facilitates the excretion of the drug.

3 The ways in which many drugs are metabolized vary from person to person and can be genetically determined. In some instances, the biochemical basis is understood. For example, persons differ in the rate at which they inactivate the antituberculosis drug isoniazid by acetylation in the liver, being either rapid or slow inactivators. Slow inactivators have an increased risk of toxic side-effects associated with isoniazid therapy. Other examples include sensitivity to the muscle relaxant succinylcholine because of abnormal or reduced plasma pseudocholinesterase activity, and the development of a severe haemolytic anaemia when given the anti-malarial drug primaquine (or a number of other drugs) due to deficiency of the enzyme glucose-6-phosphate dehydrogenase in red blood cells.

4 In some instances, genetic variation can be revealed exclusively by exposure to drugs. One such example is malignant hyperthermia. This rare disorder is associated with the use of certain anaesthetic agents and muscle relaxants in general anaesthesia.

5 A number of hereditary disorders, such as porphyria variegata and some of the haemoglobinopathies, are associated with altered response to certain drugs. With disorders such as diabetes and gout, where the aetiology is complex, biochemical evidence of variation in response to drugs suggests a genetic contribution.

6 The information from the Human Genome Project allows the possibility of the development of new drugs, or what is called pharmacogenomics, as well as the prospect of identifying the genes which result in an increased susceptibility for developing the common diseases.

7 Ecogenetics is the term used for the study of genetically determined differences between persons in their susceptibility to the action of physical, chemical and infectious agents in the environment.

Immunogenetics

IMMUNITY

The world is filled with a wide variety of infectious agents. Evolution has resulted in a series of mechanisms which defend humans against these infective agents, which is termed immunity. In order to understand the inherited disorders of immunity, it is important to have an understanding of the fundamentals of the genetic basis of immunity.

Immune defence mechanisms can be divided into two main types: *innate immunity*, which includes a number of non-specific systems which don't require or involve prior contact with the infectious agent, and *specific acquired* or *adaptive immunity* which involves a tailor-made immune response which occurs after exposure to an infectious agent. Both types can involve either *humoral immunity*, which combats extracellular infections, or *cell-mediated immunity*, which fights intracellular infections.

INNATE IMMUNITY

The first simple type of defence against infection is a mechanical barrier. The skin functions most of the time as an impermeable barrier but, in addition, the acidic pH of sweat is inhibitory to bacterial growth. The membranes lining the repiratory and gastro-intestinal tracts are protected by mucus. In the case of the respiratory tract further protection is provided by ciliary movement, while other bodily fluids contain a variety of bactericidal agents, e.g lysozymes in tears. If an organism succeeds in invading the body, phagocytosis and bactericidal agents come into effect.

HUMORAL INNATE IMMUNITY

A number of soluble factors are involved in innate immunity by helping to minimize tissue injury by limiting the spread of infectious microorganisms. These are often called the *acute phase proteins* and include C-reactive protein, mannose binding protein and serum amyloid P component. The first two act by facilitating the attachment of one of the components of complement, C3b, to the surface of the microorganism, which becomes *opsonized* (made ready) for adherence to phagocytes, while the latter binds lysosomal enzymes to connective tissues. In addition, cells when infected by a virus synthesize and secrete *interferon*, which interferes with viral replication through reducing mRNA stability and interfering with translation.

Complement

Complement is a complex series of 20 or so interacting plasma proteins which can be activated by the cell membranes of invading microorganisms, in what is termed the *alternative pathway*. The various components of complement interact in a specific cascade sequence, resulting in a localized acute inflammatory response through the action of mediators released from mast cells and tissue macrophages. These result in increased vascular permeability and the attraction of phagocytes in the process known as *chemotaxis*. In addition, the later components of the complement cascade generate a membrane attack complex which induces defects in the cell membrane resulting in the lysis of microorganisms (Fig. 12.1).

Complement can also be activated through the *classical pathway*, by the binding of antibody with antigen (see below, p. 178).

CELL MEDIATED INNATE IMMUNITY

Phagocytosis

Microorganisms are engulfed and digested by two major types of cells, either polymorphonuclear neutrophils or macrophages. Polymorphonuclear neutrophils are found mainly in the bloodstream, while macrophages occur primarily in tissues around the basement membrane of blood vessels in connective tissue, lung, liver and in the lining of the sinusoids of the spleen and the medullary

Fig. 12.1
Classical and alternative pathways of complement activation.
(Adapted from Paul W E (ed) 1993 Fundamental immunology. Raven Press, New York.)

sinuses of the lymph nodes. Surface antigens on micro-organisms result in them being engulfed and fusing with the granules of the phagocyte subjecting them to the action of the bactericidal agents of the intracellular granules which contain hydrogen peroxide, hydroxyl radicals and nitrous oxide, which leads to their destruction.

Extracellular killing

Virally infected cells can be killed by large granular lymphocytes, known as *natural killer cells*. These have carbohydrate binding receptors on their cell surface which recognize high molecular weight glycoproteins expressed on the cell surface of the infected cell as a result of the virus taking over the cellular replicative functions. Attachment of the natural killer cells to the infected cells results in the release of a number of agents resulting in damage to the membrane of the infected cell leading to cell death.

SPECIFIC ACQUIRED IMMUNITY

Many infective microorganisms have, through mutation and selective pressures, evolved strategies to overcome or evade the mechanisms associated with innate immunity. There is the need, therefore, to be able to generate specific acquired or adaptive immunity. This can, like innate immunity, be separated into both humoral and cell-mediated processes.

HUMORAL SPECIFIC ACQUIRED IMMUNITY

The main mediators of humoral specific acquired immunity are immunoglobulins or antibodies. Antibodies are able to recognize and bind to antigens of infecting microorganisms leading to the activation of phagocytes and the initiation of the *classical pathway* of complement resulting in the generation of the membrane attack complex (Fig.12.1). Exposure to a specific antigen results in the clonal proliferation of a small lymphocyte derived from the bone marrow, hence B lymphocytes, resulting in mature antibody producing cells or *plasma cells*.

Lymphocytes capable of producing antibodies express on their surface copies of the immunoglobulin for which they code, which acts as a surface receptor for antigen. Binding of the antigen results, in conjunction with other membrane associated proteins, in signal transduction leading to the clonal expansion and production of antibody. This results in the first instance in the *primary response* with production of IgM and subsequently IgG. Re-exposure to the same antigen results in enhanced antibody levels in a shorter period of time, known as the *secondary response*, reflecting what is known as antigen specific *immunological memory*.

Immunoglobulins

The immunoglobulins (Ig), or antibodies, are one of the major classes of serum proteins. Their function, both in the recognition of antigenic variability and effector activities, was initially revealed by protein and more recently by DNA studies of their structure.

Immunoglobulin structure

Papaine, a proteolytic enzyme, splits the immunoglobulin molecule into three fragments. Two of the fragments are similar, each containing an antibody site capable of combining with a specific antigen and therefore referred to as the *antigen binding fragment* or *Fab*. The third fragment can be crystallized and was therefore called *Fc*. The Fc fragment determines the secondary biological functions of antibody molecules, binding complement and Fc receptors on a number of different cell types involved in the immune response.

The immunoglobulin molecule is made up of four polypeptide chains: two 'light' (L) and two 'heavy' (H) chains of approximately 220 and 440 amino acids in length. They are held together in a Y-shape by disulphide bonds and non-covalent interactions. Each Fab fragment is composed of L chains linked to the amino-terminal portion of the H chains, whereas each Fc fragment is composed only of the carboxy-terminal portion of the H chains (Fig. 12.2).

Fig. 12.2
Model of antibody molecule structure.

Immunoglobulin isotypes, subclasses and idiotypes

There are five different types of heavy chain designated respectively as γ, μ, α, δ and ε, one each respectively for the five major antibody classes, or what are known as *isotypes*, IgG, IgM, IgA, IgD and IgE. Further analysis has revealed that the L chains are one of two types, either kappa (κ) or lambda (λ), the two types of L chain occurring in all five classes of antibodies, but with only one type of light chain occurring in each individual antibody. Thus the molecular formula for IgG will be $\lambda_2\gamma_2$ or $\kappa_2\gamma_2$. The characteristics of the various classes of antibodies are outlined in brief in Table 12.1. In addition, there are four IgG subclasses, IgG1, IgG2, IgG3 and IgG4 and two IgA subclasses, IgA1 and IgA2, which differ in their amino acid sequence and interchain disulphide bonds.

Individual antibody molecules which recognize specific antigens are known as idiotypes.

Immunoglobulin allotypes

The five classes of immunoglobulin occur in all normal individuals but allelic variants or what are known as antibody *allotypes* of these classes have also been identified. These are the *Gm* system associated with the heavy chain of IgG, the *Am* system associated with the IgA heavy chain, the *Km* and *Inv* systems associated with the κ light chain, the *Oz* system for the λ light chain and the *Em* allotype for the IgE heavy chain. The Gm and Km systems are independent of each other and are polymorphic (p. 120), the frequencies of the different alleles varying in different ethnic groups.

The generation of antibody diversity

It could seem paradoxical for a single protein molecule to exhibit sufficient structural heterogeneity to have specificity for a large number of different antigens. Different combinations of heavy and light chains could, to some extent, account for this diversity. It would require, however, thousands of structural genes for each chain type to provide sufficient variability for the large number of antibodies produced in response to the equally large number of antigens to which individuals can be exposed. Our initial understanding of how this could occur came from persons with a malignancy of antibody-producing cells, or what is known as multiple myeloma.

Multiple myeloma

Persons with *multiple myeloma* make a single or monoclonal antibody species in large abundance which is excreted in large quantities in their urine. This protein, known as *Bence Jones protein*, consists of antibody light chains. Comparisons of this protein from different myeloma patients revealed the amino-terminal ends of the molecule to be quite variable in their amino acid sequence while the carboxy-terminal ends were relatively

Table 12.1 Classes of human immunoglobulins

Class	Mol. wt	Serum concentration (mg/ml)	Antibody activity	Complement fixation	Placental transfer
IgG	150 000	8–16	Binds to microorganisms and neutralizes bacterial toxins	+	+
IgM	900 000	0.5–2	Produced in early immune response, especially in bacteraemia	+	–
IgA	160 000	1.4–4	Guards mucosal surfaces	+	–
IgD	185 000	0–0.4	On lymphocyte cell surface, involved in control of activation and suppression	–	–
IgE	200 000	trace	In parasitic and allergic reactions	–	–

constant. These are called the *variable*, or *V*, and *constant*, or *C*, regions respectively. Further detailed analysis of the amino acid sequence of the V regions of different myeloma proteins showed four regions which vary little from one antibody to another, known as *framework regions* (FR 1–4), and three markedly variable regions interspersed between these, known as *hypervariable regions* (HV I–III) (Fig. 12.2).

DNA studies of antibody diversity

As long ago as 1965, Dreyer and Bennett proposed that an antibody could be encoded by separate 'genes' in germ line cells which undergo rearrangement, or, as they termed it, 'scrambling', in lymphocyte development. Comparison of the restriction maps of the DNA segments coding for the C and V regions of the immunoglobulin λ light chains in embryonic and antibody producing cells revealed that they were far apart in the former while they were close together in the latter. More detailed analysis revealed that the DNA segments coding for the V and C regions of the light chain are separated by some 1500 bp in antibody-producing cells. The intervening DNA segment was found to code for a *joining*, or *J*, region immediately adjacent to the V region of the light chain. The κ light chain was shown to have the same structure. Cloning and DNA sequencing of heavy chain genes in germ line cells have revealed that they have a fourth region, called *diversity*, or *D*, between the V and J regions.

There are estimated to be some 60 different DNA segments coding for the V region of the heavy chain, approximately 40 DNA segments coding for the V region of the κ light chain and 30 DNA segments coding for the λ light chain V region. Six functional DNA segments code for the J region of the heavy chain, five for the J region of the κ light chain and four for the J region of the λ light chain. A single DNA segment codes for the C region of the κ light chain, seven DNA segments code for the C region of the λ light chain and 11 functional DNA

segments code for the C region of the different classes of heavy chain. There are also 27 functional DNA segments coding for the D region of the heavy chain (Fig. 12.3).

Estimation of the number of DNA segments coding for these various portions of the antibody molecule is confounded by the presence of a large number of unexpressed DNA sequences or pseudogenes (p. 15). While the coding DNA segments for the various regions of the antibody molecule can be referred to as genes, use of this term in regard to antibodies has deliberately been avoided because they could be considered to be an exception to the general rule of 'one gene–one enzyme or protein' (p. 151).

Antibody gene rearrangement

The genes for the κ and λ light chains and the heavy chains in humans have been assigned to chromosomes 2, 22 and 14 respectively. Only one of each of the relevant types of DNA segments is expressed in any single antibody molecule. The DNA coding segments for the various portions of the antibody chains on these chromosomes are separated by DNA which is non-coding. Somatic recombinational events involved in antibody production involve short conserved recombination signal sequences that flank each germ line DNA segment (Fig. 12.4). Further diversity occurs by variable mRNA splicing at the V–J junction in RNA processing and by somatic mutation of the antibody genes. These mechanisms can easily account for the antibody diversity seen in nature. Although this probably involves some form of clonal selection, it is still not entirely clear, however, how particular DNA segments are selected to produce an antibody to a specific antigen. 'Gene shuffling' of this form is also known to account for the marked variability seen in the surface antigens of the trypanosome parasite and the different mating types in yeast.

Class switching of antibodies

There is a normal switch of antibody class produced by B cells on continued or further exposure to antigen, from IgM which is the initial class of antibody produced in response to exposure to an antigen, to IgA or IgG. This process, known as *class switching*, involves retention of the specificity of the antibody to the same antigen. Analysis of class switching in a population of cells derived from a single B cell has shown that both classes of antibody have the same antigen binding sites, having the same V region, differing only in their C region. Class switching occurs by a somatic recombination event which involves DNA segments designated S (for switching) which lead to looping out and deletion of the intervening DNA. The result is to eliminate the DNA segment coding for the C region of the heavy chain of the IgM molecule and to bring the gene segment encoding the C region of

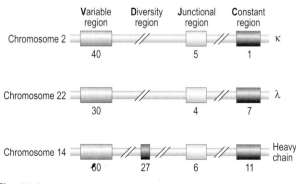

Fig. 12.3
Estimated number of the various DNA segments coding for the κ, λ and various heavy chains.

Fig. 12.4
Immunoglobulin heavy chain gene rearrangement and class switching.

the new class of heavy chain adjacent to the segment encoding the V region (Fig.12.4).

The immunoglobulin gene superfamily

Studies of the structure of other molecules involved in the immune response have shown a number to have structural and DNA sequence homology to the immuno-globulins. This involves a 110 amino acid sequence characterized by a centrally placed disulphide bridge which stabilizes a series of antiparallel β strands into what is called an antibody fold. This group of molecules with similar structure has been called the *immunoglobulin superfamily* (p. 15). It consists of eight multigene families which, in addition to the κ and λ light chains and different classes of heavy chain, include the chains of the T cell receptor (p. 18), the class I and II major histo-compatibility complex (MHC), or human leucocyte (HLA) antigens (p. 182), and β$_2$-microglobulin (p. 181). The latter is a receptor for transporting certain classes of immuno-globulins across mucosal membranes. A series of other molecules show homology to the Ig superfamily. These include the T cell CD4 and CD8 cell surface receptor molecules which cooperate with T cell receptors in anti-gen recognition and the intercellular adhesion molecules, ICAM-1, 2 and 3, which are involved in the interaction of lymphocytes with antigen presenting cells.

Antibody engineering

The techniques of genetic engineering have led to the prospect of reshaping or designing human antibodies for specific therapeutic or diagnostic purposes. These are

what are known as monoclonal antibodies. Recombinant antibodies can be constructed using the human variable region framework, the human constant regions of the heavy and light chains and the antigen binding site of a mouse antibody. Persons treated with these 'engineered' antibodies do not mount an immune response to them, a problem met with in the use of rodent hybridoma-derived monoclonal antibodies. It is hoped that the use of human-derived myeloma cells for expression of these recombinant antibodies could overcome this difficulty.

CELL-MEDIATED SPECIFIC ACQUIRED IMMUNITY

Certain microorganisms, viruses and parasites, live inside host cells. As a result a separate form of specific acquired immunity has evolved to combat intracellular infections involving lymphocytes differentiated in the thymus, hence *T cells*. T lymphocytes have specialized receptors on the cell surface, known as *T cell surface antigen receptors*, which in conjunction with the *major histocompatibility complex* on the cell surface of the infected cell, result in the involvement of *T helper cells* and *cytotoxic T cells* to combat intracellular infections by leading to the death of the infected cell.

T cell surface antigen receptor

T cells express on their surface an antigen receptor. This consists of two different polypeptide chains, linked by a disulphide bridge, which both contain two immunoglobulin-like domains, one which is relatively invariant in structure, the other highly variable like the Fab portion of an immunoglobulin. The diversity in T cell receptors required for recognition of the range of antigenic variation which can occur is generated by a similar process as seen with immunoglobulins. Re-arrangement of variable (V), diversity (D), junctional (J) and constant (C) DNA segments during T cell maturation, through a similar recombination mechanism as occurs in B cells, results in a contiguous VDJ sequence. Binding of antigen to the T cell receptor, in conjunction with an associated complex of transmembrane peptides, results in signalling the cell to differentiate and divide.

The major histocompatibility complex

The major histocompatibility complex (MHC) plays a central role in the immune system. Association of an antigen with the MHC molecule on the surface of the cells is required for recognition of the antigen by the T cell receptor which, in conjunction with the closely asso-ciated protein β$_2$-microglobulin, results in the recruitment of cytotoxic and helper T cells in the immune response. MHC molecules occur in three classes: class I molecules occurring on virtually all cells and which are responsible for recruiting cytotoxic T cells; class II molecules which occur on B cells and macrophages and are involved in signalling T helper cells to recruit further B cells and macrophages; the non-classic class III molecules which include a number of other proteins with a variety of other immunological functions. The latter include inflammatory mediators such as the tumour necrosis factor, heat shock proteins and the various components of complement (p. 177).

Structural analysis of the class I and II MHC molecules reveals them to be heterodimers with homology to immunoglobulin. The genes coding for the class I (A, B, C, E, F and G), class II (DR, DQ and DP) and class III MHC molecules, or what is also known as the *human leukocyte antigen* (HLA) system, are located on chromosome 6.

Transplantation genetics

Replacement of diseased organs by transplantation has become a routine part of clinical medicine. Except for corneal and bone grafts, the success of such transplants depends on the degree of antigenic similarity between the donor and recipient. The closer the similarity, the greater the likelihood that the transplanted organ or tissue, which is known as a *homograft*, will be accepted rather than rejected. Homograft rejection does not occur between identical twins or between non-identical twins where there has been mixing of the placental circulations before birth (p. 53). In all other instances, the antigenic similarity of donor and recipient has to be assessed by testing the donor and recipient with suitable antisera or monoclonal antibodies for antigens on donor and recipient tissues. These were originally known as transplantation antigens and are now known to be a result of the major histocompatibility complex. As a general rule a recipient will reject a graft from any person who has antigens which the recipient lacks. HLA typing of an individual is conventionally carried out by serological means, or what is known as *tissue typing*, but in most centres this is now being done by DNA methods.

The HLA system is highly polymorphic (Table 12.2). A virtually infinite number of phenotypes resulting from different combinations of the various alleles at these loci are theoretically possible. Two unrelated individuals are therefore very unlikely to have identical HLA phenotypes. The close linkage of the HLA loci means that they tend to be inherited en bloc, the term *haplotype* being used to indicate the particular HLA alleles which an individual carries on each of his two number 6 chromosomes. Thus any individual will have a 25% chance of having identical HLA antigens with a sib since there are only four possible combinations of the two paternal haplotypes (say P and Q) and the two maternal haplotypes (say R and S), i.e. PR, PS, QR and QS. The

Table 12.2   Alleles at the HLA loci

HLA locus	Number of alleles
A	57
B	111
C	34
D	228

sibs of a particular recipient are more likely to be antigenically similar than either of his/her parents, and the latter more than an unrelated person. For this reason, a brother or sister is frequently selected as a potential donor for organ or tissue transplantation.

Although crossing over does occur within the HLA region, certain alleles tend to occur together more frequently than would be expected by chance, i.e. they exhibit linkage disequilibrium (p. 124). An example is the association of the HLA antigens A1 and B8 in populations of Western European origin.

H–Y antigen

In a number of different animal species it was noted that tissue grafts from males were rejected by females of the same inbred strain. These incompatibilities were found to be due to a histocompatibility antigen, known as the H–Y antigen. The H–Y antigen seems, however, to play little part in transplantation in humans. Although the H–Y antigen seems to be important for testicular differentiation and function, its expression does not, however, necessarily correlate with the presence or absence of testicular tissue. A separate sex-determining region of the Y chromosome (*SRY*) has been isolated which is now known to be the testis-determining gene (p. 90).

HLA polymorphisms and disease associations

A finding which helps to throw light on the pathogenesis of certain diseases is the demonstration of their association with certain HLA types (Table 12.3). The best documented is that between ankylosing spondylitis and HLA B27. In the case of narcolepsy, a condition of unknown aetiology characterized by a periodic uncontrollable tendency to fall asleep, almost all affected individuals are HLA DR2. The possession of a particular HLA antigen does not mean that an individual will necessarily develop the associated disease, merely that he or she has a greater relative risk of being affected than the general population (p. 131).

Explanations for the various HLA associated disease susceptibilities include close linkage to a susceptibility gene near the HLA complex, cross-reactivity of antibodies to environmental antigens or pathogens with specific HLA antigens, and abnormal recognition of 'self' antigens

Table 12.3 Some HLA-associated diseases

Disease	HLA
Ankylosing spondylitis	B27
Coeliac disease	DR4
Haemochromatosis	A3
Insulin-dependent diabetes (type 1)	DR3/4
Myasthenia gravis	B8
Narcolepsy	DR2
Rheumatoid arthritis	DR4
Systemic lupus erythematosus	DR2/DR3
Thyrotoxicosis (Graves disease)	DR3

through defects in T cell receptors or antigen processing. These conditions are known as *autoimmune diseases*. At present, however, the mechanisms involved in most HLA disease associations are still not completely understood.

INHERITED IMMUNODEFICIENCY DISORDERS

Inherited immunodeficiency disorders are uncommon and are usually associated with severe morbidity and mortality. They can occur as a primary isolated abnormality or can be a secondary or associated finding.

PRIMARY INHERITED DISORDERS OF IMMUNITY

The manifestations of at least some of the primary immunological deficiency diseases in humans (Table 12.4) can be understood by considering whether they are disorders of innate immunity or of specific acquired immunity. Abnormalities of humoral immunity are associated with reduced resistance to bacterial infections which can lead to death in infancy. Abnormalities of specific acquired immunity which are cell-mediated are associated with increased susceptibility to virus infections

and are manifest experimentally in animals by prolonged survival of skin homografts.

Disorders of innate immunity

Primary disorders of innate immunity involving humoral and cell-mediated immunity have been described.

Disorders of innate humoral immunity

There are a variety of defects of complement which can lead to disordered innate immunity.

Disorders of complement

Defects of the third component of complement, C3, lead to abnormalities of opsonization of bacteria resulting in difficulties in combating pyogenic infections. Defects in the later components of complement involved in the formation of the membrane attack complex also result in susceptibility to a particular bacterial species, primarily *Neisseria*.

Deficiency of the C1-inhibitor results in inappropriate activation of the classical pathway of complement leading to uncontrolled production of C2a which is vasoactive resulting in fluid accumulation in soft tissue and the airways. This is known as hereditary angioneurotic oedema which is inherited as an autosomal dominant disorder.

Disorders of innate cell-mediated immunity

A very important mechanism in innate cell-mediated immunity is phagocytosis which results in subsequent cell-mediated killing of microorganisms.

Chronic granulomatous disease

Chronic granulomatous disease (CGD) is the best known example of a disorder of phagocytic function. It can be inherited as either an X-linked or autosomal recessive

Table 12.4 Some immunological deficiency diseases and their features

Disorder	Thymus gland	Lymphocytes	Cell-mediated	Plasma cells	Ig synthesis	Genetics	Treatment
Severe combined immunodeficiency	Vestigial	↓	↓	↓	↓	AR/XR	BMT, enzyme replacement for ADA deficiency
DiGeorge syndrome	Absent (parathyroids absent as well)	+	↓	+	N	Deletion	Transplantation of fetal thymus
Bruton-type agammaglobulinaemia	+	+	N	↓	↓	XR	Ig injections and antibiotics

AR = autosomal recessive; XR = X-linked recessive; BMT = bone marrow transplant; ADA = adenosine deaminase; N = normal; ↓ = reduced; + = present disorder and is in all instances caused by an inability to generate superoxide radicals leading to a loss of anti-bacterial activity of the phagocytes (Fig. 12.5). CGD is, therefore, associated with recurrent bacterial or fungal infections, often by commensal microorganisms. Until the advent of supportive treatment in the form of infection-related and prophylactic antibiotics, it was associated with a high childhood mortality. The gene for CGD was the first human disease gene cloned by positional cloning (p. 74).

Leucocyte adhesion deficiency

Individuals affected with leucocyte adhesion deficiency present with life-threatening bacterial infections of the skin and mucous membranes with impaired pus formation. The increased susceptibility to infections occurs due to the absence of the β_2 chain of the leucocyte integrins, which results in defective migration of phagocytic cells due to abnormal adhesion-related functions of chemotaxis and phagocytosis. This disorder is fatal unless antibiotics are given both for infection and prophylactically until bone marrow transplantation can be offered.

Disorders of specific acquired immunity

Again these can be considered under the categories of disorders of humoral and cell-mediated specific acquired immunity.

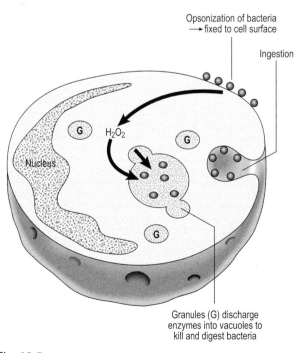

Opsonization of bacteria → fixed to cell surface

Ingestion

H_2O_2

G

G

G

Nucleus

Granules (G) discharge enzymes into vacuoles to kill and digest bacteria

Fig. 12.5
Phagocytosis and the pathways involved in intracellular killing of microorganisms.

Disorders of humoral acquired immunity

Abnormalities of immunoglobulin function lead to an increased tendency to develop bacterial infections.

Bruton-type agammaglobulinaemia

Boys with this X-linked immunodeficiency usually develop multiple recurrent bacterial infections of the respiratory tract and skin after the first few months of life, having been protected initially by placentally transferred maternal IgG. Treatment of life-threatening infections with antibiotics and the use of prophylactic intravenous immunoglobulins have improved survival prospects but children with this disorder can still die from respiratory failure through complications of repeated lung infections. The diagnosis of this type of immuno-deficiency is confirmed by demonstration of immuno-globulin deficiency and absence of B lymphocytes. The disorder has been shown to result from mutations in a tyrosine kinase specific to B cells (Btk) which result in loss of the signal for B cells to differentiate to mature antibody-producing plasma cells.

Disorders of cell-mediated specific acquired immunity

The most common inherited disorder of cell-mediated specific acquired immunity is severe combined immuno-deficiency.

Severe combined immunodeficiency

Severe combined immunodeficiency (SCID), as the name indicates, is associated with an increased susceptibility to both viral and bacterial infections because of profoundly abnormal humoral and cell-mediated immunity. Death usually occurs in infancy because of overwhelming infection, unless bone marrow transplantation is performed. SCID is genetically heterogeneous and can be inherited either as an X-linked or autosomal recessive disorder, although all forms have in common a defect in T cell function or development. The X-linked form is the most common form of SCID in males and has been shown to be due to mutations in the γ chain of the cytokine receptor for interleukin (IL)-2.

In approximately one-third to one-half of children with SCID which is not X-linked, autosomal recessive deficiency of the enzymes adenosine deaminase or purine nucleoside phosphorylase can be demonstrated. These latter two causes of SCID are, for all intents and purposes, inborn errors of metabolism (p. 165) which specifically affect the immune system through the accumulation of purine degradation products being selectively toxic to T cells. Another rare autosomal recessive form of SCID, the so-called *bare lymphocyte syndrome*, is due to absence of the class II molecules of the major histocompatibility complex.

SECONDARY OR ASSOCIATED IMMUNODEFICIENCY

There are a number of hereditary disorders in which immunological abnormalities occur as one of a number of associated features as part of a syndrome (p. 229).

DiGeorge syndrome

Children with the DiGeorge syndrome present with recurrent viral illnesses and are found to have markedly abnormal cellular immunity as characterized by severely reduced or absent T lymphocytes, as well as abnormal antibody production. This has been found to be associated with absence of their thymus gland leading to defects in cell-mediated immunity and T cell dependent antibody production. They also usually have a number of characteristic congenital abnormalities which can include heart disease and absent parathyroid glands. The latter finding can result in affected individuals presenting in the newborn period with tetany due to low serum calcium levels secondary to low parathormone levels. This syndrome has been recognized to be part of the spectrum of phenotypes caused by abnormalities of the third and fourth pharyngeal pouches as a consequence of a deletion of a particular region of the long arm of chromosome 22 (p. 225).

Ataxia telangiectasia

Ataxia telangiectasia is an autosomal recessive disorder in which children present in early childhood with difficulty in control of movement and balance (cerebellar ataxia), dilated blood vessels of the whites of the eyes (conjunctiva), ears and face (oculocutaneous telangiectasia), and a susceptibility to sinus and pulmonary infections. Persons with this disorder have low serum IgA levels and a hypoplastic thymus which are the result of a defect in the cellular response to DNA damage. The diagnosis of ataxia telangiectasia can be confirmed by demonstration of low or absent serum IgA and IgG and characteristic chromosome abnormalities on culture of peripheral blood lymphocytes, so-called chromosome instability (p. 262). In addition, individuals affected with ataxia telangiectasia have an increased risk of developing leukaemia or lymphoid malignancies.

Wiskott–Aldrich syndrome

Wiskott–Aldrich syndrome is an X-linked recessive disorder in which affected boys have eczema, diarrhoea, recurrent infections, a low platelet count (thrombocytopenia) and, usually, low serum IgM levels and impaired T cell function and numbers. Mutations in the gene responsible have been shown to result in loss of cytotoxic T cell responses and T cell help for B cell response leading to an impaired response to bacterial infections. Until the advent of bone marrow transplantation, the majority of affected boys died by mid-adolescence from haemorrhage or B cell malignancies.

Carrier tests for X-linked immunodeficiencies

Before the identification of the genes responsible for the Wiskott–Aldrich syndrome, Bruton-type hypogammaglobulinaemia and X-linked SCID, the availability of closely linked DNA markers allowed carrier testing by studies of the pattern of X-inactivation (p. 92) in the lymphocytes of females at risk. A non-random pattern of X-inactivation in the T lymphocyte population, in a female relative of a sporadically affected male with an X-linked immunodeficiency demonstrating that all her peripheral blood T lymphocytes have the same chromosome inactivated, would confirm her to be a carrier (Fig. 12.6).

The carrier (C) and non-carrier (NC) are both heterozygous for an *Hpa*II/*Msp*I restriction site polymorphism. *Hpa*II and *Msp*I recognize the same nucleotide recognition sequence but *Msp*I cuts double-stranded DNA whether it is methylated or not, while *Hpa*II will only cut unmethylated DNA, i.e. only the active X chromosome.

H/M, E = *Hpa*II/*Msp*I and *Eco*RI restriction sites
■ = mutant gene   □ = normal gene

Fig. 12.6
Non-random inactivation in T lymphocytes for carrier testing in X-linked SCID.

In the carrier female the mutation in the SCID gene is on the X chromosome on which the *Hpa*II/*Msp*I restriction site is present. *Eco*RI/*Msp*I double digests of T lymphocytes result in 6, 4 and 2 kb DNA fragments on gel analysis of the restriction fragments for both the carrier and non-carrier females. *Eco*RI/*Hpa*II double digests of T lymphocyte DNA result, however, in a single 6 kb fragment in the carrier female. This is because in a carrier the only T cells to survive will be those in which the normal gene is on the active unmethylated X chromosome. Thus in a carrier, inactivation appears non-random, although strictly speaking it is cell population survival which is non-random.

A mixed pattern of X-inactivation in the lymphocytes of the mother of a sporadically affected male is consistent with the disorder either having arisen as a new X-linked mutation or being due to the autosomal recessive form. Similar X-inactivation studies of the peripheral blood B lymphocyte population can be used to determine the carrier status of women at risk for Bruton-type agammaglobulinaemia and the Wiskott–Aldrich syndrome. This technique is being replaced by direct identification of mutations in the genes responsible.

BLOOD GROUPS

Blood groups reflect the antigenic determinants on red cells and were one of the first areas in which an understanding of basic biology led to significant advances in clinical medicine. Our knowledge of the ABO and rhesus blood groups has resulted in safe blood transfusion and the prevention of rhesus haemolytic disease of the newborn.

THE ABO BLOOD GROUPS

The ABO blood groups were discovered by Landsteiner just after the turn of the twentieth century. The transfusion of red blood cells from certain persons to others, in some instances, resulted in rapid haemolysis, in other words, their blood was incompatible. Studies revealed there to be four major ABO blood groups: A, B, AB and O. Persons who are blood group A possess the antigen A on the surface of their red blood cells, persons of blood group B have antigen B, persons who are AB have A and B antigens while persons who are blood group O have neither. Persons of blood group A have naturally occurring anti-B antibodies in their blood, persons of blood group B have anti-A and persons of blood group O have both. The alleles at the ABO blood group locus for antigens A and B are inherited in a codominant manner but are both dominant to the gene for the O antigen

Table 12.5   ABO blood group phenotypes and genotypes

Red blood cells Phenotype	Genotype	Antibodies	React with antiserum Anti-A	Anti-B
O	OO	anti-A,B	–	–
A	AA, AO	anti-B	+	–
B	BB, BO	anti-A	–	+
AB	AB	–	+	+

(p. 106). There are, therefore, six possible genotypes. The homozygous and heterozygous states for antigens A and B (i.e. AA, AO, BB, BO) can only be determined by family studies (Table 12.5).

Since individuals of blood group AB do not produce A or B antibodies they can receive a blood transfusion from individuals of all other ABO blood groups and are therefore referred to as *universal recipients*. On the other hand, since individuals of group O do not express either A or B antigens on their red cells they are referred to as *universal donors*. Antisera can differentiate two subgroups of blood group A, A1 and A2, but this is of little practical importance as far as blood transfusions are concerned.

Molecular basis of ABO blood groups

Individuals with blood groups A, B and AB possess enzymes with glycosyltransferase activity which convert the basic blood group, which is known as the H antigen, into A or B antigens. The alleles for blood groups A and B differ in seven single base substitutions which result in different A and B transferase activities, the A allele being associated with the addition of *N*-acetylgalactosaminyl groups and the B allele with the addition of D-galactosyl groups. The O allele results from a critical single base pair deletion which results in an inactive protein incapable of modifying the H antigen.

Secretor status

In the majority of persons, the ABO blood group antigens, in addition to being expressed on red blood cells, are secreted in various body fluids including saliva. This is controlled by two alleles at the so-called *secretor locus*, persons being either secretor-positive or secretor-negative, the former being dominant to the latter. *Secretor status* has been associated with a predisposition to peptic ulcer. The secretor locus has also been shown to be linked to the locus for myotonic dystrophy. Before the advent of DNA markers, family studies of secretor status were used to predict whether an asymptomatic person had inherited the gene for this disorder (p. 269).

RHESUS BLOOD GROUP

The rhesus (Rh) blood group system involves three sets of closely linked antigens, Cc, Dd and Ee. D is very strongly antigenic and persons are, for practical purposes, either Rh-positive (possessing the D antigen) or Rh-negative (lacking the D antigen).

Rhesus haemolytic disease of the newborn

A proportion of women who are Rh-negative have an increased chance of having a child who will either die in utero or be born severely anaemic because of haemolysis unless transfused in utero. This occurs for the following reason. If Rh-positive blood is given to persons who are Rh-negative, the majority will develop anti-Rh antibodies. Such sensitization occurs with exposure to very small quantities of blood and, once a person is sensitized, further exposure results in the production of very high antibody titres.

In the case of an Rh-negative mother carrying an Rh-positive fetus, red cells of fetal origin can enter the mother's circulation, for example after a miscarriage or at the time of delivery. This can induce the formation of Rh antibodies in the mother. In a subsequent pregnancy these antibodies can cross the placenta and enter the fetal circulation. This leads to haemolysis of the fetal red blood cells if the fetus is Rh-negative which can result either in fetal death, which is known as *erythroblastosis fetalis*, or a severe haemolytic anaemia of newborn infants which is called *haemolytic disease of the newborn*. Once a woman is sensitized there is a significantly greater risk that a child in a subsequent pregnancy, if Rh-positive, will be more severely affected.

To avoid sensitizing a Rh-negative woman, Rh compatible blood must always be used in any blood transfusion. Furthermore, the development of sensitization and therefore Rh incompatibility after delivery can be prevented by giving the mother an injection of Rh antibodies, so-called anti-D, so that any fetal cells which have found their way into the maternal circulation are destroyed before the mother can become sensitized.

It is routine to screen all Rh-negative women during pregnancy for the development of Rh antibodies. Despite these measures, a small proportion of women do become sensitized. If Rh antibodies appear, tests are then carried out to see if the fetus is affected. If so, then there is a delicate balance between early delivery, with the risks of prematurity and exchange transfusion, and treating the fetus in utero with blood transfusions.

Molecular basis of the Rhesus blood group

Recent biochemical evidence has shown there to be two types of Rh red cell membrane polypeptide. One corresponds to the D antigen and the other to the C and E series of antigens. Cloning of the genomic sequences responsible using Rh cDNA from reticulocytes has revealed that there are two genes coding for the Rh system, one for D and d and a second for both C and c and E and e. The D locus is present in most persons and codes for the major D antigen present in persons who are Rh-positive. Rh-negative individuals are homozygous for a deletion of the D gene. It is not, perhaps, surprising therefore that an antibody has never been raised to d!

Analysis of cDNA from reticulocytes in Rh-negative persons, who were homozygous for dCe, dcE and dce, allowed identification of the genomic DNA sequences responsible for the different antigenic variants at the second locus, revealing that they are produced by alternative splicing of the mRNA transcript. The Ee polypeptide is a full-length product of the CcEe gene, very similar in sequence to the D polypeptide. The E and e antigens differ by a point mutation in exon 5. The Cc polypeptides are, in contrast, products of a shorter length transcript of the same gene having either exons 4, 5 and 6 or 4, 5 and 8 spliced out. The difference between C and c is due to four amino acid substitutions in exons 1 and 2. These findings help explain what was an apparently complex blood group system!

OTHER BLOOD GROUPS

There are approximately another 12 'common' blood group systems of clinical importance in humans, which include Duffy, Lewis, MN and S. These are usually only of concern in cross-matching blood for persons who, because of repeated transfusions, have developed antibodies to one of these other blood group antigens. Until the advent of DNA fingerprinting (p. 67), they were used in linkage studies (p. 131) and paternity testing (p. 247).

FURTHER READING

Bell J I, Todd J A, McDevitt H O 1989 The molecular basis of HLA-disease association. Adv Hum Genet 18: 1–41
Good review of the HLA disease associations.
Dreyer W J, Bennet J C 1965 The molecular basis of antibody formation: a paradox. Proc Natl Acad Sci USA 54: 864–869
The proposal of the generation of antibody diversity.
Hunkapiller T, Hood L 1989 Diversity of the immunoglobulin gene superfamily. Adv Immunol 44: 1–63
Good review of the structure of the immunoglobulin gene superfamily.
Janeway C A, Travers P, Walport M, Capra J D 1999 Immunobiology, 4th edn. Current Biology, London
Good, well-illustrated textbook of the biology of immunology.
Lachmann P J, Peters K, Rosen F S, Walport M J 1993 Clinical aspects of immunology, 5th edn. Blackwell, Oxford
A comprehensive three-volume multiauthor text covering both basic and clinical immunology.
Roitt I 1997 Essential immunology, 9th edn. Blackwell, Oxford
Excellent basic immunology textbook.

ELEMENTS

1 The immune response in humans can be divided into two main types, innate and specific acquired or adaptive immunity. Both types can be further subdivided into humoral and cell-mediated immunity.

2 Innate humoral immunity involves acute phase proteins which act to minimize tissue injury by limiting the spread of infective organisms and through the alternative pathway of complement results in a localized inflammatory response and the attraction of phagocytes and opsonization of microorganisms. Complement, which consists of a series of inactive blood proteins which are sequentially activated in a cascade, can also be activated through the classical pathway by antibody binding to antigen.

3 Innate cell-mediated immunity involves engulfment of microorganisms by macrophages and their destruction by intracellular granules.

4 Specific acquired humoral immunity involves production of antibodies by mature B cells or plasma cells in response to antigen. Antibodies are Y-shaped molecules and each is composed of two identical heavy (H) chains and two identical light (L) chains. The antibody molecule has two parts which differ in their function: two identical antigen binding sites (Fab) and a single binding site for complement (Fc). There are five classes of antibody, IgA, IgD, IgE, IgG and IgM, each with a specific heavy chain. The light chain of any class of antibody can be made up of either kappa (κ) or lambda (λ) chains.

5 Each immunoglobulin light or heavy chain has a variable (V) region of approximately 110 amino acids at the amino-terminal end. The carboxy-terminal end consists of a constant (C) region of approximately 110 amino acids in the κ and λ light chains and three to four times that length in the heavy chain. Most of the amino acid sequence variation in both the light and heavy chains occurs within several small hypervariable regions. These are thought to be the sites of antigen binding. The immunoglobulin chains are produced from combinations of separate groups of DNA segments. These consist of one from a variable number of DNA segments coding for the constant (C), variable (V) and joining (J) regions between the V and C regions for the κ and λ light chains and the various types of heavy chains. The heavy chains also contain a diversity (D) region located between the V and J regions. The total number of possible antibodies which could be produced by various combinations of these DNA segments accounts for the antibody diversity seen in humans.

6 Cell-mediated specific acquired immunity primarily involves T cells which, through the T cell surface antigen receptor, in conjunction with the major histocompatibility complex molecules on the surface of infected cells, engage T helper cells and cytotoxic T cells to combat intracellular infections.

7 The major histocompatibility complex or human leucocyte antigen system consists of a number of closely linked loci on chromosome 6. The many different alleles which can occur at each locus mean that a very large number of different combinations of these can result. The HLA loci are inherited 'en bloc' as a haplotype. The closer the match of HLA antigens between the donor and recipient in organ transplantation, the greater the likelihood of long-term survival of the homograft. Possession of certain HLA antigens is associated with an increased relative risk of developing specific diseases.

8 An understanding of the ABO and rhesus blood groups has resulted in safe blood transfusions and the prevention of Rhesus haemolytic disease of the newborn.

The genetics of cancer

There are cancers in which environmental factors are of primary importance and heredity seems to play no part in causation. This is true of the 'industrial cancers' which result from prolonged exposure to carcinogenic chemicals. Examples include cancer of the skin in tar workers, cancer of the bladder in aniline dye workers, angiosarcoma of the liver in process workers making polyvinyl chloride (PVC), and cancer of the lung in asbestos workers. The recognition that a number of rare cancer-predisposing syndromes and that a small but significant proportion of the common cancers have a hereditary basis, has led over the last 25 years to an explosion in our understanding of the genetic basis and cellular biology of cancer in humans.

DIFFERENTIATING BETWEEN GENETIC AND ENVIRONMENTAL FACTORS IN CANCER

In many cancers the differentiation between genetic and environmental aetiological factors is not always obvious. In the majority of cancers in humans there is no clear-cut mode of inheritance nor is there any clearly defined environmental cause. In certain of the common cancers, such as breast and bowel, genetic factors play an important, but not exclusive, role in the aetiology. Evidence to help differentiate environmental and genetic factors can come from a combination of epidemiologic, family and twin studies, disease associations, biochemical factors and animal studies.

EPIDEMIOLOGIC STUDIES

Breast cancer is the most common cancer in women. Reproductive and menstrual histories are well-recognized risk factors. Women who have had children have a lower risk of developing breast cancer than nulliparous women. In addition, the younger the age at which a woman has her first pregnancy, the lower her risk of developing breast cancer. Conversely, the later the age of onset of menstrual periods, the greater the risk of developing breast cancer.

The incidence of breast cancer varies greatly between different populations, being highest in women in North America and Western Europe and up to eight times lower in women of Japanese and Chinese origin. While these differences could be attributed to genetic differences between these population groups, study of immigrant populations moving from an area with a low incidence to one with a high incidence has shown that the risk of developing breast cancer rises with time to that of the native population, supporting the view that breast cancer has a significant environmental component.

It has long been recognized that persons from the less well-off socioeconomic groups have an increased risk of developing gastric cancer. Specific dietary irritants, such as salts and preservatives, or potential environmental agents, such as nitrates, have been suggested as being possible carcinogens. Gastric cancer also shows variation in incidence in different populations, being up to eight times more common in Japanese and Chinese populations than in persons of Western European origin. Migration studies have shown that the risk of gastric cancer for immigrants from high risk populations does not fall to that of the native low risk population for two or three generations. It has been suggested previously that this could be due to exposure to environmental factors at an early critical age. There is a substantial body of evidence accumulating that early infection with *Helicobacter pylori* which causes chronic gastric inflammation is associated with a five- to sixfold increased risk of developing gastric cancer.

FAMILY STUDIES

The frequency with which other family members develop the same cancer can provide evidence supporting a genetic contribution. The lifetime risk for a woman in Western Europe of developing breast cancer is 1 in 12. Family studies have shown that the likelihood of a first-degree female relative of a woman with breast cancer developing breast cancer is between 1.8 and 3 times the risk for the general population. The risk varies depending on the age of developing breast cancer in the proband, being greater the younger the age of onset in the proband (p. 201).

Similar studies in gastric cancer have shown that first degree relatives of persons with cancer of the stomach have a two- to threefold increased risk compared to the general population of developing gastric cancer. The increased risk of developing gastric cancer in close relatives is, however, relatively small, suggesting that environmental factors are likely to be more important.

TWIN STUDIES

Concordance rates for breast cancer in twins are low for both types of twins, being only slightly greater in monozygotic female twins at 17% than 13% in dizygotic female twins, suggesting that environmental factors are likely to be more important than genetic factors. Twin studies in gastric cancer have not shown an increased concordance rate in monozygotic compared to dizygotic twins.

DISEASE ASSOCIATIONS

Blood groups are genetically determined and therefore association of a particular blood group with a disease suggests a possible genetic contribution to the aetiology. A large number of studies from a variety of countries have shown an association between blood group A and gastric cancer. It is estimated that persons with blood group A have a 20% increased risk over the general population for developing gastric cancer. Blood group A is associated with an increased risk of developing pernicious anaemia which is also closely associated with chronic gastritis. It appears, however, that pernicious anaemia has a separate association with gastric cancer. Persons with pernicious anaemia have a three- to sixfold increased risk of developing gastric cancer.

BIOCHEMICAL FACTORS

Biochemical factors can determine the susceptibility to environmental carcinogens. Examples include the association between slow acetylator status and debrisoquine metabolizer status (p. 170) and a predisposition to bladder cancer (p. 172), as well as glutathione S-transferase activity (p. 175) which influences the risk of developing lung cancer in smokers.

ANIMAL STUDIES

Certain inbred strains of mice have been developed which have a high chance of developing a particular type of tumour. The A (albino) Bittner strain is especially prone to develop tumours of the lung and breast; the C3H strain is particularly prone to develop breast tumours as well as tumours of the liver; the C58 strain is prone to develop leukaemia. Breeding experiments with mice have shown that the tendency to develop cancer is influenced by environmental factors. In strains with a high incidence of breast tumours, the frequency of these tumours is reduced by dietary restrictions and increased by high temperature.

VIRAL FACTORS

In 1908 Ellerman and Bang showed that erythroid leukaemia in chickens was transmitted by a cell-free filtrate. At that time, however, leukaemia was regarded as a blood disease rather than a cancer and the significance of these observations was only realized by the work of Peyton Rous between 1910 and 1914 who showed that crude extracts of a tumour from a Plymouth Rock hen, inoculated into healthy chickens, resulted in the growth of new tumours. Bittner subsequently showed that the susceptibility to develop breast tumours in certain strains of mice depended on a combination of genetic factors as well as a transmissible factor present in the milk known as the 'milk agent'. In high incidence strains both genetic susceptibility and the milk agent are involved, but in low incidence strains there is no milk agent. By using foster mothers from cancer-free strains to suckle newborn mice from strains with a high cancer susceptibility it is possible to reduce the incidence of breast cancer from 100% to less than 50%. Conversely, it is possible to increase the incidence in cancer-free strains by suckling the newborn mice with foster mothers from high cancer-prone strains. The milk agent was shown to be a virus which was usually transmitted by the mother's milk but could also be transmitted by the father's sperm.

Subsequent studies have shown that certain viruses are tumour-forming or *oncogenic* in humans. A limited number of DNA viruses are associated with certain types of human tumours (Table 13.1), while a variety of RNA viruses, or *retroviruses*, cause neoplasia in animals (Table 13.2). The study of the genetics and replicative processes of oncogenic retroviruses has revealed some of the cellular biological processes involved in carcinogenesis.

Retroviruses

Retroviruses have their genetic information encoded in RNA and replicate through DNA by coding for an enzyme known as reverse transcriptase (p. 57) which makes a double stranded DNA copy of the viral RNA. This DNA intermediate integrates into the host cell genome, allowing the appropriate proteins to be manufactured, resulting in repackaging of new progeny virions.

Naturally occurring retroviruses have only the three genes necessary to ensure replication: *gag*, encoding the

Table 13.1 Human DNA viruses implicated in carcinogenesis

Virus family	Type	Tumour
Papova	Papilloma (HPV)	Warts (plantar and genital), urogenital cancers (cervical, vulval and penile), skin cancer
Herpes	Epstein–Barr (EBV)	Burkitt's lymphoma*, nasopharyngeal carcinoma, lymphomas in immunocompromised hosts
Hepadna	Hepatitis B (HBV)	Hepatocellular carcinoma*

*For full oncogenicity, 'co-carcinogens' are necessary, e.g. aflatoxin B_1 in hepatitis B-associated hepatocellular carcinoma.

Table 13.2 Oncogenic retroviruses, their hosts and associated tumours

Host	Virus	Tumour/disease
Chicken	Rous sarcoma virus	Sarcoma
	Avian leucosis virus	Avian leukaemia
Mice	Murine sarcoma virus	Sarcoma
	Murine leukaemia virus	Leukaemia
	Mouse mammary tumour virus	Breast cancer
Primates	Simian sarcoma virus	Sarcoma
	Gibbon ape leukaemia virus	Leukaemia
Humans	Human T cell lymphotrophic virus 1 (HTLV1)	T cell leukaemia
	Kaposi sarcoma-associated herpes virus (KSAHV)	Kaposi's sarcoma

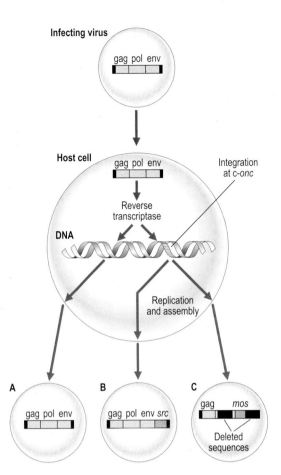

Fig. 13.1

Model for acquisition of transforming ability in retroviruses. (A) Normal retroviral replication. (B) The Rous sarcoma virus has integrated near a cellular oncogene. The transforming ability of this virus is due to the acquired homologue of the cellular oncogene, v-src. (C) A defective transforming virus carries an oncogene similar to src but is defective in the structural genes, e.g. Moloney murine sarcoma virus which carries mos.

structural proteins for the core antigens, *pol*, coding for reverse transcriptase, and *env*, the gene for the glycoprotein envelope proteins (Fig. 13.1). Study of the virus responsible for the transmissible tumour in chickens, the so-called Rous sarcoma virus, identified a fourth gene which results in *transformation* of cells in culture, a model for malignancy in vivo. This viral gene, which *transforms* the host cell, is known as an *oncogene*.

ONCOGENES

A large number of different oncogenes have been identified. They are known by three letter abbreviations which reflect their origin and/or the type of tumour with which they are associated (Table 13.3). Studies have revealed the presence in normal mammalian cells of DNA sequences homologous to the viral oncogenes which have been called *proto-oncogenes* or *cellular oncogenes*. The terms proto-oncogene and cellular oncogene are often used interchangeably, although strictly speaking the term proto-oncogene is reserved for the normal gene and the term *cellular oncogene*, or *c-onc*, refers to a mutated proto-oncogene with oncogenic properties like the *viral oncogenes*, or *v-onc*.

RELATIONSHIP BETWEEN C-*ONC* AND V-*ONC*

Cellular oncogenes are highly conserved in evolution suggesting that they have important roles as regulators of cell growth maintaining the ordered progression through the cell cycle, cell division and differentiation. Retroviral oncogenes are thought to acquire their dominant transforming activity during viral transduction through errors in the replication of the retrovirus genome following their random integration into the host DNA. The end result is a viral gene which is structurally similar to its cellular counterpart but is persistently different in its function.

Table 13.3   Some transforming retroviruses, the species affected, the tumour formed and the oncogene responsible

Virus	Species	Virus-induced tumour	Oncogene
Rous sarcoma	Chicken	Sarcoma	*src*
Avian erythroblastosis	Chicken	Erythroleukaemia	*erb*-B
Avian myeloblastosis	Chicken	Myeloblastic leukaemia	*myb*
Avian myelocytomatosis	Chicken sarcoma	Myelocytoma, sarcoma	*myc*
Abelson leukaemia	Mouse	Pre-B cell leukaemia	*abl*
FBJ murine osteosarcoma	Mouse	Osteosarcoma	*fos*
Moloney murine sarcoma	Mouse	Sarcoma	*mos*
Harvey murine sarcoma	Rat	Sarcoma	*Ha-ras*
Kirsten murine sarcoma	Rat	Sarcoma	*Ki-ras*
Simian sarcoma	Monkey	Sarcoma	*sis*

IDENTIFICATION OF ONCOGENES

Oncogenes have been identified by two types of cyto-genetic findings found in association with certain types of leukaemias and tumours in humans. These include the location of oncogenes at chromosomal translocation break-points or their amplification in double minute chromosomes or homogeneously staining regions of chromosomes. In addition, a number of oncogenes have also been identified by the ability of tumour DNA to induce tumours in vitro by DNA transfection.

Identification of oncogenes at chromosomal translocation break-points

Chromosome aberrations are common in malignant cells which often show marked variation in chromosome number and structure. Certain chromosomes seemed to be more commonly involved and it was initially thought that these changes were secondary to the transformed state rather than causal. This attitude changed when evidence suggested that chromosomal structural changes, often translocations (p. 46), resulted in rearrangements within or adjacent to proto-oncogenes. It has been found that chromosomal translocations can lead to novel chimeric genes with altered biochemical function or level of proto-oncogene activity. There are numerous examples of both types, of which chronic myeloid leukaemia is an example of the former and Burkitt's lymphoma an example of the latter.

Chronic myeloid leukaemia

In 1960, investigators in Philadelphia were the first to describe an abnormal chromosome in white blood cells from patients with chronic myeloid leukaemia. The abnormal chromosome, referred to as the Philadelphia, or Ph[1] chromosome, is an acquired abnormality found in blood or bone marrow cells but not found in other tissues from these patients. The Ph[1] is a tiny chromosome which is now known to be a chromosome 22 from

Fig. 13.2

Karyotype from a patient with chronic myeloid leukaemia, showing the chromosome 22 (arrowed) or Philadelphia chromosome which has material translocated to the long arm of one of the number 9 chromosomes (arrowed).

which material from the long arm has been reciprocally translocated to and from the long arm of chromosome 9 (Fig. 13.2), i.e. t(9;22)(q34;q11). This chromosomal re-arrangement is seen in 90% of persons with this form of leukaemia. This translocation has been found to transfer the cellular *abl* oncogene from chromosome 9 into a region of chromosome 22 known as the *break point cluster*, or *bcr*, region resulting in a chimeric transcript derived from both the c-*abl* (70%) and the *bcr* genes. This results in a chimeric gene expressing a fusion protein consisting of the *bcr* protein at the amino end and *abl* protein at the carboxy end which is associated with transforming activity.

Burkitt's lymphoma

An unusual form of neoplasia seen in children in Africa is a lymphoma which involves the jaw, known as Burkitt's lymphoma, so named after Dennis Burkitt who first described the condition in the late 1950s. Chromosomal analysis has revealed the majority (90%) of affected children to have a translocation of the c-*myc* gene from the long arm of chromosome 8 on to chromosome 14. Less commonly the c-*myc* gene is translocated to chromosome 2 or 22. The regions of chromosomes 14, 2 and 22 involved encode the genes for the immunoglobulin heavy chain and the kappa (κ) and lambda (λ) light chains respectively (p. 179). As a consequence of these translocations c-*myc* comes under the influence of the regulatory sequences of the respective immunoglobulin gene and is overexpressed tenfold or more.

Oncogene amplification

Proto-oncogenes can also be activated by the production of multiple copies of the gene or what is known as *gene amplification*, a mechanism known to have survival value when cells encounter environmental stress. For example, when leukaemic cells are exposed to the chemotherapeutic agent methotrexate, the cells acquire resistance to the drug by making multiple copies of the gene for dihydrofolate reductase, the target enzyme for methotrexate.

Gene amplification can increase the number of copies of the oncogene per cell severalfold to several hundred times, leading to greater amounts of the corresponding oncoprotein. In mammals the amplified sequence of DNA in tumour cells can be recognized by the presence of small extra chromosomes known as *double-minute chromosomes* or *homogeneously staining regions* of the chromosomes. These changes are seen in approximately 10% of tumours and are often present more commonly in the later rather than the early stages of the malignant process.

Amplification of specific proto-oncogenes appears to be a feature of certain tumours and is frequently seen with the MYC family of genes. For example, N-*myc* is amplified in approximately 30% of neuroblastomas but in advanced cases this figure rises to 50%, where gene amplification can be up to 1000-fold. Human small cell carcinomas of the lung also show amplification of c-*myc*, N-*myc*, and L-*myc*.

Amplification of c-*erb*-B2, c-*myc* and cyclin D1 is a feature in 20% of breast carcinomas where it has been suggested that it correlates with a number of well established prognostic factors such as lymph node status, oestrogen and progestogen receptor status, tumour size and histological grade.

Detection of oncogenes by DNA transfection studies

The ability of DNA from a human bladder carcinoma cell line to transform a well established mouse fibroblast cell line called NIH3T3, as demonstrated by the loss of contact inhibition of the cells in culture, or what is known as DNA *transfection*, led to the discovery of the human sequence homologous to the *ras* gene of the Harvey murine sarcoma virus. The human *ras* gene family consists of three closely related members, c-H-*ras*, c-K-*ras* and N-*ras*. The *ras* proteins are closely homologous to their viral counterparts and only differ from one another near the carboxy termini. Oncogenicity of the *ras* proto-oncogenes has been shown to arise by acquisition of point mutations in the nucleotide sequence. In approximately 50% of colorectal cancers and 95% of pancreatic cancers, as well as in a proportion of thyroid and lung cancers, a mutation in a *ras* gene can be demonstrated.

DNA transfection studies have also led to identification of other oncogenes which have not been demonstrated through retroviral studies. These include *met*, *trk*, *mas* and *ret* (Table 13.4).

Table 13.4 The functional classification of oncogenes as intracellular signalling transduction factors

Growth factors	Growth factor receptors	Proteins with GTPase activity	Post receptor tyrosine kinases	Cytoplasmic serine threonine kinases	Nuclear DNA-binding trancription factors	Cell-cycle factors
sis (PDGF)	*erb*-B	N-*ras*	*src*	*mos*	*fos*	*cyclin D1*
int (FGF-related)	*erb*-B2	Ha-*ras*	*abl*	*raf*	*jun*	*bcl*-2
hst (FGF-related)	*fms*	Ki-*ras*	*yes*	*pim*	*erb*-A	
	kit	*gsp*	*fgr*		*myb*	
	ros	*gip*	*fes*		*myc*	
	trk				N-*myc*	
	ret				L-*myc*	
	met				*ski*	
	mas				*rel*	
					ets	

FUNCTION OF ONCOGENES

Cancers have characteristics which indicate, at the cellular level, loss of the normal function of oncogene products consistent with a role in the control of cellular proliferation and differentiation in the process known as *signal transduction*. Signal transduction is a complex multistep pathway from the cell membrane, through the cytoplasm to the nucleus involving a variety of types of proto-oncogene products involved in positive and negative feedback loops necessary for accurate cell proliferation and differentiation (Fig. 13.3).

Proto-oncogenes have been highly conserved during evolution, being present in a wide variety of different species, indicating that the protein products they encode are likely to have essential biological functions. Proto-oncogenes act in three main ways in the process of signal transduction. The first is through phosphorylation of serine, threonine and tyrosine residues of proteins by the transfer of phosphate groups from ATP. This leads to alteration of the configuration activating the kinase activity of proteins and generating docking sites for target proteins resulting in signal transduction. The *ras* family

of proto-oncogenes are examples of the second type which are GTPases and which function as molecular switches through the GDP/GTP cycle as intermediates relaying the transduction signal from membrane associated tyrosine kinases to serine threonine kinases. The third type involves proteins located in the nucleus which control progress through the cell cycle, DNA replication and the expression of genes.

TYPES OF ONCOGENES

Oncogenes can be classified according to their cellular location and the function of their encoded oncoproteins in the signal transduction pathway (Table 13.4).

Growth factors

The transition of a cell from G_0 to the start of the cell cycle (p. 40) is governed by substances called *growth factors*. Growth factors stimulate cells to grow by binding to growth factor receptors. The best known oncogene which acts as a growth factor is the v-*sis* oncogene which encodes part of the biologically active platelet-derived growth factor (PDG) B subunit. When v-*sis* oncoprotein is added to the NIH 3T3 cultures, the cells are transformed, behaving like neoplastic cells, i.e. their growth rate increases and they lose contact inhibition. In vivo they form tumours when injected into nude mice. Oncogene products showing homology to fibroblast growth factors (FGFs) include *hst* and *int*-2 which are amplified in stomach cancers and in malignant melanomas respectively.

Growth factor receptors

Many oncogenes encode proteins which form growth factor receptors with tyrosine kinase activity possessing tyrosine kinase domains which allow cells to bypass the normal control mechanisms. More than 40 different tyrosine kinases have been identified and can be divided into two main types, those which span the cell membrane (growth factor receptor tyrosine kinases) and those which are located in the cytoplasm (non-receptor tyrosine kinases). Examples of tyrosine kinases include c-*erb*-B which encodes the epidermal growth factor (EGFR) receptor and the related c-*erb*-B2 oncogene. Mutations in, rearrangements of or amplification of the c-*erb*-B2 oncogene result in ligand independent activation which has been associated with cancer of the stomach, pancreas and ovary.

Intracellular signalling transduction factors

Two different types of intracellular signalling transduction factors have been identified, proteins with GTPase activity and cytoplasmic serine threonine kinases.

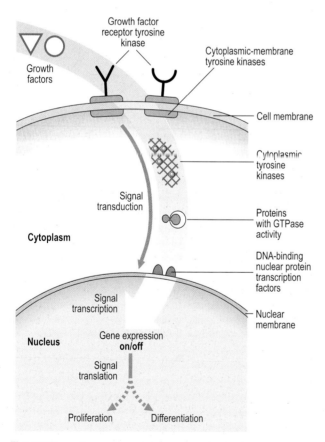

Fig. 13.3
Simplified schema of the steps in signal transduction and transcription from cell surface to nucleus. The intracellular pathway amplifies the signal by a cascade which involves one or more of the steps.

Proteins with GTPase activity

Proteins with GTPase activity are intracellular membrane proteins which bind GTP to become active and through their intrinsic GTPase activity generate GDP which inactivates the protein. Mutations in the *ras* genes result in increased or sustained GTPase activity leading to unrestrained growth.

Cytoplasmic serine threonine kinases

A number of soluble cytoplasmic gene products are recognized to be part of the signal transduction pathway. The *raf* oncogene product modulates the normal signalling transduction cascade. Mutations in the gene can result in sustained or increased transmission of a growth promoting signal to the nucleus.

DNA binding nuclear proteins

The *fos*, *jun* and *erb*-A oncogenes encode proteins which are specific transcription factors which regulate gene expression by activating or suppressing nearby DNA sequences. The function of c-*myc* and related genes remains uncertain but appears to be related to alterations in control of the cell cycle. The c-*myc* and c-*myb* oncoproteins stimulate cells to progress from the G_1 into the S phase of the cell cycle (p. 40). Their overproduction prevents cells from entering a prolonged resting phase, resulting in persistent cellular proliferation.

Cell cycle factors

Cancer cells can increase in number either by increased growth and division or accumulate through decreased cell death. Most cells in vivo are in a non-dividing state. Progress through the cell cycle (p. 40) is regulated at two points, one in G_1 when a cell becomes committed to DNA synthesis in the S phase and another in G_2 for cell division in the M (mitosis) phase, through factors known as cyclin-dependent kinases. Abnormalities in regulation of the cell cycle through growth factors, growth factor receptors, GTPases or nuclear proteins or loss of inhibitory factors leads to activation of the cyclin-dependent kinases, such as cyclin D1, resulting in cellular transformation with uncontrolled cell division. Alternatively loss of the factors which lead to normal programmed cell death, or what is known as *apoptosis* (p. 82), can result in the accumulation of cells through prolonged cell survival as a mechanism of development of some tumours. Activation of the *bcl*-2 oncogene through chromosomal rearrangements is associated with inhibition of apoptosis leading to certain types of lymphomas.

TUMOUR SUPPRESSOR GENES

While the study of oncogenes has revealed much about the cellular biology of the somatic genetic events in the malignant process, the study of hereditary cancer in humans has revealed the existence of what are known as *tumour suppressor genes*.

Studies carried out by Harris and colleagues in the late 1960s, which involved fusion of malignant cells with non-malignant cells in culture, resulted in the suppression of the malignant phenotype in the hybrid cells. The recurrence of the malignant phenotype with loss of certain chromosomes from the hybrid cells suggested that normal cells contain a gene(s) with tumour suppressor activity which, if lost or inactive, can lead to malignancy and which was acting like a recessive trait. Such genes were initially referred to as antioncogenes. This term was considered inappropriate since they do not oppose the action of the oncogenes and are more correctly known as tumour suppressor genes. The basis for our understanding of the biology of tumour suppressor genes came from the study of the eye tumour retinoblastoma.

RETINOBLASTOMA

Retinoblastoma (Rb) is a relatively rare, highly malignant childhood cancer of the developing retinal cells of the eye which usually occurs before the age of 5 years (Fig. 13.4). If diagnosed and treated at an early stage, it is associated with a good long-term outcome.

Retinoblastoma can occur either sporadically, the so-called 'non-hereditary' form, or be familial, the so-called

Fig. 13.4
Section of an eye showing a retinoblastoma in situ.

'hereditary' form, which is inherited in an autosomal dominant manner. Non-hereditary cases usually involve only one eye, whereas hereditary cases can be unilateral but are more commonly bilateral or occur in more than one site in one eye, i.e. are multifocal. The familial form also tends to present at an earlier age than the non-hereditary or sporadic form.

'Two-hit' hypothesis

In 1971, Knudson carried out an epidemiological study of a large number of cases of both types of retinoblastoma and advanced a 'two-hit' hypothesis to explain the occurrence of this rare tumour in patients with and without a positive family history. He proposed that affected individuals with a positive family history had inherited one non-functional gene which was present in all the cells of the individual, or what is known as a *germ line mutation*, with the second gene at the same locus becoming inactivated somatically in a developing retinal cell. The occurrence of a second mutation was likely given the large number of retinal cells, explaining the autosomal dominant pattern of inheritance. This would also explain the observation that in hereditary retinoblastoma the tumours were occasionally bilateral and multifocal. In contrast, in the non-heritable or sporadic form, two inactivating *somatic mutations* would need to occur independently in the same retinoblast, which was much less likely to occur, explaining the fact that tumours in these patients were often unilateral and unifocal and usually occurred at a later age than in the hereditary form.

It was also recognized, however, that approximately 5% of children presenting with retinoblastoma had other physical abnormalities along with developmental concerns. Detailed cytogenetic analysis of blood samples from these children revealed some of them to have an interstitial deletion involving the long arm of one of their number 13 chromosome pair. Comparison of the regions deleted revealed a common 'smallest region of overlap' involving the sub-band 13q14 (Fig. 13.5). The detection of a specific chromosomal region involved in the aetiology of these cases of retinoblastoma (p. 254) suggested that it could also be the locus involved in the autosomal dominant familial form of retinoblastoma. Family studies using a polymorphic enzyme, esterase D, which had previously been mapped to that region, rapidly confirmed linkage of the hereditary form of retinoblastoma to that locus.

Loss of constitutional heterozygosity

Analyses of the DNA sequences in this region of chromosome 13 in the peripheral blood and in retinoblastoma

Fig. 13.5
Two homologues of chromosome 13 from a patient with retinoblastoma showing an interstitial deletion of 13q14 in the right-hand homologue as indicated.

tumour material of children who had inherited the gene for retinoblastoma showed them to have loss of an allele at the retinoblastoma locus in the tumour material or what is known as *loss of constitutional heterozygosity* (LOCH). An example of this is shown in Figure 13.6A in which the mother transmits the retinoblastoma gene along with allele 2 at a closely linked marker locus. The father is homozygous for allele 1 at this same locus with the result that the child is constitutionally an obligate heterozygote at this locus. Analysis of the tumour tissue reveals apparent homozygosity for allele 2. In fact, there has been loss of the paternally derived allele 1, i.e. LOCH in the tumour material. This loss of heterozygosity is consistent with the 'two-hit' hypothesis leading to development of the malignancy as proposed by Knudson.

LOCH can occur through several mechanisms which include loss of a chromosome through mitotic non-disjunction (p. 254), a deletion on the chromosome carrying the corresponding allele or a cross-over between the two homologous genes leading to homozygosity for the mutant allele (Fig. 13.6B). Observation of consistent cytogenetic rearrangements in other malignancies has led to demonstration of loss of heterozygosity in a number of other cancers (Table 13.5). Subsequent to the observation of LOCH, linkage studies of familial cases can be carried out to determine if the familial cases of a specific type of malignancy are due to mutations at the same locus and thus lead to the identification of the gene responsible, as occurred with the isolation of the *RB1* gene.

Function of tumour suppressor genes

While familial retinoblastoma was classically considered to be an autosomal dominant trait, demonstration of the

Table 13.5   Syndromes and cancers which show loss of heterozygosity and their chromosomal location

Syndrome or cancer	Chromosomal location
Retinoblastoma	13q14
Osteosarcoma	13q, 17p
Wilms' tumour	11p13, 11p15, 16q
Renal carcinoma	3p25, 17p13
von Hippel–Lindau disease	3p25
Bladder carcinoma	9q21, 11p15, 17p13
Lung carcinoma	3p, 13q14, 17p
Breast carcinoma	11p15, 11q, 13q12, 13q14, 17p13, 17q21
Rhabdomyosarcoma	11p15, 17p13
Hepatoblastoma	5q, 11p15
Gastric cancer	1p, 5q, 7q, 11p, 13q, 17p, 18p
Familial adenomatous polyposis	5q21
Colorectal carcinoma	1p, 5q21, 8p, 17p13, 18q21
Neurofibromatosis I (NF1 von Recklinghausen's disease)	17q
Neurofibromatosis II (NF2)	22q
Meningioma	22q
Multiple endocrine neoplasia type 1 (MEN1)	11q
Thyroid medullary carcinoma	1p
Phaeochromocytoma	1p
Melanoma	9p21, 17q
Ovarian	16q, 17q
Pancreatic	9p21, 13q14, 17p13
Prostate cancer	1p36, 7q, 8p, 10q, 13q, 16q

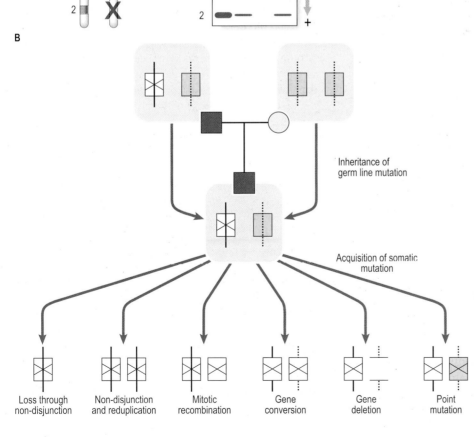

Fig. 13.6

(A) Diagrammatic representation of the loss of constitutional heterozygosity (LOCH) in the development of a tumour. The mother (M) and father (F) are both homozygous for different alleles at the same locus, 2–2 and 1–1 respectively. The child (C) will therefore be constitutionally heterozygous, 1–2. If an analysis of DNA from a tumour at that locus reveals only a single allele, 2, this is consistent with LOCH.

(B) Diagrammatic representations of the mechanisms leading to the 'second hit' leading to the development of retinoblastoma.

action of the retinoblastoma gene as a tumour suppressor gene is consistent with it being, in fact, a recessive trait, as originally suggested in the somatic cell hybridization studies carried out by Harris and his colleagues. In other words, absence of the gene product in the homozygous state leads to the development of this particular tumour. In contrast to oncogenes, tumour suppressor genes are a class of cellular genes whose normal function is to suppress inappropriate cell proliferation, i.e. the development of a malignancy is due to a loss-of-function mutation (p. 23).

The tumour suppressor activity of the retinoblastoma gene has been demonstrated in vitro in cancer cells. In addition, further support for the *RB1* gene acting as a tumour suppressor gene comes from the recognition that individuals with the hereditary form of retinoblastoma have an increased risk of developing second new malignancies later in life which include osteosarcoma, fibrosarcoma and chondrosarcomas.

The RB1 gene/p110^{RB} protein

The *RB1* gene specifies a 4.7 kb transcript which encodes a nuclear protein, p110^{RB}, which associates with DNA and is involved in the regulation of the cell cycle. Fortuitously, unrelated research on the mechanism of action of the *E1A* oncogene of human adenovirus, demonstrated that *E1A* oncoprotein forms a complex with p110^{RB} which results in its inhibition. As *E1A* is known to be a transcription regulator it is suggested that p110^{RB} is also involved in modulating the transcription of critical genes. p110^{RB} exists in a phosphorylated or unphosphorylated state. In its unphosphorylated state p110^{RB} is active in growth suppression. In its phosphorylated state it associates with a number of other factors involved in the cell cycle which includes cyclin-dependent and independent kinases allowing the cell to proceed into the S phase of the cell cycle (p. 40).

p110^{RB} interacts with several viral oncoproteins, such as the transforming proteins of SV40 (large T antigen) and papilloma virus (E7 protein), and is inactivated, thereby liberating cells from normal growth constraints.

These findings yield insight into the mechanisms of interaction between oncogenes and tumour suppressor genes. As research continues there could well be many other examples whereby oncogenes exert their influence by directly or indirectly inactivating the function of tumour suppressor gene encoded proteins or other proteins intimately involved in the cell cycle.

p53

The p53 protein was first identified as a host cell protein bound to T antigen, the dominant transforming oncogene of the DNA tumour virus SV40. After the murine p53 gene was cloned it was shown to be able to cooperate with activated *ras* and act as an oncogene transforming primary rodent cells in vitro, even though the rodent cells expressed the wild-type or normal p53. Subsequently, inactivation of p53 was frequently found in murine Friend virus-induced erythroleukaemia cells, which led to the proposal that the *Tp53* gene was, in fact, a tumour suppressor gene.

Twenty to 25% of breast and over 50% of bladder, colon and lung cancers have been found to have *Tp53* mutations which, although occurring in different codons, are clustered in highly conserved regions in exons 5 to 10. This is in contrast to p53 mutations in hepatocellular carcinoma which occur in a 'hot spot' in codon 249. The base change in this mutated codon, usually G to T, could be the result of an interaction with the carcinogen aflatoxin B1 which is associated with liver cancer in China and South Africa, or with the hepatitis B virus which is also implicated as a risk factor in hepatomas. Interestingly, aflatoxin B1, a ubiquitous food-contaminating aflatoxin in these areas, is a mutagen in many animal species and induces G to T substitutions in mutagenesis experiments. If an interaction between hepatitis B viral proteins and non-mutated p53 can be demonstrated, this will further support the role of this virus in the aetiology of hepatocellular carcinomas.

The p53 protein is a multimeric complex. Mutant p53 protein monomers are more stable than the normal p53 proteins and can form complexes with the normal wild-type p53 acting in a dominant-negative manner to inactivate it. p53 has been coined the 'guardian of the genome'. It functions as a check-point control site in the cell cycle at G_1 before the S phase interacting with other factors including cyclins and p21 preventing DNA damaged through normal 'wear and tear' from being replicated.

The Li-Fraumeni syndrome

As mutations in *Tp53* appear to be a common event in the genesis of many cancers, an inherited or germ line mutation of *Tp53* would be expected to have serious consequences. This hypothesis was substantiated with the discovery of such a defect in persons with the Li–Fraumeni syndrome. Members of families with this rare syndrome (p. 202), which is inherited as an autosomal dominant trait, are highly susceptible to developing a variety of malignancies at a relatively early age. These include sarcomas, adrenal carcinomas and breast cancer. Point mutations in highly conserved regions of the *Tp53* gene (codons 245–258) have been identified in the germ line of family members with analysis of the tumour revealing loss of the normal allele.

GENETICS OF COMMON CANCERS

It is estimated that about 5% of colorectal and breast cancer arises as a result of an inherited cancer susceptibility gene. It is likely that, with the exception of cancers where there is an obvious external factor involved, a similar proportion of many other cancers are due to genetic factors. Study of the common cancers, bowel or colorectal and breast cancer, has provided further insights into the genetics of cancer.

COLORECTAL CANCER

One in 50 persons in the developed countries of Western Europe and North America will develop cancer of the bowel or colorectal cancer. An understanding of the development of colorectal cancer has shed light on the process of carcinogenesis.

The multistage process of carcinogenesis

The majority of colorectal cancers are believed to develop from 'benign' adenomas. Conversely, only a small percentage of adenomas proceed to invasive cancer. Histologically, adenomatous polyps less than 1 cm in diameter rarely contain areas of carcinomatous changes, whereas

Fig. 13.7
Representation of the events in the multistage process of carcinogenesis in colorectal cancer.

the risk of carcinomatous change increases to 5–10% when an adenoma reaches 2 cm in diameter. The transition from a small adenomatous polyp to an invasive cancer is thought to take between 5 and 10 years. Adenomatous polyps less than 1 cm in diameter have mutations in the *ras* gene in less than 10% of cases. As the size of the polyp increases to between 1 and 2 cm the prevalence of *ras* gene mutations is in the region of 40%, rising to approximately 50% in full-blown colorectal cancers.

Similarly, allele loss of chromosome 5 markers occurs in approximately 40% of adenomatous polyps and 70% of carcinomas. Deletions on chromosome 17p in the region containing the p53 gene occur in more than 75% of carcinomas, but this is an uncommon finding in small or intermediate-sized polyps. A region on 18q is deleted in about 10% of small adenomas, rising to almost 50% when the adenoma shows foci of invasive carcinoma and in over 70% of carcinomas (Fig. 13.7).

It appears, therefore, that mutations of the *ras* and p53 genes and loss of constitutional heterozygosity on 5q and 18q accumulate during the transition from a small 'benign' adenoma to carcinoma. The accumulation of alterations, rather than the order, appears to be more important in the development of carcinoma. More than one of these four alterations is seen in only 7% of small, early adenomas. Two or more such alterations are seen, with increasing frequency, when adenomas progress in size and show histological features of malignancy. Over 90% of carcinomas show two or more such alterations and approximately 40% show three.

The multistage process of the development of cancer is likely, of course, to be an oversimplification. The distinction between oncogenes and tumour suppressor genes (Table 13.6) has not stood the test of time, e.g. the *RET* oncogene and *MEN2* (p. 88). In addition, the same mutation in some of the inherited cancer syndromes (p. 203) can result in cancers at various sites in different individuals which could be a consequence of the effect of interactions with inherited polymorphic variation in a

Table 13.6 Some familial cancers or cancer syndromes due to tumour suppressor mutations

Disorder	Gene	Locus
Retinoblastoma	*RB1*	13q14
Familial adenomatous polyposis	*APC*	5q31
Li–Fraumeni syndrome	*Tp53*	17p13
von Hippel–Lindau syndrome	*VHL*	3p25–26
Multiple endocrine neoplasia type II	*RET*	10q11.2
Breast-ovarian cancer	*BRCA1*	17q21
Breast cancer	*BRCA2*	13q12–13
Gastric cancer	*CDH1*	16q22.1
Wilms' tumour	*WT1*	11p13
Neurofibromatosis I	*NF1*	17q12–22

number of other genes or a variety of environmental agents.

Further insight into the processes involved in the development of colorectal cancer came from a rare cause of familial colon cancer known as familial adenomatous polyposis.

Familial adenomatous polyposis

Approximately 1% of persons who develop colorectal cancer do so through inheritance of an autosomal dominant disorder known as familial adenomatous polyposis (FAP). Affected persons develop polyps of the large bowel, which can involve its entirety (Fig. 13.8). There is a high risk of carcinomatous change taking place in these polyps with more than 90% of persons with FAP eventually developing bowel cancer.

The identification of an individual with FAP and an interstitial deletion of a particular region of the long arm of chromosome 5 (5q21) led to the demonstration of linkage of FAP to DNA markers in that region (p. 74). Subsequent studies led to the isolation of the adenomatous polyposis coli (APC) gene. Analyses of the markers linked to the APC gene in cancers from persons who have inherited the gene for this disorder have shown loss of constitutional heterozygosity, suggesting a similar mechanism of gene action in the development of this type of bowel cancer.

Studies in the common form of bowel cancer which is not inherited have shown similar loss of constitutional heterozygosity at 5q in the tumour material with the FAP gene being deleted in 40% and 70% of sporadically occurring adenomas and carcinomas of the colon. LOCH has also been reported at a number of different sites in colon cancer tumours which include the regions 18q21-qter and 17p12–13, the latter region including the p53 gene, as well as another gene at 5q21 known as the *'mutated in colorectal cancer'* (MCC) gene, consistent with the development of the common form of colon cancer being a multistage process.

'Deleted in colorectal cancer' (DCC)

Allele loss on chromosome 18q is seen in over 70% of colorectal carcinomas. The original candidate gene for this region, called *deleted in colorectal carcinoma*, or *DCC*, has been identified and cloned and has a high degree of homology with the family of genes encoding cell adhesion molecules. The *DCC* gene is expressed in normal colonic mucosa but is either reduced or absent in colorectal carcinomas. As with *Tp53*, somatic mutations in the *DCC* gene of the remaining allele occur in some cancers where gene expression is absent. The known homology suggests that loss of *DCC* plays a role in cell–cell and cell–basement membrane interactions, features which are lost in overt malignancy. Mutations in the DCC gene have only been found, however, in a small proportion of colon cancers. Other genes deleted in this region in colorectal tumours, including DPC4 and JV18-1, have been suggested as other possible tumour suppressor genes.

Hereditary non-polyposis colorectal cancer

A proportion of individuals with familial colon cancer are found to have fewer polyps than usually seen in persons with familial adenomatous polyposis. In addition, the colon cancer which occurs in individuals from these families occurs more frequently in the proximal or right side of the colon, or what is sometimes called 'site-specific' colon cancer. This familial cancer-predisposing

Fig. 13.8
Large bowel from a person with polyposis coli opened up to show multiple polyps throughout the colon. (Courtesy of Mr P Finan, Department of Surgery, General Infirmary, Leeds.)

syndrome is inherited as an autosomal dominant disorder and is known as hereditary non-polyposis colorectal cancer (HNPCC).

Mismatch repair genes

Comparison of polymorphic microsatellite markers in tumour tissue and constitutional cells in persons with HNPCC looking for loss of constitutional heterozygosity, somewhat surprisingly revealed the presence of new rather than less alleles in the DNA from tumour tissue. In contrast to the site-specific chromosome rearrangements seen with certain malignancies (p. 192), this phenomenon known as *microsatellite instability* or *replication error* (RER) is generalized, occurring with all microsatellite markers analysed, irrespective of their chromosomal location.

This phenomenon was recognized to be similar to that seen in association with mutations in genes known as *mutator genes*, such as the *MutHLS* genes in yeast and *E. coli*. In addition, the human homologues of the mutator genes were located in regions of the human chromosomes to which HNPCC had previously been mapped, rapidly leading to the cloning of the genes responsible for HNPCC in humans (Table 13.7). The mutator genes code for a system of 'proof-reading' enzymes and are usually known as *mismatch repair genes* which detect mismatched base pairs arising through errors in DNA replication or acquired causes, e.g. mutagens.

Individuals who inherit a mutation in one of the mismatch repair genes responsible for HNPCC are constitutionally heterozygous for a loss-of-function mutation (p. 23). Loss-of-function of the second copy through any of the mechanisms discussed in relation to LOCH (p. 196) results in defective mismatch repair leading to an increased mutation rate associated with an increased risk of developing malignancy. Although HNPCC accounts for a small proportion of colon cancers, estimated to be between 2–4%, approximately 15% of all colorectal cancers exhibit microsatellite instability, the proportion being greater in tumours from persons who develop colorectal cancer at a younger age. Some of these latter persons have been shown to have inherited constitutional mutations in one of the mismatch repair genes in the absence of a family history of colon cancer. In addition, there is an increased risk for women with HNPCC to develop endometrial cancer, estimated to be a lifetime risk of 20–40%.

BREAST CANCER

Approximately 1 in 12 women will develop breast cancer, this being the most common cancer in women between 40 and 55 years of age, with approximately 1 in 3 affected women going on to develop metastatic disease. Fifteen to 20% of women who develop breast cancer have a family history of the disorder. Family studies have shown that the risk of a woman developing breast cancer is greater the more affected female relatives she has and the earlier the age of presentation in those relatives.

Molecular studies of breast cancer tumours revealed a variety of different findings which included amplification of *erb*-B1, *erb*-B2, *myc* and *int*-2 oncogenes as well as loss of heterozygosity for a number of chromosomes at a number of sites including 1q, 3p, 11p, 13q and 17q. In many breast tumours showing loss of heterozygosity, allele loss occurs at between two and four of the sites, again suggesting that the accumulation of alterations, rather than their order, is important in the evolution of breast cancer.

BRCA1 and BRCA2 genes

Family studies of early onset or premenopausal breast cancer showed that it behaved like a dominant trait in many families. Linkage analysis in these families showed that the tendency to develop breast cancer mapped to the long arm of chromosome 17 eventually leading to identification of the *BRCA1* gene. A proportion of families with early onset breast cancer which did not show linkage to this region showed linkage to the long arm of chromosome 13 resulting in the identification of the *BRCA2* gene.

Approximately 40–50% of families with early onset autosomal dominant breast cancer have a mutation in the *BRCA1* gene and have been shown to have an 80–90% lifetime risk of developing breast cancer. Individuals with a mutation in the *BRCA1* gene also have an increased risk of developing bowel cancer, females an increased risk of developing ovarian cancer and males an increased risk of developing prostate cancer. Mutations in the *BRCA2* gene account for 30–40% of families with early onset autosomal dominant breast cancer and have a similar lifetime risk of developing breast cancer. Although initially mutations in the *BRCA2* gene were not thought to be associated with an increased risk of other cancers, women heterozygous for a mutation have a slightly increased risk of developing ovarian cancer. In

---

Table 13.7 Mismatch repair genes associated with hereditary non-polyposis colorectal cancer

Human gene	Chromosomal locus	*E. coli* homologue	HNPCC (%)
hMSH2	2p15–22	MutS	50–60
hMLH1	3p21.3	MutL	30–40
hPMS1	2q31–q33	MutL	5
hPMS2	7p22	MutL	5

some of the original families with familial breast cancer collected for linkage studies, a number had males who had developed breast cancer. Although breast cancer in males is very rare, males with mutations in the *BRCA2* gene have been shown to have a 6% lifetime risk of developing breast cancer, approximately a 100-fold increase in the population risk of breast cancer in males.

OVARIAN CANCER

One in 70 women will develop ovarian cancer during her lifetime, the incidence increasing with age. Approximately 5% of women with ovarian cancer have a family history of the disorder and it is estimated that 1% of ovarian cancer is due to an autosomal dominant gene. In families with multiple women affected with ovarian cancer, the age of presentation is some 10 to 15 years earlier than that at which ovarian cancer occurs in the general population. Mutations in *BRCA1*, the genes responsible for HNPCC and less commonly in *BRCA2* will be responsible for a proportion of these families, but a locus for a gene for susceptibility to site-specific ovarian cancer has yet to be identified.

PROSTATE CANCER

Prostate cancer is the most common cancer in men, being the most common cancer after breast cancer, with men having a lifetime risk of 10% of developing prostate cancer and a 3% chance of dying from it. Enquiries into the family history of males presenting with prostate cancer revealed a significant proportion, in the region of 15%, to have a first-degree male relative with prostate cancer. Family studies have shown that first-degree male relatives of a man presenting with prostate cancer have between two and five times the population risk of developing prostate cancer. Analysis of prostate cancer tumour material has revealed loss of heterozygosity at several chromosomal locations. Segregation analysis of family studies of prostate cancer suggested that a single dominant susceptibility locus could be responsible accounting for 9% of all prostate cancers and up to 40% of early onset prostate cancers. Linkage analysis studies have identified two major susceptibility loci, hereditary prostate cancer-1 and 2 (*HPC1* and *HPC2*), and a number of other more minor susceptibility loci. Mutations in three genes, *PTEN*, *MXI1* and *KAI1*, have been identified in a minority of families with familial prostate cancer.

Although the majority of prostate cancers occur in men after the age of 65 years, individuals with a family history of prostate cancer consistent with the possibility of a dominant gene being responsible have a significantly increased risk of developing prostate cancer at a relatively younger age. Screening by measuring prostate-specific antigen levels has been suggested but problems with specificity and sensitivity mean that this has limited value.

GENETIC COUNSELLING IN FAMILIAL CANCER

Recognition of individuals with an inherited susceptibility to cancer usually relies on taking a careful family history to document the presence or absence of other family members with similar or related cancers. The malignancies which develop in susceptible individuals are often the same as those which occur in the population in general. There are a number of other features which can suggest an inherited cancer susceptibility syndrome in a family (Table 13.8).

INHERITED CANCER-PREDISPOSING SYNDROMES

While most cancers due to an inherited cancer syndrome occur at a specific site, families have been described in which cancers occur at more than one site in an individual or at different sites in various members of the family more commonly than would be expected. These families are referred to as having a familial cancer-predisposing syndrome. The majority of the rare inherited familial cancer-predisposing syndromes currently recognized are dominantly inherited, with offspring of affected individuals having a 50% chance of inheriting the gene and therefore of being at increased risk of developing cancer (Table 13.9). There are also a number of syndromes usually inherited as autosomal recessive disorders with an increased risk of developing cancer associated with an increased number of abnormalities in their chromosomes when they are cultured, or what are known as the chromosomal breakage syndromes. These are discussed in detail in Chapter 17 (p. 262).

Persons with an inherited familial cancer-predisposing syndrome are at risk of developing a second tumour (multifocal or bilateral in the case of breast cancer), have an increased risk of developing a cancer at a relatively

---

Table 13.8 Features suggestive of an inherited cancer susceptibility syndrome in a family

Several close (first- or second-degree) relatives with a common cancer
Several close relatives with related cancers, e.g. breast and ovary or bowel and endometrial
Two family members with the same rare cancer
An unusually early age of onset
Bilateral tumours in paired organs
Synchronous or successive tumours
Tumours in two different organ systems in one individual

Table 13.9 Inherited family cancer syndromes, mode of inheritance, gene responsible and chromosomal site

Syndrome	Mode of inheritance*	Gene	Chromosomal site	Main cancer(s)
Breast/ovary families	AD	BRCA1	17q21	Breast, ovary, colon, prostate
Breast families	AD	BRCA2	13q12	Breast, ovary
Familial adenomatous polyposis	AD	APC	5q21	Colorectal, duodenal, thyroid
Turcot's	AD	APC	5q21	Colorectal, brain
		hMLH1	3p21.3	
		hMSH2	2p15–22	
Hereditary non-polyposis colorectal cancer (HNPCC)				
• Lynch I	AD	hMSH2	2p15–22	Colorectal
		hMLH1	3p21.3	
		hPMS1	2q31–33	
		hPMS2	7p22	
• Lynch II	AD	hMSH2	2p15–22	Colorectal, endometrial, urinary tract, ovarian, gastric, small bowel, hepatobiliary
		hMLH1	3p21.3	
		hPMS1	2q31–33	
		hPMS2	7p22	
Muir–Torre	AD	hMSH2	2p15–22	As Lynch II plus sebaceous tumours, laryngeal
Familial juvenile polyposis	AD	SMAD4/DPC4	18q21.1	Colorectal
Peutz–Jeghers	AD	STK11	19p13.3	Gastrointestinal, breast, uterus, ovary, testis
Familial retinoblastoma	AD	RB1	13q14	Retinoblastoma
Li–Fraumeni	AD	Tp53	17p13	Sarcoma, breast, brain, leukaemia, adrenal cortex
Multiple endocrine neoplasia (MEN) type II	AD	RET	10q11.2	Thyroid (medullary), phaeochromocytoma
von Hippel–Lindau	AD	VHL	3p25–26	CNS haemangioblastoma, renal, pancreatic, phaeochromocytoma
Dysplastic naevus syndrome (familial atypical mole melanoma, FAMM)	AD	CMM1	1p	Melanoma

*AD = autosomal dominant

younger age compared to persons with the sporadic form, and can develop tumours at different sites in the body, although one type of cancer is usually predominant.

A number of different familial cancer-predisposing syndromes have been described, depending on the patterns of cancer which occur within a family. For example, persons with the Li–Fraumeni syndrome (p. 198) are at risk of developing soft-tissue sarcomas, breast cancer, brain tumours and leukaemia. The cancer-predisposing syndrome hereditary non-polyposis colorectal cancer is clinically separated into Lynch type I, in which family members appear to only be at risk for cancer of the colon, and Lynch type II (sometimes, somewhat confusingly, known as the cancer family syndrome), in which family members are also at risk for a number of other cancers which include stomach, endometrial, breast and transitional cell cancers.

These cancer groupings are, however, not always distinct in an individual family. In addition, although it was initially thought that these groupings of cancers into separate syndromes might identify different causal genes, the division at a molecular level in some instances has turned out to be artificial, e.g. individuals from both Lynch type I and II families have been found to have mutations in any one of the mismatch repair genes (p. 201), the Turcot syndrome is due to mutations in the APC gene and two of the mismatch repair genes and the Muir-Torre syndrome results from mutations in the hMSH2 mismatch repair gene. Individuals at risk in such families should, however, be screened for the appropriate cancers (p. 204).

INHERITED SUSCEPTIBILITY FOR THE COMMON CANCERS

The majority of persons at an increased risk of developing cancer because of their family history do not have one of the cancer-predisposing syndromes. The level of risk for persons with a family history of one of the common cancers such as bowel or breast cancer depends on a number of factors. These include the number of persons with cancer in the family, how closely related the person at risk is to the affected individuals and the age at which the affected family member(s) developed cancer. A few families with a large number of members affected with one of the common cancers are consistent with a dominantly inherited cancer susceptibility gene. In most instances there are only a few individuals with cancer in a family and there is doubt about whether a cancer susceptibility gene is responsible or not. In such an instance one relies on empirical data gained from epidemiological studies to provide risk estimates (Tables 13.10 and 13.11).

SCREENING FOR FAMILIAL CANCER

Prevention or early detection of cancer is the ultimate goal of screening individuals at risk of familial cancer. The means of prevention for certain cancers can include a change in lifestyle or diet, drug therapy, prophylactic surgery or screening.

Screening of persons at risk for familial cancer is usually directed at detecting the phenotypic expression of the genotype, i.e. surveillance for a particular cancer or its precursor. Screening can also include diagnostic tests which indirectly reveal the genotype, looking for other clinical features which are evidence of the presence or absence of the gene. For example, individuals at risk for familial adenomatous polyposis can be screened for evidence of the *APC* gene by retinal examination looking for areas of *congenital hypertrophy of the retinal pigment epithelium* or what is known as CHRPE. The finding of CHRPE increases the likelihood of an individual at risk being heterozygous for the *APC* gene and therefore developing polyposis and malignancy. More recently, however, it has been recognized that CHRPE is seen in persons with FAP when mutations occur in the first part of the *APC* gene, an example of a genotype–phenotype correlation (p. 24).

More recently, identification of the gene responsible for a number of the cancer-predisposing syndromes, and determination of the genotypic status, i.e. presymptomatic testing (p. 290), of an individual at risk allows more efficient delivery of surveillance screening for the phenotypic expression, e.g. polyposis and consequently cancer of the bowel in persons with a mutation in the *APC* gene. It also avoids unnecessary surveillance of those who have not inherited the gene. As more genes for cancer susceptibility are discovered there will be an increasing number of conditions for which DNA testing will enable presymptomatic determination of genotypic status (p. 291).

While the potential for prevention of cancer through screening persons at high risk is considerable, it is important to remember that the impact on the overall rate of cancer in the population in general will be small as only a minority of all cases of cancer are due to a

Table 13.10   Lifetime risk of colorectal cancer for an individual according to the family history of colorectal cancer

Population risk	1 in 50
One first-degree relative affected	1 in 17
One first-degree relative and one second-degree relative affected	1 in 12
One relative aged under 45 affected	1 in 10
Two first-degree relatives affected	1 in 6
Three or more first-degree relatives affected	1 in 2

From Houlston R S, Murday V, Harocopos C, Williams C B, Slack J 1990 Screening and genetic counselling for relatives of patients with colorectal cancer in a family screening clinic. Br Med J 301: 366–368

Table 13.11   Lifetime risk of breast cancer in females according to the family history of breast cancer

Population risk	1 in 12
Sister diagnosed 65–70 years of age	1 in 8
Sister diagnosed under 40 years of age	1 in 4
Two first–degree relatives affected under 40 years of age	1 in 3

mutation in a gene for a cancer-predisposing syndrome or for a common cancer.

Familial cancer-predisposing syndromes

Many familial cancer-predisposing syndromes are inherited as autosomal dominant traits which are fully penetrant, with the consequent risk for heterozygotes of developing cancer approaching 100%. This level of risk means that more invasive means of screening with more frequent and earlier initiation of screening protocols are justified than would be acceptable for the population in general (Table 13.12).

Inherited susceptibility for the common cancers

Screening for the common cancers arising from inherited susceptibility has only relatively recently been established and by its very nature involves a long-term undertaking for the individual at risk as well as his/her physician or surgeon. It is important to emphasize that the natural enthusiasm for screening needs to be balanced with the paucity of hard data in many instances on the relative benefits and risks. Recommended screening protocols at present are often based on current opinion rather than on formal evidence-based medicine (Table 13.13).

Who should be screened?

In the case of the rare dominantly inherited single gene familial cancer-predisposing syndromes such as FAP, those

Table 13.12 Suggested guidelines for screening persons at risk for the familial cancer-predisposing syndromes or for one of the common cancers

Condition/Cancer	Screening test	Frequency	Starting age
Familial susceptibility for the common cancers			
Breast cancer			
Breast	Mammography	Annual	35 (2 yearly from 50)
Breast/Ovary			
Breast	Mammography	Annual	35 (2 yearly from 50)
Ovary	US/Doppler, CA125	Annual	25
Familial cancer-predisposing syndromes			
Familial adenomatous polyposis	Retinal examination (CHRPE)*		Childhood
Colorectal	Sigmoid/colonoscopy*+	Annual	12
Duodenal	Gastroscopy	3 yearly	20
Thyroid (women)	None/US?	Annual	20
HNPCC–Lynch I			
Colorectal	Colonoscopy	3–5 yearly	35
HNPCC–Lynch II			
Colorectal	Colonoscopy	3–5 yearly	35
Endometrial	US	Annual	35
Ovary	US	Annual	25
Renal tract	US	Annual	35
Gastric	Gastroscopy	1–2 yearly	35
Small bowel	None		
Hepatobiliary	None		
Breast	Mammography	Annual	35 (2 yearly from 50)
Li–Fraumeni			
Breast	Mammography	Annual	35? (2 yearly from 50)
Sarcoma	None		
Brain	None		
Leukaemia	None		
Adrenal cortex	None		
Multiple endocrine neoplasia type II	Calcitonin provocation test*		10 years of age
Medullary thyroid	US	?	10
Phaeochromocytoma	Urinary VMA	Annual	10
Parathyroid adenoma	Ca²⁺, PO₄, PTH	Annual	10
von Hippel–Lindau			
Retinal angioma	Retinal examination*	Annual	5
Haemangioblastoma	CNS CT/MRI	3 yearly	15 (5 yearly from 40 years)
Phaeochromocytoma	Urinary VMA	Annual	10
Renal	Abdominal CT	3 yearly	20
	Abdominal US	Annual	20

*Test to detect heterozygous state.
+ In individuals found to be affected, annual colonoscopy prior to colectomy and lifelong 4–6 monthly surveillance of the rectal stump, after subtotal colectomy.
US = ultrasound; CHRPE = congenital hypertrophy of the retinal pigment epithelium; CT = computed tomography; MRI = magnetic resonance imaging; PTH = parathyroid hormone; VMA = vanillyl mandelic acid.

who should be screened can be identified on a simple Mendelian basis. For persons with a family history of the common cancers, such as bowel or breast cancer, the risk levels at which screening is recommended and below which screening is not likely to be of benefit will vary. At each extreme of risk the decision is usually straightforward, but with intermediate level risks there can be doubt as to relative benefits and risks of screening.

What age and how often?

Cancer in persons with a familial cancer-predisposing syndrome tends to occur at a relatively earlier age than in the population in general and screening programmes must reflect this. With the exception of familial adenomatous polyposis, in which it is recommended that sigmoidoscopy to detect rectal polyps should start in the teenage years, most cancer screening programmes do not start until 25 years of age or later. The age band during which the risk of developing cancer for most inherited susceptibilities is greatest is from 35 to 50 years but, because cancer can still develop in those at risk at a later age, screening is usually continued thereafter. In some families the age of onset of cancer can be especially early and it is recommended that screening of persons at risk in these families is begun 5 years before the age of onset in the earliest affected member of the family.

Table 13.13   Requirements of a screening test for persons at risk for a familial cancer-predisposing syndrome or at increased risk for the common cancers

The test should detect a malignant or premalignant condition at a stage prior to it producing symptoms with high sensitivity and specificity

The treatment of persons detected by screening should improve the prognosis

The benefit of early detection should outweigh potential harm from the screening test

The test should preferably be non-invasive since most at risk individuals require long-term surveillance

Adequate provision for prescreening counselling and follow-up should be available

The recommended interval between repeating screening procedures should be determined from the natural history of the particular cancer. The development of colorectal cancer from an adenoma is believed to take place over a number of years and as a result it is thought that 5-yearly screening intervals will suffice. If, however, a polyp is found, then the interval between screening procedures is usually brought down to 3 years. Breast cancer is not detectable in a premalignant stage and early diagnosis is critical if there is to be a good prognosis. Annual mammography for females at high risk is therefore recommended from the age of 35.

What sites should be screened?

Having decided who is at risk within a family, one has to judge which types of cancer are most likely to occur and which systems of the body should be screened.

Familial cancer-predisposing syndromes

This can be a very difficult problem with some of the family cancer syndromes, such as the Lynch type II syndrome, in which a person at risk can develop cancer at a number of different sites. Screening for every possible cancer which could occur would mean frequent investigation by a variety of different specialists and/or investigations. This would result in an unwieldy and unpleasant protocol. Persons at risk for Lynch types I and II should have regular colonoscopy while females at risk for Lynch type II should also be offered pelvic screening for gynaecological malignancies. Some of the other cancers which can occur in persons at risk for Lynch type II, such as stomach cancer, are not seen in every family and so screening is usually restricted in persons from those families to those cancers which have affected at least one family member. In persons at risk for the Li-Fraumeni syndrome, a wide spectrum of cancers

can occur. The available screening protocol is, as yet, of unproven benefit with the possible exception of regular mammography.

Inherited susceptibility for the common cancers

Colorectal cancer

Colorectal carcinoma holds the greatest promise for prevention by screening. Endoscopy provides a sensitive and specific means of examination of the colorectal mucosa and polypectomy can be carried out with relative ease so that screening, diagnosis and treatment can take place concurrently. While colonoscopy is the preferred screening method, it requires a skilled operator and, as it is an invasive procedure, it has a small but consequent morbidity.

Failure to visualize the right side of the colon with colonoscopy necessitates a barium enema to view this region, particularly in persons at risk for the hereditary non-polyposis colorectal cancer (HNPCC) syndrome, in which proximal right-sided involvement commonly occurs. For persons with a moderately increased risk of developing colorectal cancer, the majority of cancers occur in the distal colon and at a relatively later age. Flexible sigmoidoscopy, which is much less invasive than colonoscopy, provides an adequate screening tool for persons in this risk group and can be employed from the age of 50 years.

Breast cancer

In the United Kingdom screening of women aged 50 and over for breast cancer by regular mammography has become established as a national programme as a result of studies demonstrating improved survival of women detected as having early breast cancer. For women with an increased risk of developing breast cancer because of their family history, there is conflicting evidence of the relative benefit of screening with respect to the frequency of mammography and the chance of developing breast cancer in the interval between the screening procedures, or what is termed *interval cancer*.

It is also argued that the radiation exposure associated with annual mammography could be detrimental if started at an early age, leading to an increased risk of breast cancer through the screening when carried out over a long period of time. This is of particular concern in families with the Li–Fraumeni syndrome because mutations in the *Tp53* gene have been shown experimentally in vitro to impair the repair of DNA damaged by X-irradiation. The present view is, however, that there is a greater relative benefit than risk in identifying and treating breast cancer in women from this high risk group, although formal evaluation of such screening programmes is underway at present.

Mammography is usually only offered to women at increased risk of breast cancer after the age of 35 years, since interpretation of mammograms is difficult before this age because of the density of the breasts. As a consequence women at increased risk of developing breast cancer should be taught breast self-examination and undergo regular clinical examination.

Ovarian cancer

Ovarian cancer in the early stages is frequently asymptomatic and often incurable by the time a woman presents with symptoms. Early diagnosis of ovarian cancer in individuals at high risk is vital, with prophylactic oophorectomy being the only logical, if radical, alternative. The position of the ovaries within the pelvis makes screening difficult. Ultrasound imaging provides the most sensitive means of screening. Transvaginal scanning is more sensitive than conventional transabdominal scanning, and the use of colour Doppler blood flow imaging further enhances screening of women at increased risk. If a suspicious feature is seen on scanning and confirmed on further investigation, then laparoscopy or a laparotomy is usually required to confirm the diagnosis. Screening should be carried out annually as interval cancers can develop if screening is carried out less frequently.

Measuring the levels of CA125, an antigenic determinant of a glycoprotein that is present in increased levels in the blood of women with ovarian cancer, can be also be used as a screening test for women at increased risk of developing ovarian cancer. CA125 levels are not specific to ovarian cancer since they are also increased in women with a number of other disorders, such as endometriosis. In addition, there are problems with sensitivity (p. 313), since CA125 levels are not necessarily elevated in all women with ovarian cancer. Because of the problems outlined with these various screening modalities, many women who have an increased risk of developing ovarian cancer, often choose to have their ovaries removed prophylactically once they have had their family.

WHAT TREATMENT IS APPROPRIATE?

Surgical intervention for persons at risk for some of the familial cancer-predisposing syndromes, or for persons with a high risk due to an inherited susceptibility for one of the common cancers, is an accepted option, e.g. for persons at increased risk of developing colon cancer. In a number of the familial cancer-predisposing syndromes and for women at increased risk of developing breast cancer in whom the only option is prophylactic mastectomy, the management is much more controversial and alternative non-surgical treatments are under evaluation. These include dietary changes, such as the use of non-digestible starch or the use of drugs such as the aspirin-like non-steroidal anti-inflammatory sulindac in persons at risk for FAP and the anti-oestrogen drug tamoxifen or avoidance of the oral contraceptive or hormone replacement therapy in women at increased risk for breast cancer (Table 13.14).

Persons at an increased risk of developing cancer, especially if it is one of the single gene dominant cancer-predisposing syndromes or one of the single gene causes of the common cancers find themselves in an unenviable situation concerning both their health and the possibility of transmitting the condition to their children. Unfortunately they are also likely in future to experience increasing difficulties in other areas of life, such as insurance and employment (p. 340).

Table 13.14   Conditions in which prophylactic surgery is an accepted treatment and treatments which are under evaluation as an option for the familial cancer-predisposing syndromes or individuals at increased risk for the common cancers

Disorder	Treatment
Accepted treatment	
Familial adenomatous polyposis	Total colectomy
Ovarian cancer families	Oophorectomy
Breast cancer families	Bilateral mastectomy
MENII	Total thyroidectomy
Under evaluation	
Familial adenomatous polyposis	Non-digestible starch — to delay onset of polyposis
	Sulindac — to reduce rectal and duodenal adenomas
Breast cancer families	Tamoxifen — to prevent development of breast cancer
	Avoidance of the oral contraceptive, hormone replacement therapy

ELEMENTS

❶ Cancer has both genetic and environmental causes.

❷ Genetic and environmental factors in the aetiology of cancer can be differentiated by epidemiologic, family and twin studies and by analysis of disease, biochemical and viral associations.

3 Studies of tumour viruses have revealed genes present in humans known as oncogenes which are involved in carcinogenesis by altering cellular control mechanisms.

4 Study of rare dominantly inherited tumours in humans, such as retinoblastoma, has led to the identification of tumour suppressor genes consistent with the hypothesis that the development of cancer involves a minimum of two 'hits'. Persons at risk of familial cancer inherit the first 'hit' in the germ cell, the second 'hit' occurring in somatic cells in mitosis. In persons with sporadically occurring cancer both 'hits' occur in somatic cells.

5 Five per cent of the common cancers, such as breast and bowel cancer, arise as a result of an inherited cancer susceptibility. Familial susceptibility for cancer can occur as an inherited susceptibility for a single type of cancer or for a number of different types of cancer as part of a familial cancer-predisposing syndrome.

6 Persons at risk of an inherited cancer susceptibility can be screened for associated features of a familial cancer-predisposing syndrome or for particular cancers.

FURTHER READING

Cowell J K (ed) 1995 Molecular genetics of cancer. βios Scientific, Oxford
A multiauthor text covering the cancer family syndromes and the common cancers.

Eeles R A, Ponder B A J, Easton D F, Horwich A (eds) 1996 Genetic predisposition to cancer. Chapman & Hall, London
A good multiauthor text reviewing the various cancer-predisposing syndromes and the common familial cancers, as well as the accepted and controversial areas of their management.

Harris H, Miller O J, Klein G, Worst P, Tachibam T 1969 Suppression of malignancy by cell fusion. Nature 350: 377–378
Studies which eventually led to the concept of tumour suppressor genes.

Hodgson S V, Maher E R 1999 A practical guide to human cancer genetics, 2nd edn. Cambridge University Press, Cambridge
An up-to-date second edition of this text covering the developing field of human cancer genetics.

King R A, Rotter J I, Motulsky A G (eds) 1992 The genetic basis of common diseases. Oxford University Press, Oxford
Six chapters of this text cover the basic biology, epidemiology and familial aspects of cancer.

Knudson A G 1971 Mutation and cancer: statistical study of retinoblastoma. Proc Natl Acad Sci USA 68: 820–823
Proposal of the 'two-hit' hypothesis for the development of retinoblastoma.

Li F P, Fraumeni J F 1969 Soft tissue sarcomas, breast cancer, and other neoplasms: a familial syndrome? Ann Intern Med 71: 747–752
The original description of the Li–Fraumeni syndrome.

Lynch H T 1967 'Cancer families': adenocarcinomas (endometrial and colon carcinoma) and multiple primary malignant neoplasms. Recent Results Cancer Res 12: 125–142
The description of the cancer family syndrome now known as Lynch II.

Offit K 1998 Clinical cancer genetics. Wiley-Liss, Chichester
Text covering the clinical aspects of the various familial cancer-predisposing syndromes as well as the common cancers, along with the basic cellular biology and ethical and legal aspects.

Volgelstein B, Kinzler K W 1998 The genetic basis of human cancer. McGraw-Hill, London
Very comprehensive book covering in detail the cellular biology of cancer and the clinical aspects of the familial cancer-predisposing syndromes and the familial common cancers.

CHAPTER 14

Genetic factors in common diseases

Medical genetics usually concentrates on the study of rare unifactorial chromosomal and single gene disorders. Diseases such as diabetes, cancer, cardiovascular and coronary artery disease are responsible, however, for the majority of the morbidity and mortality in developed countries. These so-called *common diseases* are likely to be of even greater importance in the future with the elderly accounting for an increasing proportion of the population.

The common diseases do not usually show a simple pattern of inheritance. Instead the contributing genetic factors are often multiple, interacting with each other and environmental factors in a complex manner. In fact, it is uncommon for either genetic or environmental factors to be entirely responsible for a particular common disorder or disease in a single individual. In most instances both genetic and environmental factors are contributory, although sometimes one can appear more important than the other (Fig. 14.1).

At one extreme are diseases such as Duchenne muscular dystrophy; these are exclusively genetic in origin and the environment plays little or no direct part in the aetiology. At the other extreme are infectious diseases which are almost entirely the result of environmental factors. Between these two extremes are the common diseases and disorders such as diabetes mellitus, hypertension, cerebrovascular and coronary artery disease, schizophrenia, the common cancers and the congenital abnormalities, in which both genetic and environmental factors are involved.

GENETIC SUSCEPTIBILITY TO COMMON DISEASE

For many of the common diseases a small but significant proportion of cases have single gene causes but the major proportion of the genetic basis of common diseases can be considered to be the result of an inherited predisposition or genetic susceptibility. Common diseases result from a complex interaction of the effects of multiple different genes, or what is known as *polygenic inheritance*, with environmental factors and influences, due to what is known as *multifactorial inheritance* (p. 127).

Fig. 14.1
Human disease represented as being on a spectrum ranging from those which are largely environmental in causation to those which are entirely genetic.

TYPES AND MECHANISMS OF GENETIC SUSCEPTIBILITY

Genetic susceptibility for a particular disease can occur through single gene inheritance of an abnormal gene product involved in a particular metabolic pathway, e.g. early coronary artery disease arising from familial hypercholesterolaemia (FH) (p. 160). In an individual with a mutation in the FH gene, the genetic susceptibility is the main determinant of the development of coronary artery disease but this can be modified by environmental alteration, e.g. reduction in dietary cholesterol and avoidance of other risk factors such as obesity, lack of exercise and smoking.

Inheritance of a single gene susceptibility does not, however, necessarily lead to development of a disease. For some diseases exposure to specific environmental factors will be the main determinant in the development of the disease, e.g. smoking or occupational dust exposure in the development of pulmonary emphysema in persons with α_1-antitrypsin deficiency (p. 174).

In other instances the mechanism of the genetic susceptibility is less clear-cut. This can involve inheritance of a single gene polymorphism (p. 120) which leads to differences in susceptibility to a disease, e.g. acetaldehyde dehydrogenase activity and alcoholism (p. 173). In addition, inherited single gene polymorphisms appear to determine the response to as yet undefined environmental factors, for example the antigens of the major histocompatibility (HLA) complex and specific disease associations (p. 182), such as insulin-dependent diabetes, rheumatoid arthritis and coeliac disease. Lastly, genetic susceptibility can determine differences in responses to medical treatment, e.g. isoniazid inactivation status in the treatment of tuberculosis (p. 170).

APPROACHES TO DEMONSTRATE GENETIC SUSCEPTIBILITY TO COMMON DISEASES

In attempting to understand the genetics of a particular condition, the investigator can approach the problem in a number of ways (Table 14.1). These can include comparing the prevalence and incidence in various different population groups, the effects of migration, studying the incidence of the disease among relatives in family studies, comparing the incidence in identical and non-identical twins, determining the effect of environmental changes by adoption studies and studying the association of the disease with various other characteristics, such as the blood groups and biochemical or DNA polymorphisms. In addition, study can be made of the pathological components or biochemical factors of the disease in relatives, e.g. serum lipids among the relatives of patients with coronary artery disease. Study of diseases in animals which are homologous to diseases which occur in humans can also be helpful (p. 313). Before considering the use of these different approaches in a number of the common diseases in humans, specific aspects of some of these approaches will be discussed in more detail.

Population/migration studies

Differences in the incidence of a particular disease in different population groups suggest the possibility of genetic factors being important. They could, however, also be explained by differences in environmental factors. Studies of migrant groups moving from a population group with a low incidence of a disease to one with a high incidence, in which the incidence of the disease in the migrant group rises to that of its new population group, would suggest that environmental factors are more important. Conversely, maintenance of a low incidence of the disease in the migrant group would suggest that genetic factors are more important.

Family studies

A genetic susceptibility to a disease can be suggested by the finding of a higher frequency of a family history of the disease in relatives than in the general population. The proportion of affected relatives of a specific relationship, e.g. first degree, second degree, etc., can provide information for empiric recurrence risks in genetic counseling (p. 300), as well as evidence supporting a genetic contribution (p. 97). Familial aggregation does not, however, prove a genetic susceptibility since families share a common environment. The frequency of the disease in spouses, who share the same environment but who will usually have a different genetic background, can be used as a control, particularly for possible environmental factors in adult life.

Twin studies

If both members of a pair of identical twins have the same trait this could be thought to prove that the trait is

---

Table 14.1 Types of genetic approach to the common diseases

Population/migration studies
Family studies
Twin studies
Adoption studies
Polymorphism associations
Biochemical studies
Animal models

hereditary. This is not necessarily so. Since twins tend to share the same environment it is possible they will be exposed to the same environmental factors. For example, if one of a twin pair contracts a contagious disease such as impetigo, it is likely that the other twin will also become affected. This problem can be partly resolved by comparing differences in the frequency of a disease or disorder between non-identical or dizygotic (DZ) and identical or monozygotic (MZ) twin pairs.

Both members of a pair of twins are said to be *concordant* when either both are affected or neither is affected. The term *discordant* is used when only one member of a pair of twins is affected. Both types of twins will have a tendency to share the same environment but, whereas identical twins have identical genotypes, non-identical twins are no more similar genetically than brothers and sisters. If a disease is entirely genetically determined then, apart from rare events such as chromosome non-disjunction or a new mutation occurring in one of a twin pair, both members of a pair of identical twins will be similarly affected but non-identical twins can differ. If a disease is entirely caused by environmental factors, then identical and non-identical twins will have similar concordance rates.

Although all twins tend to share the same environment, it is probable that this is more likely in identical twins than in non-identical twins. Similarities between identical twins can therefore reflect their shared environment as much as their identical genotypes. One way of getting round this difficulty is to study differences between identical twin pairs who, through unusual family circumstances, have been reared apart from an early age. If a particular disease is entirely genetically determined then, if one identical twin is affected, the other will also be affected even if they have been brought up in different environments. It is rare, however, for identical twins to be separated from early childhood and so only a limited number of studies for any one disorder exist. In one study of identical twins reared separately, the data clearly showed that each pair of twins differed little in height but differed considerably in body weight. These observations suggest that heredity could play a bigger part in determining stature than it does in determining body weight.

Adoption studies

Another approach which helps to differentiate between genetic and environmental factors is to compare the frequency of a disease in individuals who remain with their biological parents with those who are adopted out of their biological family. Adopted individuals take their genes with them to a new environment. If the frequency of a disease in the individuals adopted out of a family is similar to that seen in those who remain with their biological parents, then genetic factors are likely to be more important. If, conversely, the frequency of the disease in the adopted individuals is similar to that of their adoptive parents, then environmental factors are likely to be more important.

Polymorphism association studies

The widespread existence of inherited biochemical, protein, enzyme and DNA polymorphisms (p. 120), allows the possibility of determining whether particular polymorphic variants occur more commonly in individuals affected with a particular disease than in the population in general, or what is known as a polymorphism association. Although demonstration of a polymorphic association can suggest that the inherited variation is involved in the aetiology of the disorder, e.g. the demonstration of HLA associations in the immune response in the causation of the autoimmune disorders (p. 182), it may only reflect that a gene nearby in linkage disequilibrium (p. 124) is involved in causation of the disorder. Much store is being put in studies at the level of differences in single nucleotide polymorphisms (SNPs) (p. 67) in the identification of the genetic factors in the causation and possible therapeutic intervention (p. 174) of the common diseases.

Biochemical studies

Analysis of metabolite or enzyme activity levels in biochemical or metabolic pathways likely to be involved in the causation of a particular disorder can provide evidence of genetic contribution to some of the common diseases, e.g. the hormones involved in the control of blood pressure in hypertension or the regulation of lipid levels in atherosclerosis. However, in disorders where we have a limited understanding of the biological basis, e.g. schizophrenia, this approach has been of very little use.

Animal models

Recognition of the same disease/disorder which occurs in humans in another species, e.g. the mouse, allows the possibility of experimental studies which are often not possible in humans. In many instances, however, the disorder in the animal model will have a single gene basis which has been identified or bred for. Nevertheless, spontaneously occurring or transgenic animal models (p. 323) experimentally induced for mutations in single genes involved in the metabolic processes or disease pathways of common diseases will provide vital insights into the genetic contribution to these disorders.

DIABETES MELLITUS

There are two main forms of diabetes mellitus which are clinically distinct. Type 1 or *insulin-dependent diabetes mellitus* (IDDM) accounts for 5–10% of diabetes. IDDM has a peak age of onset in adolescence and is therefore often also know as juvenile onset diabetes. As the name suggests, it can only be controlled by regular injection of insulin. The second more common and less severe form is known as type 2 or *non-insulin-dependent diabetes mellitus* (NIDDM). NIDDM usually affects older persons and often responds to simple dietary restriction of carbohydrate intake, although many persons with NIDDM require oral hypoglycaemic medication, and some require insulin.

An additional 1–2% of persons with diabetes develop non-insulin-dependent diabetes in their early twenties and have what is known as *maturity onset diabetes of the young (MODY)*.

Lastly, 1–3% of women develop glucose intolerance during pregnancy. This is known as *gestational diabetes*. Their abnormal glucose tolerance usually reverts to normal after the pregnancy, although approximately one-half to three-quarters of these women go on to develop diabetes later in life.

Diabetes can also occur secondary to a variety of other rare genetic syndromes and non-genetic disorders. For example, it is well recognized that individuals with the autosomal dominant muscle disorder myotonic dystrophy (p. 269) have an increased risk of developing diabetes. Diabetes mellitus is therefore aetiologically heterogeneous.

EVIDENCE FOR GENETIC FACTORS

Diabetes can affect up to 5% of the population in developed countries with the prevalence varying between different population and ethnic groups. For example, IDDM is 20 times more common in North America than in China. While migration studies are consistent with a significant environmental contribution, particularly in NIDDM, the evidence from family and twin studies suggests that there is a significant genetic contribution to the aetiology of diabetes mellitus.

Family studies

Between 25% and 50% of diabetics have a family history of diabetes as opposed to less than 15% in the general population. A variety of formal family studies have shown a prevalence of diabetes in relatives which ranges from 10% to 30% compared to between 1% and 6% in relatives of non-diabetics (Table 14.2). The criteria for the diagnosis of diabetes used in the different studies have not, however, always been the same, ranging from frank clinical diabetes through formal glucose tolerance tests to random blood sugars. In addition, while some studies looked at risks in relatives dependent on the type or age of onset of the diabetes in the proband, many of the studies considered all ages of onset and different types of diabetes together. These factors can account, to some extent, for the differences seen in the percentage of affected relatives in the various studies.

Twin studies

A number of surveys have shown that between 45% and 96% of identical twins are concordant for diabetes whereas between only 3% and 37% of non-identical twins are. More recent twin studies in which the concordance rates for insulin-dependent and non-insulin-dependent diabetes have been looked at separately have shown concordance rates in identical twins for the former to be in the region of 30–50% while for the latter they have been in excess of 90%. These data indicate that genetic factors are important in both forms of diabetes. The fact that a significant proportion of the identical twins were discordant for IDDM suggests that environmental factors have a significant influence in that form of diabetes. The very high concordance rate of MZ twins for NIDDM suggests that the primary determining factor is genetic, although a diabetogenic diet is necessary for the susceptibility to be expressed.

Table 14.2 Population and recurrence risks for NIDDM and IDDM

Group	%
NIDDM	
Population	4–5 (ages 20–74)
First-degree relatives	10–15
IDDM	
Population	0.2
1 high risk allele (DR3 or DR4)	0.25
HLA DR3/3 or HLA DR4/4	0.75
HLA DR3/4	2.5
Relatives	
Siblings	7
No antigens shared	1
1 antigen shared	5
2 antigens shared	16
2 antigens shared — DR3/4	20–25
Offspring	4
Offspring of affected female	2–2.5
Offspring of affected male	5

From Rotter J I, Vadhein C M, Rimoin D L Diabetes mellitus, Chapter 21 in King, Rotter and Motulsky 1992.

POSSIBLE SINGLE GENE MODELS OF INHERITANCE

Attempts to see if simple single gene modes of inheritance could explain the familial data for diabetes have been undertaken. If diabetes were due to a recessive allele (d) and an affected person (dd) had two unaffected parents, the parents must have the genotype Dd and it would be expected that, on average, 25% of their offspring would be affected. If one parent of a diabetic was also a diabetic, then the mating must be dd × Dd and 50% of their offspring should be affected. Finally, if both parents are diabetic then all of their offspring should be affected. The ratios of affected offspring in these three types of mating would therefore be 1/4:1/2:1 or 1:2:4. Some studies have reported results which agree with these expected ratios. It must be pointed out, however, that from the data obtained in family studies it is estimated that about 5% of the general population would be homozygous for this gene! Population surveys have shown, however, that only about 1% of the population is diabetic. Therefore if diabetes mellitus were due to a recessive gene, then the gene cannot be fully penetrant and only about 20% of those who are presumed to be homozygous will actually develop diabetes. Some investigators who support the idea that diabetes mellitus is due to a recessive gene have suggested that the severe childhood form of the disease represents the homozygous state, whereas non-insulin-dependent diabetes represents the heterozygous state. Family studies do not, however, fit this model. Similar attempts to fit the family data to an autosomal dominant gene exhibiting reduced penetrance have not met with obvious success. Not surprisingly, suggestions of mixed models of dominant and recessive genes have also been made.

ASSOCIATED RISK FACTORS

The alternative approach of considering diabetes to be multifactorial in origin together with the concept of genetic susceptibility has led to the identification of associated risk factors (p. 131).

IDDM

Persons with IDDM are recognized to have an increased risk of developing autoimmune disorders such as autoimmune thyroiditis, pernicious anaemia and Addison's disease. A significant proportion of persons with IDDM also develop pancreatic islet cell antibodies. Not surprisingly, perhaps, IDDM has been found to be associated with specific HLA antigens, with 95% of persons with IDDM having the HLA DR3 and/or DR4 antigens. The reported peak of onset of IDDM in the autumn and winter seasons along with the autoimmune observations have suggested the possibility that viral infections, such as mumps, Coxsackie B or cytomegalovirus infection, act as a trigger in genetically susceptible individuals.

Siblings with IDDM have HLA haplotypes (p. 131) in common more frequently than would be expected by chance. An individual with either the DR3 or DR4 HLA antigens has a slightly increased risk of developing IDDM compared to the general population (Table 14.2). The presence of either of these two antigens in siblings of an individual with IDDM increases their chance of developing diabetes significantly and if a sibling has both high risk antigens the risk is greatly increased. Linkage studies have show that the HLA susceptibility locus (IDDM1) has the major role in IDDM, accounting for between 30–40% of the genetic predisposition. A large number of other loci have been identified as candidate susceptibility genes for IDDM, the only significant one being a VNTR (p. 132) 5′ to the insulin gene on the short arm of chromosome 11 which accounts for around 10% of the genetic susceptibility (p. 132).

NIDDM

NIDDM is characterized initially by relative insulin resistance with subsequent defective secretion of insulin and is frequently associated with obesity. A number of candidate susceptibility genes for NIDDM have been suggested by the relative preservation of pancreatic islet β cell function and insulin resistance which include the insulin and insulin receptor genes and the glucokinase and glycogen synthase genes. Although preliminary studies in individual populations suggested that each of these genes possibly contribute to NIDDM, there have not been consistent findings in studies in different populations. Genome scanning linkage studies have demonstrated evidence of three loci conferring susceptibility to NIDDM on chromosomes 2 (NIDDM1), 12 (NIDDM2) and 20 (NIDDM3). Again, however, the relative importance of these susceptibility loci has varied in studies in different populations.

Maturity onset diabetes of the young

The initial description of MODY resulted in reports of a number of families where the inheritance of the disorder was compatible with an autosomal dominant gene. Further studies have indicated that only a proportion of families are consistent with it being due to a dominant gene. There are a few reports of associated risk factors for MODY. The initial reports of chlorpropamide-alcohol-induced flushing (p. 173) as a marker for MODY have not been substantiated in most families.

213

Linkage studies in MODY families with what could be considered obvious candidate genes, such as the insulin, insulin receptor and the glucose transport protein genes, have been negative. Linkage of MODY to markers on the long arm of chromosome 20 near the adenosine deaminase gene has been demonstrated in a proportion of MODY families. This has been called the MODY1 locus and some families have been shown to have mutations in the hepatocyte nuclear factor-4-α gene in that region of chromosome 20. A significant proportion of families which did not show linkage to MODY1 have been shown to be linked to the glucokinase gene on chromosome 7, the MODY2 locus. Mutations in the glucokinase gene in that region of chromosome 7 have been identified in a number of such families. A further locus, MODY3, has been identified on the long arm of chromosome 12 in a proportion of MODY families, some of which have been shown to have a mutation in the hepatic transcription factor-1 gene. Evidence for another locus(i) has been provided by families with MODY which do not show linkage to any of the existing loci. This resulted in the mapping of two further loci, MODY4 and MODY5 to chromosomes 13 and 17. Mutations in the insulin promoter factor-1 and hepatic transcription factor-2 genes in those regions of chromosomes 13 and 17 have been demonstrated in a proportion of families.

Gestational diabetes

While gestational diabetes was originally suggested to be a pre-type 2 or non-insulin-dependent form of diabetes, it appears to be genetically heterogeneous, showing association with HLA antigens DR3 and DR4, pancreatic islet cell antibodies and autoimmune disorders.

Predisposition to diabetic complications

Persons with diabetes are at risk of developing complications in a number of systems, specifically the kidneys, the retina and large blood vessels in the form of early coronary artery and peripheral vascular disease. While the development of complications in these systems has been thought to relate primarily to the duration and control of the diabetes, there is preliminary evidence to suggest that there could be specific genetic factors determining the predisposition to these complications. For example, there is evidence that individuals with IDDM who are homozygous for the I (insertion) allele in the angiotensin I converting enzyme (ACE) (p. 216) have a reduced risk of developing renal complications, while the presence of the D (deletion) allele in persons with NIDDM is associated with an increased risk of coronary artery disease.

ANIMAL MODELS FOR DIABETES

A number of spontaneously occurring animal models for diabetes have been identified which include the non-obese diabetic (nod) mouse for IDDM and the obese diabetic (ob) mouse and GK rat for NIDDM. Studies of the genetics of the tendency to diabetes in these animal models are consistent with a minimum of two and up to six or more genes being involved, suggesting that orthologous regions for genes for which linkage is shown would be candidate regions for genes leading to diabetes susceptibility in humans.

HYPERTENSION

Various studies have shown that between 10% and 25% of the population is hypertensive but the prevalence is age dependent with up to 40% of 75–79-year-olds being hypertensive. Hypertension leads to an increased morbidity and mortality through a greater risk of stroke, coronary artery and renal disease. There is substantial evidence that treatment of hypertension prevents the development of these complications.

Persons with hypertension fall into two groups. In one the onset is usually in early adult life and is a consequence of another disorder such as kidney disease or abnormalities of certain endocrine glands. This is referred to as secondary hypertension. In the second more common group, hypertension usually begins in middle age and there is no recognized cause. This is known as essential hypertension. The following discussion is concerned with only essential hypertension.

ENVIRONMENTAL FACTORS IN HYPERTENSION

Environmental factors, such as high sodium levels in the diet, obesity, alcohol intake and reduced exercise, are recognized as being associated with an increased risk of hypertension. Hypertension is also more prevalent in persons from poorer socioeconomic groups. Studies of adopted children have shown lower correlation of their blood pressure with their biological parents than with children remaining with their biological parents. In addition, migration studies involving persons moving from a population with a low prevalence to one with a high prevalence of hypertension have shown that the immigrant group acquires the frequency of hypertension of their new population group during the course of 1 to 2 generations. This suggests that environmental factors are of major importance in the aetiology of hypertension.

GENETIC FACTORS IN HYPERTENSION

Family and twin studies have shown that hypertension is familial (Table 14.3) and that blood pressure correlates with the degree of relationship (Table 14.4). These findings suggest the importance of genetic factors in the aetiology of hypertension. In addition, there are differences in the prevalence of hypertension between populations, hypertension being more common in persons of Afro-Caribbean origin and less common in Eskimos, Australian Aborigines and Central and South American Indians.

POSSIBLE SINGLE GENE MODELS OF INHERITANCE

If blood pressure measurements are made on a large enough number of persons, the results are normally distributed and show no evidence of any bimodality. Hypertension could therefore be considered to represent one extreme of the normal distribution curve and to be due to the action of many genes which interact with environmental factors consistent with a multifactorial or polygenic basis.

Another school of thought considers that essential hypertension could be due to a common dominant gene. It is argued that if essential hypertension is a disorder of middle age resulting from the action of a dominant gene, it would be expected that the sibs of hypertensive patients would segregate into two groups: those who inherit the gene for hypertension and those who do not. Analysis of blood pressure readings from sibs of persons known to have hypertension, excluding as far as possible cases of secondary hypertension by choosing all cases from the age group 45–60 years, showed that the blood pressure values of the sibs were not normally distributed but had a bimodal distribution with two peaks corresponding to systolic blood pressures of 130 and 160 mmHg (Fig. 14.2). This suggested that those with systolic blood pressure values around 130 mmHg had inherited the normal gene whereas those with systolic blood pressure values around 160 mmHg had inherited the gene for hypertension.

Much of the controversy between these two schools of thought concerning the hereditary nature of hypertension revolves around the definition of bimodality. Critics of the single gene theory claim that what others have interpreted as bimodality are merely irregularities in the distribution curve which are of no significance. It is argued that with small sample sizes the distribution curve of any variable can show small dips and irregularities and that if a large enough sample is taken then the resultant distribution curve would be less likely to show any evidence of bimodality.

BIOCHEMICAL STUDIES

Biochemical studies supported the possibility of a common autosomal dominant gene being responsible for hypertension. Dietary salt has long been recognized as a contributory factor in hypertension and a salt-free diet has been used in its treatment. In some persons with hypertension there appeared to be defective extrusion of sodium from red cells because of an abnormality in the sodium–potassium cotransport in the red cell membrane resulting in an increased intracellular sodium. This defect was proposed as a major biochemical determinant

Table 14.3	Recurrence risks for hypertension
Group	%
Population	5
2 Normotensive parents	4
1 Hypertensive parent	8–28
2 Hypertensive parents	25–45

From Burke W, Motulsky A G Hypertension. Chapter 10 in King, Rotter and Motulsky 1992.

Table 14.4 Coefficient of correlation for blood pressure in various relatives	
Group	Correlation coefficient
Siblings	0.12–0.34
Parent/child	0.12–0.37
Dizygotic twins	0.25–0.27
Monozygotic twins	0.55–0.72

From Burke W, Motulsky A G Hypertension. Chapter 10 in King, Rotter and Motulsky 1992.

Fig. 14.2
Distribution of systolic blood pressures in 252 sibs of persons aged 45–60 with hypertension. (After Platt R 1959 Lancet ii: 57, with permission.)

of hypertension on the basis that this could reflect a generalized membrane abnormality in vessel walls. Family studies showed that this abnormality appeared to be inherited in an autosomal dominant manner.

In communities which use little salt the incidence of hypertension is less than, for example, among the Japanese who eat large amounts of salty foods. It was proposed that individuals with a defect in sodium–potassium cotransport can eat little salt and develop hypertension. Conversely, persons with normal cotransport can eat large amounts of salt yet remain normotensive.

A second assay of red cell ion transport was developed, known as the sodium–lithium countertransport system. This involved loading red blood cells with lithium and measuring the rate of efflux of lithium from the red cells in high and low sodium concentrations. Increased sodium–lithium countertransport correlated positively with hypertension. Studies of the correlation of sodium–lithium countertransport in different types of biological relatives of hypertensives were compatible with a genetic rather than an environmental basis. Segregation analysis testing different models of inheritance suggested that sodium–lithium countertransport was compatible with a recessive gene of major effect on a polygenic background.

Studies in North American individuals of Afro-Caribbean origin suggested that differences in sodium–lithium countertransport were not as important a factor in that population as in other population groups even though they were twice as likely to develop hypertension as North Americans of Caucasian origin. This emphasized the importance of possible differences between various population groups in genetic susceptibility.

A third assay, known as the ouabain-sensitive sodium–potassium ATPase system, was investigated as a possible indicator of genetic susceptibility. Attempts to correlate the findings from these various assay systems have not been straightforward and it is fair to say that these findings have not provided clear evidence for the role of a single gene of major importance in determining predisposition to essential hypertension.

ASSOCIATED RISK FACTORS

The renin–angiotensin system is integrally involved in the biological control of blood pressure and would seem to provide an obvious series of candidate susceptibility genes for hypertension

The renin–angiotensin system

Renin catalyses the cleavage of angiotensinogen to angiotensin I, which is converted to angiotensin II by the angiotensin I converting enzyme (ACE).

Renin gene

The renin–angiotensin system is rate limiting in angiotensin II production. Although one study has shown that approximately one-third of persons with essential hypertension have elevated renin levels compared to normotensive controls, no association between renin gene polymorphisms or renin levels and hypertension has been demonstrated in a number of different studies.

Angiotensinogen gene

Angiotensinogen is the substrate for renin. Correlation between angiotensinogen levels and blood pressure suggested that it could have a role in hypertension. Two studies of a microsatellite dinucleotide polymorphism in the 3′ end of the angiotensinogen gene in hypertensive sib-pairs in the United States and France showed a significant frequency of allele sharing in hypertensive sib-pairs. A polymorphic sequence variant has been identified in the angiotensinogen gene which leads to methionine or threonine being present at position 235 in the angiotensinogen protein. The threonine variant has been found to be associated with increased angiotensinogen levels and hypertension in a number of different studies.

Angiotensin I gene

There is evidence that the angiotensin I gene contributes to the normal control of blood pressure as well as polymorphic variants in the gene being associated with hypertension in studies of some populations.

Angiotensin I converting enzyme

Angiotensin I converting enzyme (ACE) converts angiotensin I into angiotensin II and inactivates bradykinin. ACE levels can vary as much as fivefold between different individuals. The variation in ACE levels is, in part, associated with the presence or absence of a polymorphic DNA deletion (D)/insertion (I) in the ACE gene (p. 214), with individuals homozygous for the D allele having ACE levels twice as high as those homozygous for the I allele. A number of different association studies of the ACE polymorphisms with hypertension have not shown consistent results, suggesting they do not play a major role in determining blood pressure.

Angiotensin II type 1 receptor

The angiotensin II type 1 receptor mediates the biological and physiological effects of the renin–angiotensin system and is, therefore, an obvious candidate gene for genetic susceptibility to hypertension. Increased activity of the receptor could lead to hypertension. Preliminary studies have shown a possible association between hypertension and polymorphic variants in the angiotensin II type 1 receptor.

PREGNANCY-INDUCED HYPERTENSION

Women who develop pre-eclampsia in pregnancy were thought to have an increased risk of hypertension after the pregnancy. A familial tendency to pre-eclampsia is well recognized. Hormonal influences, such as the elevated oestrogen levels of pregnancy, are associated with stimulation of angiotensinogen expression. Preliminary evidence of inherited variation in the angiotensinogen gene has been demonstrated in familial pre-eclampsia.

ANIMAL MODELS

Animal models of hypertension, such as the SA locus and the α-adducin gene, identified from strains of genetically hypertensive rats, have led to the suggestion that the orthologous regions could contain susceptibility loci for hypertension in humans.

SUSCEPTIBILITY GENES

To date there is fairly good evidence for three loci contributing to the predisposition to hypertension, one on the long arm of chromosome 17 (HYT1), another on chromosome 16 which is homologous to the SA locus in rats (HYT3) and a third on the long arm of chromosome 15 (HYT2).

CORONARY ARTERY DISEASE

Coronary artery disease is a major cause of morbidity and mortality, accounting for up to 50% of deaths in many of the developed countries. It results from atherosclerosis, a process taking place over many years which involves deposition of lipid in the subendothelial space (intima) of arteries with a consequent narrowing of their lumen. The first stage involves the deposition of lipid in the arterial wall which is determined by haemodynamic factors. Monocytes adhere to areas of the endothelial surface of arterial walls with lipid deposits and enter the vessel wall, proliferate and differentiate into macrophages. The macrophages scavenge the lipids producing the classical fatty streaks and through the action of cytokines, growth factors and adhesion molecules induce smooth muscle proliferation and the formation of extracellular matrix which results in the development of the fibrous atherosclerotic plaques. The narrowing of the coronary arteries compromises the metabolic needs of the heart muscle leading to myocardial ischaemia, which, if severe, results in myocardial infarction.

LIPID METABOLISM

The metabolic pathways by which the body absorbs, synthesizes, transports and catabolizes dietary and endogenous lipids are complex. Lipids are packaged in intestinal cells as a complex with various proteins known as *apolipoproteins* to form triglyceride-rich chylomicrons. These are secreted into the lymph and transported to the liver, where, in association with endogenous synthesis of triglyceride and cholesterol, they are packaged and secreted into the circulation as triglyceride-rich very low density lipoproteins (VLDLs). VLDL is degraded to intermediate density lipoprotein (IDL) which is further broken down into cholesterol-rich low density lipoprotein (LDL). High density lipoproteins (HDLs) are formed from lipoproteins secreted by the liver, chylomicrons and VLDL remnants.

High levels of LDLs are associated with an increased risk of coronary artery disease. Conversely, levels of high density lipoproteins are inversely correlated with a risk of coronary artery disease. Consequently the LDL:HDL ratio has been used as a risk predictor for coronary artery disease and as an indicator for therapeutic intervention.

EPIDEMIOLOGY OF CORONARY ARTERY DISEASE

The incidence of coronary artery disease varies greatly between different population groups, being one-sixth as common in Japan as in many Western countries. These differences can, in part, be attributed to well-known environmental risk factors. Support for this comes from the results of migration studies which show that persons moving from populations with a low risk of coronary artery disease to areas with a high risk acquire the higher risk of their new population group within 10–20 years.

Coronary artery disease can occur secondary to other diseases, such as diabetes mellitus and hypertension. It is also more common in males than in females. After the menopause, the risk for females increases and approaches that of males within 10–15 years as a result of the associated hormonal changes.

Although there are well-recognized environmental factors associated with an increased risk of developing coronary artery disease, it is clear that genetic factors are also important in its aetiology.

FAMILY AND TWIN STUDIES

The familial nature of coronary artery disease has been recognized since the early part of the twentieth century. The risk to a first-degree relative of a person with premature coronary artery disease, defined as occurring before age 55 in males and age 65 in females, varies between two and seven times that for the general population (Table 14.5). Twin studies of concordance for coronary artery disease vary from 15% to 25% for dizygotic twins and from 39% to 48% for monozygotic twins. Although these figures support the involvement of genetic factors, the low concordance rate for monozygotic twins clearly supports the importance of environmental factors.

SINGLE GENE DISORDERS OF LIPID METABOLISM LEADING TO CORONARY ARTERY DISEASE

Although there are a number of individually rare inherited disorders of specific lipoproteins, levels of the various lipoproteins and the hyperlipidaemias are determined by a complex interaction of genetic and environmental factors. Family studies of some of the hyperlipidaemias are, however, consistent with a single gene being a major factor determining genetic susceptibility.

Familial combined hyperlipidaemia

The most common disorder of lipid metabolism associated with an increased risk of early coronary artery disease is familial combined hyperlipidaemia (FCH). FCH affects 1 in 200 of the population, is inherited as an autosomal dominant disorder, is associated with elevated triglyceride and cholesterol levels and accounts for approximately 10% of premature coronary artery disease. It has been shown to be genetically heterogeneous with at least four loci being involved.

Familial hypercholesterolaemia

The best known disorder of lipid metabolism is familial hypercholesterolaemia (FH) (p. 160). FH is associated with a significantly increased risk of early coronary artery disease and is inherited as an autosomal dominant disorder. It has been estimated that about 1 person in 500 in the general population, and about 1 in 20 persons presenting with early coronary artery disease, are heterozygous for a mutation in the gene for FH. Molecular studies in FH have revealed that it is due to a variety of defects in the number, function or processing of the LDL receptors on the cell surface (p. 162).

ASSOCIATED RISK FACTORS

For the majority of persons their risk of coronary artery disease is multifactorial or polygenic in origin. A variety of different genetic and environmental risk factors have been identified which predispose to early onset of the atherosclerotic process. Well-publicized environmental risk factors include lack of exercise, dietary cholesterol

Table 14.5 Recurrence risks for premature coronary artery disease

Proband	Relative risk
Male (< 55 years)	
Brother	5
Sister	2.5
Female (< 65 years)	
Sibs	7

Data from Slack J, Evans K A 1966 The increased risk of death from ischaemic heart disease in first degree relatives of 121 men and 96 women with ischaemic heart disease. J Med Genet 3: 239–257.

and smoking. The advice with respect to the potential for prevention of developing coronary artery disease for these factors is obvious.

Lipoprotein polymorphisms

A number of inherited polymorphisms of the apolipoproteins of the plasma lipoproteins involved in the transport of lipids have been found to be associated with an increased risk of coronary artery disease.

Apolipoprotein E

Apolipoprotein E (apo E) is a major protein constituent of two of the classes of plasma lipoprotein involved in the transport and metabolism of lipids. It binds with the LDL receptors on cell surfaces which are responsible for cholesterol uptake by the cell. Polymorphic variants of apo E have been shown to be associated with elevated cholesterol levels and an increased risk of early coronary artery disease.

Lipoprotein a

Lipoprotein a (Lp(a)) is a glycoprotein which binds to apolipoprotein B (apo B). Apo B is the principal apolipoprotein constituent of LDL, the major lipoprotein involved in cholesterol transport. Lp(a) is highly polymorphic and also shows variation in levels of up to 1000-fold in the population. Elevated Lp(a) levels and certain Lp(a) polymorphic variants are associated with elevated plasma cholesterol levels and an increased risk of early coronary artery disease. Of interest is that Lp(a) has sequence homology with one of the fibrinolytic enzymes, plasminogen.

Angiotensin I converting enzyme

Individuals assessed as being at low risk for coronary artery disease by the common associated risk factors such as environmental and lipoprotein polymorphisms who have had a history of myocardial infarction are more likely to be homozygous for the D (deletion) allele of the angiotensin I converting enzyme (ACE) (p. 216) than to be heterozygous or homozygous for the I (insertion) allele.

ANIMAL MODELS FOR CORONARY ARTERY DISEASE

The demonstration that the Watanabe heritable hyper-lipidaemic (WHHL) rabbit is due to a mutation in the LDL receptor has allowed its use for the evaluation of various therapeutic modalities including hepatocyte grafts and gene therapy. Although Lp(a) is present only in primates, the generation of a transgenic mouse, allowed the demonstration that the major effect of Lp(a) is the inhibition of the conversion of plasminogen to plasmin resulting in reduced fibrinolysis and this is probably the basis of the increased risk of coronary artery disease.

SCHIZOPHRENIA

Schizophrenia is a serious psychotic illness with an onset usually in late adolescence or early adult life. It is characterized by grossly disorganized thought processes and behaviour together with a marked deterioration of social and occupational functioning and can be accompanied by hallucinations and delusions.

EPIDEMIOLOGY

Schizophrenia is a principal cause of chronic mental illness. There is a 1% lifetime risk for a person to develop schizophrenia and at any one time approximately 0.2% of the population is affected. Schizophrenia occurs more commonly in individuals of poorer socioeconomic status and has an earlier age of onset and worse prognosis in males. There is an excess of winter births in schizophrenic individuals which has suggested that environmental factors, such as certain viral infections or nutritional factors, could be contributory.

EVIDENCE FOR GENETIC FACTORS

The nature and extent of the genetic contribution to schizophrenia is not clear. This is partly because of past and continuing controversy concerning the definition of schizophrenia and the term schizoid. The latter term refers to the schizophrenia-like traits often seen in relatives of schizophrenics. The problem arises because clinical criteria to distinguish schizoid from normal personality are lacking. For the sake of simplicity we can regard the term schizoid as referring to a person with the fundamental symptoms of schizophrenia but in a milder form. It has been estimated that roughly 4% of the general population have schizophrenia or a schizoid personality disorder.

Family and twin studies

The results of several studies of the prevalence of schizophrenia and schizoid disorder among the relatives of schizophrenics are summarized in Table 14.6. If only schizophrenia is considered, the concordance rate for identical twins is only 50%, suggesting the importance of environmental factors. If, however, schizophrenia and schizoid personality disorder are considered together, then almost 90% of identical co-twins are concordant.

Adoption studies

Other evidence which provides compelling support for genetic factors in the causation of schizophrenia is

Table 14.6 Proportions (%) of first-degree relatives of individuals with schizophrenia who are similarly affected or have a schizoid disorder

Relatives	Proportion (%) of relatives		
	Schizophrenia*	Schizoid	Total schizophrenia + schizoid
Identical twins	46	41	87
Offspring (of 1 schizophrenic)	16	33	49
Sibs	14	32	46
Parents	9	35	44
Offspring (of 2 schizophrenics)	34	32	66
General population	1	3	4

*Age corrected.
From Heston L L 1970 The genetics of schizophrenia and schizoid disease. Science 167: 249–256.

provided by the results of adoption studies. The nature of schizophrenia can result in disruption of the family, with children being placed with adoptive parents. Any differences in the frequency of schizophrenia between individuals adopted away from their biological parents and their siblings can help to differentiate genetic and environmental influences.

In one study of 47 offspring of schizophrenic mothers separated shortly after birth, five of the offspring developed schizophrenia compared to none of 50 offspring of age- and sex-matched control mothers. Another study looked at the prevalence of schizophrenia in the relatives of adoptees who were schizophrenic as compared to matched-control adoptees who were not schizophrenic. This showed a fivefold increase in the prevalence of schizophrenia in the biological relatives of the schizophrenic adoptees compared to biological relatives of the control adoptees, the prevalence in the latter group being the same as that seen in the adoptive relatives in both groups. Another study showed similar concordance rates of schizophrenia in identical twin offspring born to a schizophrenic parent, whether reared together or separated at birth. These findings provide compelling evidence that genetic factors are important in the causation of schizophrenia.

POSSIBLE SINGLE GENE MODELS OF INHERITANCE

What interpretation can be put on these results? The simplest would be that schizophrenia and schizoid disorders are both inherited as an autosomal dominant trait with almost complete penetrance. The idea that schizophrenia and schizoid disorders represent a single genetic disease is supported by their clinical similarity and the fact that both occur with almost equal frequency in identical co-twins of schizophrenics. If the two conditions are considered together, then the proportion of affected first-degree relatives fits well with the hypothesis of autosomal dominant inheritance, with 50% of first degree relatives of an affected individual and 75% of the offspring of two affected individuals being affected. However, the proportion of more distant relatives being affected does not fit this mode of inheritance so well.

Schizophrenia has been associated with a number of complex traits such as body build and intelligence. It is clear from twin studies and other findings that environmental factors also play an important part in the aetiology of schizophrenia. The prevalence of schizophrenia among close relatives could partly be the result of sharing a common environment but most investigators consider that schizophrenia is, in fact, determined in a multifactorial manner, the genetic contribution being on a polygenic basis.

LINKAGE AND ASSOCIATION STUDIES

The report of a proband and his maternal uncle with schizophrenia, both of whom had an unbalanced translocation leading to partial trisomy for part of the long arm of chromosome 5, led molecular geneticists to look for linkage to that region of the genome in schizophrenia. There were, however, conflicting results. In several Icelandic and two English families with schizophrenia there was evidence supporting linkage of schizophrenia to DNA markers on the long arm of chromosome 5, but studies in Swedish, Scottish and North American families did not show linkage to this locus (SCZD1). It is not clear whether the observation of linkage in the original study was a chance finding or a consequence of genetic heterogeneity with different major predisposing loci in the various populations. A number of other cytogenetic abnormalities have been reported with familial schizophrenia, most of which appear to have been coincidental rather than causal, although a locus on the long arm of chromosome 11 (SCZD2) has been reported to be associated with a predisposition to schizophrenia in a number of studies.

The observation of differences in concentrations of neurotransmitter substances, such as dopamine or 5-hydroxytryptamine (serotonin), in various parts of the brains of schizophrenics at autopsy and the pharmacological action of antipsychotic drugs has suggested that genes for CNS neurotransmitter substances and their receptors could be possible candidate genes for linkage studies. No definite evidence of linkage has been found, although some studies have shown evidence of possible associations with particular allelic variants, e.g. the 5-hydroxytryptamine type 2a receptor.

Systematic genome searches have provided evidence of linkage to the short arm of chromosome 6 (SCZD3) and the long arm of chromosome 22 (SCZD4). Analysis of the results suggests that these loci could contain major susceptibility genes for schizophrenia. The locus on the long arm of chromosome 22 is of special interest, in view of the reported higher incidence of schizophrenia in individuals with the Shprintzen syndrome, a microdeletion syndrome involving the long arm of chromosome 22 (p. 254). A further two loci predisposing to schizophrenia have been reported in one or more studies.

ANTICIPATION

More recently, observations in several studies of an earlier age of onset and an increase in severity in affected individuals in subsequent generations in familial schizophrenia have suggested the possibility of anticipation (p. 107). Although care has to be taken with regard to possible ascertainment bias, these observations introduce unstable mutations (p. 22) as a possible mutational mechanism.

AFFECTIVE DISORDERS

Affective disorders include purely depressive or *unipolar* illness and manic-depressive or *bipolar* illness. Both are episodic disorders characterized by a persistent lowering of feeling, emotion and desire resulting in difficulty in performing routine tasks at the usual rate and expected quality. The manic phase of bipolar illness is characterized by elevation of affect, euphoric emotions, pathological desire and rapid speech. Manic-depressive illness is associated with a significant risk of suicide. Bipolar and unipolar illness show differences in the length and number of episodes and age of onset.

EPIDEMIOLOGY

Affective disorders are universal, occurring in all societies. The lifetime risk of developing bipolar depressive illness is between 0.5% and 1% while unipolar depressive illness ranges from 2% to 25%, the latter variation probably being due to different cultural and environmental influences.

FAMILY STUDIES

Familial occurrence of affective disorders has been reported in a number of studies. Relatives of persons with unipolar and bipolar affective disorders have an increased risk of similar problems compared to the general population. Although there is a tendency for recurrence of the same type of affective disorder in affected relatives, unipolar depressive illness is the most common disorder in first-degree relatives of persons with both unipolar and bipolar affective disorder.

TWIN STUDIES

Concordance rates in monozygotic and dizygotic twins are 67% and 20% respectively, being slightly higher for bipolar illness and lower for unipolar illness. Although concordance for the polarity of the affective disorder occurs in the majority of the familial recurrences, approximately one-quarter are for unipolar affective disorder when the proband has bipolar affective disorder and vice versa.

ADOPTION STUDIES

The results of adoption studies, which have shown a high prevalence of affective disorder in the biological parents and other relatives of adoptees with bipolar affective disorder, support the concept that the majority of affective disorders have a genetic basis.

POSSIBLE SINGLE MODELS OF INHERITANCE

The possibility of autosomal dominant, autosomal recessive and X-linked modes of transmission for affective disorders has been proposed in various different studies over the years. The results of segregation and population studies support the likelihood of affective disorders being genetically heterogeneous rather than being explained by a simple single gene mode of inheritance. The excess of females with, and a deficiency of male to male transmission in, manic-depressive illness have suggested the possibility of a subgroup due to X-linked dominant inheritance. It has been suggested, however, that the lack of increased severity of the disorder in hemizygous males (p. 102) and the fact that affected males are less likely to reproduce do not provide formal support for this mode of inheritance.

LINKAGE AND ASSOCIATION STUDIES

Although the first suggestion of linkage in affective disorders was the observation of an increased rate of shared HLA haplotypes in sib-pairs with depressive illness, further studies separately analysing unipolar and bipolar illness revealed less clear-cut findings. Analysis of families with manic-depressive illness in the Old Order Amish in Lancaster County in Pennsylvania suggested linkage to a locus on the short arm of chromosome 11. Subsequent reanalysis of the results of the families originally reported with further clinical follow-up and analysis of additional individuals resulted in the loss of the apparent linkage. Studies in other populations have failed to find linkage of manic-depressive illness to the short arm of chromosome 11.

Support for the possibility of X-linked inheritance of bipolar illness was first provided by reports of possible linkage to two loci on the different arms of the X chromosome, i.e. the colour blindness (p. 103) and the Xg blood group loci. Further studies of G6PD polymorphisms and DNA markers on the long arm of the X chromosome have reported linkage covering a region of some 30–40 cM from Xq26 to Xq28.

More recently, there have been reports of possible linkage to loci on both the long and short arms of chromosome 18. Further studies are required to determine whether these observations are substantiated or suffer the fate of previous reports of linkage in affective disorders.

BIOCHEMICAL STUDIES

A number of the neurotransmitters and their respective receptors have been suggested as possible candidate genes for affective disorders. These include the receptor for the major inhibitory neurotransmitter gamma-aminobutyric acid on the long arm of chromosome 15 and one of the 5-hydroxytryptamine receptor genes on the long arm of chromosome 11 in the region in which linkage in the Old Order Amish was reported as well as a number of the dopamine receptors.

ANTICIPATION

Analysis of the age of onset and severity in familial bipolar illness has shown more severe illness and an earlier age of onset consistent with anticipation (p. 107), suggesting the possibility of unstable triplet repeat mutations being involved in the aetiology of the disorder (p. 22).

ALZHEIMER'S DISEASE

Dementia is characterized by an irreversible and progressive global impairment of intellect, memory, social skills and control of emotional reactions in the presence of normal consciousness. Dementia is aetiologically heterogeneous occurring secondary to both a variety of non-genetic causes, such as vascular disease and infections such as AIDS, as well as genetic causes. Alzheimer's disease (AD) is the most common cause of dementia in persons with either early onset dementia (less than the age of 60 or presenile) or late onset (greater than age 60 or senile). The classical neuropathological finding in persons with AD is the presence at postmortem examination of amyloid deposits in neurofibrillary tangles and neuronal or senile plaques. In addition, individuals with Down's syndrome have an increased risk of developing dementia (p. 251) which, at postmortem, has identical CNS findings to those seen in persons with typical AD.

EPIDEMIOLOGY

Limited numbers of studies of the incidence and prevalence of AD are available due to problems of ascertainment. Although it has been suggested that environmental factors could have a role in aetiology, the risk of developing AD increases dramatically with age (Table 14.7).

TWIN STUDIES

Differences in the age of onset of AD in identical twins are consistent with the importance of environmental factors.

FAMILY STUDIES

There are difficulties with family studies in AD. Many studies are based on a clinical diagnosis. A significant proportion of persons with a clinical diagnosis of AD are found to have other causes at postmortem, such as cerebrovascular atherosclerotic disease. Attempts to confirm diagnoses in relatives who have died previously are often unsuccessful. Obviously, given the age of onset, it is generally neither practical nor possible to obtain funding for prospective studies of the risk to offspring. Therefore, family studies of the risk to siblings are the only practical type of family study to provide reliable data. Although there are numerous retrospective reports of families with AD which are consistent with autosomal dominant inheritance, recurrence risks in a number of studies for first-degree relatives are less than 10%. The risks are age-related and greater the younger the age of the diagnosis in the affected individual.

BIOCHEMICAL STUDIES

The amyloid deposits in the neurofibrillary tangles and neuronal plaques have been shown to consist of the amyloid β A4 precursor protein (APP). The major protein component of the neurofibrillary tangles has been shown to be derived from a microtubule-associated protein (MAP) called tau (τ). Along with other MAPs, it interacts with β-tubulin to stabilize microtubules.

LINKAGE STUDIES

The identification of APP in the amyloid deposits of the neuronal plaques, its mapping in or near to the critical region of the distal part of the long arm of chromosome 21 associated with the phenotypic features of Down's syndrome (p. 251), along with the increased risk of AD in

Table 14.7 Estimates of age-specific cumulative prevalence of dementia	
Age interval (years)	Prevalence (%)
< 70	1.3
70–74	2.3
75–79	6.4
80–84	15.3
85–89	23.7
90–94	42.9
> 95	50.9

From Heston L L Alzheimer's disease, Chapter 39 in King, Rotter and Motulsky 1992.

persons with Down's syndrome, led to the suggestion that duplication of the APP gene could be a cause of AD. This mechanism as a cause for familial AD has been found to be the exception rather than the rule, although a small proportion of families with early onset AD show linkage to the APP locus (AD1). Of these families, only a limited number have been found to have mutations in the APP gene, which has led to the suggestion that another gene near the APP gene on chromosome 21 could be responsible for the AD in the remaining families. There is, however, controversy as to whether there is definite evidence for this second locus on chromosome 21.

Late onset AD, the most frequent form of the disease, presented problems in comparison with the early onset form of AD for linkage studies in the collection of families for analysis. Late onset AD was thought to be familial, but it was not clear if this was an ascertainment artefact due to AD being a common disease. Linkage studies identified a susceptibility locus to late onset AD in a region of the long arm of chromosome 19 (AD2) which was known to contain the apolipoprotein E gene (p. 218).

Evidence of linkage was found for another locus for early onset AD mapping to the long arm of chromosome 14 (AD3). Mutations were identified in a proportion of affected individuals in one of a novel class of genes, known as presenilin-1. A second gene, presenilin-2, with homology to presenilin-1 was mapped to chromosome 1 and has been shown to have mutations in a limited number of families with AD (AD4). Presenilin-1 and -2 are integral membrane proteins containing multiple transmembrane domains which localize to the endoplasmic reticulum and the Golgi complex. A large number of mutations in the presenilin-1 gene have been identified and appear to account for up to 70% of early onset Alzheimer's disease.

ASSOCIATION STUDIES

The apolipoprotein E gene is polymorphic with three major protein isoforms, ε2, ε3 and ε4. A number of studies in various populations and ethnic groups have shown an increased frequency of heterozygosity and homozygosity for the ε4 allele in persons with both sporadic and late onset familial AD. In addition, the ε2 allele has been shown to be associated with a decreased risk of developing AD. The finding of apolipoprotein E in senile plaques and neurofibrillary tangles, along with its role in lipid transport possibly in relation to the nerve injury and regeneration seen in AD, provides further evidence for a possible role in the acceleration of the neurodegenerative process in AD.

In addition, there is an association with polymorphisms in the α-2 macroglobulin gene and the low density lipoprotein-related protein, both of which interact with components involved in the clearance and degradation of amyloid protein.

Although it is clear that the APOE ε4 allele is the most significant risk factor for late onset AD, accounting for up to 40% of late onset Alzheimer's disease, it is neither necessary nor sufficient for the development of AD, emphasizing the importance of other genetic and environmental aetiological factors. This underlies the recommendation of the US National Institute on Aging and the Alzheimer's Association Working Group that APOE testing is not used to predict whether an asymptomatic person is likely to develop AD.

ANIMAL MODELS

Transgenic mice with mutations in the presenilin-1 and -2 genes resulting in their overexpression showed an increase in the rate of deposition of amyloid in the brain, suggesting that mutations in the presenilin genes could cause AD through a gain-of-function. Generation of a transgenic mouse expressing the APP gene will allow a better understanding of the pathogenesis of AD and the assessment of possible therapeutic interventions.

ELEMENTS

1 Both genetic and environmental factors are involved in the aetiology of many of the common diseases affecting humans. The genetic factors can be considered to be due to an inherited predisposition or genetic susceptibility.

2 The genetic contribution in a particular condition can be assessed by studying the incidence of disease in relatives, comparing concordance rates in identical and non-identical twins, studying differences between populations and the effects of migration, studying the effects of adoption, biochemical studies, evaluating any possible association with other inherited factors and studying animal models.

3 For common disorders, such as diabetes mellitus, hypertension, coronary artery disease, peptic ulcer, schizophrenia, the common cancers and the common congenital abnormalities, a multifactorial mode of inheritance is most likely. However, it is also becoming clear that many of these conditions are heterogeneous, that is, they are caused by a variety of genetic and environmental factors.

4 Prevention of the common diseases involves determining causative environmental agents as well as identifying those individuals who are genetically susceptible to such agents.

FURTHER READING

Heston L L 1966 Psychiatric disorders in foster home reared
children of schizophrenic mothers. Br J Psychiatry 112: 819–825
*A classic paper demonstrating genetic factors in the aetiology of
schizophrenia.*

Jameson J L (ed) 1998 Principles of molecular medicine. Humana
Press, Totawa, New Jersey
A large multiauthor text covering in detail the molecular basis of the
common diseases as well as many of the more common single gene and
chromosome disorders.

King R A, Rotter J I, Motulsky A G (eds) 1992 The genetic basis of
common diseases. Oxford University Press, Oxford
*An excellent multiauthor text covering the principles of analysis with
an extensive review of the genetic basis of the common diseases plus an
exhaustive reference list.*

Plomin R, De Fries J C, McClearn G E, Rutter M 1997 Behavioral
genetics. W H Freeman, New York
*A multiauthor text covering the approaches to studying behavioural
genetics.*

CHAPTER 15

Genetics and congenital abnormalities

The formation of a human being, a process sometimes known as *morphogenesis*, involves an extremely complicated and as yet very poorly understood interaction of genetic and environmental factors. Given the extraordinary complexity of this process it is not surprising that on occasion it can go wrong. Nor is it surprising that in many congenital abnormalities genetic factors can clearly be implicated. In this chapter we shall consider the overall impact of abnormalities in morphogenesis by reviewing:

1. The incidence of abnormalities at various stages from conception onwards.
2. Their nature and the ways in which they can be classified.
3. Their causes, when known, with particular emphasis on the role of genetics.

INCIDENCE

SPONTANEOUS FIRST-TRIMESTER PREGNANCY LOSS

It has been estimated that around 50% of all human conceptions are lost either before implantation at 5–6 days post conception or shortly afterwards before the mother realizes that she is pregnant. Among recognized pregnancies at least 15% end in spontaneous miscarriage before 12 weeks gestation. Even if material from the abortus can be obtained it is often very difficult to establish why a pregnancy loss has occurred. However, careful study of large numbers of spontaneously aborted embryos has shown that gross structural abnormalities are present in between 80% and 85%. These abnormalities vary from complete absence of an embryo in the developing pregnancy sac, or what is known as a 'blighted ovum', to a very distorted body shape, or a specific abnormality in a single body system.

Chromosome abnormalities such as trisomy, monosomy or triploidy are found in 50% of all spontaneous abortions.

This incidence rises to 60% when a gross structural abnormality is present (p. 249).

CONGENITAL ABNORMALITIES AND PERINATAL MORTALITY

Perinatal mortality figures include all infants who are stillborn after 28 weeks gestation plus all babies who die during the first week of life. Studies undertaken in several centres in Europe and North America have shown that between 25% and 30% of all perinatal deaths occur as a result of a serious structural abnormality. In 80% of these cases genetic factors can be implicated, with a recurrence risk to future pregnancies equal to 1% or greater. The relative contribution of structural abnormalities to perinatal mortality is lower in developing countries where environmental factors play a much greater role.

NEWBORN INFANTS

Surveys reviewing the incidence of both major and minor anomalies in newborn infants have been undertaken in many parts of the world. A major anomaly is defined as one which has an adverse outcome on either the function or social acceptability of the individual (Table 15.1). In contrast, minor abnormalities are of neither medical nor cosmetic importance (Table 15.2).

These surveys have consistently shown that between 2% and 3% of all newborns have at least one major abnormality apparent at birth. The true incidence, taking into account abnormalities which present later in life, such as brain malformations, is probably close to 5%. Minor abnormalities are found in approximately 10% of all newborn babies. If two or more minor abnormalities are present in a newborn infant, then there is a risk of between 10% and 20% that the baby will also have a major malformation.

The long-term outlook for a baby with a major abnormality obviously depends on the nature of the specific birth defect and whether it can be treated successfully. Taken together the overall prognosis for this

Table 15.1 Examples of major congenital structural abnormalities

System and abnormality	Incidence per 1000 births
Cardiovascular	10
Ventricular septal defect	2.5
Atrial septal defect	1
Patent ductus arteriosus	1
Fallot's tetralogy	1
Central nervous system	10
Anencephaly	1
Hydrocephaly	1
Microcephaly	1
Lumbo-sacral spina bifida	2
Gastro-intestinal	4
Cleft lip/palate	1.5
Diaphragmatic hernia	0.5
Oesophageal atresia	0.3
Imperforate anus	0.2
Limb	2
Transverse amputation	0.2
Urogenital	4
Bilateral renal agenesis	2
Polycystic kidneys (infantile)	0.02
Bladder exstrophy	0.03

Table 15.2 Examples of minor congenital structural abnormalities

Preauricular pit or tag
Epicanthic folds
Lacrimal duct stenosis
Brushfield spots in the iris
Lip pits
Single palmar crease
Fifth finger clinodactyly
Syndactyly between second and third toes
Supernumerary nipple
Umbilical hernia
Hydrocele
Sacral pit or dimple

Table 15.3 The incidence of structural abnormalities

Incidence	(%)
Spontaneous miscarriages	
First trimester	80–85
Second trimester	25
All babies	
Major abnormality	
Apparent at birth	2–3
Apparent later	2
Minor abnormality	10
Deaths in perinatal period	25
Deaths in first year of life	25
Deaths from 1 to 9 years	20
Deaths from 10 to 14 years	7.5

carriages, it is evident that at least 15% of all recognized human conceptions are structurally abnormal (Table 15.3). It is probable that genetic factors are involved in the causation of at least 50% of all structural abnormalities.

group of newborns is relatively poor, with 25% dying in early infancy, 25% having subsequent mental or physical disability and the remaining 50% having a fair to good outlook after treatment.

CHILDHOOD MORTALITY

Congenital abnormalities make a significant contribution to mortality throughout childhood. During the first year of life approximately 25% of all deaths are the result of major structural abnormalities. This figure falls to 20% between the ages of 1 and 10 years and to around 7.5% for children aged between 10 and 15 years.

Taking into account the incidence of major and minor abnormalities noted in newborn surveys and the high incidence of defects observed in early spontaneous mis-

DEFINITIONS AND CLASSIFICATION OF BIRTH DEFECTS

So far in this chapter the terms 'congenital abnormality' and 'birth defect' have been used in a general sense to describe all types of structural abnormality which can occur in an embryo, fetus or newborn infant. While these terms are perfectly acceptable for the purpose of lumping together all these abnormalities when studying their overall incidence, they do not provide any insight into possible underlying mechanisms. More specific definitions have been devised which have the added advantage of providing a combined clinical and aetiological classification.

SINGLE ABNORMALITIES

Malformation

A *malformation* is a primary structural defect of an organ or part of an organ which results from an inherent abnormality in development. This used to be known as a primary or intrinsic malformation. The presence of a malformation implies that the early development of a particular tissue or organ has been arrested or misdirected. Common examples of malformations include congenital heart abnormalities such as ventricular or atrial septal defects, cleft lip and/or palate (p. 130), and neural tube defects such as anencephaly or lumbo-sacral myelomeningocele (Fig. 15.1). Most malformations involving only a single organ show multifactorial inheritance, implying an interaction of many genes with environmental factors (p. 129).

Fig. 15.1
Child with a large thoraco-lumbar myelomeningocele consisting of protruding spinal cord covered by meninges.

A

B

Fig. 15.2
(A) Hand and (B) foot of a baby with digital amputations due to amniotic bands showing residual strands of amnion. (Courtesy of Dr Una MacFadyen, Leicester Royal Infirmary.)

Disruption

The term *disruption* refers to an abnormal structure of an organ or tissue as a result of external factors disturbing the normal developmental process. This used to be known as a secondary or extrinsic malformation. Extrinsic factors which can disrupt normal development include ischaemia, infection and trauma. An example of a disruption is the effect seen on limb development when a strand or band of amnion becomes entwined around a baby's forearm or digits (Fig. 15.2). By definition a disruption is not genetic, although occasionally genetic factors can predispose to disruptive events. For example, a small proportion of amniotic bands are caused by an underlying, genetically determined defect in collagen which weakens the amnion making it more liable to tear or rupture spontaneously.

Deformation

A *deformation* is a defect which results from an abnormal mechanical force which distorts an otherwise normal structure. Well-recognized examples include dislocation of the hip and mild 'positional' talipes ('club foot') (Fig. 15.3), both of which can be caused by lack of amniotic fluid (oligohydramnios) or intra-uterine crowding due to twinning or a structurally abnormal uterus. Deformations

Fig. 15.3
The lower limbs of a baby with talipes equinovarus.

usually occur late in pregnancy and convey a good prognosis with appropriate treatment, e.g. gentle splinting for talipes, since the underlying organ is fundamentally normal in structure.

Dysplasia

A *dysplasia* is an abnormal organization of cells into tissue. Usually the effects are seen in all parts of the body in which that particular tissue is present. For example, in a skeletal dysplasia such as thanatophoric dysplasia, which is caused by mutations in *FGFR3* (p. 87), almost all parts of the skeleton are affected (Fig. 15.4). Similarly, in an ectodermal dysplasia, widely dispersed tissues of ectodermal origin such as hair, teeth and nails are involved (Fig. 15.5). Most dysplasias are caused by single gene defects and are associated with high recurrence risks for siblings and/or offspring.

A

B

Fig. 15.4
(A) Infant with thanatophoric dysplasia; (B) X-ray of the infant showing short ribs, flat vertebral bodies and curved femora.

A

B

Fig. 15.5
(A) Hair and (B) teeth of a male with ectodermal dysplasia.

MULTIPLE ABNORMALITIES

Sequence

The most logical and easily understood pattern of multiple abnormalities is the concept of a *sequence*. This describes the findings which occur as a consequence of a cascade of events initiated by a single primary factor. This can often be a single organ malformation. In the 'Potter' sequence, chronic leakage of amniotic fluid or defective urinary output results in oligohydramnios (Fig. 15.6). This, in turn, leads to fetal compression, resulting in squashed facial features, dislocation of the hips, talipes and usually life-threatening pulmonary hypoplasia (Fig. 15.7).

Syndrome

In practice the term *syndrome* is used very loosely (e.g. the amniotic band 'syndrome'), but in theory it should be reserved for consistent patterns of abnormalities for which there will often be a known underlying cause. These underlying causes can include chromosome abnormalities, as in Down's syndrome, or single gene defects, as in the Van der Woude syndrome in which cleft lip and/or palate occurs in association with pits in the lower lip (Fig. 15.8).

Several thousand multiple malformation syndromes are now recognized. This field of study is known as *dysmorphology*. The diagnosis of individual syndromes has been greatly helped by the development of computerized databases (see appendix). It is possible to obtain a list of differential diagnoses by providing the computer with details of key abnormal clinical features. Even with the help of this extremely valuable diagnostic tool, there are, unfortunately, many dysmorphic children for whom no diagnosis can be reached, so that it can be very difficult to provide accurate information about the likely prognosis and recurrence risk (p. 293).

Association

The term *association* has been introduced in recognition of the fact that certain malformations tend to occur together more often than would be expected by chance, yet this non-random occurrence of abnormalities cannot be explained on the basis of a sequence or a syndrome. The main differences from a syndrome are the lack of consistency of abnormalities from one affected individual

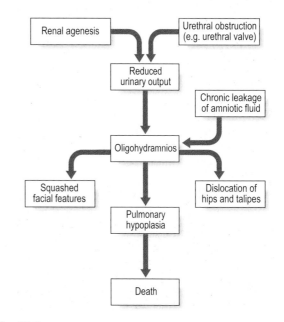

Fig. 15.6
The 'Potter' sequence showing the cascade of events leading to and resulting from oligohydramnios (reduced volume of amniotic fluid).

Fig. 15.7
Facial appearance of a baby with Potter sequence due to oligohydramnios as a consequence of bilateral renal agenesis. Note the squashed appearance caused by in utero compression.

Fig. 15.8
A posterior cleft palate and lower lip pits in a child with Van der Woude syndrome.

GENETIC CAUSES OF MALFORMATIONS

There are many recognized causes of congenital abnormalities although it is notable that in up to 50% of all cases no clear explanation can be established (Table 15.4).

CHROMOSOME ABNORMALITIES

These account for approximately 6% of all recognized congenital abnormalities. As a general rule any perceptible degree of autosomal imbalance, such as duplication, deletion, trisomy or monosomy, will result in severe structural and developmental abnormality. If very severe this can lead to early spontaneous miscarriage. Common chromosome syndromes are described in detail in Chapter 17. It is not known whether malformations caused

to another and the absence of a satisfactory underlying explanation. The names of associations are often acronyms devised by juggling the first letters of the organs or systems most commonly involved; for example the VATER association features <u>V</u>ertebral, <u>A</u>nal, <u>T</u>racheo-<u>E</u>sophageal and <u>R</u>enal abnormalities. Associations convey a low risk of recurrence and are generally thought not to be genetic in origin even though the underlying cause is usually unknown.

It is recognized that this classification of birth defects is not perfect. It will be readily apparent that it is far from being either fully comprehensive or mutually exclusive. For example, bladder outflow obstruction caused by a primary malformation such as a urethral valve will result in the oligohydramnios or Potter sequence, leading to secondary deformations such as dislocation of the hip and talipes. To complicate matters further, the absence of both kidneys, which will result in the same sequence of events, is usually erroneously referred to as Potter's syndrome. Despite this semantic confusion, adherence to this classification is important since it serves as an aid to understanding and ensures that correct information is given about recurrence risks (p. 293).

Table 15.4	Causes of congenital abnormalities
Cause	**%**
Genetic	
Chromosomal	6
Single gene	7.5
Multifactorial	20–30
Subtotal	30–40
Environmental	
Drugs and chemicals	2
Infections	2
Maternal illness	2
Physical agents	1
Subtotal	5–10
Unknown	50
Total	100

by a significant chromosome abnormality, such as a trisomy, are the result of dosage effects of the individual genes involved ('additive' model) or general developmental instability caused by a large number of abnormal developmental gene products ('interactive' model).

SINGLE GENE DEFECTS

These account for approximately 7.5% of all congenital abnormalities. Some of these are isolated, i.e. they involve only one organ or system (Table 15.5). Other single gene defects result in multiple congenital abnormality syndromes involving many organs or systems which do not have any obvious underlying embryological relationship. For example, ectrodactyly (Fig. 15.9) in isolation can be inherited as an autosomal dominant trait. It can also occur as one manifestation of the EEC syndrome (Ectodermal dysplasia, Ectrodactyly and Cleft lip/palate), which also shows autosomal dominant inheritance. There is abundant evidence from the study of dysmorphology that several different mutations, allelic or non-allelic, can cause similar if not identical malformations.

The importance of identifying birth defects which show single gene inheritance is twofold. From the family's point of view it is essential that correct counselling is available so that close relatives can be alerted to possible risks. From the academic point of view, the identification

of a molecular defect causing an isolated single gene abnormality in a particular organ can provide a clue as to the locus of a susceptibility gene for similar malformations affecting the same organ which show multifactorial inheritance.

MULTIFACTORIAL INHERITANCE

This accounts for the majority of congenital abnormalities in which genetic factors can clearly be implicated. These include most isolated ('non-syndromal') malformations involving the heart, central nervous system and kidneys (Table 15.6). For many of these conditions empiric risks have been derived (p. 301) based on large family studies, so that it is usually possible to provide the parents of an affected child with a clear indication of the likelihood that a future child will be similarly affected. Risks to the

Fig. 15.9
Appearance of the feet in a child with ectrodactyly.

Table 15.5 Congenital abnormalities which can be caused by single gene defects

Isolated	Inheritance
Central nervous system	
Hydrocephalus	XR
Megalencephaly	AD
Microcephaly	AD/AR
Ocular	
Aniridia	AD
Cataracts	AD/AR
Microphthalmia	AD/AR
Limb	
Brachydactyly	AD
Ectrodactyly	AD
Polydactyly	AD
Other	
Infantile polycystic kidneys	AR

Syndromes		
Syndrome	Inheritance	Abnormalities
Apert	AD	Craniosynostosis, syndactyly
EEC	AD	Ectodermal dysplasia, ectrodactyly, cleft lip/palate
Meckel	AR	Encephalocoele, polydactyly, polycystic kidneys
Roberts	AR	Cleft lip/palate, phocomelia
Van der Woude	AD	Cleft lip/palate, lip pits

AD = autosomal dominant; AR = autosomal recessive;
XR = sex-linked recessive.

Table 15.6 Isolated (non-syndromal) malformations which show multifactorial inheritance

Cardiac
Atrial septal defect
Fallot's tetralogy
Patent ductus arteriosus
Ventricular septal defect

Central nervous system
Anencephaly
Encephalocoele
Spina bifida

Genitourinary
Hypospadias
Renal agenesis
Renal dysgenesis

Other
Cleft lip/palate
Congenital dislocation of hips
Talipes

offspring of patients who were themselves treated successfully in childhood are becoming available. These are usually similar to the risk figures which apply to siblings as would be predicted by the multifactorial model (p. 129).

GENETIC HETEROGENEITY

It has long been recognized that specific congenital malformations can have many different causes, hence the importance of trying to distinguish between syndromal and isolated cases. This causal diversity has become increasingly apparent as developments in molecular biology have led to the identification of highly conserved families of genes which play crucial roles in early embryogenesis.

This subject is discussed at length in Chapter 5. In this chapter two specific malformations, holoprosencephaly and neural tube defects, shall be considered to demonstrate the rate of progress in this field and the extent of the challenge which lies ahead before full understanding is achieved.

Holoprosencephaly

This severe and often lethal malformation is caused by a failure of cleavage of the embryonic forebrain or prosencephalon. Normally this divides transversely into the telencephalon and the diencephalon. The telencephalon divides in the sagittal plane to form the cerebral hemispheres and the olfactory tracts and bulbs. The diencephalon develops to form the thalamic nuclei, the pineal gland, the optic chiasm and the optic nerves. In holoprosencephaly there is incomplete or partial failure of these developmental processes and in the severe alobar form this results in an abnormal facial appearance (Fig. 5.1) and profound neurodevelopmental impairment.

Aetiologically holoprosencephaly can be classified as chromosomal, syndromal or isolated. Chromosomal causes account for around 30–40% of all cases with the most common abnormality being trisomy 13 (p. 252). Other chromosomal causes include duplication or deletion of 13q, deletion of 2p and triploidy (p. 256). Syndromal causes of holoprosencephaly are numerous and include relatively well known conditions such as the DiGeorge/Shprintzen syndromes (p. 185) and a host of much rarer multiple malformation syndromes many of which show autosomal recessive inheritance. One of these, the Smith–Lemli–Opitz syndrome, is associated with low levels of cholesterol which is relevant in that it is known that cholesterol is necessary for normal functioning of the *hedgehog* development gene family (p. 82).

This leads conveniently to the third group consisting of isolated holoprosencephaly which until recently was largely unexplained. However over the last few years three genes have been identified which, when mutated, can cause very variable degrees of holoprosencephaly, ranging from mild 'microforms' with minimal features such as anosmia to the full-blown lethal alobar form. These three genes are *sonic hedgehog* (*SHH*) on chromosome 7q36, *ZIC2* on chromosome 13q32 and *SIX3* on chromosome 2p21. Of these *SHH* is thought to make the greatest contribution accounting for up to 20% of all familial cases and between 1 and 10% of isolated cases.

The fact that so many familial cases remain unexplained indicates that many important holoprosencephaly genes await identification. The extent of causal heterogeneity shown by this condition is further illustrated by its association with poorly controlled maternal insulin-dependent diabetes mellitus (p. 236).

Neural tube defects (NTDs)

Neural tube defects, such as spina bifida and anencephaly, illustrate many of the underlying principles of multifactorial inheritance and emphasize the importance of trying to identify possible adverse environmental factors. These conditions result from defective closure of the developing neural tube during the first month of embryonic life. A defect occurring at the upper end of the developing neural tube results in either anencephaly or an encephalocele (Fig. 15.10). A defect occurring at the lower end of the developing neural tube leads to a spinal lesion such as a lumbo-sacral myelocele or meningomyelocele (Fig. 15.1). Most NTDs have serious consequences. Anencephaly is not compatible with survival for more than a few hours after birth. Large lumbo-sacral lesions usually cause partial or complete paralysis of the lower limbs with impaired bladder and bowel continence.

As with many malformations neural tube defects can be classified aetiologically under the headings of chromosomal, syndromal and isolated. Chromosomal causes include trisomy 13 and trisomy 18 in both of which NTDs show an incidence of around 5–10%. Syndromal causes include the relatively rare autosomal recessive disorder Meckel's syndrome in which an encephalocele occurs in association with polycystic kidneys and polydactyly. However most NTDs represent isolated malformations in otherwise normal infants and most isolated NTDs are believed to show multifactorial inheritance.

The empiric recurrence risks to first-degree relatives (siblings and offspring) vary according to the local population incidence and are as high as 4–5% in areas where NTDs are common. The incidence in the United Kingdom is highest in people of Celtic origin. If such individuals move from their country of origin to another part of the world, the incidence of NTDs in their offspring declines but remains higher than amongst the indigenous population. These observations suggest that there is a

Fig. 15.10
A baby with a large occipital encephalocoele.

relatively high incidence of adverse susceptibility genes in the Celtic populations.

No definite NTD susceptibility genes have been identified in humans, although there is some evidence that a specific mutation in the gene coding for methylenetetrahydrofolate reductase (MTHFR) can be a contributory factor. Reduction in MTHFR activity results in decreased plasma folate levels which are known to be causally associated with NTDs (see below). Research efforts have also focused on developmental genes, such as the *PAX* family (p. 84), which are expressed in the embryonic neural tube and vertebral column. To date understanding of the processes involved in humans is very limited. In contrast, studies in mice have revealed that an interaction between mutations of *PAX1* and the platelet-derived growth factor α gene (*Pdgfra*) results in severe NTDs in 100% of double mutant embryos. This rare example of *digenic inheritance* serves as a useful illustration of the difficulties posed by a search for susceptibility genes in a multifactorial disorder.

Environmental factors involved in the aetiology of NTDs which have been identified include poor socioeconomic status, multiparity and valproic acid embryopathy. Firm evidence has also emerged that periconceptional multivitamin supplementation reduces the risk of recurrence by a factor of 70–75% when a woman has had one affected child. Several studies have shown that folic acid is likely to be the effective constituent in multivitamin preparations. In both the United Kingdom and the United States it is recommended that all women who have had a previous child with an NTD should take 4–5 mg of folic acid daily both before and during the early stages of all subsequent pregnancies. Similarly in the United Kingdom it has been recommended that all women who are trying to conceive should take 0.4 mg folic acid daily. In the United States, where bread is fortified with folic acid, this recommendation applies to all women of reproductive age throughout their reproductive years. In the United Kingdom this recommendation has not as yet resulted in a noticeable decline in the incidence of NTDs although a longer time period may be necessary to show any such effect.

ENVIRONMENTAL AGENTS (TERATOGENS)

An agent which can cause a birth defect by interfering with normal embryonic or fetal development is known as a *teratogen*. Many teratogens have been identified and exhaustive tests are now undertaken before any new drug is approved for use by pregnant women. The potential effects of any particular teratogen will usually depend on the dosage and timing when it is administered during the pregnancy along with the susceptibility of both the mother and her unborn baby.

An agent which conveys a high risk of teratogenesis, such as the rubella virus or thalidomide, will usually be identified relatively quickly. Unfortunately, it is much more difficult to detect a low grade teratogen which causes an abnormality in only a small proportion of cases. This is because of the relatively high background incidence of congenital abnormalities and also because many pregnant women take medication at some time in pregnancy, often for an ill-defined 'flu-like' illness. Despite extensive study, controversy still surrounds the use of a number of drugs in pregnancy. The antinausea drug Debendox has been the subject of successful litigation in the United States despite the absence of firm evidence to support a definite teratogenic effect.

DRUGS AND CHEMICALS

Drugs and chemicals which have a proven teratogenic effect in humans are listed in Table 15.7. Overall these account for approximately 2% of all congenital abnormalities.

Table 15.7   Drugs with a proven teratogenic effect in humans

Drug	Effects
ACE inhibitors	Renal dysplasia
Alcohol	Cardiac defects, microcephaly, characteristic facies
Chloroquine	Chorioretinitis, deafness
Diethylstilboestrol	Uterine malformations, vaginal adenocarcinoma
Lithium	Cardiac defects (Ebstein's anomaly)
Phenytoin	Cardiac defects, cleft palate, digital hypoplasia
Retinoids	Ear and eye defects, hydrocephalus
Streptomycin	Deafness
Tetracycline	Dental enamel hypoplasia
Thalidomide	Phocomelia, cardiac and ear abnormalities
Valproic acid	Neural tube defects, characteristic facies
Warfarin	Nasal hypoplasia, stippled epiphyses

Many other drugs have been proposed as possible teratogens but the relatively small numbers of reported cases make it difficult to confirm that they are definitely teratogenic. This applies to many anticancer drugs, such as methotrexate and chlorambucil, and to anticonvulsants, such as carbamazepine and primadone. Exposure to environmental chemicals is also an area of widespread concern. Organic mercurials ingested in contaminated fish in Minamata, Japan, as a result of industrial pollution caused a 'cerebral palsy-like' syndrome in babies who had been exposed in utero. Controversy surrounds the use of agents used in warfare such as dioxin (Agent Orange) in Vietnam and various nerve gases in the Gulf War.

The thalidomide tragedy

Thalidomide was used widely in Europe during the years 1958 to 1962 as a sedative. In 1961 an association with severe limb anomalies in babies whose mothers had taken the drug during the first trimester was recognized and the drug was subsequently withdrawn from use. It has been estimated that during this short period over 10 000 babies were damaged by this drug. Review of these babies' records indicated that the critical period for fetal damage was between 20 and 35 days from conception, i.e. 34–50 days after the beginning of the last menstrual period.

The most characteristic abnormality caused by thalidomide was phocomelia (Fig. 15.11). This is the name given to a limb which is malformed due to absence of some or all of the long bones, with retention of digits giving a 'flipper' or 'seal-like' appearance. Other external abnormalities included ear defects, microphthalmia and cleft lip/palate. In addition, approximately 40% of 'thalidomide babies' died in early infancy as a result of severe internal abnormalities affecting the heart, kidneys or gastro-intestinal tract.

The thalidomide tragedy focused attention on the importance of avoiding all drugs in pregnancy as far as is possible, unless absolute safety has been established. Drug manufacturers undertake extensive research trials before releasing a drug for general use and invariably urge caution about the use of any new drug in pregnancy. Monitoring systems have been set up in most Western countries so that it is unlikely that an 'epidemic' on the scale of the thalidomide tragedy could ever happen again.

The fetal alcohol syndrome

Children born to mothers who have consistently consumed large quantities of alcohol during pregnancy tend to show a distinctive facial appearance with short palpebral fissures (eye apertures) and a long smooth philtrum (upper lip). They also show mild developmental delay and are often hyperactive and clumsy in later childhood.

Fig. 15.11
A child with thalidomide embryopathy. There is absence of the upper limbs (amelia). The lower limbs show phocomelia and polydactyly. (Courtesy of Emeritus Professor R W Smithells, University of Leeds.)

This condition is referred to as the fetal alcohol syndrome. There is uncertainty about the level of alcohol consumption which is 'safe' in pregnancy and there is evidence that even mild to moderate ingestion can be harmful. Generally it is advised that all women should try to abstain from alcohol intake completely throughout pregnancy.

MATERNAL INFECTIONS

Several infectious agents can interfere with embryogenesis and fetal development (Table 15.8). The developing brain, eyes and ears are particularly susceptible to damage by infection.

Rubella

The rubella virus, which damages between 15% and 25% of all babies infected during the first trimester, also causes cardiovascular malformations such as patent ductus arteriosus and peripheral pulmonary artery stenosis. Congenital rubella infection can be prevented by the widespread use of immunization programmes based on administration of either the measles, mumps, rubella (MMR) vaccine in early childhood or the rubella vaccine alone to young adult women.

Cytomegalovirus

At present no immunization is available against the cytomegalovirus (CMV) and naturally occurring infection does not always produce long term immunity. The risk of abnormality is greatest if infection occurs during the first trimester. Overall this virus causes damage in only 5% of infected pregnancies.

Toxoplasmosis

Maternal infection with the parasite causing toxoplasmosis conveys a risk of 20% that the fetus will be infected during the first trimester, rising to 75% in the second and third trimesters. Vaccines against toxoplasmosis are not available.

If a woman is exposed to any of these infectious agents during pregnancy then an attempt can be made to establish whether the fetus has been infected by sampling fetal blood to look for specific IgM antibodies. Fetal blood analysis can also reveal generalized evidence of infection such as abnormal liver function and thrombocytopenia.

There is some evidence to suggest that maternal infection with listeriosis can cause a miscarriage and a definite association has been established between maternal infection with this agent and neonatal meningitis. Maternal infection with parvovirus can cause severe anaemia in the fetus resulting in hydrops fetalis and pregnancy loss.

PHYSICAL AGENTS

Women who have had babies with congenital abnormalities are often understandably anxious that exposure to agents such as radiowaves, ultrasound or magnetic fields could have caused their babies' problems. Unfortunately, it is difficult to prove or disprove any of these possibilities as exposure to these physical agents is almost universal.

However, there is evidence that two specific physical agents, ionizing radiation and prolonged hyperthermia, can have teratogenic effects.

Ionizing radiation

Heavy doses of ionizing radiation, far in excess of those used in routine diagnostic radiography, can cause microcephaly and ocular defects in the developing fetus. The most sensitive time of exposure is from 2 to 5 weeks after conception. Ionizing radiation can also have mutagenic (p. 24) and carcinogenic effects, and although the risks associated with low dose diagnostic procedures are minimal, radiography should always be avoided during pregnancy if at all possible.

Prolonged hyperthermia

There is evidence that prolonged hyperthermia in early pregnancy can cause microcephaly and microphthalmia as well as neuronal migration defects. Consequently it is recommended that care should be taken to avoid excessive use of hot baths and saunas during the first trimester.

MATERNAL ILLNESS

A number of maternal illnesses are associated with an increased risk of an untoward pregnancy outcome.

Table 15.8 Infectious teratogenic agents	
Infection	**Effects**
Viruses	
Cytomegalovirus	Chororetinitis, deafness, microcephaly
Herpes simplex	Microcephaly, microphthalmia
Rubella	Microcephaly, cataracts, retinitis, cardiac defects
Varicella zoster	Microcephaly, chorioretinitis, skin defects
Bacteria	
Syphilis	Hydrocephalus, osteitis, rhinitis
Parasites	
Toxoplasmosis	Hydrocephalus, microcephaly, cataracts, chorioretinitis, deafness

Diabetes mellitus

Maternal insulin-dependent diabetes mellitus is associated with a two- to threefold increase in the incidence of congenital abnormalities in offspring. Malformations which occur most commonly in such infants include congenital heart disease, neural tube defects, sacral agenesis, femoral hypoplasia, holoprosencephaly and sirenomelia ('mermaidism'). The likelihood of an abnormality is inversely related to the quality of the control of the mother's blood glucose levels during early pregnancy. This can be assessed by regular monitoring of blood glucose and glycosylated haemoglobin levels. Non-insulin-dependent diabetes and gestational diabetes do not convey an increased risk for congenital malformations in offspring.

Phenylketonuria

The other main maternal metabolic condition which conveys a risk to offspring is untreated phenylketonuria (p. 155). A high serum level of phenylalanine in a pregnant woman with phenylketonuria who is not on a special diet will almost invariably result in serious damage to the fetus with the incidence of mental retardation in the offspring close to 100%. Structural abnormalities can include microcephaly and congenital heart defects. All women with phenylketonuria should be strongly advised to adhere to a strict low phenylalanine diet both before and during pregnancy.

Maternal epilepsy

There has been considerable interest in whether or not maternal epilepsy leads to congenital abnormalities. There have been a number of studies of this problem and it seems that maternal epilepsy itself is not associated with an increased risk of congenital abnormalities. Treatment of the mother with one of the anticonvulsants can, however, be associated with teratogenic effects on the fetus. Phenytoin is associated with a risk of cleft lip and/ or palate of about 1–2%, while with sodium valproate there is a risk of anencephaly or spina bifida of about 2%. Of course, potential risks to the fetus have to be weighed against the dangers of stopping treatment and risking seizures during pregnancy. Medical advice, at present, is that if the patient has been seizure-free for at least 2 years she can be offered withdrawal of anticonvulsant treatment before proceeding with a pregnancy. If therapy is essential, then single drug treatment is preferred, since a combination of several anticonvulsants appears to carry a greater risk of fetal abnormality.

MALFORMATIONS OF UNKNOWN CAUSE

In up to 50% of all congenital abnormalities no clear cause can be established. This applies to many relatively common conditions such as isolated diaphragmatic hernia, tracheo-oesophageal fistula, anal atresia and single limb reduction defects. For an isolated limb defect, such as absence of a hand, it is reasonable to postulate that loss of vascular supply at a critical time during the development of the limb bud leads to developmental arrest with formation of only vestigial digits. It is much more difficult to envisage how vascular occlusion could result in an abnormality such as oesophageal atresia with an associated tracheo-oesophageal fistula.

While it is obviously frustrating for the parents of a child with one of these abnormalities that no factual explanation can be given, they can at least be reassured that the empiric risk of recurrence for siblings is very low. It is worth noting that this does not necessarily mean that genetic factors are irrelevant. Some 'unexplained' malformations and syndromes could well be due to new dominant mutations (p. 100), submicroscopic micro-deletions (p. 253) or uniparental disomy (p. 108).

All of these would convey negligible recurrence risks to future siblings, although those cases due to new mutations or microdeletions would be associated with a significant risk to offspring of affected individuals. There is optimism that molecular techniques will provide at least some of the answers to these many unresolved issues.

FURTHER READING

Aase J 1990 Diagnostic dysmorphology. Plenum, London
A detailed text of the art and science of dysmorphology.
Graham J M 1988 Smith's recognizable patterns of human deformation, 2nd edn. Saunders, Philadelphia
An illustrated guide to human deformations and how they are caused.
Hanson J W 1997 Human teratology. In: Rimoin D L, Connor J M, Pyeritz R E (eds) Principles and practice of medical genetics, 3rd edn. Churchill Livingstone, New York, pp. 697–724
A comprehensive balanced overview of known and suspected human teratogens.
Jones K L 1996 Smith's recognizable patterns of human malformation, 5th edn. Saunders, Philadelphia
The standard paediatric textbook guide to syndromes.
Smithells R W, Newman C G H 1992 Recognition of thalidomide defects. J Med Genet 29: 716–723
A comprehensive account of the spectrum of abnormalities caused by thalidomide.
Spranger J, Benirschke K, Hall J G et al 1982 Errors of morphogenesis: concepts and terms. Recommendations of an international working group. J Pediatr 100: 160–165
A short paper providing a classification and clarification of the terms used in describing birth defects.
Stevenson R E, Hall J G, Goodman R M 1993 Human malformations and related anomalies. Oxford University Press, New York
The definitive guide, in two volumes, to human malformations.

ELEMENTS

1 Congenital abnormalities are apparent at birth in 1 in 40 of all newborn infants. They account for 20–25% of all deaths occurring in the perinatal period and in childhood up to the age of 10 years.

2 A single abnormality can be classified as a malformation, a deformation, a dysplasia or a disruption. Multiple abnormalties can be classified as a sequence, a syndrome or an association.

3 Congenital abnormalities can be caused by chromosome imbalance, single gene defects, multifactorial inheritance or non-genetic factors. Most isolated malformations, including isolated congenital heart defects and neural tube defects, show multifactorial inheritance, whereas most dysplasias have a single gene aetiology.

4 Many congenital malformations, including cleft lip/palate, congenital heart defects and neural tube defects, show aetiological heterogeneity, so that when counselling it is important to establish whether these malformations are isolated or are associated with other abnormalities.

5 Many environmental agents have been shown to have a teratogenic effect and, if at all possible, great care should be taken to avoid exposure to these agents during pregnancy.

CLINICAL GENETICS

Genetic counselling

Any couple who have had a child with a serious abnormality must inevitably reflect on why this has happened and whether any child(ren) they choose to have in future could be similarly affected. Similarly, individuals who have a family history of a serious disorder are likely to be concerned that they could either develop the disorder or transmit it to future generations.

Realization of the needs of such individuals and couples together with awareness of the importance of providing them with accurate and appropriate information has led to the widespread introduction of genetic counselling clinics in parallel with the establishment of clinical genetics as a recognized medical specialty.

DEFINITION

Since the first introduction of genetic counselling services approximately 40 years ago many attempts have been made to devise a satisfactory and all-embracing definition. A theme common to all is the concept of genetic counselling being a process of communication and education which addresses concerns relating to the development and/or transmission of a hereditary disorder.

An individual who seeks genetic counselling is known as a *consultand*. During the genetic counselling process it is widely agreed that the counsellor should try to ensure that the consultand is provided with information which enables him or her to understand:

1. The medical diagnosis and its implications in terms of prognosis and possible treatment.
2. The mode of inheritance of the disorder and the risk of developing and/or transmitting it.
3. The choices or options available for dealing with the risks.

It is also agreed that genetic counselling should include a strong communicative and supportive element, so that those who seek information are able to reach their own fully informed decisions without undue pressure or stress (Table 16.1).

ESTABLISHING THE DIAGNOSIS

The most crucial step in any genetic consultation is that of establishing the diagnosis. If this is incorrect, then inappropriate and totally misleading information could be given with potentially tragic consequences.

Reaching a diagnosis in clinical genetics usually involves the three fundamental steps of any medical consultation, i.e. taking a history, carrying out an examination and undertaking appropriate investigations. Often information about the consultand's family history will have been obtained by a skilled genetics nurse or counsellor as part of a preclinic home visit. Further information about the consultand's family and personal medical history often emerges at the clinic visit, when a full examination can be undertaken and appropriate investigations initiated. These can include chromosome and molecular studies as well as referral on to specialists in other fields such as neurology and ophthalmology.

It cannot be overemphasized that genetic counselling should only be undertaken when facilities exist to ensure that an accurate diagnosis can be made.

Even when a firm diagnosis has been made, problems can arise if the disorder in question shows aetiological heterogeneity. Common examples include hearing loss and non-specific mental retardation, both of which can be caused by either environmental or genetic factors. In these situations empiric risks can be used (p. 300) although these are not as satisfactory as risks based on a precise and specific diagnosis.

A disorder is said to show genetic *heterogeneity* if it can be caused by more than one genetic mechanism (p. 101).

Table 16.1   Steps in genetic counselling

Diagnosis — based on history, examination and investigations
Risk assessment
Communication
Discussion of options
Long-term contact and support

Many such disorders are recognized and counselling can be extremely difficult if the heterogeneity extends to different modes of inheritance. Commonly encountered examples include the various forms of Ehlers–Danlos syndrome (Fig. 16.1), Charcot–Marie–Tooth disease (p. 271) and retinitis pigmentosa, all of which can show autosomal dominant, autosomal recessive and sex-linked recessive inheritance (Table 16.2). Fortunately, progress in molecular genetics is providing solutions to some of these problems. For example, mutations in the gene which codes for rhodopsin, a retinal pigment protein, are found in approximately 30% of families showing autosomal dominant inheritance of retinitis pigmentosa (Fig. 16.2) and the molecular basis of the most common forms of Charcot–Marie–Tooth disease, also known as hereditary motor and sensory neuropathy (HMSN), is now understood (ch.18).

CALCULATING AND PRESENTING THE RISK

In some counselling situations, calculation of the recurrence risk is relatively straightforward and requires little more than a reasonable knowledge of Mendelian inheritance. However, many factors such as delayed age of onset, reduced penetrance and the use of linked DNA markers can result in the calculation becoming much more complex. The theoretical aspects of risk calculation are considered in more detail in Chapter 20.

The provision of a recurrence risk does not simply involve conveying a stark risk figure in isolation. It is very important that information which is provided is understood and that parents are given as much background information as possible to help them reach their own decision. As a working rule of thumb, recurrence risks should be quantified, qualified and placed in context.

QUANTIFICATION — THE NUMERICAL VALUE OF A RISK

Most prospective parents will be familiar to some degree with the concept of risks, but not everyone is comfortable with probability theory and the alternative ways of expressing risk, such as in the form of odds or as a percentage. Thus, for example, a risk of 1 in 4 can be presented as an odds ratio of 3 to 1 against or numerically as 25%. Consistency and clarity are important if confusion is to be avoided. It is also essential to emphasize that a

Table 16.2 Hereditary disorders which can show different patterns of inheritance

Disorder	Inheritance patterns
Cerebellar ataxia	AD, AR
Charcot–Marie–Tooth disease (HMSN)	AD, AR, XR
Congenital cataract	AD, AR, XR
Ehlers–Danlos syndrome	AD, AR, XR
Ichthyosis	AD, AR, XR
Microcephaly	AD, AR
Polycystic kidney disease	AD, AR
Retinitis pigmentosa	AD, AR, XR, M
Sensorineural hearing loss	AD, AR, XR, M

AD = autosomal dominant; AR = autosomal recessive;
XR = sex-linked recessive; M = mitochondrial.

Fig. 16.1
Child with one of the Ehlers–Danlos syndromes showing hyperextensible skin of the face.

Fig. 16.2
Fundus showing typical pigmentary changes of retinitis pigmentosa.

risk applies to **each** pregnancy and that chance does not have a memory. For example the fact that parents have just had a child with an autosomal recessive disorder (recurrence risk equals 1 in 4) does not mean that their next three children will be unaffected. A useful analogy is that of the tossed coin which cannot be expected to remember whether it landed heads or tails at the last throw and cannot therefore be expected to know what it should do at the next throw.

It is also important that genetic counsellors should not be seen exclusively as prophets of doom. Continuing the penny analogy, the good side of the coin should also be emphasized, particularly if the odds strongly favour a successful outcome. For example a couple faced with a probability of 1 in 25 that their next baby will have a neural tube defect should be reminded that there are 24 chances out of 25 that their next baby will **not** be affected.

QUALIFICATION — THE NATURE OF A RISK

Several studies have indicated that the factor which most influences parents when deciding whether or not to have another child is the nature of the long term burden associated with a risk rather than its precise numerical value. Therefore a 'high' risk of 1 in 2 for a trivial problem such as an extra digit (polydactyly) will deter very few parents. In contrast a 'low' risk of 1 in 25 for a disabling condition such as a neural tube defect can have a very significant deterrent effect. Other factors, such as whether a condition can be successfully treated, whether it is associated with pain and suffering, and whether prenatal diagnosis is available, will all be relevant to the decision-making process.

PLACING RISKS IN CONTEXT

Prospective parents seen at a genetic counselling clinic should be provided with information which enables them to put their risks in context so as to be able to decide for themselves whether a risk is 'high' or 'low'. For example, it can be helpful to point out that approximately 1 in 40 of all babies has a congenital malformation or handicapping disorder. Therefore an additional quoted risk of 1 in 50, while initially alarming, might on reflection be perceived as relatively low. As an arbitrary guide, risks of 1 in 10 or greater tend to be regarded as high, 1 in 20 or less as low, and intermediate values as moderate.

DISCUSSING THE OPTIONS

Having established the diagnosis and discussed the risk of occurrence/recurrence, the counsellor is then obliged to ensure that the consultands are provided with all of the information necessary for them to make their own informed decisions. This should include details of all the choices open to them. For example, if relevant, the availability of prenatal diagnosis should be discussed, together with details of the techniques, limitations and risks associated with the various methods employed (ch. 21). Mention will sometimes be made of other reproductive options. These can include alternative approaches to conception such as artificial insemination using donor sperm (AID), the use of donor ova and preimplantation genetic diagnosis (p. 306). These techniques can be used when one partner is infertile, as in the case of Klinefelter's syndrome and Turner's syndrome (ch. 17), or simply to obviate the possibility that one or other partner will transmit his or her disadvantageous gene(s) to the baby.

These are issues which should be broached with great care and sensitivity. For some couples the prospect of prenatal diagnosis followed by selective termination of pregnancy is unacceptable, whereas others view this as their only means of ensuring that any children they do have will be healthy. Whatever the personal views of the counsellor, the consultands are entitled to knowledge of those prenatal diagnostic procedures which are both technically feasible and legally permissible.

COMMUNICATION AND SUPPORT

The ability to communicate is essential in genetic counselling. Communication is a two-way process. Not only does the counsellor provide information, but he or she also has to be receptive to the fears and aspirations, expressed or unexpressed, of the consultand. A readiness to listen is a key attribute for anyone involved in genetic counselling, as is an ability to present information in a clear, sympathetic and appropriate manner.

Often an individual or couple will be extremely upset when first made aware of a genetic diagnosis. The delivery of potentially distressing information cannot be carried out in isolation. Genetic counsellors need to take into account the complex psychological and emotional factors which can influence the counselling dialogue. The setting should be agreeable, private and quiet with ample time for discussion and questions. When possible, technical terms should be avoided or, if used, fully explained. Questions should be answered openly and honestly, and if information is lacking it is certainly not a fault or sign of weakness to admit that this is so. Most couples respect and recognize the truth, and some parents of children whose condition cannot be diagnosed derive a curious pleasure from knowing that their child appears to be unique and has bamboozled the medical profession (unfortunately this is not particularly difficult!).

Despite all these measures, a counselling session can be so intense and intimidating that the amount and accuracy of information retained on follow-up at a later date can be very limited. For this reason a letter summarizing the topics discussed at a counselling session is usually sent to the family afterwards. In addition, they are often contacted at a later date by a member of the counselling team, either by telephone or by a home visit, thereby providing an opportunity for clarification of any confusing issues and for further questions to be answered.

It would be wrong to simply convey information of a distressing nature without offering an opportunity for further discussion and long-term support. Most genetic counselling centres maintain informal contact with relevant families through a network of genetic associates or nurse specialists who are familiar with the family and their particular circumstances. This is especially valuable for prospective parents who subsequently request specific prenatal diagnostic investigations and for presymptomatic adults who are shown to be at high risk of developing late onset autosomal dominant disorders such as Alzheimer's disease and Huntington's disease (p. 267). Genetic registers (p. 319) provide a very useful means of ensuring that effective contact can be maintained with all such relevant family members.

PATIENT SUPPORT GROUPS

Finally, mention should be made of the widespread network of support groups which now exists. These organizations have usually been established by highly motivated and well-informed parents who can provide enormous support and companionship for parents whose child is newly diagnosed with a particular genetic condition or syndrome. When confronted by a new diagnosis of a rare disorder many families feel very isolated, so that if at all possible they should be given an opportunity to meet with other parents who have shared similar experiences. Referral to an appropriate support group would now be viewed as an essential integral component of the genetic counselling process. As well as providing support and information for families these groups have often been very successful in fostering research.

GENETIC COUNSELLING — DIRECTIVE OR NON-DIRECTIVE?

It has already been emphasized that genetic counselling should be viewed as a communication process which provides information. The ultimate goal is to ensure that an individual or couple can reach their own decisions based on full information about risks and options. There is universal agreement that genetic counselling should be **non-directive** with no attempt being made to steer the consultand along a particular course of action. In the same spirit the genetic counsellor should also strive to be **non-judgemental**, even if a decision is reached which seems ill-advised or is contrary to the counsellor's own beliefs. Thus the role of the genetic counsellor is to facilitate and enhance individual autonomy rather than give advice or recommend a particular course of action.

Genetic counsellors are sometimes asked what they themselves would do if placed in the consultand's position. Generally it is preferable to avoid being drawn into expressing an opinion, opting instead to suggest that the consultand try to imagine how he or she might feel in the future having pursued each of the available options. This approach, sometimes referred to as 'scenario-based decision counselling', provides individuals with an opportunity for careful reflection. This is particularly important if one of the options under consideration involves a potentially irreversible reproductive decision such as sterilization. There is a well-established maxim that it is the consultands and not the counsellors who have to live with the consequences of their decisions.

OUTCOMES IN GENETIC COUNSELLING

The issue of defining outcomes in genetic counselling is difficult, topical and contentious. The difficulty arises because of the rather nebulous nature of genetic counselling, which in contrast to most medical activities does not have any easily quantified end points, such as rate of infection or survival after surgery. The issue is topical because of the increasing pressure being applied by funding authorities with emphasis on demonstrable quality and effectiveness.

Finally the issue is contentious because it raises serious questions about the purpose of genetic counselling and whether this should be viewed as simply the provision of information or whether there should be identified benefits for society in terms of a reduction in the incidence of genetic disease.

In practice the three main outcome measures which have been assessed are recall, impact on subsequent reproductive behaviour and patient satisfaction. Most studies have shown that the majority of individuals who have attended a genetic counselling clinic have a reasonable recall of the information given, particularly if this was reinforced by a personal letter or follow-up visit. Nevertheless, confusion can arise and as many as 30% of counsellees have difficulty in remembering a precise risk figure. Studies which have focused on the subsequent reproductive behaviour of couples who have attended a genetic counselling clinic have shown that approximately 50% have been influenced to some extent. Those factors which have been shown to be influential are the severity of the disorder, the desire of the parents to have children and whether prenatal diagnosis and/or treatment are available. Finally studies which have attempted to assess patient satisfaction have struggled to address the problem of how this should best be defined. For example, an individual could be very satisfied with the way in which they were counselled but remain very dissatisfied by lack of a precise diagnosis or availability of subsequent prenatal diagnostic tests.

In an increasingly cost-conscious society it is not surprising that the purchasers of health care, whether privately or state funded, are keen to identify quantifiable targets with which they can assess the 'effectiveness' of genetics services and genetic counselling in particular. Outcomes such as the number of abnormal pregnancies terminated or individuals screened can seem attractive to administrators and politicians who are preoccupied with balancing budgets and cost–benefit analyses. In contrast clinical geneticists and non-medical counsellor colleagues universally reject the use of these outcome criteria on the grounds that they hint at a eugenics philosophy which is totally unacceptable in a society in which individual choice is paramount. Instead they emphasize the benefits of an educated informed community with enhanced individual autonomy. The goals of satisfaction as expressed by the users of genetic services and their ability to make informed decisions are seen as much more acceptable than a reduction in the financial and personal burdens caused by genetic disease.

In the future it is likely that an outcome measure such as 'perceived personal control' will be developed. This will almost certainly incorporate both information and satisfaction criteria, together with an assessment of whether individuals have been able to understand the information and come to terms with their situation, thereby enabling them to make appropriate life decisions with which they are comfortable.

SPECIAL PROBLEMS IN GENETIC COUNSELLING

There are a number of special problems which can arise in genetic counselling.

CONSANGUINITY

A consanguineous relationship is one between blood relatives who have at least one common ancestor no more remote than a great-great grandparent. Consanguineous marriage is widespread in many parts of the world (Table 16.3). In Arab populations the most common type of consanguineous marriage occurs between first cousins who are the children of two brothers, whereas in the Indian subcontinent uncle–niece marriages are the most commonly encountered form of consanguineous relationship. While there is in these communities some recognition of the potential disadvantageous genetic effects of consanguinity, there is also a strongly held view that these are greatly outweighed by social advantages such as greater family and marital stability.

Many studies have shown that among the offspring of consanguineous marriages there is an increased incidence of both congenital malformations and other conditions which will present later, such as hearing loss and mental retardation. For the offspring of first cousins the incidence of congenital malformations is increased to approximately $2\frac{1}{2}$ times that which is seen in the offspring of unrelated parents. Almost all of this increase in morbidity and

Table 16.3 Worldwide incidence of consanguineous marriage

Country	Incidence (%)
Kuwait	54
Saudi Arabia	54
Jordan	50
Pakistan	40–50
India	5–60
Syria	33
Egypt	28
Lebanon	25
Algeria	23
Japan	2–4
France, UK, USA	2

Data adapted from various sources including Jaber L, Halpern G J, Shohat M 1998 The impact of consanguinity worldwide. Community Genet 1: 12–17.

mortality is attributed to homozygosity for autosomal recessive disorders, a finding consistent with Garrod's original observation that 'the mating of first cousins gives exactly the conditions most likely to enable a rare, and usually recessive, character to show itself' (p. 100).

On the basis of studies of children born to consanguineous parents it has been estimated that the average human carries between 1 and 2 genes for a harmful autosomal recessive disorder, together with several mutations for conditions which result in lethality before birth. Most prospective consanguineous parents are concerned primarily with the risk that they will have a handicapped child and fortunately the overall risks are usually relatively small. When estimating a risk for a particular consanguineous relationship it is generally assumed that each common ancestor carried one deleterious recessive mutation.

Therefore, for first cousins, the probability that their first child will be homozygous for their common grandfather's deleterious gene will be 1 in 64 (Fig. 16.3). Similarly, the risk that this child will be homozygous for the common grandmother's recessive gene will also be 1 in 64. This gives a total probability that the child will be homozygous for one of the grandparent's deleterious genes of 1 in 32. This risk should be added to the general population risk of 1 in 40 that any baby will have a major congenital abnormality (p. 225), to give an overall risk of approximately 1 in 20 that a child born to first cousin parents will be either malformed or handicapped in some way.

Risks arising from consanguinity for more distant relatives are much lower.

For consanguineous marriages there is also a slightly increased risk that a child will have a multifactorial disorder. In practice this risk is usually very small. In contrast a close family history of an autosomal recessive disorder can convey a relatively high risk that a consanguineous couple will have an affected child. For example, if the sibling of someone with an autosomal recessive disorder marries a first cousin, the risk that their first baby will be affected equals 1 in 24 (p. 293).

INCEST

Incestuous relationships are those which occur between first-degree relatives (in other words, brother/sister or parent/child — see Table 16.4). Marriage between first-degree relatives is forbidden, both on religious grounds and by legislation in almost every culture. Incestuous relationships are associated with a very high risk of abnormality in offspring, with less than half the children of such unions being entirely healthy (Table 16.5).

ADOPTION AND GENETIC DISORDERS

The issue of adoption can arise in several situations relating to genetics. Firstly, parents at high risk of having a child

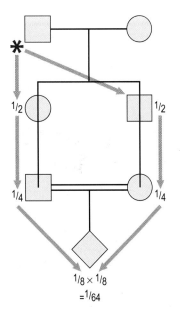

Fig. 16.3
Shows the probability that the first child of first cousins will be homozygous for the deleterious allele (*) carried by the common great-grandfather. A similar risk of 1 in 64 will apply to the deleterious allele belonging to the common great-grandmother, giving a total risk of 1 in 32.

Table 16.4 Genetic relationship between relatives and risk of abnormality in their offspring

Genetic relationship	Proportion of shared genes	Risk of abnormality in offspring (%)
First degree Parent/child Brother/sister	$\frac{1}{2}$	50
Second degree Uncle/niece Aunt/nephew Double first cousins	$\frac{1}{4}$	5–10
Third degree First cousins	$\frac{1}{8}$	3–5

Table 16.5 Frequencies of the three main types of abnormality in the children of incestuous relationships

Abnormality	Frequency (%)
Mental retardation Severe	25
Mild	35
Autosomal recessive disorder	10–15
Congenital malformation	10

with a serious abnormality often express interest in adopting rather than running the risk of having an affected baby. In genetic terms this is a perfectly reasonable option, although in practice the number of couples wishing to adopt usually far exceeds the number of babies and children available for adoption.

The physician with a knowledge of genetics can also be called upon to try to determine whether a child who is being placed for adoption will develop a genetic disorder. For the offspring of consanguineous or incestuous matings, risks can be given as outlined previously (Tables 16.4 and 16.5). Adoption societies sometimes also wish to place a child with a family history of a particular hereditary disorder. This raises the difficult ethical dilemma of predictive testing in childhood for conditions showing onset in adult life (p. 339). Increasingly it is felt that such testing should not be undertaken unless this will be of direct medical benefit to the child. In practice, even when a child is actually affected by a genetic disorder, suitable adoptive parents can usually be found.

Concern about the possible misuse of genetic testing in neonates and young children who are up for adoption has prompted the American Society of Human Genetics and the American College of Medical Genetics to issue joint recommendations. These are based on the best interests of the child. They can be summarized as supporting genetic testing in such children only when the testing would be appropriate for all children of that age and when the tests are undertaken for disorders which manifest during childhood and for which preventive measures can be undertaken during childhood. The joint statement does not support testing for untreatable disorders of adult onset or for detecting predispositions to 'physical, mental or behavioral traits within the normal range'.

DISPUTED PATERNITY

This presents a difficult problem for which the help of a clinical geneticist is sometimes sought. Until recently paternity could never be proved with absolute certainty, although it could be disproved or excluded in two ways. If a child was found to possess a blood group or other polymorphism not present in either the mother or the putative father, then paternity could be confidently excluded. For example, if the mother and putative father both lacked blood group B, but this was present in the child, then the putative father could be excluded. Similarly, if a child lacked a marker which the putative father would have had to transmit to all of his children, then once again paternity could be excluded. As an example, a putative father with blood group AB could not have a child with blood group O.

Until recently attempts to establish paternity were based on analysis of several different polymorphic systems such as blood groups, isoenzymes and HLA haplotypes. The

Fig. 16.4

Genetic fingerprint obtained using two minisatellite probes with DNA from a mother (M), father (F) and their twins (1 and 2). The twins have an identical set of bands and each band in the twins originates from one of the parents. Reproduced with permission from the American Journal of Medical Genetics. (Courtesy of Dr Raymond Dalgleish and Professor Sir Alec Jeffreys, University of Leicester, reproduced from Young I D, Dalgleish R, Mackay E H, MacFadyen U M 1988 Discordant expression of the G syndrome in monozygotic twins. Am J Med Genet 29: 863–869.)

results of these studies can be consistent with paternity but cannot give absolute proof of it. Depending on the number of polymorphic systems analysed and their frequencies in the general population, it is possible to calculate the relative probability that a particular male is the father as compared with any male taken at random from the general population.

The limitations of these approaches have been overcome by the development of genetic fingerprinting using minisatellite repeat sequence probes (p. 16). The pattern of DNA fragments generated by these probes is so highly polymorphic that the restriction map obtained is unique to each individual, with the exception of identical twins (Fig. 16.4). If DNA from the child and the mother is analysed then the bands inherited from the biological father can be analysed and compared with those present in DNA from the putative father(s). If these match, this gives an extremely high mathematical probability that the putative and biological fathers are the same individual.

FURTHER READING

ASHG/ACMG. Statement 2000. Genetic testing in adoption. Am J Hum Genet 66: 761–767
The joint recommendations of the American Society of Human Genetics and the American College of Medical Genetics on genetic testing in young children who are being placed for adoption.

Clarke A (ed) 1994 Genetic counselling. Practice and principles. Routledge, London
A thoughtful and provocative multiauthor text which addresses difficult issues such as predictive testing, screening, prenatal diagnosis and confidentiality.

Clarke A, Parsons E, Williams A 1996 Outcomes and process in genetic counseling. Clin Genet 50: 462–469
A critical review of previous studies of the outcomes of genetic counselling.

Frets P G, Niermeijer M F 1990. Reproductive planning after genetic counselling: a perspective from the last decade. Clin Genet 38: 295–306
A review of studies undertaken between 1980 and 1989 to determine which factors are most important in influencing reproductive decisions.

Harper P S 1998 Practical genetic counselling, 5th edn. Butterworth-Heinemann, Oxford
An extremely useful practical guide to all aspects of genetic counselling.

Jaber L, Halpern G J, Shohat M 1998 The impact of consanguinity worldwide. Community Genet 1: 12–17
A review of the incidence and consequences of consanguinity in various parts of the world.

Jeffreys A J, Brookfield J F Y, Semeonoff R 1985 Positive identification of an immigration test-case using human DNA fingerprints. Nature 317: 818–819
A clever demonstration of the value of genetic fingerprinting in analysing alleged family relationships.

ELEMENTS

1 Genetic counselling may be defined as a communication process which deals with the risk of developing or transmitting a genetic disorder.

2 The most important steps in genetic counselling are the establishment of a diagnosis, estimation of a recurrence risk, communication of relevant information and the provision of long term support.

3 Genetic counselling should be non-directive and the genetic counsellor should be non-judgemental. The goal of genetic counselling is to provide accurate information which enables counsellees to make their own fully informed decisions.

4 Marriage between blood relatives conveys an increased risk for an autosomal recessive disorder in future offspring. The probability that first cousins will have a child with an autosomal recessive condition is approximately 3%, although this risk can be greater if there is a family history of a specific genetic disorder.

5 The most sensitive technique for paternity testing is genetic fingerprinting. Other polymorphic systems can disprove paternity but cannot establish with such a high statistical probability that a particular male is the biological father.

Chromosome disorders

The development of a reliable technique for chromosome analysis in 1956 soon led to the discovery that several previously described conditions were due to an abnormality in chromosome number. Within 3 years the causes of Down's syndrome (47,XX/XY, +21), Klinefelter's syndrome (47,XXY) and Turner's syndrome (45,X) had been established. Shortly afterwards other autosomal trisomy syndromes were recognized and gradually over the ensuing years many other multiple malformation syndromes were described in which there was loss or gain of chromosome material.

To date around 1000 chromosome syndromes have been reported. While on an individual basis most of these are rare, together they make a major contribution to human morbidity and mortality. Chromosome abnormalities account for a large proportion of spontaneous pregnancy loss and childhood disability and also contribute to the genesis of a significant proportion of malignancy in both childhood and adult life as a consequence of acquired somatic chromosome aberrations.

In Chapter 3 the basic principles of chromosome structure and function were described. Details of chromosome behaviour during cell division were also provided along with a theoretical account of the nature of chromosome abnormalities and how these can both arise and be transmitted in families. In this chapter the medical aspects of chromosome abnormalities are considered and specific chromosome abnormality syndromes are described.

INCIDENCE OF CHROMOSOME ABNORMALITIES

Chromosome abnormalities are present in at least 10% of all spermatozoa and 25% of mature oocytes. Between 15% and 20% of all recognized pregnancies end in spontaneous miscarriage and many more zygotes and embryos are so abnormal that survival beyond the first few days or weeks after fertilization is not possible. Approximately 50% of all spontaneous miscarriages have a chromosome abnormality (Table 17.1) and the incidence

of chromosomal abnormalities in morphologically normal embryos is around 20%. These observations indicate that chromosome abnormalities account for the loss of a very high proportion of all human conceptions.

From conception onwards the incidence of chromosome abnormalities falls rapidly. By birth it has declined to a level of 0.5–1%, although the total is much higher (5%) if only stillborn infants are considered. Table 17.2 lists the

Table 17.1 Chromosome abnormalities in spontaneous abortions (percentage figures relate to total of chromosomally abnormal abortuses)

Abnormality		Incidence (%)
Trisomy	13	2
	16	15
	18	3
	21	5
	Other	25
Monosomy X		20
Triploidy		15
Tetraploidy		5
Other		10

Table 17.2 Incidence of chromosome abnormalities in the newborn

Abnormality	Incidence per 10 000 births
Autosomal	
Trisomy 13	2
18	3
21	15
Sex chromosomes	
Female births	
45,X	1–2
47,XXX	10
Male births	
47,XXY	10
47,XYY	10
Other unbalanced rearrangements	10
Balanced rearrangements	30
Total	90

incidence figures for chromosome abnormalities based on newborn surveys. It is notable that among the commonly recognized aneuploidy syndromes there is also a high proportion of spontaneous pregnancy loss (Table 17.3). This is illustrated by comparison of the incidence of conditions such as Down's syndrome at the time of chorionic villus sampling (11–12 weeks), amniocentesis (16 weeks) and term (Fig. 17.1).

DISORDERS OF THE AUTOSOMES

DOWN'S SYNDROME (TRISOMY 21)

This condition derives its name from Dr Langdon Down who first described it in the Clinical Lecture Reports of the London Hospital in 1866. The chromosomal basis of Down's syndrome was not established until 1959 by Lejeune and his colleagues in Paris.

Table 17.3   Spontaneous pregnancy loss in commonly recognized aneuploidy syndromes

Disorder	Proportion undergoing spontaneous pregnancy loss (%)
Trisomy 13	95
Trisomy 18	95
Trisomy 21	80
Monosomy X	98

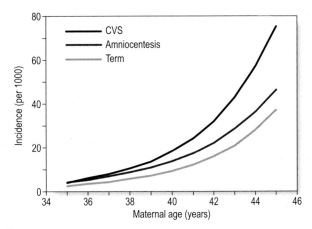

Fig. 17.1
Approximate incidence of trisomy 21 at the time of chorionic villus sampling (CVS) (11–12 weeks), amniocentesis (16 weeks) and delivery. (Data from Hook E B, Cross P K, Jackson L, Pergament E, Brambati B 1988 Maternal age-specific rates of 47, +21 and other cytogenetic abnormalities diagnosed in the first trimester of pregnancy in chorionic villus biopsy specimens. Am J Hum Genet 42: 797–807; and Cuckle H S, Wald N J, Thompson S G 1987 Estimating a woman's risk of having a pregnancy associated with Down's syndrome using her age and serum alpha-fetoprotein level. Br J Obstet Gynaecol 94: 387–402.)

Incidence

The overall incidence, when adjusted for the impact of antenatal screening, is approximately 1 in 650 to 1 in 700. In the United Kingdom approximately 50% of Down's syndrome cases are detected prenatally. There is a strong association between the incidence of Down's syndrome and advancing maternal age (Table 17.4).

Clinical features

These are summarized in Table 17.5. The most common finding in the newborn period is severe hypotonia. Usually the facial characteristics of upward sloping

Table 17.4   Incidence of Down's syndrome in relation to maternal age

Maternal age at delivery (years)	Incidence of Down's syndrome
20	1 in 1500
25	1 in 1350
30	1 in 900
35	1 in 400
36	1 in 300
37	1 in 250
38	1 in 200
39	1 in 150
40	1 in 100
41	1 in 85
42	1 in 65
43	1 in 50
44	1 in 40
45	1 in 30

Adapted from Cuckle H S, Wald N J, Thompson S G 1987 Estimating a woman's risk of having a pregnancy associated with Down's syndrome using her age and serum alpha-fetoprotein level. Br J Obstet Gynaecol 94: 387–402.

Table 17.5   Common findings in Down's syndrome

Newborn period
Hypotonia, sleepy, excess nuchal skin

Craniofacial
Brachycephaly, epicanthic folds, protruding tongue, small ears, upward sloping palpebral fissures

Limbs
Single palmar crease, small middle phalanx of fifth finger, wide gap between first and second toes

Cardiac
Atrial and ventricular septal defect, common atrioventricular canal, patent ductus arteriosus

Other
Anal atresia, duodenal atresia, Hirschsprung's disease, short stature, strabismus

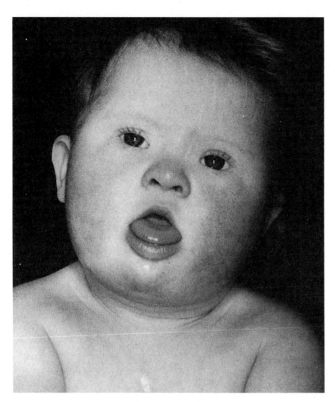

Fig. 17.2
A child with Down's syndrome.

Fig. 17.3
Close-up view of the eyes and nasal bridge of a child with Down's syndrome showing upward sloping palpebral fissures, Brushfield spots and bilateral epicanthic folds.

Fig. 17.4
The hands of an adult with Down's syndrome. Note the single palmar crease in the left hand plus bilateral short curved fifth fingers (clinodactyly).

palpebral fissures, small ears and protruding tongue (Figs 17.2 and 17.3) prompt rapid suspicion of the diagnosis, although this can be delayed in very small or premature babies. Single palmar creases are found in 50% of Down's syndrome children (Fig. 17.4) in contrast to 2–3% of the general population. Congenital cardiac abnormalities are present in 40–45% of babies with Down's syndrome with the three most common lesions being atrioventricular canal defects, ventricular septal defects and patent ductus arteriosus.

Natural history

Affected children show a broad range of intellectual ability with IQ scores ranging from 25 to 75. The average IQ of young adults with Down's syndrome is around 40 to 45. Social skills are relatively well advanced and most children with Down's syndrome are happy and very affectionate. Adult height is usually around 150 cm. In the absence of a severe cardiac anomaly, which leads to early death in 15–20% of cases, average life expectancy is 50–60 years. Most affected adults develop Alzheimer's disease in later life, possibly because of a gene dosage effect as the locus for the amyloid precursor protein gene is on chromosome 21. This gene has been implicated in some familial cases of Alzheimer's disease (p. 223)

Table 17.6 Chromosome abnormalities in Down's syndrome

Abnormality	Frequency (%)
Trisomy	95
Translocation	4
Mosaicism	1

Chromosome findings

These are listed in Table 17.6. In cases resulting from trisomy 21, the additional chromosome is maternal in origin in over 90% of cases, and DNA studies have shown that this arises most commonly as a result of non–disjunction in maternal meiosis I (p. 45). Robertsonian translocations (p. 48) account for approximately 4% of all cases, in roughly one–third of which one of the parents is found to be a carrier of the translocation. Children with mosaicism are often less severely affected than in the full syndrome.

Efforts have been made to correlate the various clinical features in Down's syndrome with trisomy for specific regions of chromosome 21, by studying children with partial trisomy for different regions. There is some support for a Down's syndrome 'critical region' at the distal end of the long arm (21q22) as children with trisomy for this region usually have typical Down's syndrome facial features. Chromosome 21 is a 'gene poor' chromosome with a high ratio of AT to GC sequences (p. 37). At present the only reasonably well-established genotype–phenotype correlation in trisomy 21 is the high incidence of Alzheimer's disease which is attributed to an amyloid precursor protein gene dosage effect.

Recurrence risk

For straightforward trisomy 21 the recurrence risk is related to maternal age and is usually of the order of $\frac{1}{200}$ to $\frac{1}{100}$. In translocation cases similar figures apply if neither parent is a carrier. In familial translocation cases, the recurrence risks vary from around 1–3% for male carriers up to 10–15% for female carriers, with the exception of very rare carriers of a 21q21q translocation for whom the recurrence risk is 100% (p. 49).

Prenatal diagnosis can be offered based on analysis of chorionic villi or cultured amniotic cells. Prenatal screening programmes have been introduced based on the so-called 'triple' or 'quadruple' tests of maternal serum at 16 weeks' gestation (p. 314).

PATAU'S SYNDROME (TRISOMY 13) AND EDWARDS' SYNDROME (TRISOMY 18)

These very severe conditions were first described in 1960 and share many features in common (Figs 17.5 and 17.6). They both show incidence figures of approximately 1 in 5000 and convey a very poor prognosis with most affected infants dying during the first few weeks of life. In the unusual event of long-term survival there is severe mental retardation. Cardiac abnormalities occur in at least 90% of all cases.

Usually chromosome analysis reveals straightforward trisomy. Both of these disorders show an association

Fig. 17.6
A baby with trisomy 18. Note the prominent occiput and tightly clenched hands.

Fig. 17.5
Facial view of a child with trisomy 13 showing severe bilateral cleft lip and palate.

between increasing incidence and advanced maternal age, and in both the additional chromosome is usually of maternal origin (Table 3.4, p. 44). Approximately 10% of cases are caused by mosaicism or unbalanced rearrangements, particularly Robertsonian translocations in cases of Patau's syndrome.

CHROMOSOME DELETION SYNDROMES

Microscopically visible deletions of the terminal portions of chromosomes 4 and 5 cause the Wolf–Hirschhorn (4p–) (Fig. 17.7) and Cri du chat (5p–) (Fig. 17.8) syndromes respectively. In both conditions there is severe mental retardation, often in association with failure to thrive. The Cri du chat syndrome derives its name from the characteristic cat-like cry of affected neonates which results from underdevelopment of the larynx. Both conditions are very rare with estimated incidences of approximately 1 in 50 000 births. In some children with clinical features of one of these syndromes but apparently normal chromosomes, the presence of a very subtle deletion can be demonstrated by FISH (p. 34) using locus-specific probes for 4p or 5p (Fig. 17.9).

MICRODELETION SYNDROMES

Through a combination of high resolution prometaphase banding (p. 32) and FISH (p. 34), several previously unexplained syndromes have been shown to be due to

Fig. 17.8
Facial view of a 2-year-old boy with the Cri du chat syndrome.

Fig. 17.9
FISH showing failure of a chromosome 4p locus specific probe (red) to hybridize to one number 4 chromosome in a child with the Wolf–Hirschhorn syndrome. The yellow probe acts as a marker for the centromere of each number 4 chromosome. (Courtesy of Nigel Smith, City Hospital, Nottingham.)

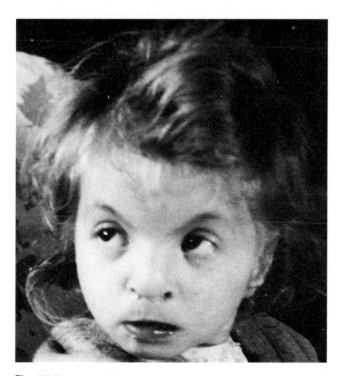

Fig. 17.7
Facial view of a 3-year-old child with the Wolf–Hirschhorn syndrome.

submicroscopic or 'micro-'deletions. Some of these *microdeletions* involve loss of only a few genes at closely adjacent loci, resulting in what are known as *contiguous gene syndromes*. For example, several boys with Duchenne muscular dystrophy (DMD) have been described who also have other X-linked disorders such as retinitis pigmentosa and glycerol kinase deficiency (p. 74). The loci for these disorders are known to be very close to the DMD locus on Xp21.

In several other microdeletion syndromes it is likely that more than a few loci are involved. Examples are given in Table 17.7. Even when considered together these conditions are rare, but improvements in molecular technology will probably reveal that microdeletion syndromes, and possibly microduplication syndromes also, are more common than is realized. Many malformations and syndromes have been described for which there is as yet no recognized cause (p. 236).

Lessons from microdeletion syndromes

Retinoblastoma

The first clue to the location of the gene for retinoblastoma was provided by the discovery that approximately 5% of children presenting with the condition had other abnormalities including mental retardation. In several of these children a constitutional interstitial deletion of a region of the long arm of chromosome 13 was identified. The smallest region of overlap was 13q14 which was subsequently shown to be the position of the locus for the autosomal dominant form of retinoblastoma. This in turn led to the cloning of the gene and identification of the gene product (pp. 195, 197).

Wilms' tumour

A proportion of children who develop the rare renal embryonal neoplasm known as Wilms' tumour (or

hypernephroma) also have Aniridia (= absent iris, see Fig. 5.4, p. 85), Genitourinary abnormalities and Retardation of growth and development. This combination of findings is referred to as the WAGR syndrome. Chromosome analysis in these children reveals an interstitial deletion of chromosome 11p13 (Fig. 17.10). Molecular studies have identified several genes within this deletion. Loss of one of these, *PAX6*, is responsible for the aniridia (Fig. 17.11). Loss of another, known as *WT1*, causes the development of Wilms' tumour. This knowledge can now be used to predict whether a newly diagnosed child with an 11p13 deletion is at high risk of developing a Wilms' tumour. This is achieved by FISH using *WT1* as a locus specific probe. Failure of *WT1* to hybridize to the deletion site indicates that the risk for developing Wilms' tumour is high (Fig. 17.12).

It is important to note that in contrast to retinoblastoma the genetic aspects of Wilms' tumour have proved to be extremely complicated with several different autosomal loci involved. Nevertheless these discoveries based on the study of microdeletion syndromes have proved to be extremely valuable in leading to the isolation of genes which cause these two embryonal tumours.

Angelman and Prader–Willi syndromes

Recent developments in these disorders have generated particular interest. Children with Angelman's syndrome (Fig. 6.20, p. 110) show inappropriate laughter with

Table 17.7 **Microdeletion syndromes**	
Syndrome	**Chromosome**
Williams	7
Langer–Giedion	8
WAGR*	11
Anglelman	15
Prader–Willi	15
Rubinstein–Taybi	16
Miller–Dieker	17
Smith–Magennis	17
DiGeorge/Shprintzen	22

*WAGR = Wilms' tumour, Aniridia, Genitourinary malformations and Retardation of growth and development.

Fig. 17.10
Metaphase spread showing the number 11 chromosomes (arrowed). The chromosome indicated by the single arrow has an interstitial deletion in the short arm. See Figs 17.11 and 17.12. (Courtesy of Meg Heath, City Hospital, Nottingham.)

Fig. 17.11
FISH showing failure of a *PAX6* locus specific probe (red) to hybridize to the deleted number 11 chromosome shown in Figure 17.10 from a child with WAGR syndrome. The green probe acts as a marker for the centromere of each number 11 chromosome. (Courtesy of Dr John Crolla, Salisbury and Dr Veronica van Heyningen, Edinburgh.)

Fig. 17.12
FISH showing failure of a *WT1* locus specific probe (red) to hybridize to the deleted number 11 chromosome shown in Figure 17.10 from a child with WAGR syndrome. The green probe acts as a marker for the centromere of each number 11 chromosome. (Courtesy of Dr John Crolla, Salisbury and Dr Veronica van Heyningen, Edinburgh.)

convulsions, poor coordination (ataxia) and mental retardation. Children with the Prader–Willi syndrome (Fig. 6.19, p. 109) are extremely floppy (hypotonic) in early infancy and develop quite marked obesity with mild to moderate mental retardation in later years. A large proportion of children with these disorders have a microdeletion involving the proximal part of the long arm of chromosome 15q (15q11–12).

It is now known that if the deletion occurs de novo on the paternally inherited number 15 chromosome the child will have the Prader–Willi syndrome. In contrast, a deletion occurring at the same region on the maternally inherited number 15 chromosome causes Angelman's syndrome. Non-deletion cases also exist and are often due to uniparental disomy (p. 108), with both number 15 chromosomes being paternal in origin in Angelman's syndrome and maternal in origin in the Prader–Willi syndrome. Thus loss of a critical region from a paternal number 15 chromosome causes the Prader–Willi syndrome. Loss of an identical or similar region from a maternally inherited number 15 chromosome causes Angelman's syndrome. These observations are fundamental to the concept of imprinting (p. 109) and illustrate how new technological developments coupled with clinical observation have helped identify new underlying genetic mechanisms.

DiGeorge and Shprintzen syndromes

The DiGeorge syndrome is a rare disorder, usually occurring sporadically, characterized by a high incidence of heart malformations, particularly those involving the cardiac outflow tract, along with thymic and parathyroid hypoplasia (p. 185). Molecular and FISH studies have shown that most if not all cases are due to a micro-deletion involving the proximal long arm of chromosome 22 (22q11–2).

Curiously, it has emerged that most children and adults with what was thought to be a separate syndrome known as Shprintzen's syndrome show a similar defect. This condition is characterized by similar cardiac malformations, cleft palate and a recognizable facial appearance (Fig. 17.13). Several families showing apparent autosomal dominant inheritance have been described. It is possible that in Shprintzen's syndrome there is a smaller deletion which does not convey such a high risk for a life-threatening malformation, although variation in severity within families has been noted.

Perhaps even more curiously it has emerged that some families showing apparent clustering of isolated cardiac malformations, previously believed to be multifactorial in origin, are also segregating a 22q microdeletion. This was one of the first demonstrations of an important dominantly inherited susceptibility locus in an apparent multifactorial disorder.

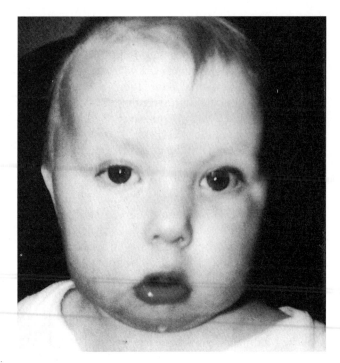

Fig. 17.13
Facial view of a child with the DiGeorge/Shprintzen syndrome with a deletion of one number 22 chromosome.

TRIPLOIDY

Triploidy (69,XXX, 69,XXY, 69,XYY) is a relatively common finding in material cultured from spontaneous abortions, but is seen only rarely in a liveborn infant. Such a child will almost always show severe intra-uterine growth retardation with relative preservation of head growth at the expense of a small thin trunk. Syndactyly involving the third and fourth fingers and/or the second and third toes is a common finding. Cases of triploidy due to a double paternal contribution usually miscarry in early to mid-pregnancy and are associated with partial hydatidiform changes in the placenta (p. 90). Cases with a double maternal contribution survive for longer but rarely beyond the early neonatal period.

Hypomelanosis of Ito

Several children with mosaicism for diploidy/triploidy have been identified. These can demonstrate the clinical picture seen in full triploidy but in a milder form. An alternative presentation is as the condition known as hypomelanosis of Ito. In this curious disorder the skin shows alternating patterns of normally pigmented and depigmented streaks which correspond to the embryological developmental lines of the skin known as Blaschko's lines (Fig. 17.14). Most children with hypomelanosis of Ito are moderately retarded and have convulsions which can be particularly difficult to treat. There is increasing evidence that this clinical picture represents a non-specific embryological response to cell or tissue mosaicism. A similar pattern of skin pigmentation is sometimes seen in women with one of the rare X-linked dominant disorders (p. 104) with skin involvement, such as incontinentia pigmenti. Such women can be considered as being mosaic, as some cells will be expressing the normal gene whereas others will be expressing only the mutant gene.

DISORDERS OF THE SEX CHROMOSOMES

KLINEFELTER'S SYNDROME (47,XXY)

First described in 1942, this relatively common condition with an incidence of 1 in 1000 male live births, was shown to be due to the presence of an additional X chromosome in 1959.

Clinical features

In childhood the diagnosis can be suspected in a male presenting with clumsiness or mild learning difficulties, particularly in relation to verbal skills. The overall verbal IQ is reduced by 10–20 points below that of unaffected siblings and controls. Adults with Klinefelter's syndrome tend to be slightly taller than average with long lower limbs. Approximately 30% of adult males with Klinefelter's

Fig. 17.14
Mosaic pattern of skin pigmentation on the arm of a child with hypomelanosis of Ito. (Reproduced with permission from Jenkins D, Martin K, Young I D 1993 Hypomelanosis of Ito associated with mosaicism for trisomy 7 and apparent 'pseudomosaicism' at amniocentesis. J Med Genet 30: 783–784.)

syndrome show moderately severe gynaecomastia (enlargement of the breasts) and all are infertile with small soft testes. There is an increased incidence of leg ulcers, osteoporosis and carcinoma of the breast in adult life. Treatment with testosterone from puberty onwards is beneficial for the development of secondary sexual characteristics and the long-term prevention of osteoporosis. Males with Klinefelter's syndrome are usually infertile due to the absence of sperm in their semen (*azoospermia*), although fertility has been achieved for a small number of affected males using the technique known as ICSI (*intra-cytoplasmic sperm injection*).

Chromosome findings

Usually the karyotype shows an additional X chromosome. Molecular studies have shown that there is a roughly equal chance that this will have been inherited from the mother or from the father. The maternally derived cases are associated with advancing maternal age. A small proportion of cases show mosaicism, i.e. 46,XY/47,XXY. Rarely, a male with more than two X chromosomes can be encountered, e.g. 48,XXXY or 49,XXXXY. These individuals are usually quite severely retarded.

TURNER'S SYNDROME (45,X)

This condition was first described in 1938. The absence of a Barr body, consistent with the presence of only one X chromosome, was noted in 1954 and cytogenetic confirmation was forthcoming in 1959. While common at conception and in spontaneous abortions (Table 17.1),

the incidence in liveborn female infants is low, with estimates ranging from 1 in 5000 to 1 in 10 000.

Clinical features

Presentation can be at any time from pregnancy to adult life. Increasingly Turner's syndrome is being detected during the second trimester as a result of routine detailed ultrasound scanning which can reveal either generalized oedema (hydrops) or swelling localized to the neck (nuchal cyst or thickened nuchal pad) (Fig. 17.15). At birth many babies with Turner's syndrome look entirely normal. Others show the residue of intra-uterine oedema with puffy extremities (Fig. 17.16) and neck webbing. Other findings can include a low posterior hair-line, increased carrying angles at the elbows, short fourth metacarpals, widely spaced nipples and coarctation of the aorta which is present in 15% of cases.

Intelligence in Turner's syndrome is normal. The two main medical problems are short stature and ovarian failure. The short stature becomes apparent by mid-childhood, and without growth hormone treatment the average adult height is 145 cm. This short stature is due, at least in part, to haploinsufficiency for the *SHOX* gene

Fig. 17.16
The foot of an infant with Turner's syndrome showing oedema and small nails.

Fig. 17.15
Ultrasound scan at 18 weeks' gestation showing hydrops fetalis. Note the halo of fluid surrounding the fetus. (Courtesy of Dr D Rose, City Hospital, Nottingham.)

which is located in the pseudoautosomal region (p. 105). Ovarian failure commences during the second half of intra-uterine life and almost invariably leads to primary amenorrhoea and infertility. Oestrogen replacement therapy should be initiated at adolescence for development of secondary sexual characteristics and long-term prevention of osteoporosis. In vitro fertilization using donor eggs offers the prospect of pregnancy for women with Turner's syndrome.

Chromosome findings

These are summarized in Table 17.8. The most common finding is 45,X, sometimes erroneously referred to as 45,XO. It has been shown that Turner's syndrome arises in 80% of instances through a sex chromosome (X or Y) being lost in paternal meiosis.

XXX FEMALES

Birth surveys have shown that approximately 0.1% of all females have a 47,XXX karyotype. These women usually have no physical abnormalities but can show a mild reduction of between 10 and 20 points in intellectual skills. This is rarely of sufficient severity to require special education. Studies have shown that the additional X chromosome is of maternal origin in 95% of cases and usually arises from an error in meiosis I. Women with a 47,XXX karyotype usually show normal fertility and have children with normal karyotypes.

As with males who have more than two X chromosomes, women with more than three X chromosomes show a high incidence of mental retardation, the severity of which is directly related to the number of X chromosomes present.

XYY MALES

This condition shows an incidence of 1 in 1000 in males in newborn surveys but is found in 2–3% of males who are in institutions because of mental retardation or antisocial criminal behaviour. However, it is important to stress that most 47,XYY men are neither mentally retarded nor in possession of a criminal record, although they can show emotional immaturity and impulsive behaviour.

Physical appearance is normal and stature is usually above average. Intelligence is mildly impaired with an overall IQ score of 10–20 points below a control sample. The additional Y chromosome must arise as a result of non-disjunction in paternal meiosis II or as a post-zygotic event.

THE FRAGILE X SYNDROME

This condition, which could equally well be classified as a single gene disorder rather than a chromosome abnormality, has the unique distinction of being both the most common inherited cause of mental retardation and the first disorder in which a dynamic mutation was identified (p. 22). First described in 1969, the significance of the chromosome abnormality was not really fully realized until 1977 and it was only in 1991 that the underlying molecular defect was discovered.

Incidence

The Fragile X syndrome affects approximately 1 in 2000 males and accounts for 4–8% of all males with mental retardation.

Clinical features

Older boys and adult males usually have a recognizable facial appearance with high forehead, large ears, long face and prominent jaw (Fig. 17.17). After puberty most affected males have large testes (macro-orchidism). There can also be evidence of connective tissue weakness with hyperextensible joints, stretch marks on the skin (striae) and mitral valve prolapse. The mental retardation is moderate to severe and many affected boys show autistic features and/or hyperactive behaviour. Speech tends to be halting and repetitive. Female carriers can show some of the facial features and approximately 50% of women with the full mutation show mild to moderate retardation.

The Fragile X chromosome

The Fragile X syndrome takes its name from the appearance of the X chromosome which shows a *fragile site* close to the telomere at the end of the long arm at Xq27.3 (Fig. 17.18). A fragile site is a non-staining gap usually involving both chromatids at a point at which the chromosome is liable to break. In this condition, detection of the fragile site involves the use of special culture techniques such as folate or thymidine depletion, which

Table 17.8 Chromosome findings in Turner's syndrome	
Karyotype	Frequency (%)
Monosomy X — 45,X	50
Mosaicism — e.g. 45,X/46,XX	20
Isochromosome — 46,X,i(Xq)	15
Ring — 46,X,r(X)	5
Deletion — 46,X,del(Xp)	5
Other	5

Fig. 17.17
Facial view of a boy with the Fragile X syndrome.

can result in the fragile site being detectable in up to 50% of cells from affected males. Demonstration of the fragile site in female carriers is much more difficult and cytogenetic studies alone are not a reliable means of carrier detection, in that although a positive result confirms carrier status, the absence of the fragile site does not exclude a woman from being a carrier.

The molecular defect

In gene mapping the Fragile X locus is known as *FRAXA*. The *FRAXA* mutation consists of an increase in the size of a region in the 5'-untranslated region of the Fragile X mental retardation (FMR-1) gene. This region contains a long CGG trinucleotide repeat sequence. In the DNA of a normal person there are between 10 and 50 copies of this triplet repeat and these are inherited in a stable fashion. However, a small increase to between 50 and 200 renders this repeat sequence unstable, a condition in which it is referred to as *premutation*.

A man who carries a premutation is known as a 'normal transmitting male'. All of his daughters will inherit the premutation and will be of normal intelligence, but when these daughters come to have sons there is a high risk that the premutation will undergo a further increase in size during meiosis. If this reaches a critical size of greater than 200 CGG triplets it becomes a full mutation. This process is sometimes referred to as *expansion* of the triplet repeat sequence.

The full mutation is unstable not only during female meiosis but also in somatic mitotic divisions. Consequently in an affected male, gel electrophoresis shows a 'smear' of DNA consisting of many different sized alleles rather than a single band (Fig. 17.19). Note that a premutation can be identified by PCR, whereas Southern blotting is necessary to detect full mutations as the long GCC expansion is refractory to PCR amplification. At the molecular level a full mutation suppresses transcription of the FMR-1 gene by hypermethylation, and this in turn is thought to be responsible for the clinical features seen in males, and in some females with a large expansion (Table 17.9). The FMR-1 gene contains 17 exons which encode a cytoplasmic protein which plays a crucial role in the development and function of cerebral neurones. The FMR-1 protein can be detected in blood using specific monoclonal antibodies.

Table 17.9   The Fragile X syndrome — genotype–phenotype correlations

Number of triplet repeats (Normal range = 10–50)	Fragile site detectable	Intelligence
Males		
50–200 (premutation)	No	Normal (normal transmitting male)
200–2000 (full mutation)	Yes (in up to 50% of cells)	Moderate to severe mental retardation
Females		
50–200 (premutation)	No	Normal
200–2000 (full mutation)	Yes (usually < 10% of cells)	50% normal, 50% mild mental retardation

Fig. 17.18
X chromosome from several males with Fragile X syndrome. (Courtesy of Ashley Wilkinson, City Hospital, Nottingham.)

greater than 100 CGG repeats almost invariably increasing in size to become full mutations.

For a woman who carries a full mutation there is a risk of 1 in 2 that each of her sons will be affected with the full syndrome and that each of her daughters will inherit the full mutation. Since approximately 50% of females with the full mutation are mildly retarded, the risk that a female carrier of a full mutation will have a retarded daughter equals $\frac{1}{2} \times \frac{1}{2}$, i.e. $\frac{1}{4}$. Prenatal diagnosis can be offered based on analysis of DNA from chorionic villi but in the event of a female fetus with a full mutation accurate prediction of phenotype cannot be made.

The Fragile X syndrome is a condition for which population screening could be offered, either among selected high risk groups such as mentally retarded males, or on a widespread general population basis. Such programmes will have to surmount major ethical, financial and logistical concerns if they are to achieve widespread acceptance (p. 342).

Fig. 17.19
Southern blot of DNA from a family showing expansion of the CGG triplet repeat being passed from a normal transmitting male through his obligate carrier daughter to her son with Fragile X mental retardation. (Courtesy of Dr G Taylor, St James's Hospital, Leeds.)

Another fragile site closely adjacent to *FRAXA* has been identified at Xq28. This is known as *FRAXE*. The expansion mutations at *FRAXE* also involve CGG triplet repeats and occur at approximately one-thirtieth the frequency of FRAXA mutations. Males with these mutations show either normal intelligence or mild mental retardation. These men are usually ascertained through the discovery of a fragile site on chromosome analysis with a normal result on *FRAXA* mutation analysis. A third fragile site, *FRAXF*, has recently been identified close to *FRAXA* and *FRAXE*. This does not seem to cause any clinical abnormality.

Genetic counselling and the Fragile X syndrome

This common cause of mental retardation presents a major counselling problem. Inheritance can be regarded as modified or atypical X-linked. All the daughters of a normal transmitting male will carry the premutation. Their male offspring are at risk of inheriting either the premutation or a full mutation. This risk is dependent on the size of the premutation in the mother, with mutations

DISORDERS OF SEXUAL DIFFERENTIATION

The process of sexual differentiation has been described in Chapter 5 (p. 90). Given the complexity of the sequential cascade of events which take place between 6 and 14 weeks of embryonic life it is not surprising that errors can occur. Many of these errors can lead to sexual ambiguity or to discordance between the chromosomal sex and the appearance of the external genitalia. These disorders are also sometimes referred to as various forms of *intersex* (Table 17.10).

Table 17.10   Disorders of sexual differentiation and development

Seminiferous tubule dysgenesis (Klinefelter's syndrome)
47,XXY, 48,XXXY, 48,XXYY, 49,XXXXY

Ovarian dysgenesis (Turner's syndrome)
45,X, 46,X,i(Xq), 46,X,del(Xp), 46,X,r(X)

True hermaphroditism
46,XX with Y-derived sequences
46,XX/46,XY chimerism

Male pseudohermaphroditism
Androgen insensitivity
Complete — testicular feminization
Incomplete — Reifenstein syndrome
Inborn errors of testosterone biosynthesis
e.g. 5α-reductase deficiency
45,X/46,XY mosaicism

Female pseudohermaphroditism
Congenital adrenal hyperplasia
Maternal androgen ingestion or androgen secreting tumour

TRUE HERMAPHRODITISM

In this extremely rare condition an individual has both testicular and ovarian tissue, often in association with ambiguous genitalia. When an exploratory operation is carried out in these patients an ovary can be found on one side and a testis on the other. Alternatively, there can be a mixture of ovarian and testicular tissue in the gonad which is known as an ovotestis. Most patients with true hermaphroditism have a 46,XX karyotype and in many of these individuals the paternally derived X chromosome carries Y chromosome-specific DNA sequences as a result of illegitimate crossing over between the X and Y chromosomes during meiosis I in spermatogenesis (Fig. 17.20).

A small proportion of patients with true hermaphroditism are found to be chimeras with both 46,XX and 46,XY cell lines, a situation analogous to freemartins in cattle (p. 53).

MALE PSEUDOHERMAPHRODITISM

In pseudohermaphroditism there is gonadal tissue of only one sex. The external genitalia can be ambiguous or of the sex opposite to that of the chromosomes. Thus in male pseudohermaphroditism there is a 46,XY karyotype with ambiguous or female genitalia.

The most widely recognized cause of male pseudohermaphroditism is androgen insensitivity (p. 160). In this condition, which is also known as the testicular feminization syndrome, the karyotype is normal male and the external phenotype is essentially that of a normal female. Internally the vagina ends blindly and the uterus and Fallopian tubes are absent. Testes are located in the abdomen or in the inguinal canal where they can be mistaken for inguinal herniae. This condition is caused by the absence of androgen receptors in the target organs, so that although testosterone is formed normally, its peripheral masculinizing effects are blocked. These androgen receptors are coded for by a gene on the X chromosome in which both deletions and point mutations have been identified. Curiously, expansion of a CAG repeat in the first exon of this androgen receptor gene causes a neurological disorder known as Kennedy's disease. This is a rare example of the phenomenon referred to as a 'gene within a gene' (p. 15).

Other causes of male pseudohermaphroditism include:

1. An incomplete form of androgen insensitivity known as Reifenstein syndrome in which affected males have hypospadias, small testes and gynaecomastia.
2. Enzyme defects in testosterone synthesis such as 5α-reductase deficiency in which the external genitalia are ambiguous at birth but undergo masculinization (virilization) at puberty.
3. Chromosome mosaicism (45,X/46,XY) in which most individuals are normal males but a small proportion have ambiguous or female external genitalia.
4. Campomelic dysplasia which is caused by mutations in the *SOX9* gene on chromosome 17. *SOX9* is believed to be an important gene in the regulatory pathway by which *SRY* causes masculinization of the undifferentiated fetal gonads (p. 84).
5. The Smith–Lemli–Opitz syndrome which is caused by deficiency of 7-dehydrocholesterol reductase, an enzyme involved in cholesterol biosynthesis. Some severely affected male infants have female external genitalia.

FEMALE PSEUDOHERMAPHRODITISM

In female pseudohermaphroditism, the karyotype is female and the external genitalia are virilized so that they either resemble those of a normal male or are ambiguous.

Congenital adrenal hyperplasia is by far the most important cause of female pseudohermaphroditism (p. 158). This can be caused by several different enzyme defects in the adrenal cortex, all of which show autosomal recessive inheritance. Reduced cortisol production leads to an increase in ACTH secretion which in turn causes hyperplasia of the adrenal glands. In the most common form of congenital adrenal hyperplasia due to 21-hydroxylase deficiency, hormone synthesis switches from the manufacture of cortisol and aldosterone to the androgen pathway (Fig. 10.5, p. 159), leading to striking virilization of a female fetus (Fig. 10.6, p. 160). The lack

Fig. 17.20
FISH showing hybridization of a Y chromosome paint to the short arm of an X chromosome in a 46,XX male. (Courtesy of Nigel Smith, City Hospital, Nottingham.)

of cortisol and aldosterone usually leads to rapid collapse shortly after birth which can prove fatal unless appropriate hormone and electrolyte supplementation are initiated (p. 160).

Rarer causes of female pseudohermaphroditism include an androgen secreting tumour and maternal androgen ingestion during pregnancy.

CHROMOSOME BREAKAGE SYNDROMES

Constitutional and acquired chromosome abnormalities which predispose to malignancy are considered in Chapter 13. In addition to these conditions, it is recognized that a small number of hereditary disorders are characterized by an excess of chromosome breaks and gaps as well as an increased susceptibility to neoplasia.

ATAXIA TELANGIECTASIA

This is an autosomal recessive disorder which presents in early childhood with ataxia, oculocutaneous telangiectasia (Fig. 17.21), radiation sensitivity and susceptibility to sinus and pulmonary infection (p. 185). There is a 10–20% risk of leukaemia or lymphoma. Cells from patients show an increase in spontaneous chromosome abnormalities, such as chromatid gaps and breaks, which are enhanced by radiation. The gene for ataxia telangiectasia is called *ATM* (*M* = mutation) and maps to chromosome 11q23. The protein product is thought to act as a 'check-point' protein kinase which interacts with the *Tp53* and *BRCA1* gene products to arrest cell division and thereby allow repair of radiation induced chromosome breaks before the S phase in the cell cycle.

BLOOM'S SYNDROME

Children with this autosomal recessive disorder are small with a light-sensitive facial rash and reduced immunoglobulin levels (IgA and IgM). The risk of lymphoreticular malignancy is approximately 20%. Cultured cells show an increased frequency of chromosome breaks, particularly if they are exposed in vitro to ultraviolet light. The gene for Bloom's syndrome maps to chromosome 15q26 where it encodes one member of a group of enzymes called the DNA helicases (p. 13). These are responsible for unwinding double stranded DNA prior to replication, repair and recombination. Normally the Bloom's syndrome gene plays a major role in maintaining genome stability. When defective in the homozygous state, DNA repair is impaired and the rate of recombination between sister chromatids is increased dramatically. This can be demonstrated by looking for sister chromatid exchanges — see below.

Fig. 17.21
Ocular telangiectasia in a child with ataxia telangiectasia.

Fig. 17.22
Bilateral radial aplasia with absent thumbs in an infant with Fanconi's anaemia.

FANCONI'S ANAEMIA

This autosomal recessive disorder is associated with upper limb abnormalities involving the radius and thumb (Fig. 17.22), increased pigmentation and bone marrow failure leading to deficiency of all types of blood cells, i.e. pancytopenia. There is also an increased risk of neoplasia, particularly leukaemia, lymphoma and hepatic carcinoma. Multiple chromosomal breaks are observed in cultured cells (Fig. 17.23) and the basic defect lies in the repair of DNA strand cross-links. There are five known subtypes of Fanconi's anaemia, each caused by recessive mutations at different autosomal loci. The commonest, type A, maps to chromosome 16q24. It is not known how any of the Fanconi anaemia genes are involved in maintaining the integrity of DNA cross-links.

Fig. 17.23
Multiple chromosome breaks and gaps in a metaphase spread prepared from a child with Fanconi's anaemia.

XERODERMA PIGMENTOSA

This exists in at least seven different forms, all of which show autosomal recessive inheritance. Patients present with a light-sensitive pigmented rash and usually die of skin malignancy in sun-exposed areas before the age of 20 years. Cells cultured from these patients only show chromosome abnormalities after exposure to ultraviolet light. These disorders are due to defects in the nucleotide excision repair pathway. This involves endonuclease cleavage 5′ and 3′ to each damaged nucleotide, excision of the damaged nucleotide(s) and finally restoration of the damaged strand using the intact opposite strand as a template.

CHROMOSOME BREAKAGE AND SISTER CHROMATID EXCHANGE

Strong evidence of increased *chromosome instability* is provided by the demonstration of an increased number of *sister chromatid exchanges* (SCEs) in cultured cells. An SCE is an exchange (crossing-over) of genetic material between the two chromatids of a chromosome in mitosis, in contrast to recombination in meiosis I which is between homologous chromatids. SCEs can be demonstrated by differences in the uptake of certain stains by the two chromatids of each metaphase chromosome after two rounds of cell division in the presence of the thymidine

analogue 5-bromodeoxyuridine (BudR), which becomes incorporated in the newly synthesized DNA (Fig. 17.24). There are normally about 10 SCEs per cell but the number is greatly increased in cells from patients with Bloom's syndrome and xeroderma pigmentosa. In the latter condition this is only apparent after the cells have been exposed to ultraviolet light.

At present it is not clear how SCEs relate to the increase in chromosome breakage observed in these two disorders, but it is thought that the explanation could involve one of the steps in DNA replication. It is also of interest that the number of SCEs in normal cells is increased on exposure to certain carcinogens and chemical mutagens. For this reason the frequency of SCEs in cells in culture has been suggested as a useful in vitro test of the carcinogenicity and mutagenicity of chemical compounds (p. 27).

INDICATIONS FOR CHROMOSOME ANALYSIS

It should be apparent from the contents of this chapter that chromosome abnormalities can present in many different ways. Consequently it is appropriate to consider the indications for chromosome analysis under a number of different headings (Table 17.11).

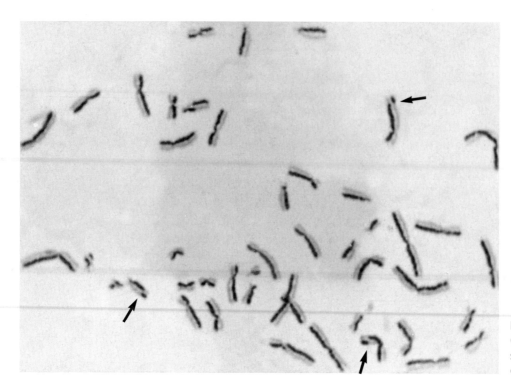

Fig. 17.24
Chromosome preparation
showing sister chromatid
exchanges (arrowed).

Table 17.11   Indications for chromosome analysis

Multiple congenital abnormalities
Unexplained mental retardation
Sexual ambiguity or abnormality in sexual development
Infertility
Recurrent miscarriage
Unexplained stillbirth
Malignancy and chromosome breakage syndromes

MULTIPLE CONGENITAL ABNORMALITIES

Every child with multiple congenital abnormalities should have chromosome studies undertaken. This is important for several reasons:

1. Establishing a chromosomal diagnosis will prevent further potentially unpleasant investigations being undertaken.

2. Information about the prognosis can be provided along with details of the relevant support group and an offer of contact with other families.

3. A chromosomal diagnosis should facilitate the provision of accurate information about the recurrence risk for future siblings.

Although it can be very distressing for parents to be told that their child has a chromosome abnormality they will often be relieved that an explanation for their child's problems has been found.

UNEXPLAINED MENTAL RETARDATION

Chromosome abnormalities cause at least one-third of the 50% of mental retardation which is attributable to genetic factors. While most children with a chromosome abnormality will have other features such as growth retardation and physical anomalies, this is not always so. If the Fragile X syndrome is a possibility it is important that the cytogenetics laboratory is informed so that the correct culture conditions are used (p. 258), although in most centres the Fragile X syndrome is now diagnosed by molecular methods rather than chromosome analysis.

SEXUAL AMBIGUITY

The birth of a child with ambiguous genitalia should be regarded as a medical emergency not only because of the inevitable parental anxiety, but also because of the importance of ruling out the potentially life-threatening diagnosis of salt-losing congenital adrenal hyperplasia (p. 159). A chromosome analysis should be among the first investigations undertaken.

Disorders of sexual development presenting in later life with problems such as delayed puberty, primary amenorrhoea or male gynaecomastia are also strong indications for chromosome analysis as a first-line investigation. This can provide a diagnosis such as Turner's syndrome (45,X) or Klinefelter's syndrome (47,XXY). Alternatively a normal karyotype will stimulate a search for other possible explanations such as an endocrine abnormality.

INFERTILITY AND RECURRENT MISCARRIAGE

Unexplained involuntary infertility should prompt a request for chromosome studies, particularly if investigations reveal evidence of azoospermia in the male partner. At least 5% of such men are found to have Klinefelter's syndrome. More rarely a complex chromosome rearrangement such as a translocation can cause such severe mechanical disruption in meiosis that complete failure of gametogenesis ensues.

At least 15% of all recognized pregnancies end in spontaneous miscarriage and in 50% of cases this is because of a chromosome abnormality (pp. 225, 249). Unfortunately, some couples experience recurrent pregnancy loss, which is usually defined as three or more spontaneous miscarriages. Often no explanation is ever found and many such couples go on to have successful pregnancies. However, in 3–6% of such couples, one partner is found to carry a chromosome rearrangement which predisposes to severe imbalance through malsegregation at meiosis (p. 47). Consequently it is now standard practice to offer chromosome analysis to all couples who have experienced three or more spontaneous pregnancy losses.

UNEXPLAINED STILLBIRTH/NEONATAL DEATH

The presence of growth retardation and at least one congenital abnormality in a stillbirth or neonatal death would be an indication for chromosome studies based on analysis of blood or skin collected from the baby before or as soon after death as possible. Skin fibroblasts continue to be viable for several days after death. Chromosome abnormalities account for 5% of all stillbirths and neonatal deaths and not all of these babies have multiple abnormalities which would immediately suggest a chromosomal cause.

MALIGNANCY AND CHROMOSOME BREAKAGE SYNDROMES

Certain types of leukaemia (p. 192) and many solid tumours, such as retinoblastoma (p. 195) and Wilms' tumour (p. 254), are associated with specific chromosomal abnormalities which can be of both diagnostic and prognostic value. Clinical features suggestive of a chromosome breakage syndrome (p. 262), such as a combination of photosensitivity and short stature, should also lead to appropriate chromosome fragility studies, such as analysis of sister chromatid exchanges.

FURTHER READING

De Grouchy J, Turleau C 1984 Clinical atlas of human chromosomes, 2nd edn. John Wiley, Chichester
A lavishly illustrated atlas of known chromosomal syndromes.
Gardner R J M, Sutherland G R 1996 Chromosome abnormalities and genetic counselling, 2nd edn. Oxford University Press, Oxford
A useful updated guide to genetic counselling in families with a chromosome disorder.
Hagerman R J, Silverman A C (eds) 1991 Fragile X syndrome. Diagnosis, treatment and research. Johns Hopkins University Press, Baltimore
A detailed account of the clinical and genetic aspects of the Fragile X syndrome.
Jacobs P A, Browne C, Gregson N, Joyce C, White H 1992 Estimates of the frequency of chromosome abnormalities detectable in unselected newborns using moderate levels of banding. J Med Genet 29: 103–108
A review of the results of over 14 000 prenatal diagnoses with estimates of the incidence of chromosome abnormalities in term infants.
Schinzel A 1994 Human cytogenetics database. Oxford University Press, Oxford
A regularly updated computerized database of all known chromosome abnormalities. This is an invaluable aid to diagnosis and counselling.

ELEMENTS

1 Chromosome abnormalities account for 50% of all spontaneous miscarriages and are present in 0.5–1.0% of all newborn infants.

2 Down's syndrome is the most common autosomal chromosomal syndrome and shows a strong association between increasing incidence and advancing maternal age. 95% of all cases are caused by trisomy 21. Chromosome studies are necessary in all cases so that the rare but important cases due to unbalanced familial Robertsonian translocations can be identified.

3 An increasing number of chromosome microdeletion syndromes are being recognized. These have helped in gene mapping and in enhancing understanding of underlying genetic mechanisms such as imprinting. Microdeletions of chromosome 15 are found in both Angelman's and the Prader–Willi syndrome and are maternally and paternally derived respectively.

④ Triploidy is a common finding in spontaneously aborted products of conception but rare in a live-born infant. Some children with diploidy/triploidy mosaicism present with mental retardation and areas of depigmentation, a condition known as hypomelanosis of Ito.

⑤ Sex chromosome abnormalities include Klinefelter's syndrome (47,XXY), Turner's syndrome (45,X), the XYY syndrome (47,XYY) and the triple X syndrome (47,XXX). In all of these conditions intelligence is either normal or only mildly impaired. Infertility is the rule in Klinefelter's and Turner's syndromes. Fertility is normal in the XYY and the triple X syndrome.

⑥ The Fragile X syndrome is the most common inherited cause of mental retardation. It is associated with a fragile site on the long arm of the X chromosome and shows modified X-linked inheritance. Affected males are moderately to severely mentally retarded; carrier females can show mild mental retardation. At the molecular level there is expansion of a CGG triplet repeat which can exist as a premutation or a full mutation.

⑦ Disorders of sexual differentiation include true and pseudohermaphroditism. True hermaphroditism is extremely rare. Male pseudohermaphroditism is caused most commonly by androgen insensitivity, an X-linked disorder involving formation of androgen receptors. The most common cause of female pseudohermaphroditism is congenital adrenal hyperplasia, in which virilized infants can collapse with adrenal failure during the first week of life.

⑧ The chromosome breakage syndromes are rare autosomal recessive disorders characterized by increased chromosome breakage in cultured cells and an increased tendency to neoplasia such as leukaemia and lymphoma. They are caused by underlying defects in DNA repair.

Single gene disorders

To date over 10 000 single gene traits and disorders have been identified. Most of these are individually rare but together they affect between 1% and 2% of the general population at any one time. The management of these disorders in affected individuals and in their extended families presents a major challenge for clinical genetics and allied relevant specialties.

In this chapter some of the most common and important single gene disorders will be described, with particular emphasis on their basic molecular defects. Each of these disorders illustrates important genetic principles and for many the identification of the mutational basis and isolation of the associated protein product represent some of the most notable scientific achievements of the last decade.

HUNTINGTON'S DISEASE

Huntington's disease (HD), also known as Huntington's chorea, derives its eponymous title from Dr George Huntington who described multiple affected individuals in a large North American kindred in 1872. George Huntington's paper, which was published in the Philadelphia journal, *The Medical and Surgical Reporter*, gave a graphic description of the progressive neurological disability which has endowed HD with the unenviable reputation of being one of the most feared and unpleasant hereditary disorders encountered in humans. The natural history is characterized by slowly progressive selective cell death in the central nervous system, for which there is no effective treatment or cure. The prevalence in most parts of the world is approximately 1 in 15 000, although in some areas, such as Tasmania and the Lake Maracaibo region of Venezuela, much higher figures have been noted.

Generally HD is a disorder of middle to late adult life. There is, however, a rare juvenile form which presents at a much younger age with different clinical features. This is one of several enigmatic aspects of HD which have been explained, at least in part, by the relatively recent discovery of the underlying molecular defect.

CLINICAL FEATURES

In the common adult onset form of HD the disease course is characterized by a slowly progressive movement disorder and an insidious impairment of intellectual function with psychiatric disturbance and eventual dementia. The average age of onset is around 40 years and the mean duration of the illness is approximately 15 years. Chorea is the most common movement abnormality. This takes the form of subtle involuntary movements such as facial grimacing, twitching of the face and limbs, folding of the arms and crossing of the legs. As the disease progresses the gait becomes very unsteady and speech becomes unclear.

Intellectual changes in the early stages of HD include memory impairment and poor concentration span. Anxiety, aggressive behaviour, paranoia and alcohol abuse can also occur. There is a gradual deterioration in intellectual function leading eventually to total incapacitation and dementia.

Juvenile Huntington's disease

In approximately 10% of cases the disorder presents before the age of 20 years. Instead of chorea there is rigidity with slowing of voluntary movement and clumsiness. A decline in school performance heralds the onset of a severe progressive dementia, often in association with epileptic seizures. The average duration of the illness is around 10–15 years.

GENETICS

Traditionally HD has been said to show autosomal dominant inheritance with a variable age of onset, close to complete penetrance, and a very low mutation rate. In addition, it has been noted that the disorder often shows anticipation whereby the onset is at a younger age in succeeding generations, particularly when transmitted by a male. The recent discovery of the HD gene has provided an explanation for some of these observations.

Mapping and isolation of the HD gene

HD was one of the first disorders to be mapped by linkage analysis using polymorphic DNA markers when, in 1983, the disorder was found to show close linkage with a probe known as G8 on the short arm of chromosome 4. This initial search for the HD locus was helped enormously by the collection of blood samples from a huge pedigree containing over 100 affected subjects living on the shores of Lake Maracaibo in Venezuela. As well as providing the first means of predictive testing for HD, this work also revealed that HD homozygotes are no more severely affected than heterozygotes. This is in contrast to most other autosomal dominant disorders (p. 100). Ten years later, in 1993, the gene itself was isolated and found to contain a highly polymorphic CAG repeat sequence located in the 5′ region. The messenger RNA codes for a protein of approximately 350 kDa, known as *huntingtin*. Huntingtin is expressed in many different cells throughout the central nervous system although its function remains unclear. One proposed role, as yet unproven, is that it is involved in apoptosis, i.e. cell death.

The mutation in HD

Almost all individuals with HD possess an expansion of a CAG polyglutamine repeat sequence located in the 5′ region of the HD gene. HD is thus an example of a disorder caused by expansion of a triplet repeat (p. 22), a mutational mechanism which was first identified in humans in contrast to almost all other types of mutation which were first reported in other species such as *Drosophila* and mice. A recent joint working party of the American College of Medical Genetics and the American Society of Human Genetics recommended that HD genes should be categorized under four headings on the basis of CAG repeat length (Table 18.1).

Normal alleles

Alleles containing 26 or fewer CAG repeats are not associated with disease manifestations and are stable in meiosis.

Mutable alleles

Allele sizes of 27 to 35 CAG repeats do not cause disease but show meiotic instability with a potential to increase or decrease in size. These 'mutable' alleles thus constitute a reservoir for new mutations. When an affected individual presents with what appears to be a new mutation, it usually emerges that the father carries a mutable allele. Furthermore there is evidence that mutable alleles which expand are associated with a particular haplotype as identified by intragenic and flanking DNA markers. This implies that certain haplotypes are more mutable than others.

Reduced penetrance alleles

This third category consists of alleles containing 36 to 39 CAG repeats. These are associated with either late onset disease or complete absence of disease expression, i.e. non-penetrance.

Disease alleles

The final group of HD genes contains 40 or more CAG repeats. These are invariably associated with disease, although sometimes this may not develop until the eighth or ninth decade. There is a direct relationship between length of repeat and disease expression, with

Table 18.1   Comparison of genetic aspects of Huntington's disease and myotonic dystrophy

	Huntington's disease		Myotonic dystrophy
Inheritance	Autosomal dominant		Autosomal dominant
Chromosome locus	4p16.3		19q13.3
Trinucleotide repeat	CAG in 5′ translated region		CTG in 3′ untranslated region
Repeat sizes	Normal	≤ 26	Normal < 37
	Mutable	27–35	
	Reduced penetrance	36–39	Full mutation 50–2000+
	Fully penetrant	≥ 40	
Protein product	Huntingtin		MD protein kinase (MDPK)
Early onset form	Juvenile		Congenital
	Usually paternally transmitted		Usually maternally transmitted

the average age of onset for repeat sizes of 40, 45 and 50 being 57, 37 and 26 years respectively. Most affected adults have repeat sizes of between 36 and 55, whereas juvenile cases often have an expansion greater than 60 repeats.

Parent of origin effect in disease transmission

Autosomal dominant inheritance is well established with an offspring risk of 1 in 2 regardless of whether the affected parent is male or female. However, for reasons which are not understood, meiotic instability appears to be much greater in spermatogenesis than in oogenesis. This is reflected in anticipation occurring mainly when the mutant allele is transmitted by a male. Juveniles with the rigid form of HD have almost always inherited the mutant allele from their more mildly affected father.

Several possible explanations have been suggested for this preferential transmission of expanded alleles by the male. One possibility is that expansion caused by slippage (p. 22) of DNA polymerase simply reflects the number of mitoses undergone during gametogenesis. In Chapter 3 it was pointed out that spermatogenesis involves a much larger number of mitotic divisions than oogenesis (p. 43). An alternative possibility is based on the observation that huntingtin is expressed in oocytes so that there could be selection against oocytes with large expansions as a consequence of preferential apoptosis.

CLINICAL APPLICATIONS AND FUTURE PROSPECTS

The discovery of the HD gene has meant that accurate predictive testing is possible, although there is universal agreement that this should only be offered as part of a well-planned and carefully monitored counselling package. Experience to date indicates that more women than men take up the offer of predictive testing, with the degree of psychological disturbance in those given positive results being less than was expected. Prenatal diagnosis is also possible for those couples who feel that this is acceptable. Obviously there are considerable emotional and ethical issues associated with termination of pregnancy on the grounds that a child could go on to develop a neurodegenerative disease in middle age. This will be particularly pertinent when effective therapeutic strategies have been devised. One appealing approach is based on the observation that large CAG repeats result in intracellular accumulation of huntingtin 'aggregates', which are cleaved by a protease known as caspase to form a toxic product which causes cell death (apoptosis). Caspase inhibitors have been shown to have a beneficial effect in an HD mouse model. Other suggested therapeutic approaches include injection of fetal stem cells into regions of the brain, such as the caudate nucleus

and putamen, which become atrophic in the early stages of the disease.

MYOTONIC DYSTROPHY

Myotonic dystrophy (MD) is the most common form of muscular dystrophy seen in adults, with an overall incidence of approximately 1 in 8000. MD shares many features in common with HD (Table 18.1). In particular both disorders show autosomal dominant inheritance with anticipation and an early onset form with rather different clinical features. However, in MD the early onset form is transmitted almost exclusively by the mother and presents at birth, in contrast to juvenile HD which is generally paternally transmitted with an age of onset in the teens.

CLINICAL FEATURES

In contrast to most forms of muscular dystrophy, these are not limited exclusively to the neuromuscular system. Most commonly persons with MD present in adult life with slowly progressive weakness and myotonia. This latter term refers to tonic muscle spasm with prolonged relaxation which can manifest as a delay in releasing the grip on shaking hands. Other clinical abnormalities can include cataracts (Fig. 18.1), cardiac conduction defects, disturbed gastrointestinal peristalsis, frontal balding and testicular atrophy. The age of onset can be very variable and the disorder usually runs a relatively benign course. However, in the 'congenital' form affected babies present

Fig. 18.1
Refractile lens opacities in an asymptomatic person with myotonic dystrophy. (Courtesy of Mr R Doran and Mr M Geall, Department of Ophthalmology, General Infirmary, Leeds.)

at birth with hypotonia, talipes and respiratory distress which can prove life threatening. Children who survive tend to show a lack of facial expression ('myopathic facies') with delayed motor development and mild mental retardation.

The diagnosis of MD used to be based on the finding of myotonic discharges seen on electromyography (p. 290). This unpleasant investigation has now been superseded by mutation analysis.

GENETICS

It has long been recognized that MD shows autosomal dominant inheritance with increasing severity in succeeding generations. At one time it was thought that this phenomenon of anticipation (p. 107) was a reflection of ascertainment bias, caused by the greater likelihood of detecting a mildly affected parent having a severely affected child rather than the other way round. Recent studies have confirmed that anticipation is a real phenomenon in MD.

Mapping and isolating the MD gene

Genetic linkage of MD to the secretor and Lutheran blood group loci was established in 1971, and the MD locus was mapped to chromosome 19 in 1982. As with HD, 10 years elapsed before the gene itself was isolated. This was achieved by an international collaborative effort whereby most of the relevant region of chromosome 19 was cloned. The mutational basis of MD was shown in 1992 to be instability in a CTG repeat sequence which is present in the 3' untranslated region of a protein kinase gene (DMPK).

Genotype–phenotype correlation in MD

In unaffected persons the CTG sequence lying 3' to the DMPK gene consists of up to 37 repeats (Table 18.1). Affected individuals have an expansion of at least 50 copies of the CTG sequence. There is a close correlation between disease severity and the size of the expansion, which can exceed 2000 repeats. The severe congenital cases show the largest repeat copy number with almost invariable inheritance from the mother. Thus meiotic or germ line instability is greater in the female for alleles containing a large number of sequences. Curiously expansion of a relatively small number of repeats appears to occur more commonly in the male and most MD mutations are thought to have occurred originally during meiosis in the male. One possible explanation for these observations is that mature spermatozoa can only carry small expansions whereas ova can accommodate much larger expansions; hence congenital onset cases are almost exclusively maternally transmitted.

Yet another puzzling feature of MD is the reported tendency for healthy individuals who are heterozygous for MD alleles in the normal size range to preferentially transmit alleles which are greater than 19 CTG repeats in size. This possible example of meiotic drive (p. 120) could explain the relatively high frequency of MD with constant replenishment of a reservoir of potential MD mutations.

The MD protein kinase

At present it is not known how or indeed if the MD protein kinase causes muscular weakness or the other clinical problems. Rather surprisingly it has been shown that mice with both overexpression and underexpression of DMPK do not show the typical clinical features of MD. This has led to the suggestion that abnormal protein kinase activity is not the main cause of MD, but that instead the RNA produced by the mutant DMPK gene somehow interferes with the cellular processing of RNA produced by other genes. This would be an example of a 'dominant-negative' effect mediated at the RNA level instead of the more usual protein level (p. 24). Another possibility is that expansion of the CTG sequence in the 3' region of the DMPK gene influences expression not only of the protein kinase but also of other closely adjacent genes, such as the recently identified homeobox containing gene known as DMAHP (= DM locus associated homeodomain protein).

CLINICAL APPLICATIONS AND FUTURE PROSPECTS

The development of a reliable molecular diagnostic test for MD has meant that both presymptomatic testing and prenatal diagnosis can be offered to those families for whom it is appropriate and acceptable. This is particularly relevant for couples who have had a child with the severe congenital form for whom it is known that the risk of recurrence is relatively high. As in Huntington's disease, presymptomatic testing should not be undertaken without an offer of long term support and medical care, and in both HD and MD the possibility of difficulty in obtaining both life and health insurance should be discussed before predictive testing is undertaken (p. 340).

Important components of the management of MD include regular surveillance for cardiac conduction defects and the provision of information about risks associated with general anaesthesia. Logical approaches to gene therapy will almost certainly have to await a better understanding of the mechanism whereby expansion of the repeat sequence in the 3' untranslated region of the DMPK gene causes such diverse and variable clinical abnormalities.

HEREDITARY MOTOR AND SENSORY NEUROPATHY

Hereditary motor and sensory neuropathy (HMSN) comprises a group of clinically and genetically heterogeneous disorders characterized by slowly progressive distal muscle weakness and wasting. Other names for these disorders include Charcot–Marie–Tooth disease and peroneal muscular atrophy. Their overall incidence is approximately 1 in 2500.

HMSN can be classified on the basis of the results of motor nerve conduction velocity (MNCV) studies. In HMSN type I MNCV is reduced and nerve biopsies from patients show segmental demyelination accompanied by hypertrophic changes with 'onion bulb' formation. In HMSN type II MNCV is normal or only slightly reduced and nerve biopsies show axonal degeneration.

CLINICAL FEATURES

In autosomal dominant HMSN I, which is the most common form, there is onset of slowly progressive distal muscle weakness and wasting in the lower limbs between the ages of 10 and 30 years. Similar changes occur later in the upper limbs in many patients, often in association with ataxia and tremor. The appearance of the lower limbs has been likened to that of an 'inverted champagne bottle' (Fig. 18.2). With age, locomotion becomes more difficult and the feet tend to show exaggeration of their normal arch, known as 'pes cavus'. Despite these quite striking changes most patients retain reasonable muscle strength and are not too seriously disabled. Other faculties such as vision, hearing and intellect are not impaired. In keeping with the pathological changes of hypertrophy, palpable thickening of peripheral nerves can be detected in around one-third of cases.

The clinical features in other forms of HMSN are relatively similar but differ in the age of onset, rate of progression and presence of other neurological involvement. For example, in HMSN II onset is later than in HMSN I and the disease course is milder to the extent that some affected individuals are asymptomatic. In contrast in HMSN III, which is very rare, onset is in early childhood and there is severe delay in achieving motor milestones.

GENETICS

HMSN can show autosomal dominant, autosomal recessive or X-linked inheritance, although autosomal dominant forms are by far the most common. In over 90% of cases of HMSN I the disorder arises as the result

Fig. 18.2
Lower limbs of a male with hereditary motor and sensory neuropathy (HMSN) showing severe muscle wasting below the knees.

of a duplication of 1.5 megabases of genomic DNA on the short arm of chromosome 17. This is seen both in familial cases and in most sporadic cases, implying a common causal mechanism with a high mutation rate. Located within this 1.5 megabase region on 17p is the gene which codes for a 22 kDa glycoprotein known as peripheral myelin protein-22 (PMP-22). This is present in the myelin membranes of peripheral nerves where it plays a major role in arresting Schwann cell division. Changes in this protein cause a peripheral neuropathy in a mutant strain of mice known as 'trembler'. HMSN I in humans is thought to be the result of a *PMP-22* dosage effect. Point mutations have been identified in the *PMP-22* gene in a small number of non-duplication HMSN I patients.

Recent studies have shown that the HMSN I duplication is generated by misalignment and subsequent recombination between homologous sequences which flank the *PMP-22* gene (Fig. 18.3). For reasons which are not understood this recombination event usually occurs in male gametogenesis, rather than in the female as is the case in Duchenne muscular dystrophy (p. 281). The

Fig. 18.3
Mechanism by which misalignment and recombination with unequal crossing over lead to the formation of the duplication and deletion which cause hereditary motor and sensory neuropathy type I (HMSN I) and hereditary liability to pressure palsies (HLPP). X and Y represent homologous sequences flanking the *PMP-22* gene.

reciprocal deletion product of this unequal crossing-over event causes a relatively mild disorder known as hereditary liability to pressure palsies, in which minor nerve trauma causes focal numbness and weakness. The mechanism whereby duplication and deletion products result from misalignment and recombination is identical to that which produces Hb Lepore and anti-Lepore (Fig. 9.3, p. 141).

Other forms of HMSN

In a small proportion of families with typical features of HMSN I, linkage analysis indicated that the disease locus was on chromosome 1 rather than on chromosome 17. This led to chromosome 17 cases being referred to as HMSN Ia and chromosome 1 cases as HMSN Ib. It is now known that HMSN Ib is caused by mutations in the gene which codes for another major myelin protein, known as protein zero (P_0). This plays a crucial role as an adhesion molecule in the compaction of myelin in peripheral nerves.

A rare form of HMSN shows X-linked inheritance with males having typical HMSN I features and females being more mildly affected. This form of HMSN is caused by mutations in the gene which encodes a gap junction protein called connexin 32. Previously it was not known that gap junctions existed in peripheral nerves and the role of connexin 32 in causing HMSN is not fully understood at present.

FUTURE PROSPECTS

The discovery of the chromosome 17 duplication in HMSN Ia has dramatically improved diagnostic precision and has removed the need for nerve conduction studies as a presymptomatic test for family members at risk. Unfortunately successful treatment remains elusive. Efforts at gene therapy in mouse models such as 'trembler' will almost certainly be directed at trying to achieve a reduction in gene dosage by switching off or 'downregulating' *PMP-22* expression.

NEUROFIBROMATOSIS

References to the clinical features of neurofibromatosis (NF) first appeared in the eighteenth century medical literature, but historically the disorder is most commonly associated with the name Von Recklinghausen, a German pathologist, who coined the term 'neurofibroma' in 1882.

Neurofibromatosis is now known to be one of the most common genetic disorders in humans and gained public notoriety when it was suggested that Joseph Merrick, the 'elephant man' was probably affected. However, subsequent review of Merrick's photographs and skeleton led to the conclusion that he did not have neurofibromatosis but instead had a much rarer disorder known as the Proteus syndrome.

There are two main types of neurofibromatosis, NF1 and NF2. NF1 is by far the more common with an incidence at birth of approximately 1 in 3000. NF2 has an incidence of approximately 1 in 35 000 and a prevalence of around 1 in 200 000.

CLINICAL FEATURES

The most notable features of NF1 are small pigmented skin lesions, known as café-au-lait spots, and small soft fleshy growths known as neurofibromata (Fig. 18.4). Café-au-lait spots first appear in early childhood and continue to increase in both size and number until puberty. A minimum of six café-au-lait spots at least 5 mm in diameter are required to support the diagnosis in childhood. Neurofibromata are benign tumours which arise most commonly in the skin. They usually appear in late childhood and adult life and show an increase in number with age.

Fig. 18.4
A patient with neurofibromatosis type I showing truncal freckling, café-au-lait spots and multiple neurofibromata.

Fig. 18.5
Lisch nodules seen in neurofibromatosis type I. (Courtesy of Mr R Doran, Department of Ophthalmology, General Infirmary, Leeds.)

Other clinical findings in NF1 include axillary freckling, macrocephaly (large head), mild developmental delay, and Lisch nodules. These are small harmless raised pigmented hamartomata of the iris (Fig. 18.5). Most individuals with NF1 enjoy a normal healthy life and are not unduly inconvenienced by their condition. Unfortunately a small number of patients develop one or more major complications such as epilepsy, a central nervous system tumour or a scoliosis.

In NF2 both café-au-lait spots and neurofibromata can occur, but these are much less common than in NF1. The most characteristic feature of NF2 is the development in early adult life of tumours involving the eighth cranial nerves. These used to be called acoustic neuromas and are now known as vestibular Schwannomas.

GENETICS

NF1 shows autosomal dominant inheritance with almost complete penetrance by the age of 5 years. Expression is very variable and affected members of the same family can show quite striking differences in disease severity. The features in affected identical twins are usually very similar so that variable expression in family members, who must have the same mutation, is probably due to the effects of modifying genes at other loci. Approximately 50% of cases of NF1 are due to new mutations, with the estimated mutation rate being approximately 1 per 10 000 gametes. This is around 100 times greater than the average mutation rate per generation per locus in humans.

There are a few reports of multiple affected children born to unaffected healthy parents. These probably represent examples of parental gonadal mosaicism (p. 108). Somatic mosaicism in NF1 can manifest with features limited to a particular part of the body. This is referred to as segmental NF.

Mapping and isolating the NF1 gene

The application of polymorphic DNA markers for each autosome, coupled with the willingness of large numbers of families to participate in research, led to the successful mapping of the NF1 gene on chromosome 17 in 1987. Refined mapping using multipoint linkage analysis (p. 123) pinpointed the NF1 locus to the long arm of chromosome 17 closely adjacent to the centromere.

Isolation of the NF1 gene was aided by the identification of two patients who had both NF1 and a balanced translocation with a break-point at 17q11.2. A cosmid clone was identified containing both translocation breakpoints and a search for transcripts from this region yielded four genes, one of which was shown to be the NF1 gene. This spans over 350 kb of genomic DNA and contains at least 59 exons which encode a messenger RNA of 11–13 kb. The other three genes identified in this region were found to lie within a single intron of the NF1 gene where they are transcribed in the opposite direction from the complementary strand (p. 17).

The NF1 gene product

Sequence analysis of the NF1 gene has shown that it encodes a protein, known as *neurofibromin*. This shows structural homology to the GTPase activating protein (GAP), which plays an important role in signal transduction (p. 193) by downregulating *RAS* activity. Loss of heterozygosity for chromosome 17 markers has been observed in several malignant tumours in patients with NF1, as well as in a small number of benign neurofibromata. These observations indicate that the NF1 gene functions as a tumour suppressor. It has been shown to contain a GAP-related domain (GRD) which interacts with the *RAS* proto-oncogene product. A mRNA editing site exists in the NF1 gene and edited transcript causes GRD protein truncation which inactivates the tumour suppressor function. A higher range of editing is seen in more malignant tumours.

Other genes, including p53 on the short arm of chromosome 17 (p. 198), are also involved in tumour development and progression in NF1. Conversely it is also known that the NF1 gene is implicated in the development of sporadic tumours not associated with NF, including carcinoma of the colon, neuroblastoma and malignant melanoma. These observations confirm that the NF1 gene plays an important role in cell growth and differentiation.

Genotype–phenotype correlation

Over 100 different mutations have been identified in the NFI gene. These include deletions, insertions, duplications and point substitutions. Most of these mutations lead to severe truncation of the protein or complete absence of gene expression. To date there is little evidence for a clear relationship between specific mutations and clinical features. This is consistent with reports of quite striking intrafamilial variation and points to the effects of modifier genes. Patients with large deletions which include the entire NF1 gene tend to be severely affected with more severe intellectual impairment than is usual in NF1 as well as a larger than average number of cutaneous neurofibromata.

NF2

The NF2 locus was mapped to chromosome 22q by linkage analysis in 1987. The gene was cloned in 1993 and found to span 110 kb with 17 exons. The gene product is known as *merlin* and is thought to be a cytoskeleton protein which acts as a tumour suppressor.

CLINICAL APPLICATIONS AND FUTURE PROSPECTS

Mapping of the NF1 gene has provided a means of offering both presymptomatic and prenatal diagnosis using either linkage or direct mutation analysis. In practice very few families express a wish to pursue either of these options, partly because they do not perceive NF1 as a serious illness and partly because mutation analysis does not help in predicting disease severity.

At present there is no cure for NF1. Drug therapy aimed at upregulating neurofibromin GAP activity or downregulating *RAS* activity could prove beneficial in the absence of effective gene therapy. However, it is difficult to envisage how this could be applied to diverse target tissues including the central nervous system. In the short term the major impact of the cloning of the NF1 and NF2 genes will probably be in the achievement of better understanding of the processes involved in the development of the nervous system and in tumour formation rather than the imminent introduction of effective gene therapy.

HUMAN PRION DISEASES

Prion diseases consist of a relatively small number of transmittable neurodegenerative disorders. Unlike the other conditions considered in this chapter, human prion diseases are extremely rare, with an estimated overall incidence in the world of approximately one person per million per year. However despite this rarity they have been the focus of intense interest over the last decade, initially because of the novel concept of transmission of a disease by protein inoculation and more recently because of the widely publicized concern that bovine spongiform encephalopathy (BSE) could lead to an epidemic of prion disease in many Western populations.

Human prion diseases can be considered under the three headings of inherited, sporadic and acquired (Table 18.2). The large majority of cases in humans are sporadic, with around 15% of cases being inherited. However, it is the relatively small number of new variant Creutzfeldt-Jakob disease (CJD) cases and their possible association with BSE which have led human prion diseases to become an area of major research interest and public concern.

INHERITED

The human prion protein gene (*PRNP*) is located on the short arm of chromosome 20 where it spans 16 kb and contains two exons. Normally it encodes a protein PrP which has an unknown function in cells where it exists in a particular cellular isoform PrP^C. A conformational change in PrP^C leads to an abnormal isoform PrP^{Sc} which constitutes a pathological transmittable agent. The term *prion* was originally coined by Stanley Prusiner to describe 'proteinaceous infectious particles', a discovery for which he subsequently won the Nobel Prize for Medicine and Physiology in 1997.

Table 18.2 Human prion diseases

Form	Disease	Cause
Inherited	Familial CJD Fatal familial insomnia Gerstmann-Sträussler	Germ line mutation in *PRNP*
Sporadic	Typical and atypical CJD	? Somatically acquired mutations in *PRNP*
Acquired	CJD Kuru New variant CJD	Corneal transplant, cadaver derived growth hormone Cannibalism Bovine spongiform encephalopathy (BSE)

CJD = Creutzfeldt-Jakob disease.

Inherited human prion diseases are caused by mutations in the *PRNP* gene. The various disorders which have been described (Table 18.2) involve deterioration in neurological function with no known effective treatment. The most common of these, CJD, has a peak onset in the sixth decade of life and presents with a rapidly progressive dementing illness associated with a movement disorder. Death usually follows within a period of 3–6 months. A diagnosis is confirmed on the basis of postmortem changes in the brain consisting of spongiform vacuolation, astrocytic proliferation and neuronal loss. Inherited human prion diseases are unusual in that they can show quite remarkable variation in severity within a family, so that the same mutation can result in classical CJD in one family member and in a much milder and much more slowly progressive form of dementia in a close relative.

SPORADIC

Most prion diseases in humans represent sporadic events and are of unknown cause. It is generally thought that these cases arise from somatic mutations in *PRNP* or as a result of spontaneous conversion of PrP^C to PrP^{Sc}. An alternative explanation based on the observation that transgenic mice with high levels of prion gene expression develop neuromuscular disease is that sporadic prion diseases in humans result from overexpression of *PRNP*, possibly as a result of gene amplification (p. 193) or formation of a novel chimeric transcript (p. 192).

ACQUIRED

These have long been the subject of intense interest but it was not until 1966 that it was confirmed that human diseases such as kuru could be transmitted by intracerebral inoculation. Kuru is a severe neurodegenerative disorder characterized by progressive cerebellar ataxia leading to death within a period of around 12 months from time of onset. It was known for many years that this condition was particularly common among the remotely situated eastern islanders of Papua New Guinea, who traditionally practised ritualistic cannibalism in that they consumed the remains of their close relatives shortly after death. Subsequently it was shown that acquired CJD could be transmitted as a result of corneal grafting or injection of human pituitary derived growth hormone.

It is now believed that these acquired forms of human prion disease result from the transmission of an abnormal isoform of the prion protein, PrP^{Sc}, which, unlike the normal PrP^C, is partially protease resistant. It appears that a direct interaction occurs between PrP^{Sc} and PrP^C which catalyses the conversion of PrP^C to PrP^{Sc} with its subsequent replication. This process is more likely to occur if the recipient is homozygous for a particular polymorphism in the *PRNP* gene. Genetic susceptibility to both sporadic and acquired prion diseases is now well established and has been shown to be based on homozygosity for a particular polymorphism in residue 129 in the *PRNP* gene. Heterozygotes are protected in that they show a lower incidence of both sporadic and acquired prion diseases, and in the event that they inherit a germ line mutation for a condition such as familial CJD then the age of onset tends to be delayed.

Thus acquired prion diseases in humans are unique in that they result from replication of a protein which lacks any obvious replicative process. The key factor in determining sensitivity is the so-called 'species barrier' which probably relates to the degree of homology between the prion protein molecules in the host and in the inoculating agent.

NEW VARIANT CJD AND BOVINE SPONGIFORM ENCEPHALOPATHY (BSE)

For many years it was considered that the epidemic of spongiform encephalopathy which occurred in cattle in the United Kingdom and elsewhere did not constitute a serious health risk for humans. This was based to some extent on the knowledge that a similar condition known as scrapie which affects sheep and goats has been recognized for over 200 years with no evidence that it can be transmitted to humans. However in 1995 two cases of apparent sporadic CJD were reported in the UK in teenagers and shortly afterwards a handful of other cases were recognized. These young people were diagnosed as having a 'new variant' form of CJD which differed both clinically and pathologically from the inherited and acquired forms. Strong evidence that this new variant form of Creutzfeldt-Jakob disease is caused by BSE was provided by close resemblance of the molecular characteristics of prion proteins in the two conditions.

At present the link between BSE and new variant CJD awaits absolute scientific confirmation although it is generally accepted that the two conditions are probably aetiologically related. The relatively small number of affected human cases suggests that there is likely to be an effective species barrier between cattle and humans with the small number of affected young people representing a genetically susceptible subpopulation. Concern about the possibility of a major human epidemic prompted the widespread slaughter of affected herds in the United Kingdom with an embargo on the export of British beef which continues to generate controversy, despite its recent withdrawal. Most human prion diseases have a very long incubation period so that the possibility of a major epidemic of new variant CJD in years to come is still a very real concern. A possible ray of hope is provided by the recent discovery that a group of drugs known as phthalocyanines can interfere with the generation of the mutant protease-resistant form of prion protein.

CYSTIC FIBROSIS

Cystic fibrosis (CF) was first recognized as a discrete entity in 1936 and used to be known as 'mucoviscidosis' because of the accumulation of thick mucous secretions which lead to blockage of the airways and secondary infection. Although antibiotics and physiotherapy have been very effective in increasing the average life expectancy of a child with CF from less than 5 years in 1955 to around 30 years at present, CF remains a significant cause of chronic ill health and mortality in childhood and early adult life.

CF is one of the most common autosomal recessive disorders encountered in individuals of Western European origin, in whom the incidence varies from 1 in 2000 to 1 in 3000. The incidence is slightly lower in Eastern and Southern European populations and much lower in African-Americans (1 in 15 000) and Asian-Americans (1 in 31 000).

CLINICAL FEATURES

The organs most commonly affected in CF are the lungs and the pancreas. Chronic lung disease caused by recurrent infection eventually leads to fibrotic changes in the lungs with secondary cardiac failure, a condition known as *cor pulmonale*. When this complication occurs the only hope for long term survival rests in a successful heart–lung transplant.

In 85% of persons with CF pancreatic function is impaired with reduced enzyme secretion due to blockage of the pancreatic ducts by inspissated secretions. This leads to malabsorption with an increase in the fat content of the stools. This complication of CF is readily amenable to treatment with oral supplements of pancreatic enzymes.

Other problems which are commonly encountered in CF include nasal polyps, rectal prolapse, cirrhosis and diabetes mellitus. Around 10% of children with CF present in the newborn period with obstruction of the small bowel due to thickened meconium, a condition known as *meconium ileus*. Almost all males with CF are sterile because of congenital bilateral absence of the vas deferens (CBAVD). It is now recognized that a small subset of males have a very mild form of CF in which CBAVD is the only significant clinical problem. Other rare presentations of CF include chronic pancreatitis, diffuse bronchiectasis and bronchopulmonary allergic aspergillosis.

GENETICS

CF shows autosomal recessive inheritance. Other autosomal recessive disorders, such as haemochromatosis which causes tissue iron overload, show a higher incidence, but CF is by far the most serious autosomal recessive disorder encountered in children of Western European origin. Possible explanations which have been proposed for this high incidence include multiple CF loci, a high mutation rate, meiotic drive and heterozygote advantage. This latter explanation, possibly mediated by increased heterozygote resistance to chloride-secreting bacterial-induced diarrhoea, is thought to be the most likely although absolute proof is lacking.

Mapping and isolation of the CF gene

The CF locus was mapped to chromosome 7q31 in 1985 by the demonstration of linkage to the gene for a polymorphic enzyme known as paraoxanase. Shortly afterwards two polymorphic DNA marker loci, known as MET and D7S8, were shown to be closely linked flanking markers. The region between these markers was scrutinized for the presence of HTF or CpG islands, which are known to be present close to the 5′ end of many genes (p. 73). This led to the identification of several new DNA markers which were shown to be very tightly linked to the CF locus with recombination frequencies of less than 1%. These loci were found to be in linkage disequilibrium (p. 124) with the CF locus, and the CF mutation was found to be associated with one particular haplotype in 84% of cases. This discovery of linkage disequilibrium was consistent with the concept of a single original mutation being responsible for a large proportion of all CF genes. The identification of loci tightly linked to the CF locus narrowed its location down to a region of approximately 500 kb. Genes expressed in tissues involved in CF, such as lung and pancreas, and conserved between species were identified. The CF gene was eventually cloned by two groups of scientists in North America in 1989 by a combination of chromosome jumping, physical mapping, isolation of exon sequences and mutation analysis. It was named the CF transmembrane conductance regulator (CFTR) gene and was shown to span a genomic region of approximately 250 kb and to contain 27 exons.

The CFTR protein

The structure of *CFTR* is consistent with a protein product containing 1480 amino acids with a molecular weight of 168 kDa. It is believed to consist of two transmembrane (TM) domains which anchor it to the cell membrane, two nucleotide binding folds (NBF) which bind ATP, and a regulatory (R) domain, which is phosphorylated by protein kinase-A (Fig. 18.6).

The primary role of the CFTR protein is to act as a chloride channel. Activation by phosphorylation of the regulatory domain, followed by binding of ATP to the NBF domains, opens the outwardly rectifying chloride channel and exerts a negative effect on intracellular sodium absorption by closure of the epithelial sodium channel. The net effect is to reduce the level of intracellular sodium chloride, which improves the quality of cellular mucus secretions.

Mutations in the CFTR gene

The first mutation to be identified in *CFTR* was a deletion of three adjacent base pairs at the 508th codon which results in the loss of a phenylalanine residue. This mutation is known as ΔF508 (Δ for deletion and F for phenylalanine) and it has been shown to account for approximately 70% of all mutations in *CFTR* with the highest incidence of 88% being in Denmark (Table 18.3). The ΔF508 mutation can be demonstrated relatively simply by PCR (p. 58) using primers which flank the 508th codon (Fig. 18.7).

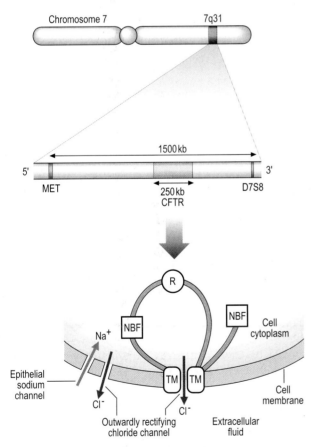

Fig. 18.6
The cystic fibrosis locus, gene and protein product which influences closely adjacent epithelial sodium and outwardly rectifying chloride channels. R = regulatory domain; NBF = nucleotide binding fold; TM = transmembrane domain.

Table 18.3   Contribution of ΔF508 mutation to all CF mutations

Country	%
Denmark	88
Netherlands	79
United Kingdom	78
Ireland	75
France	75
United States	66
Germany	65
Poland	55
Italy	50
Turkey	30

Data from European Working Group on CF Genetics (EWGCFG) Gradient of distribution in Europe of the major CF mutation and of its associated haplotype. Hum Genet 1990 85: 436–441, and Worldwide survey of the ΔF508 mutation – report from the cystic fibrosis genetic analysis consortium. Am J Hum Genet 1990 47: 354–359.

Fig. 18.7
PCR amplification of 98 and 95 bp DNA fragments surrounding the ΔF508 mutation site in the CF gene from a child with cystic fibrosis and his parents. The child, II₁, is homozygous for ΔF508. His parents, I₁ and I₂, are heterozygous, as is his sister II₂, confirming her carrier status.

Over 800 other mutations in *CFTR* have been identified. These include missense, frameshift, splice-site, nonsense and deletion mutations. Most of these are extremely uncommon, although a few can account for a small but significant proportion of mutations in a particular population. For example, the G542X and G551D mutations account for 12% and 3% of all CF mutations in the Ashkenazi Jewish and North American Caucasian populations respectively. A multiplex PCR technique has been developed which detects approximately 85% of all carriers. Using this it is possible to reduce the carrier risk for a healthy individual from a population risk of 1 in 22 to less than 1 in 140 (p. 297).

Genotype–phenotype correlation

Mutations in *CFTR* can influence the function of the protein product by:

1. causing a complete or partial reduction in its synthesis, e.g. G542X and IVS8-6(5T)
2. preventing it from reaching the epithelial membrane, e.g. ΔF508
3. causing it to function incorrectly when it reaches its final location, e.g. G551D and R117H.

The net effect of all these mutations is to reduce the normal functional activity of the CFTR protein. The extent to which normal CFTR protein activity is reduced correlates well with the clinical phenotype. Levels of less than 3% are associated with severe 'classic' CF, sometimes referred to as the PI type because of associated pancreatic insufficiency. Levels of activity between 3% and 8% cause a milder 'atypical' form of CF in which there is respiratory disease but relatively normal pancreatic function. This is referred to as the PS (pancreatic sufficient) form. Finally, levels of activity between 8% and 12% cause the mildest CF phenotype, in which the only clinical abnormality is CBAVD in males.

The relationship between genotype and phenotype is complex. Homozygotes for ΔF508 almost always have severe classical CF, as do compound heterozygotes with ΔF508 and G551D. The outcome for other compound heterozygote combinations can be much more difficult to predict. The complexity of the interaction between *CFTR* alleles is illustrated by the IVS8-6 mutation/ polymorphism. This contains a polythymidine tract in intron 8 which influences the splicing efficiency of exon 9 resulting in reduced synthesis of normal CFTR protein. Three variants consisting of 5T, 7T and 9T have been identified. The 9T variant is associated with normal activity. The 5T variant (i.e. IVS8-6(5T)) is the most common *CFTR* mutation seen in patients with CBAVD and is generally associated with a mild phenotype. Curiously it has been shown that the number of thymidine residues influences the effect of another mutation, R117H. When R117H is in *cis* with 5T (i.e. in the same allele) it causes severe CF when another CF mutation is present on the other allele. However when R117H is in *cis* with 7T it causes only CBAVD when present with another CF mutation. The diversity of known CF mutations and the complexity of their interactions at the molecular and protein levels can make it very difficult to predict the clinical outcome when counselling the parents of a compound heterozygote identified prenatally.

CLINICAL APPLICATIONS AND FUTURE PROSPECTS

Prior to the mapping of the CF locus and the subsequent isolation of *CFTR*, it was not possible to offer either carrier detection or reliable prenatal diagnosis. Now parents of an affected child can almost always be offered prenatal diagnosis, either by direct mutational analysis of DNA from chorionic villi, or by linkage analysis using polymorphic intragenic markers if one or both of the mutations in the affected child cannot be identified. Similarly, knowledge of one or both of the mutations in an affected child now permits the offer of carrier detection to close family relatives. In many parts of the world it is now standard practice to offer what is known as *cascade screening* to all families in which a mutation has been identified. Population screening for carriers of CF (p. 318) and neonatal screening for CF homozygotes

(p. 317) have been widely implemented and are discussed elsewhere.

CF is a prime candidate for gene therapy because of the relative accessibility of the crucial target organs, i.e. the lungs. Gene transfer studies carried out using adenoviruses and *CFTR* cDNA liposome complexes have resulted in the restoration of chloride secretion in CF transgenic mice. Several clinical trials have been undertaken in small groups of volunteer CF patients. Although there has been experimental evidence of *CFTR* expression in the treated patients, this has generally been transient. Problems have been encountered with poor vector efficiency and inflammatory reactions, particularly when adenoviruses have been used as the vector. Despite these initial problems there is cautious optimism that effective gene therapy for CF will be developed within the next decade.

SPINAL MUSCULAR ATROPHY

Spinal muscular atrophy (SMA) is the term used to describe a clinically and genetically heterogeneous group of disorders which are among the most common genetic causes of death in childhood. The disease is characterized by degeneration of the anterior horn cells of the spinal cord leading to progressive muscle weakness and ultimately death.

Three common childhood forms of SMA are recognized with a collective incidence of approximately 1 in 10 000 and carrier frequency of 1 in 50. Of these type I SMA is the most common and the most severe.

CLINICAL FEATURES

Type I SMA (Werdnig–Hoffmann disease)

Children with type I SMA present at birth or in the first 6 months of life with severe hypotonia and lack of spontaneous movement. Sometimes the mother will have noticed that intra-uterine fetal movements were reduced in both strength and frequency. These children show normal intellectual activity but their profound muscle weakness, which affects swallowing and respiratory function, leads to death within the first 2 years of life. The diagnosis is confirmed by electromyography and there is no effective means of treating the disorder or even delaying its rate of progression.

Type II SMA

This is less severe than type I with an age of onset being between 6 and 18 months. As in type I SMA, muscle weakness and hypotonia are the main presenting features. These children are able to sit unaided but are never able to achieve independent locomotion. The rate of progression is slow and most affected children survive into early adult life.

Type III SMA (Kugelberg–Welander disease)

In this relatively mild form of childhood or juvenile onset SMA the age of onset is after 18 months and all patients are able to walk without support. Slowly progressive muscle weakness results in many affected individuals having to use a wheelchair by early adult life. Long-term survival can be jeopardized by recurrent respiratory infection and the development of a scoliosis caused by weakness of the spinal muscles.

GENETICS

All three types of childhood onset SMA show autosomal recessive inheritance. Several other much rarer forms of spinal muscular atrophy have been described, and among these all forms of Mendelian inheritance have been noted. Type I SMA generally shows a high degree of intrafamilial concordance with affected siblings showing an almost identical clinical course. In types II and III SMA, intrafamilial variation can be quite marked.

Mapping the SMA locus

Using linkage analysis all three childhood forms of SMA were mapped to the long arm of chromosome 5 in 1990. Subsequently linkage analysis and physical mapping narrowed the disease locus down to a region of approximately 1000 kb which has been shown to consist of a 500 kb inverted duplication (Fig. 18.8). This region of chromosome 5q is notable for its high rate of instability with several DNA duplications and a relatively large number of pseudogenes (p. 15).

Isolating the SMA gene(s)

The search for the childhood SMA gene(s) within this 500 kb inverted duplication region has yielded confusing and conflicting results. However, two distinct genes have been isolated which show a high incidence of deletion in SMA patients. Each of these is present as two almost identical copies. One, the survival motor neurone (*SMN*) gene shows homozygous deletion of exons 7 and 8 in the telomeric copy (*SMN^T*) in around 95% of all childhood onset SMA patients. Point mutations in *SMN^T* have been identified in some of the 1–2% of childhood SMA patients who do not show *SMN^T* deletions. A closely adjacent gene known as *NAIP*, which codes for the neuronal apoptosis inhibitory protein, is deleted in

Fig. 18.8
The inverted duplication with the *SMN* and *NAIP* genes, which are deleted in childhood spinal muscular atrophy. *SMN* = survival motor neurone; *NAIP* = neuronal apoptosis inhibitory protein.

approximately 45% of individuals with type I SMA and up to 20% of those with type II and type III SMA. These observations suggest that most cases of childhood SMA result from homozygous deletions involving the telomeric copy of *SMN* and possibly extending to involve the closely adjacent *NAIP*ᵀ gene. This interpretation of the results observed in several studies has been questioned by the description of a small number of carrier parents and unaffected siblings of patients who have been found to be homozygous for deletions of *NAIP*ᵀ and/or *SMN*ᵀ. These apparent contradictions indicate that other modifying genes may play a role in disease expression. This would be consistent with the clinical observation that types II and III SMA can show intrafamilial discordance in siblings.

CLINICAL APPLICATIONS AND FUTURE PROSPECTS

On the one hand the discovery of *SMN* and *NAIP* deletions in SMA has raised the possibility of prenatal diagnosis for those families who feel that this is appropriate. On the other hand the confusion surrounding the occasional demonstration of homozygous deletions in apparently unaffected siblings and parents has created concern that prenatal diagnosis based on deletion analysis would not always be 100% accurate. Carrier detection based on deletion analysis is difficult because of the presence of other copies of *SMN* and *NAIP* in the inverted duplication. Successful therapeutic intervention will almost certainly have to await a fuller understanding of the underlying molecular mechanisms and identification of the relevant protein product(s). Overexpression, by upregulation, of the centromeric copy of *SMN* has been proposed as an attractive but as yet unachievable treatment option.

DUCHENNE MUSCULAR DYSTROPHY

Duchenne muscular dystrophy (DMD) is the commonest and most severe form of muscular dystrophy. The eponymous title is derived from the French neurologist, Guillaume Duchenne, who described a case in 1861. A similar but milder condition known as Becker muscular dystrophy (BMD) is caused by mutations in the same gene. The incidences of DMD and BMD are approximately 1 in 3500 males and 1 in 20 000 males respectively. There is no effective cure for either of these disorders.

CLINICAL FEATURES

Males with DMD usually present between the ages of 3 and 5 years with slowly progressive muscle weakness resulting in an awkward gait, inability to run quickly and difficulty in rising from the floor which can be achieved only by pushing on, or 'climbing up', the legs and thighs (Gowers' sign). Most affected boys have to use a wheelchair by the age of 11 years because of severe proximal muscle weakness in the lower limbs. Subsequent deterioration leads to a lumbar lordosis, joint contractures and cardio-respiratory failure leading to death at a mean age of 18 years.

On examination boys with DMD show an apparent increase in the size of the calf muscles which is actually due to replacement of muscle fibres by fat and connective tissue. This is referred to as *pseudohypertrophy* (Fig. 18.9) and DMD is sometimes known as pseudohypertrophic muscular dystrophy. In addition, approximately one-third of boys with DMD show mild to moderate intellectual impairment with the mean IQ of all cases being 83.

In BMD the clinical picture is very similar but the disease process runs a much less aggressive course. The mean age of onset is 11 years and many patients remain ambulant until well into adult life. Overall life expectancy is only slightly reduced. A few patients with proven mutations in the DMD/BMD gene have been asymptomatic in their fifth or sixth decade.

GENETICS

Both DMD and BMD show X-linked recessive inheritance. Males with DMD rarely, if ever, reproduce. Therefore as genetic fitness equals zero, the mutation rate equals the incidence in affected males divided by 3

The probable location of the DMD gene at Xp21 was soon confirmed by the discovery of affected males with visible microdeletions involving Xp21 and by linkage analysis using polymorphic DNA markers from the Xp21 region. This led to the next phase of the isolation of the gene whereby intragenic probes were used to identify conserved sequences in muscle cDNA libraries which were shown to consist of exons from the actual DMD gene. The full transcribed sequence was isolated in 1987 in a series of overlapping cDNA clones.

The DMD gene was found to be the largest yet identified in humans. It consists of 2.3 megabases of genomic DNA, of which only 14 kb are transcribed into mRNA. The gene contains 79 exons and is transcribed not only in muscle but also in brain which probably explains why some boys with DMD show learning difficulties. The very large size of the gene probably explains its high mutation rate and why a number of women with X-autosome translocations were identified.

Mutations in the DMD gene

Deletions of part or all of the gene account for two-thirds of all mutations. These differ in their size and in their position. They arise almost exclusively in maternal meiosis, probably due to unequal crossing over. A small number of affected males with duplications have also been described. Two deletion 'hot spots' exist, one involving the first 20 exons and the other in the centre of the gene around exons 45–53. One of the deletion break-point 'hot spots' in intron 7 contains a cluster of transposon-like repetitive DNA sequences which could facilitate misalignment in meiosis with a subsequent cross-over leading to deletion and duplication products.

The size of the deletion does not correlate with disease severity. However, deletions which cause DMD usually disturb the translational reading frame (p. 23). In contrast deletions seen in males with BMD usually do not alter the reading frame so that the amino acid sequence of the protein product of the DMD gene downstream of the deletion is normal. This probably explains why the clinical features in BMD are relatively mild. In clinical practice deletions are usually detected by a multiplex-PCR technique in which several exons are amplified simultaneously. The presence of a deletion is then confirmed by Southern blotting.

Mutations identified in the remaining one-third of affected boys include stop codons, frameshift mutations, altered splicing signals and promoter mutations. Most point mutations in DMD lead to premature translational termination resulting in the production of little if any protein product. In contrast to deletions, point mutations in the DMD gene usually arise in paternal meiosis, most probably due to a copy error in DNA replication.

Fig. 18.9
Lower limbs of an adult male with Becker muscular dystrophy showing proximal wasting and calf pseudohypertrophy.

(p. 117), which approximates to 1 in 10 000. This is one of the highest known mutation rates in humans.

Isolation of the DMD gene

The isolation of the DMD gene represented a major scientific achievement and is an excellent example of a successfully applied positional cloning strategy. The initial clue to the site of the DMD locus was provided by reports of several females affected with DMD who had a balanced X-autosome translocation with a common X chromosome break-point at Xp21. In these women those cells in which the derivative X chromosome is randomly inactivated are at a major disadvantage due to inactivation of the autosomal segment (Fig. 6.14, p. 104). Consequently cells in which the normal X chromosome has been randomly inactivated are more likely to survive. The net result is that the derivative X-autosome is active in most cell lines and if the break-point has damaged an important gene, such as the DMD gene, then the woman will be affected by whatever disease results from interruption of that gene.

The gene product – dystrophin

The DMD gene encodes a 427 kDa protein known as *dystrophin*. This is located close to the muscle membrane where it links intracellular actin with extracellular laminin. Absence of dystrophin, as occurs in males with DMD, results in gradual muscle cell degeneration. The presence of dystrophin in a muscle biopsy sample can be assessed by immunofluorescence. Levels of less than 3% are diagnostic of DMD. In muscle biopsies from males with BMD the dystrophin shows qualitative rather than gross quantitative abnormalities.

Dystrophin binds to a glycoprotein complex in the muscle membrane through its C-terminal domain (Fig. 18.10). This glycoprotein complex consists of several subunits, abnormalities of which cause other rare genetic muscle disorders including several different types of autosomal recessive and congenital muscular dystrophy.

Carrier detection

Until molecular methods were available carrier detection was based on pedigree analysis combined with creatine kinase assay in serum (p. 288). Creatine kinase is grossly elevated in the serum of boys with DMD and is marginally increased in approximately two-thirds of all carriers (Fig. 19.1, p. 288). Creatine kinase assay is still used occasionally as an adjunct in carrier detection and family studies, but its lack of sensitivity has led to it being superseded by DNA analysis.

Accurate carrier detection can now be achieved for most female relatives of affected DMD/BMD males by direct mutation/deletion analysis or indirectly by linkage studies using polymorphic intragenic markers. If a microsatellite maps to the site of a deletion, then study of the segregation of the microsatellite marker in a family will often provide conclusive evidence of carrier status in relevant female relatives (Fig. 19.2, p. 289). Care

has to be taken when using linkage for carrier detection because there is a high recombination rate of 12% across the DMD gene.

PROSPECTS FOR TREATMENT

At present there is no cure for DMD or BMD, although physiotherapy is beneficial for maintaining mobility and preventing muscle spasm and joint contractures.

Gene therapy offers the only realistic hope of a cure in the short to medium term. Several approaches have been tried experimentally in transgenic and naturally occurring mutant mice with dystrophin-negative muscular dystrophy. These include direct injection of recombinant DNA, myoblast implantation and transfection with retroviral or adenoviral vectors carrying a dystrophin *minigene* containing only those sequences which code for the important functional domains. The fact that mice with dystrophin-negative muscular dystrophy can show spontaneous muscle repair indicates that there could be a way of switching on an alternative compensatory protein such as utrophin. This is expressed in the fetus instead of dystrophin with which it shares a large degree of homology. Genetically engineered mice which are deficient for both dystrophin and utrophin develop a typical Duchenne-like form of muscular dystrophy. If the utrophin gene could be reactivated as in the dystrophin-negative mouse, this could have a striking beneficial therapeutic effect in affected boys.

HAEMOPHILIA

There are two forms of haemophilia — A and B. Haemophilia A is the most common severe inherited coagulation disorder with an incidence of 1 in 5000 males. It is caused by a deficiency of factor VIII which, together with factor IX, plays a critical role in the intrinsic pathway activation of prothrombin to thrombin. Thrombin then converts fibrinogen to fibrin which forms the structural framework of clotted blood. The existence of haemophilia was recognized in the Talmud and the tendency for males to be affected much more often than females was acknowledged by the Jewish authorities 2000 years ago when they excused from circumcision the sons of the sisters of a mother who had an affected son. Queen Victoria was a carrier and as well as having an affected son, Leopold Duke of Albany, she transmitted the disorder through two of her daughters to most of the royal families of Europe (Fig. 18.11).

Haemophilia B affects approximately 1 in 40 000 males and is caused by deficiency of factor IX. It is also known as Christmas disease whereas haemophilia A is sometimes referred to as 'classical haemophilia'.

Fig. 18.10
Probable structure of the dystrophin protein molecule, which is depicted as a dimer linking intracellular actin with extracellular laminin. (Adapted from Ervasti J M, Campbell K P 1991 Membrane organization of the dystrophin–glycoprotein complex. Cell 66: 1121–1131.)

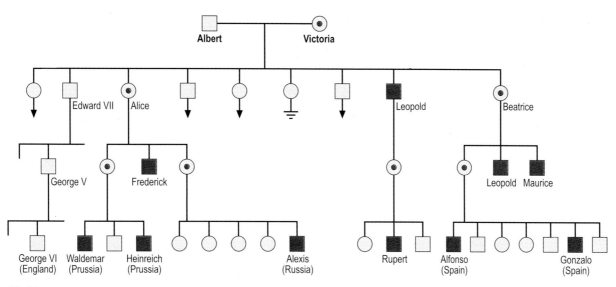

Fig. 18.11

Pedigree showing the segregation of haemophilia among Queen Victoria's descendants.

CLINICAL FEATURES

These are similar in both forms of haemophilia and vary from mild bleeding following major trauma or surgery to spontaneous haemorrhage into muscles and joints. The degree of severity shows a close correlation with the reduction in factor VIII or IX activity. Levels below 1% are usually associated with a severe haemorrhagic tendency dating from birth. Haemorrhage into joints causes severe pain and swelling which, if recurrent, causes a progressive arthropathy with severe disability (Fig. 18.12). Affected family members generally show the same degree of severity.

GENETICS

Both forms of haemophilia show sex-linked recessive inheritance. The loci lie close together near the distal end of the long arm of the X chromosome.

Haemophilia A

The factor VIII gene is relatively large spanning 186 kb with 26 exons and a 9 kb mRNA transcript. Deletions account for 5% of all cases and usually cause complete absence of factor VIII expression. Frameshift, nonsense and missense mutations have also been described, as have insertions and a 'flip' inversion which represented a new form of mutation when first identified in haemophilia A in 1993. These inversions account for 50% of all severe cases, i.e. those cases with less than 1% factor VIII activity. They are caused by recombination between a small gene called A located within intron 22 of the factor VIII gene and other copies of the A gene which are located upstream near the telomere (Fig. 18.13). This

Fig. 18.12

The lower limbs of a male with haemophilia showing the effect of recurrent haemorrhage into the knees. (Courtesy of Dr G Dolan, University Hospital, Nottingham.)

inversion results in disruption of the factor VIII gene and very low factor VIII activity. It can be detected relatively simply by Southern blotting in contrast to the numerous

Fig. 18.13
How intrachromosomal recombination causes the 'flip' inversion which is the most common mutation found in severe haemophilia A. (Adapted from Lakich D, Kazazian H H, Antonarakis S E, Gitschier J 1993 Inversions disrupting the factor VIII gene are a common cause of severe haemophilia A. Nat Genet 5: 236–241.)

other heterogeneous mutations which require more complex methods of analysis such as SSCP, DGGE and chemical mismatch cleavage (p. 63).

Recent studies have shown that, as in Duchenne muscular dystrophy, point mutations usually originate in male germ cells whereas deletions arise mainly in the female, probably as a consequence of unequal crossing over. The 'flip' inversions show a greater than tenfold higher mutation rate in male than in female germ cells. This is probably because the long arm of the X chromosome does not pair with a homologous chromosome in male meiosis, so that there is much greater opportunity for intra-chromosomal recombination to occur via looping of the distal end of the long arm (Fig. 18.13).

Carrier detection used to be based on assay of the ratio of factor VIII coagulant activity to the level of factor VIII antigen, but, as with creatine kinase estimation in Duchenne muscular dystrophy, this does not provide clear discrimination between carriers and non-carriers. This approach has been superseded by linkage analysis, using polymorphic intragenic markers, and specific mutation analysis. Prenatal diagnosis is sometimes requested in families with severe haemophilia A. This can usually be achieved by mutation or linkage analysis.

Haemophilia B

The gene for factor IX is 34 kb long and contains eight exons. Over 400 different point mutations, deletions and insertions have been reported, for which a complete international database is maintained in a central registry. By analysing only 2.2 kb of the gene it is possible to detect the mutation in 96% of all patients. The remaining mutations can be identified by sequencing the rest of the gene.

A rare variant form known as haemophilia B-Leyden shows the extremely unusual characteristic of age-dependent expression. During childhood the disease is very severe with factor IX levels of less than 1%. After puberty these levels rise to around 50% of normal and the condition resolves to become asymptomatic. Haemophilia B-Leyden has been shown to be caused by mutations in the promoter region.

Factor IX levels are now rarely used in carrier detection and prenatal diagnosis, both of which are achieved much more reliably by linkage analysis or direct mutation analysis.

TREATMENT

Both forms of haemophilia have been treated successfully for many years using plasma-derived factor VIII or factor IX. Factor VIII is concentrated in the cryoprecipitate fraction of plasma and has been used widely for replacement therapy. It has a half-life of 8 hours so that repeated infusions are necessary for elective surgery or major trauma.

Two major disadvantages emerged using this approach. The first was that the purification process for preparation of cryoprecipitate did not prevent transmission of viral infection such as hepatitis B and HIV, with the inevitable disastrous consequence that many males with haemophilia contracted the acquired immune deficiency syndrome (AIDS). This problem of viral contamination was overcome by better purification and screening processes. In addition recombinant factor VIII became available in 1994, although expense has been a limiting factor in its widespread introduction.

The second disadvantage was that around 10% of patients with both forms of haemophilia developed inhibitory antibodies to the relevant factor which their immune systems recognized as a foreign agent. This problem can sometimes be overcome using porcine factor VIII or by immunosuppression.

Haemophilia A and B are excellent candidates for gene therapy as only a slight increase in the plasma level of the relevant factor is of major clinical benefit. Studies in dogs and mice with haemophilia B have shown encouraging results using an adeno-associated viral vector expressing factor IX which is injected into skeletal muscle. The early results of similar studies in severely affected humans are encouraging with evidence that severe disease can be converted to a much milder form.

FURTHER READING

Biros I, Forrest S 1999 Spinal muscular atrophy: untangling the knot? J Med Genet 36: 1–8
A contemporary account of current understanding of the genetic basis of childhood spinal muscular atrophy.

Brown T, Schwind E L 1999 Update and review: cystic fibrosis. J Genet Counseling 8: 137–162
A useful review of recent genetic developments in cystic fibrosis.

Collinge J 1997 Human prion diseases and bovine spongiform encephalopathy (BSE). Hum Mol Genet 6: 1699–1705
A clear account of human prion diseases and their known causes with particular reference to BSE.

Emery A E H 1993 Duchenne muscular dystrophy, 2nd edn. Oxford University Press, Oxford.
A detailed monograph reviewing the history, clinical features and genetics of Duchenne and Becker muscular dystrophy.

Harper P S 1991 Huntington's disease. W B Saunders, London
A comprehensive review of the clinical aspects of Huntington's disease.

Huson S M, Hughes R A C (eds) 1994 The neurofibromatoses. Chapman & Hall, London
A very thorough description of the different types of neurofibromatosis. Includes a chapter on the 'Elephant Man'.

Karpati G, Pari G, Molnar M J 1999 Molecular therapy for genetic muscle diseases — status 1999. Clin Genet 55: 1–8
An optimistic review of possible approaches to gene therapy for inherited muscle disorders such as Duchenne muscular dystrophy.

Kay M A, Manno C S, Ragni, M V et al 2000 Evidence for gene transfer and expression of factor IX in haemophilia B patients treated with an AV vector. Nat Genet 24: 257–261
Report of provisional encouraging results of gene therapy in patients with haemophilia B.

Lakich D, Kazazian H H, Antonarakis S E, Gitschier J 1993 Inversions disrupting the factor VIII gene are a common cause of severe haemophilia A. Nat Genet 5: 236–241
The first report showing how the common 'flip' inversion is generated.

ELEMENTS

1 Huntington's disease is an autosomal dominant disorder characterized by choreiform movements and progressive dementia. The disease locus has been mapped to the short arm of chromosome 4 and the mutational basis involves expansion of a CAG triple repeat sequence. Meiotic instability is greater in the male than in the female, which probably explains why the severe 'juvenile' onset form is almost always inherited from a more mildly affected father.

2 Myotonic dystrophy shows autosomal dominant inheritance and is characterized by slowly progressive weakness and myotonia. The disease locus has been mapped to chromosome 19 and the mutational basis involves expansion of an unstable CTG triple repeat sequence. The range of meiotic expansion is greater in the female than in the male, which almost certainly accounts for the almost exclusive maternal inheritance of the severe 'congenital' form.

3 Hereditary motor and sensory neuropathy (HMSN) includes several clinically and genetically heterogeneous disorders characterized by slowly progressive distal muscle weakness and wasting. HMSN Ia has been mapped to chromosome 17 and is usually caused by duplication of a gene (*PMP-22*) which encodes a protein present in the myelin membrane of peripheral nerve. The reciprocal deletion product of the unequal cross-over event which generates a duplication causes a mild disorder known as hereditary liability to pressure palsies.

4 Neurofibromatosis type I (NF1) shows autosomal dominant inheritance with complete penetrance and variable expression. The NF1 gene has been mapped to chromosome 17 where it encodes a protein known as neurofibromin. This normally acts as a tumour suppressor by inactivating the *RAS*-mediated signal transduction of mitogenic signalling.

5 Human prion diseases are rare, progressive, fatal disorders of the central nervous system caused by the deposition of a modified prion protein PrP^{Sc} which is transmittable and has the unique ability to replicate itself by associating with normal host-encoded prion protein PrP^C. Most cases in humans are sporadic and probably result from acquired somatic mutations in the prion protein gene *PRNP*.

6 Cystic fibrosis (CF) shows autosomal recessive inheritance and is characterized by recurrent chest infection and malabsorption. The CF locus has been mapped to chromosome 7, where the gene (*CFTR*) encodes the cystic fibrosis transmembrane receptor protein. This acts as a chloride channel and controls the level of intracellular sodium chloride, which in turn influences the viscosity of mucous secretions.

7 The childhood forms of spinal muscular atrophy (SMA) are characterized by hypotonia and progressive muscle weakness. They show autosomal recessive inheritance and the disease locus has been mapped to chromosome 5q13. This region shows a high incidence of instability with duplication of a 500 kb fragment containing two genes (*SMN, NAIP*) which are deleted in a high proportion of patients.

8 Duchenne muscular dystrophy (DMD) shows X-linked recessive inheritance, with most carriers being entirely healthy. The DMD locus has been mapped to chromosome Xp21 and is the largest known in humans. The gene product, dystrophin, links intracellular actin with extracellular laminin. The commonest mutational mechanism is a deletion which disturbs the translational reading frame. Deletions which maintain the reading frame cause the milder Becker form of muscular dystrophy.

9 Haemophilia A is the most common severe inherited coagulation disorder in humans. It shows X-linked recessive inheritance and is caused by a deficiency of factor VIII. The most common mutation in severe haemophilia A is caused by a 'flip' inversion which disrupts the factor VIII gene at intron 22. Treatment with factor VIII replacement therapy is very effective and the results of gene therapy in animal models offer hope that this will soon be possible in humans.

Carrier detection and presymptomatic diagnosis

If it was easy to recognize carriers of autosomal and X-linked recessive disorders and persons who are heterozygous for autosomal dominant disorders which show reduced penetrance or a late age of onset, much doubt and uncertainty would be removed when providing information in genetic counselling. A number of tests of different types are available to detect carriers for autosomal and X-linked recessive disorders and for presymptomatic diagnosis of heterozygotes for autosomal dominant disorders.

CARRIER TESTING FOR AUTOSOMAL RECESSIVE AND X-LINKED DISORDERS

In a number of autosomal recessive disorders, such as some of the inborn errors of metabolism, e.g. Tay-Sachs disease (p. 163), and the haemoglobinopathies, e.g. sickle-cell disease (p. 142), carriers can be recognized with a high degree of certainty using biochemical or haematological techniques. In other single gene disorders, it is possible to detect or confirm carrier status by biochemical means in a proportion of carriers, e.g. the presence of abnormal coagulation studies in a woman at risk of being a carrier for haemophilia (p. 284). A significant proportion of obligate carriers of haemophilia will have normal coagulation, however, so that a normal result in a woman at risk does not exclude her from being a carrier.

There are several possible ways in which carriers of genetic diseases can be recognized.

CLINICAL MANIFESTATIONS IN CARRIERS

Occasionally, carriers for certain disorders can have mild clinical manifestations of the disease (Table 19.1), particularly with some of the X-linked disorders. These manifestations are usually so slight that they will only be apparent on careful clinical examination. Such mani-

Table 19.1 Clinical and biochemical abnormalities used in carrier detection of X-linked disorders

Disorder	Abnormality
Clinical	
Ocular albinism	Mosaic retinal pigmentary pattern
Retinitis pigmentosa	Mosaic retinal pigmentation, abnormal electroretinogram
Anhidrotic ectodermal dysplasia	Sweat pore counts reduced, dental anomalies
Lowe's syndrome	Lens opacities
Alport's syndrome	Haematuria
Biochemical	
Haemophilia A	Reduced factor VIII activity:antigen ratio
Haemophilia B	Reduced levels of factor IX
G6PD deficiency	Erythrocyte G6PD activity reduced
Lesch–Nyhan syndrome	Reduced hypoxanthine-guanine phosphoribosyl transferase activity in skin fibroblasts
Hunter's syndrome	Reduced sulphoiduronate sulphatase activity in skin fibroblasts
Vitamin D-resistant rickets	Serum phosphate level reduced
Duchenne muscular dystrophy	Elevated serum creatine kinase level
Becker muscular dystrophy	Elevated serum creatine kinase level
Fabry's disease	Reduced α-galactosidase activity in hair root follicles

festations, even though minimal are unmistakably pathological, e.g. the mosaic pattern of retinal pigmentation seen in manifesting female carriers of X-linked ocular albinism. Unfortunately, in most autosomal and X-linked recessive disorders there are either no manifestations at all in carriers or they overlap with variation seen in the general population. An example would be female carriers of haemophilia, who have a tendency to bruise easily. This would not, however, be a reliable sign of carrier status as a significant proportion of the general population have this tendency. Thus clinical manifestations are only of importance in detecting carriers when they are unmistakably pathological, and this is the exception rather than the rule with most single gene disorders.

BIOCHEMICAL ABNORMALITIES IN CARRIERS

By far the most important approach to determining the carrier status for autosomal recessive and X-linked disorders has been the demonstration of detectable biochemical abnormalities in carriers of certain diseases (Table 19.1). In some disorders the biochemical abnormality seen is a direct product of the gene and the carrier status can be tested for with confidence. For example, in carriers of Tay–Sachs disease the range of enzyme activity is intermediate between levels found in normal and affected persons. In many inborn errors of metabolism, however, the enzyme activity levels in carriers overlap with the normal range so that it is not possible to reliably distinguish between carriers and normal individuals.

In many single gene disorders, however, the biochemical abnormality used in the diagnosis of the disorder in the affected individual is not a direct result of action of the gene product but the consequence of a secondary or downstream process. Such abnormalities are further from the primary action of the gene and consequently are usually even less likely to be useful in distinguishing carriers from the general population. For example, in Duchenne muscular dystrophy (DMD) there appears to be an increased permeability of the muscle membrane as a result of the dystrophic process which results in an escape of muscle enzymes into the blood. An elevated serum creatine kinase (CK) is used as one of the clinical investigations to confirm the diagnosis of DMD in a boy presenting with features of the disorder (p. 280). Obligate carrier females of DMD have, on average, serum CK levels which are elevated when compared to the general female population (Fig. 19.1). There is, however, an overlap of CK values between normal and obligate carrier females. This information can, however, be used in conjunction with pedigree risk information (p. 298) and the results of linked DNA markers (p. 68) to help predict the likelihood of a woman being a carrier for this disorder.

There is another reason for difficulty with carrier testing in the case of X-linked recessive disorders. Random inactivation of the X chromosome in females (p. 92) means that many, often the majority, of female carriers of X-linked disorders cannot be reliably detected by biochemical methods. An exception to this involves analysis of individual clones to look for evidence of two populations of cells, as can be done with peripheral blood lymphocytes in female carriers of some of the X-linked immunodeficiency syndromes (p. 185).

LINKAGE BETWEEN A DISEASE LOCUS AND A POLYMORPHIC MARKER

Demonstration of linkage between the gene for a hereditary disorder and a polymorphic marker (p. 68) can

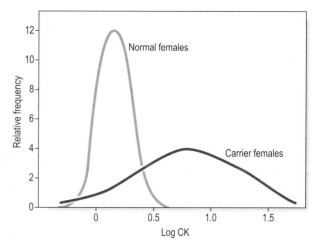

Fig. 19.1
Creatine kinase levels in obligate carrier females of Duchenne muscular dystrophy and women from the general population. (Adapted from Tippett P A, Dennis N R, Machin D, Price C P, Clayton B E 1982 Creatine kinase activity in the detection of carriers of Duchenne muscular dystrophy: comparison of two methods. Clin Chim Acta 121: 345–359.)

be used in determining the carrier status of persons at risk in a family.

Biochemical and blood group polymorphic markers

The close linkage between the loci for glucose-6-phosphate dehydrogenase (G6PD) deficiency (p. 171) and haemophilia A (p. 282) could provide a possible means of determining carrier status for females at risk of being carriers for haemophilia A. Unfortunately, polymorphisms at the G6PD locus are not commonly found in most populations so that use of this approach is usually uninformative for determining carrier status of females at risk. The small number of conventional biochemical and blood group polymorphisms which are informative has meant they have been of limited use in determining carrier status.

DNA polymorphic markers

Developments in recombinant DNA technology have revolutionized the approach to carrier detection. The large number of different types of DNA sequence variants (p. 16) in the human genome means that if sufficient numbers of families are available, linkage of any disease with a polymorphic DNA marker is possible. The demonstration of linkage between a DNA sequence variant and a disease locus overcomes the need to identify a biochemical defect or protein marker and the necessity for it to be expressed in accessible tissues. In addition, use of markers at the DNA level also overcomes the difficulties which occur in carrier detection due to X-inactivation for women at risk for X-linked disorders (p. 92).

Linked polymorphic DNA markers are frequently used in determining the carrier status of females in families at risk for Duchenne muscular dystrophy. An example is shown in Figure 19.2 in which individual III₃ presents for genetic counselling wanting to know whether she is a carrier and therefore at risk for having sons affected with DMD. Analysis of the pedigree reveals that her mother, II₄, along with her sister, II₁, and their mother, I₂, are all obligate carriers of DMD. The family is informative for a polymorphic CA dinucleotide repeat (p. 16) in the closely flanking region 5′ to the dystrophin gene known as Dys 5′ II which can be demonstrated by PCR (p. 58). The mutation in the dystrophin gene in the family is segregating with allele 1 and, since individual III₃ has inherited this allele from her mother, she is likely to be a carrier. Linked polymorphic DNA markers can be used for prenatal diagnosis to predict whether a male fetus is likely to be affected with DMD, even in the absence of identifying a specific mutation in the dystrophin gene in the affected male(s) in the family (p. 282).

Fig. 19.2
Family with Duchenne muscular dystrophy showing segregation of the CA repeat 5′ to the dystrophin gene known as Dys 5′ II. (Courtesy of J Rowland, Yorkshire Regional DNA Laboratory, St James's Hospital, Leeds.)

Potential pitfalls with linked polymorphic DNA markers

There are a number of potential pitfalls to keep in mind with the use of linked polymorphic DNA markers.

Recombination

The first potential pitfall is the chance of recombination occurring between the polymorphic DNA marker and the disease locus to which linkage has been shown. The risk of a recombination can be minimized, in most instances, by the identification of either intragenic or closely linked markers on either side of the disease locus, or what are termed *flanking* markers. In some instances such as with the dystrophin locus, however, there is a 'hot spot' for recombination (p. 282). Even with closely flanking or intragenic markers there appears to be a minimal chance of approximately 12% that recombination will occur in any meiosis in a female. The uncertainty introduced by this possibility needs to be taken into account when combining the results of linked polymorphic DNA markers with pedigree risks and the results of CK testing for women at risk of being carriers of DMD (p. 299).

Sample availability

The use of linked polymorphic DNA markers means that samples from the appropriate family members are required and therefore their cooperation is essential. This can prove difficult depending on relationships within the family and the need to maintain confidentiality of individual family members. In addition, families and physicians with individuals affected with lethal inherited disorders, such as DMD and the severe form of the autosomal recessive disorder spinal muscular atrophy (Werdnig–Hoffmann disease), need to have the foresight to arrange for DNA to be banked from the affected individual(s). For example, it is not unusual that by the time a younger sister of a male with DMD seeks advice about her carrier status, the affected male will no longer be alive. If the family structure is suitable, e.g. there are one or more unaffected males in the pedigree, it is often possible to 'reconstruct' the likely alleles of the linked polymorphic DNA markers in the affected male. This will, however, affect the risk estimation in the pedigree as the phase of the marker in the affected male cannot be known with certainty (p. 299).

Polymorphic variation

Another problem which can be encountered in the use of linked DNA markers is whether the family possesses the necessary variation in a linked marker to be what is known as *informative*. This is now very rare with the large number of different types of DNA sequence variants in the human genome available, especially the variable number tandem repeat sequences such as CA dinucleotide repeats (p. 16). It will also become less of a problem as specific mutational analysis becomes available for an increasingly greater number of single gene disorders.

PRESYMPTOMATIC DIAGNOSIS OF AUTOSOMAL DOMINANT DISORDERS

There are a number of single gene disorders inherited in an autosomal dominant manner which either have a delayed age of onset (p. 295) or exhibit reduced penetrance (p. 295). The results of clinical examination, specialist investigations, biochemical studies and family DNA studies can allow one to predict whether a person has inherited the gene before the onset of symptoms or signs. This is known as *presymptomatic diagnosis* or *predictive testing* (Table 19.2).

CLINICAL EXAMINATION

In a number of dominantly inherited disorders simple clinical means can be used for presymptomatic diagnosis, taking into account possible pleiotropic effects of a gene (p. 97). For example, persons with the dominantly inherited disorder known as neurofibromatosis type I (NF1) can have a number of different clinical features (p. 272). It is not unusual to examine an apparently unaffected relative of someone with NF1 who has had no medical problems, only to discover that they have sufficient numbers of a diagnostic feature, such as café-au-lait spots or cutaneous neurofibroma(ta), to confirm that they are affected.

SPECIALIST INVESTIGATION

Evidence of clinical involvement of multiple different systems of the body with a number of autosomal dominantly inherited disorders can be utilized as a means of presymptomatic diagnosis. For example, in

---

Table 19.2 Autosomal disorders which show a delayed age of onset or exhibit reduced penetrance in which linked DNA markers or specific mutational analysis can be used to offer presymptomatic diagnosis

Adult onset polycystic kidney disease
Familial adenomatous polyposis
Familial hypercholesterolaemia
Hereditary motor and sensory neuropathy type I
Huntington's disease
Marfan's syndrome
Myotonic dystrophy
Neurofibromatosis type I
Neurofibromatosis type II
Retinitis pigmentosa
Tuberous sclerosis
von Hippel–Lindau disease

---

persons at risk for inheriting NF1, the presence of characteristic areas of pigmentation in the iris, known as Lisch nodules, would suggest that they have inherited the gene. 15% of the general population, however, have Lisch nodules, so that their presence in a person at risk for NF1 does not confirm that they have inherited the NF1 gene. The presence of other clinical features of NF1, such as café-au-lait spots or cutaneous neurofibroma(ta), would be needed to confirm the diagnosis (p. 272).

Persons affected with the dominantly inherited disorder known as tuberous sclerosis (TSC) usually have evidence of involvement in a number of systems of the body. This can include intracranial calcification in the central nervous system (Fig. 19.3) and cysts or a disordered growth in the kidneys known as an angiomyolipoma(ta) (Fig. 19.4). Use of relatively non-invasive tests such as computerized axial tomography of the central nervous system or renal ultrasound in relatives of persons with TSC can detect evidence of the TSC gene in asymptomatic persons.

In myotonic dystrophy, a dominantly inherited muscle disorder, in which affected persons have an inability to relax muscles normally, an electromyogram (EMG) can be used to confirm the diagnosis by detecting the presence of an abnormal spontaneous discharge of electrical activity which occurs with the insertion of the

Fig. 19.3
Intracranial calcification (arrowed) in an asymptomatic person with tuberous sclerosis.

electrode into the muscle. This discharge does not occur in muscle from unaffected persons (Fig. 19.5). In persons at risk of inheriting myotonic dystrophy, an EMG can be used as a presymptomatic test, although this is rapidly being replaced by specific DNA mutational analysis looking for expansion of the CTG triplet repeat in the 3' end of the gene (pp. 23, 278).

Persons with myotonic dystrophy are also at an increased risk of developing early cataracts. The type of cataract seen in myotonic dystrophy is different from the common, so-called senile cataract and can often be detected in the early stages only by slit-lamp examination of the lens which shows refractile opacities. The presence of this type of cataract in an asymptomatic person at risk

for myotonic dystrophy would confirm that they had inherited the gene (Fig. 18.1, p. 269).

It is important to point out, however, that the absence of these findings on clinical or specialist investigation does not exclude the diagnosis of the disorder being tested for but does reduce the likelihood of the person concerned having inherited the gene. If the relative frequencies of such findings in persons with the disorder and in persons from the general population are known, it is possible to give the person at risk a residual relative likelihood of having inherited the gene. This information can be used in conjunction with other information, such as the pedigree risk, in genetic counselling (pp. 242, 293).

BIOCHEMICAL TESTS

In a number of autosomal dominant disorders biochemical tests can determine whether or not a person at risk has inherited a gene. Examples include the use of serum cholesterol levels in persons at risk for familial hyper-cholesterolaemia (p. 160) and assay of the appropriate urinary porphyrins or the specific enzyme deficiency in the various dominant porphyrias (p. 165).

LINKED MARKERS

Linked biochemical or DNA polymorphic markers can be used in presymptomatic diagnosis of dominantly inherited disorders.

Biochemical and blood group markers

The linkage of secretor status for the ABO blood group to myotonic dystrophy was one of the first examples of the use of this approach (p. 186). Unfortunately most individuals from families at risk for myotonic dystrophy are uninformative for this polymorphism. In addition, there is a significant chance of a cross-over occurring in meiosis between the two loci with the consequence that this approach is of little practical use.

Fig. 19.4
Renal ultrasound of an asymptomatic person with tuberous sclerosis showing abnormal echogenicity due to presumed angiomyolipomata (arrowed).

Fig. 19.5
An electromyogram from a person with myotonic dystrophy showing the characteristic abnormal spontaneous electrical discharge seen with insertion of the electrode into the muscle which decreases with time. (Courtesy of Dr A DaCosta, Department of Neurophysiology, St James's Hospital, Leeds.)

DNA markers

The availability of linked DNA markers has found widespread use in presymptomatic or predictive testing for a number of single gene disorders inherited in an autosomal dominant manner. The cloning of the gene responsible means that direct mutational analysis, as has occurred for persons at risk for Huntington's disease, has, for the most part, replaced the use of linked polymorphic DNA markers.

ETHICAL CONSIDERATIONS IN CARRIER DETECTION AND PREDICTIVE TESTING

There are often clear advantages in being able to determine the carrier status for a person at risk of being a carrier for an autosomal or X-linked recessive disorder. These primarily centre around a couple being able to make an informed choice when having children (p. 241).

In those at risk for the late onset autosomal dominant disorders, there can in some instances be a clear advantage in presymptomatic diagnosis. For example, in persons at risk for familial adenomatous polyposis (p. 200), colonoscopy looking for the presence of colonic polyps can be offered as a regular screening procedure to those who have been shown to be at high risk of developing colonic cancer by molecular studies. Conversely, individuals who have been shown not to have inherited a mutation in the APC gene do not need to be screened.

In contrast, in persons at risk for Huntington's disease in which there is as yet no effective treatment to delay the onset or progression of the disorder, the benefit of predictive testing is not immediately obvious. While choice is often considered to be of paramount importance in genetic counselling for persons at risk for inherited disorders, it is important to remember that those considering presymptomatic or predictive testing should only proceed if they can give truly informed consent and are free from coercion from any outside influence. It is increasingly likely that employers, life insurance companies and society in general will put indirect and, on occasion, direct pressure on persons at risk for inherited disorders to have such testing (p. 340).

Another problem raised by the development of predictive or presymptomatic testing is that it can, in theory, be carried out on children. The issue of predictive testing in childhood is very contentious, with many persons arguing, particularly when no obvious advantage accrues to the child in carrying out such testing, that it is best left until they can make the choice to undergo predictive testing for themselves unless there are potential health concerns for the child (p. 339).

ELEMENTS

1 Determination of carrier status for autosomal recessive and X-linked disorders can involve detailed clinical examination looking for specific minor features, specialist clinical investigations, biochemical tests or family studies using linked biochemical, blood group or DNA polymorphic markers.

2 Presymptomatic or predictive testing for persons at risk for autosomal dominant disorders with reduced penetrance or a delayed age of onset can also be carried out by detailed clinical examination for specific features, specialist investigations, biochemical testing and the use of linked biochemical or DNA polymorphisms.

3 Consideration should be given to the advantages and disadvantages of presymptomatic or predictive testing both from a practical and an ethical point of view.

FURTHER READING

Bakker E, Hofker M H, Goor N et al 1985 Prenatal diagnosis and carrier detection of Duchenne muscular dystrophy with closely linked RFLPs. Lancet i: 655–658
A paper which illustrates in more detail the principle of the use of linked DNA polymorphisms in carrier detection.

Harper P S 1998 Practical genetic counselling, 5th edn. Butterworth-Heinemann, Oxford
As the title suggests, a practical book which serves as a good starting point in almost every aspect of genetic counselling including carrier testing.

Pauli R, Motulsky A G 1981 Risk counselling in autosomal dominant disorders with undetermined penetrance. J Med Genet 18: 340–343
A paper which considers the problem of counselling for autosomal dominant disorders with reduced penetrance.

Pembrey M E, Davies K E, Winter R M, Elles R G, Williamson R, Fazzone T E, Walker C 1984 Clinical use of DNA markers linked to the gene for Duchenne muscular dystrophy. Arch Dis Child 59: 208–216
A useful discussion of how DNA markers can be used for carrier detection in Duchenne muscular dystrophy.

CHAPTER 20

Risk calculation

One of the most important aspects of genetic counselling is the provision of a risk figure. This is often referred to as a recurrence risk. Estimation of the recurrence risk will usually require careful consideration and take into account:

1. the diagnosis and its mode of inheritance
2. analysis of the family pedigree
3. the results of tests which can include linkage studies using DNA markers.

Sometimes the provision of a risk figure can be quite easy, but in a surprisingly large number of situations complicating factors arise which can make the calculation very difficult. For example, the mother of a boy who is an isolated case of a sex-linked recessive disorder could very reasonably wish to know the recurrence risk for her next child. This is a very simple question, but the solution is far from straightforward, as will become clear later in this chapter.

Before proceeding any further, it is necessary to clarify what we mean by probability and review the different ways in which it can be expressed. The probability of an outcome can be defined as the number or, more correctly, the proportion of times it occurs in a large series of events. Conventionally, probability is indicated as a proportion of one, so that a probability of zero implies that an outcome will never be observed, whereas a probability of one implies that it will always be observed. Therefore a probability of 0.25 indicates that, on average, a particular outcome or event will be observed on 1 in 4 or 25% of occasions. The probability that the outcome will not occur is 0.75, which can also be expressed as 3 chances out of 4, or 75%. Alternatively, this probability could be expressed as odds of 3 to 1 against or 1 to 3 in favour of this particular outcome being observed. In this chapter fractions will be used where possible as these tend to be more easily understood than proportions of 1 expressed as decimals.

PROBABILITY THEORY

In order to calculate genetic risks it is necessary to have a basic understanding of probability theory. This will be discussed in so far as it is relevant to the skills required for genetic counselling.

LAWS OF ADDITION AND MULTIPLICATION

When considering the probability of two different events or outcomes, it is essential to clarify whether they are mutually exclusive or independent. If the events are mutually exclusive then the probability that *either* one or the other will occur equals the sum of their individual probabilities. This is known as the *law of addition*.

If, however, two or more events or outcomes are independent, then the probability that *both* the first and the second will occur equals the product of their individual probabilities. This is known as the *law of multiplication*.

As a simple illustration of these laws consider parents who have embarked upon their first pregnancy. The probability that the baby will be *either* a boy *or* a girl equals 1, i.e. $\frac{1}{2} + \frac{1}{2}$. If the mother is found on ultrasound scan to be carrying twins who are non-identical, then the probability that *both* the first *and* the second twin will be boys equals $\frac{1}{4}$, i.e. $\frac{1}{2} \times \frac{1}{2}$.

BAYES' THEOREM

Bayes' theorem, which was first devised by the Reverend Bayes and published after his death in 1763, is used widely in genetic counselling. Essentially it provides a very valuable method for determining the overall probability of an event or outcome, such as carrier status, by considering all initial possibilities, e.g. carrier or non-carrier, and then modifying or 'conditioning' these by incorporating information, such as test results, which indicates which is the more likely.

The initial probability of each event is known as its *prior probability*, which is based on ancestral or *anterior information*. The observations which modify these prior probabilities allow *conditional probabilities* to be determined. In genetic counselling these are usually based on numbers of offspring and/or the results of tests. This is *posterior information*. The resulting probability for each event or outcome is known as its *joint probability*. The final probability for each event is known as its *posterior* or *relative probability* and is obtained by dividing the joint probability for that event by the sum of all the joint probabilities.

This is not an easy concept to grasp! To try to make it a little more comprehensible, consider a pedigree with two males, I_3 and II_1, who have a sex-linked recessive disorder (Fig. 20.1). The sister, II_2, of one of these men wishes to know the probability that she is a carrier. Her mother, I_2, must be a carrier as she has both an affected brother and an affected son, i.e. she is an obligate carrier. Therefore the prior probability that II_2 is a carrier equals $\frac{1}{2}$. Similarly the prior probability that II_2 is not a carrier equals $\frac{1}{2}$.

The fact that II_2 already has three healthy sons must be taken into consideration, as intuitively this makes it rather unlikely that she is a carrier. Bayes' theorem provides a way to quantify this intuition. These three healthy sons provide posterior information. The conditional probability that II_2 would have three healthy sons if she is a carrier equals $\frac{1}{2} \times \frac{1}{2} \times \frac{1}{2}$, which equals $\frac{1}{8}$. These values of $\frac{1}{2}$ are multiplied as they are independent events in that the health of one son is not influenced by the health of his brother(s). The conditional probability that II_2 would have three healthy sons if she is not a carrier equals 1.

This information is now incorporated into a Bayesian calculation (Table 20.1). From this table the posterior probability that II_2 is a carrier equals $\frac{1}{16} / (\frac{1}{16} + \frac{1}{2})$ which reduces to $\frac{1}{9}$. Similarly the posterior probability that II_2 is not a carrier equals $\frac{1}{2} / (\frac{1}{16} + \frac{1}{2})$ which reduces to $\frac{8}{9}$. Another way to obtain these results is to consider that the odds for II_2 being a carrier versus not being a carrier are $\frac{1}{16}$ to $\frac{1}{2}$, i.e. 1 to 8 which equals 1 in 9. Thus by taking into account the fact that II_2 has three healthy sons, we have been able to reduce her risk of being a carrier from 1 in 2 to 1 in 9.

Perhaps by now the use of Bayes' theorem will be a little more clear. Try to remember that the basic approach is to draw up a table showing all of the possibilities (e.g. carrier, not a carrier), then establish the background (prior) risk for each possibility, next determine the chance (conditional possibility) that certain observed events (e.g. healthy children) would have happened if each possibility is true, then work out the combined (joint) likelihood for each possibility, and finally weigh up each

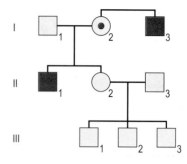

Fig. 20.1

A pedigree showing sex-linked recessive inheritance. When calculating the probability that II_2 is a carrier it is necessary to take into account her three unaffected sons.

Table 20.1   Bayesian calculation for II_2 in Figure 20.1

Probability	II_2 is a carrier	II_2 is not a carrier
Prior	$\frac{1}{2}$	$\frac{1}{2}$
Conditional Three healthy sons	$(\frac{1}{2})^3 = \frac{1}{8}$	$(1)^3 = 1$
Joint	$\frac{1}{16}$	$\frac{1}{2} (= \frac{8}{16})$
Expressed as odds	1 to	8
Posterior	$\frac{1}{9}$	$\frac{8}{9}$

of the joint probabilities to calculate the exact (posterior) probability for each of the original possibilities. If this is still confusing some of the following worked examples may bring a little more clarity!

AUTOSOMAL DOMINANT INHERITANCE

For someone with an autosomal dominant disorder, the risk that each of his or her children will inherit the mutant gene equals 1 in 2. This will apply whether the affected individual inherited the disorder from a parent or developed the condition as the result of a new mutation. Therefore the provision of risks for disorders showing autosomal dominant inheritance is usually straightforward as long as there is a clear family history, the condition is characterized by being fully penetrant and there is a reliable means of diagnosing heterozygotes. However, if penetrance is incomplete or if there is a delay in the age of onset so that heterozygotes cannot always be diagnosed, then risk calculation becomes more complicated. Two examples will be discussed to illustrate the sort of problems which can arise.

REDUCED PENETRANCE

A disorder is said to show reduced penetrance when it has clearly been demonstrated that individuals who must possess the abnormal gene, who by pedigree analysis must be obligate heterozygotes, show absolutely no manifestations of the condition (p. 99). For example, if someone who was completely unaffected had both a parent and a child with the same autosomal dominant disorder, then this would be an example of non-penetrance. Penetrance is usually quoted as a percentage, e.g. 80%, or as a proportion of 1, e.g. 0.8. This would imply that 80% of all heterozygotes express the condition in some way.

For a condition showing reduced penetrance, the risk that the child of an affected individual will be affected equals $\frac{1}{2}$, i.e. the probability that the child will inherit the mutant allele, × P, the proportion of heterozygotes who are affected. Therefore for a disorder such as hereditary retinoblastoma, an embryonic eye tumour (p. 195) which shows dominant inheritance in some families with a penetrance of P = 0.8, the risk that the child of an affected parent will develop a tumour equals $\frac{1}{2}$ × 0.8 which equals 0.4.

A more difficult calculation arises when a risk is sought for the future child of someone who is healthy but whose parent has or had an autosomal dominant disorder showing reduced penetrance (Fig. 20.2).

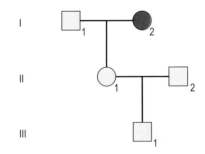

Fig. 20.2

I_2 has an autosomal dominant disorder which shows reduced penetrance. The probability that III_1 will be affected has to take into account the possibility that his mother (II_1) is a non-penetrant heterozygote.

Table 20.2 Bayesian calculation for II_1 in Figure 20.2

Probability	II_1 is heterozygous	II_1 is not heterozygous
Prior	$\frac{1}{2}$	$\frac{1}{2}$
Conditional Not affected	$1 - P$	1
Joint	$\frac{1}{2}(1 - P)$	$\frac{1}{2}$

Let us assume that the penetrance, P, equals 0.8. Calculation of the risk that III_1 will be affected can be approached in two ways. The first simply involves a little logic. The second utilizes Bayes' theorem.

1. Imagine that I_2 has 10 children. On average five children will inherit the gene but as P = 0.8 only four will be affected (Fig. 20.3). Therefore six out of the 10 children will be unaffected, one of whom has the mutant allele with the remaining five having the normal allele. II_1 is unaffected so that there is therefore a probability of 1 in 6 that she is, in fact, a heterozygote. Consequently the probability that III_1 will both inherit the mutant gene and be affected equals $\frac{1}{6} \times \frac{1}{2} \times P$ which equals $\frac{1}{15}$ if P is 0.8.

2. Now consider II_1 in Figure 20.2. The prior probability that she is a heterozygote equals $\frac{1}{2}$. Similarly the prior probability that she is not a heterozygote equals $\frac{1}{2}$. Now a Bayesian table can be constructed to determine how these prior probabilities are modified by the fact that II_1 is not affected.

The posterior probability that II_1 is a heterozygote equals $\frac{1}{2}(1 - P)/[\frac{1}{2}(1 - P) + \frac{1}{2}]$ which reduces to $\frac{1-P}{2-P}$. Therefore, the risk that III_1 will both inherit the mutant allele and be affected equals $(\frac{1-P}{2-P}) \times \frac{1}{2} \times P$ which reduces to $\frac{(P - P^2)}{(4 - 2P)}$. If P equals 0.8, this expression equals $\frac{1}{15}$ or 0.067.

By substituting different values of P in the above expression, it can be shown that the maximum risk for III_1 being affected equals 0.086, approximately $\frac{1}{12}$, which is obtained when P equals 0.6. This maximal risk figure can be used when counselling persons at risk for late onset autosomal disorders with reduced penetrance who have an affected grandparent and unaffected parents.

DELAYED AGE OF ONSET

Many autosomal dominant disorders do not present until well into adult life (p. 290). Healthy members of families in which these disorders are segregating often

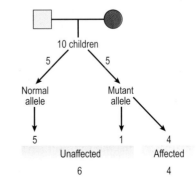

Fig. 20.3

The expected genotypes and phenotypes in ten children born to an individual with an autosomal dominant disorder with penetrance equal to 0.8.

wish to know whether they themselves will develop the condition and/or pass it on to their children. Risks for these individuals can be calculated in the following way.

Consider someone who has died with a confirmed diagnosis of Huntington's disease (Fig. 20.4). This is a late onset autosomal dominant disorder. The son of I_2 is entirely healthy at age 50 years and wishes to know the probability that his 10-year-old daughter, III_1, will develop Huntington's disease in later life. In this condition the first signs usually appear between the ages of 30 and 60 years, and approximately 50% of all heterozygotes have shown signs by the age of 50 years (Fig. 20.5).

The probability that II_1 has inherited the gene, given that he shows no signs of the condition, can be determined by a simple Bayesian calculation (Table 20.3).

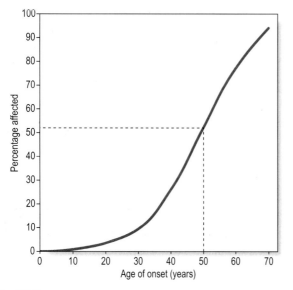

Fig. 20.4
I_2 had an autosomal dominant disorder showing delayed age of onset. When calculating the probability that III_1 will develop the disorder it is necessary to determine the probability that II_1 is a heterozygote who is not yet clinically affected.

Fig. 20.5
Graph showing age of onset in years of clinical expression in Huntington's disease heterozygotes. Approximately 50% show clinical signs or symptoms by age 50 years. (Data from Newcombe R G 1981 A life table for onset of Huntington's chorea. Ann Hum Genet 45: 375–385.)

The posterior probability that II_1 is heterozygous equals $\frac{1}{4}/(\frac{1}{4} + \frac{1}{2})$ which equals $\frac{1}{3}$. Therefore the prior probability that his daughter III_1 will have inherited the disorder equals $\frac{1}{3} \times \frac{1}{2}$, or $\frac{1}{6}$.

There is a temptation when doing calculations such as this to conclude that the overall risk for II_1 being a heterozygote simply equals $\frac{1}{2} \times \frac{1}{2}$, i.e. the prior probability that he will have inherited the mutant gene times the probability that a heterozygote will be unaffected at age 50 years, giving a risk of $\frac{1}{4}$. This is correct in as much as it gives the joint probability for this possible outcome, but it does not take into account the possibility that II_1 is not a heterozygote. Consider the possibility that I_2 has four children. On average two will inherit the mutant allele, one of whom will be affected by the age of 50 years. The remaining two children will not inherit the mutant allele. By the time these children have grown up and reached the age of 50 years, on average one will be affected and three will not. Therefore, on average one-third of the healthy 50-year-old offspring of I_2 will be heterozygotes. Hence the correct risk for II_1 is $\frac{1}{3}$ and not $\frac{1}{4}$.

AUTOSOMAL RECESSIVE INHERITANCE

With an autosomal recessive condition, the parents of an affected child are both heterozygotes. There are two possible exceptions, both of which are very rare. These arise when only one parent is a heterozygote, in which case a child can be affected if either a new mutation occurs on the gamete inherited from the other parent, or uniparental disomy occurs resulting in the child inheriting two copies of the heterozygous parent's mutant allele (p. 108). For practical purposes it is usually assumed that both parents of an affected child are carriers.

CARRIER RISKS FOR THE EXTENDED FAMILY

When both parents are heterozygotes, the risk that each of their children will be affected equals 1 in 4. On average

Table 20.3 Bayesian calculation for II_1 in Figure 20.4

Probability	II_1 is heterozygous	II_1 is not heterozygous
Prior	$\frac{1}{2}$	$\frac{1}{2}$
Conditional Unaffected at age 50 years	$\frac{1}{2}$	$\underline{1}$
Joint	$\frac{1}{4}$	$\frac{1}{2}$

three of their four children will be unaffected, of whom, on average, two will be carriers (Fig. 20.6). Therefore the probability that the healthy sibling of someone with an autosomal recessive disorder will be a carrier equals $\frac{2}{3}$. Carrier risks can be derived for other family members starting with the assumption that both parents of an affected child are carriers (Fig. 20.7).

When calculating risks in autosomal recessive inheritance the underlying principle is to establish the probability that each prospective parent is a carrier, and then multiply the product of these probabilities by $\frac{1}{4}$, this being the risk that any child born to two carriers will be affected. Therefore, in Figure 20.7, if the sister, III_3, of the affected boy was to marry her first cousin, III_4, then the probability that their first baby would be affected would equal $\frac{2}{3} \times \frac{1}{4} \times \frac{1}{4}$, i.e. the probability that III_3 is a carrier

times the probability that III_4 is a carrier times the probability that a child of two carriers will be affected. This gives a total risk of $\frac{1}{24}$.

If this same sister, III_3, was to marry a healthy unrelated individual, the probability that their first child would be affected would equal $\frac{2}{3} \times 2pq \times \frac{1}{4}$, i.e. the probability that III_3 is a carrier times the carrier frequency in the general population (p. 117) times the probability that a child of two carriers will be affected. For a condition such as cystic fibrosis, with a disease incidence of approximately 1 in 2000, $q^2 = \frac{1}{2000}$ and therefore $q = \frac{1}{44}$ and thus $2pq = \frac{1}{22}$. Therefore, the final risk would be $\frac{2}{3} \times \frac{1}{22} \times \frac{1}{4}$ or 1 in 132.

MODIFYING A CARRIER RISK BY MUTATION ANALYSIS

Cystic fibrosis is one of several autosomal recessive disorders for which population screening is being actively considered (p. 318). Over 800 different mutations have been identified in the cystic fibrosis gene, so that carrier detection by DNA mutation analysis is not straightforward. However, a relatively simple test has been developed for the most common mutations which enables 85% of all carriers of Western European origin to be detected. What is the probability that a healthy individual who has no family history of cystic fibrosis and who tests negative on the common mutation screen is a carrier?

The answer is obtained once again by drawing up a simple Bayesian table (Table 20.4). The prior probability that this healthy member of the general population is a carrier equals $\frac{1}{22}$: therefore the prior probability that he or she is not a carrier equals $\frac{21}{22}$. If this individual is a carrier, then the probability that the common mutation test will be normal is 0.15 as only 15% of carriers do not have a common mutation. The probability that someone who is not a carrier will have a normal common mutation test result is 1.

This gives a joint probability for being a carrier of $\frac{3}{440}$ and for not being a carrier of $\frac{21}{22}$. Therefore the

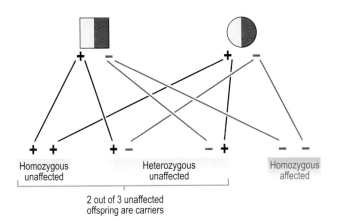

Fig. 20.6
The possible genotypes and phenotypes in the offspring of parents who are both carriers of an autosomal recessive disorder. On average two out of three healthy offspring are carriers.

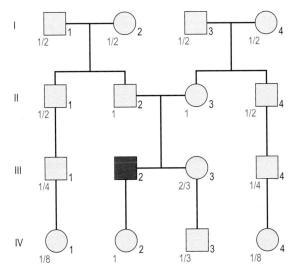

Fig. 20.7
Autosomal recessive inheritance. The probabilities that various family members are carriers are indicated as fractions.

Table 20.4 Bayesian table for cystic fibrosis carrier risk if common mutation screen is negative

Probability	Carrier	Not a carrier
Prior	$\frac{1}{22}$	$\frac{21}{22}$
Conditional		
Normal result on common mutation screening	<u>0.15</u>	<u>1</u>
Joint	$\frac{3}{440}$	$\frac{21}{22}$

posterior probability that this individual is a carrier equals $\frac{3}{440} / (\frac{3}{440} + \frac{21}{22})$ which equals $\frac{1}{141}$. Thus the normal result on common mutation testing has reduced the carrier risk from $\frac{1}{22}$ to $\frac{1}{141}$.

SEX-LINKED RECESSIVE INHERITANCE

This pattern of inheritance tends to generate the most complicated risk calculations when counselling for Mendelian disorders. In severe sex-linked conditions, affected males are often unable to have their own children. Consequently these conditions are usually transmitted only by healthy female carriers. The carrier of a sex-linked recessive disorder transmits the gene on average to half of her daughters who are therefore carriers, and to half of her sons who will thus be affected. If an affected male does have children, then he will transmit his Y chromosome to all of his sons who will be unaffected, and his X chromosome to all of his daughters who will be carriers (Fig. 20.8).

An example of how the birth of unaffected sons to a possible carrier of a sex-linked disorder results in a reduction of her carrier risk has already been discussed in the introductory section on Bayes' theorem (p. 294). In this section we shall consider two further factors which can complicate risk calculation in sex-linked recessive disorders.

THE ISOLATED CASE

If a woman has only one affected son, then in the absence of a positive family history there are three possible ways in which this can have occurred:

1. The woman is a carrier of the mutant allele, in which case there is a risk of $\frac{1}{2}$ that any future son will be affected.

2. The disorder in the son arose as a new mutation which occurred during meiosis in the gamete which led to his conception. The recurrence risk in this situation is negligible.

3. The woman is a gonadal mosaic for the mutation which occurred in an early mitotic division during her own embryonic development. The recurrence risk will be equal to the proportion of ova which carry the mutant allele, i.e. between 0% and 50%.

In practice it is often very difficult to distinguish between these three possibilities unless reliable tests are available for carrier detection. If a woman is found to be a carrier then risk calculation is straightforward. If the tests indicate that she is not a carrier, then the recurrence risk is probably low, but not negligible because of the possibility of gonadal mosaicism.

For example, in Duchenne muscular dystrophy it has been estimated that among the mothers of isolated cases approximately two-thirds are carriers, 5–10% are gonadal mosaics and in the remaining 25–30% the disorder has arisen as a new mutation in meiosis.

INCORPORATING CARRIER TEST RESULTS

Several biochemical tests are available for detecting carriers of sex-linked recessive disorders (p. 288). Unfortunately there is often overlap in the values obtained for controls and women known to be carriers, i.e. obligate carriers. Although an abnormal result in a potential carrier would suggest that she is likely to be a carrier, a normal test result does not exclude a woman being a

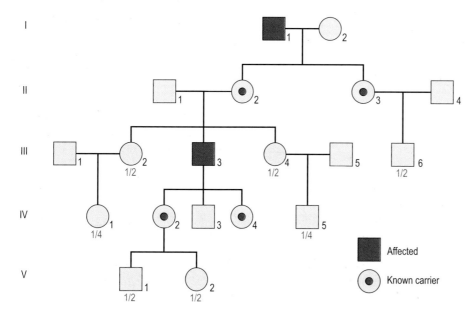

Fig. 20.8
The probabilities of male relatives being affected and female relatives being carriers of an X-linked recessive disorder. All the daughters of an affected male are obligate carriers.

■ Affected

◉ Known carrier

carrier. While for many sex-linked recessive disorders this problem can be overcome by using linked DNA markers (p. 289), the difficulties presented by overlapping biochemical test results arise sufficiently often to justify further consideration.

For example, in Duchenne muscular dystrophy, serum creatine kinase is elevated in approximately two out of three obligate carriers (Fig. 19.1, p. 288). Therefore, if a possible carrier such as II_2 in Figure 20.1 is found to have a normal level of creatine kinase, this would provide further support for her not being a carrier. The test result therefore provides a conditional probability, which is included in a new Bayesian calculation (Table 20.5).

The posterior probability that II_2 is a carrier equals $\frac{1}{48}/(\frac{1}{48} + \frac{1}{2})$ or $\frac{1}{25}$. Consequently by taking into account firstly this woman's three healthy sons and secondly her normal creatine kinase test result it has been possible to reduce her carrier risk from 1 in 2 to 1 in 9 and then to 1 in 25.

THE USE OF LINKED MARKERS

As a result of the developments which have taken place in molecular biology over the last 15 years, most of the more common single gene disorders have been mapped to the human genome (p. 76). For many conditions the gene has been isolated and characterized so that specific mutation analysis is available.

This now applies to disorders such as Huntington's disease and cystic fibrosis, and is also the case for many families in which Duchenne muscular dystrophy is present. However, in conditions such as Duchenne muscular dystrophy in which each family usually has its own unique mutation, direct mutation analysis is not always possible if, for example, there are no surviving affected males. In these families DNA markers at a locus closely linked to the disease locus can be used to assist in carrier detection.

As an illustration of the potential value of this approach, consider the sister of a boy affected with Duchenne muscular dystrophy (DMD), whose mother is an obligate carrier as she herself had an affected brother (Fig. 20.9).

A DNA marker with alleles A and B is available and is known to be closely linked to the DMD disease locus with a recombination fraction (θ) equal to 0.05 (pp. 121, 289). The disease allele must be in coupling with the A marker allele in II_2 as this woman has inherited both the A allele and the DMD allele on the X chromosome from her mother (she must have inherited the B allele from her father, so the A allele must have come from her mother). Therefore, if III_3 inherits this A allele from her mother, the probability that she will also inherit the

Table 20.5 Bayesian calculation for II_2 in Figure 20.1

Probability	II_2 is a carrier	II_2 is not a carrier
Prior	$\frac{1}{2}$	$\frac{1}{2}$
Conditional		
Three healthy sons	$\frac{1}{8}$	1
Normal creatine kinase	$\frac{1}{3}$	1
Joint	$\frac{1}{48}$	$\frac{1}{2}$

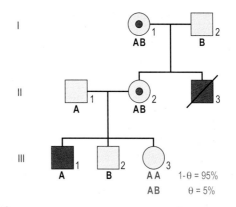

Fig. 20.9
A pedigree showing sex-linked recessive inheritance. A and B represent alleles at a locus closely linked to the disease locus.

disease allele and be a carrier equals $1 - \theta$, i.e. the probability that a cross-over will not have occurred between the disease and marker loci in the meiosis of the ova which resulted in her conception. For a value of θ equal to 0.05 this gives a carrier risk of 0.95 or 95%. Similarly the probability that III_3 will be a carrier if she inherits the B allele from her mother equals 0.05 or 5%.

Closely linked DNA markers are now available for most single gene disorders and these are widely used in genetic counselling for carrier detection and prenatal diagnosis when direct mutation testing is not available. The smaller the value of θ, then the smaller the likelihood of a predictive error. If DNA markers are available which 'bridge' or 'flank' the disease locus, this greatly reduces the risk of a predictive error as only a double cross-over will go undetected, and the probability of a double cross-over is extremely low.

BAYES' THEOREM AND PRENATAL SCREENING

As a further illustration of the potential value of Bayes' theorem in risk calculation and genetic counselling, an example from prenatal screening shall be illustrated.

Consider the situation which arises when a woman aged 20 years presents at 20 weeks gestation with a fetus which has been shown on ultrasound scanning to have duodenal atresia. Duodenal atresia is known to be a characteristic finding in Down's syndrome (p. 250), in which it shows an incidence of approximately 1 in 20. In contrast the incidence in babies not affected with Down's syndrome equals approximately 1 in 5000. In other words duodenal atresia is 250 times more common in Down's syndrome than in unaffected babies.

Question. Does this mean that the odds are 250 to 1 that this unborn baby has Down's syndrome? Answer. No! This risk, or more precisely odds ratio, would only be correct if the prior probabilities that the baby would be affected or unaffected were equal. In reality the prior probability that the baby will be unaffected is much greater than the prior probability that it will have Down's syndrome.

Actual values for these prior probabilities can be obtained by reference to a table showing maternal age specific risks for Down's syndrome (Table 17.4, p. 250). For a woman aged 20 years the incidence of Down's syndrome is approximately 1 in 1500: hence the prior probability that the baby will be unaffected equals $\frac{1499}{1500}$. If these prior probability values are used in a Bayesian calculation then it can be shown that the posterior probability that the unborn baby will have Down's syndrome is approximately 1 in 7 (Table 20.6). Obviously this is much lower than the conditional odds of 250 to 1 in favour of the baby being affected.

In practice the demonstration of duodenal atresia on ultrasound in a fetus would usually prompt an offer of definitive chromosome analysis by placental biopsy, amniocentesis or fetal blood sampling (ch. 21). This example of duodenal atresia has been used to emphasize that an observed conditional probability ratio should always be combined with a knowledge of the prior probabilities to obtain a correct indication of the actual risk.

EMPIRIC RISKS

Up to this point risks have been calculated for single gene disorders using knowledge of basic Mendelian genetics and applied probability theory. In many counselling situations it is not possible to arrive at an accurate risk figure in this way, either because the disorder in question does not show single gene inheritance or because the clinical diagnosis with which the family has been referred shows causal heterogeneity (pp. 101, 242). In these situations it is usually necessary to resort to the use of observed or *empiric risks*. These are based on observations derived from family studies rather than theoretical calculations.

MULTIFACTORIAL DISORDERS

One of the basic principles of multifactorial inheritance is that the risk of recurrence in first-degree relatives, siblings and offspring, equals the square root of the incidence of the disease in the general population (p. 130), i.e. $P^{\frac{1}{2}}$ where P equals the general population incidence. For example, if the general population incidence equals $\frac{1}{1000}$, then the theoretical risk to a first-degree relative equals the square root of $\frac{1}{1000}$ which approximates to 1 in 32 or 3%. The theoretical risks for second- and third-degree relatives can be shown to approximate to $P^{\frac{3}{4}}$ and $P^{\frac{7}{8}}$ respectively. Therefore, if there is strong support for multifactorial inheritance, it is reasonable to use these theoretical risks when counselling close family relatives.

However, when using this approach it is important to remember that the confirmation of multifactorial inheritance will often have been based on the study of observed recurrence risks. Consequently it is generally more appropriate to refer back to the original family studies and counsel on the basis of the risks derived in these (Table 20.7).

Ideally reference should be made to local studies as recurrence risks can differ quite substantially in different communities, ethnic groups, and geographical locations. For example, the recurrence risk for neural tube defects in siblings is quoted as 4%. This is essentially an average risk. The actual risk varies from 2–3% in south-east England up to 8% in Northern Ireland, and also shows an inverse relationship with the family's socioeconomic status, being greatest for mothers in poorest circumstances.

Table 20.6 Bayesian calculation to show the posterior probability that a fetus with duodenal atresia conceived by a 20-year-old mother will have Down's syndrome

Probability	Fetus unaffected	Fetus affected
Prior	$\frac{1499}{1500}$	$\frac{1}{1500}$
Conditional		
Duodenal atresia	1	250
Joint	$\frac{1499}{1500} = 1$	$\frac{1}{6}$
Expressed as odds	6 to	1
Posterior	$\frac{6}{7}$	$\frac{1}{7}$

Table 20.7 Empiric recurrence risks for common multifactorial disorders

Disorder	Incidence (per 1000)	Sex ratio (M:F)	Unaffected parents having a second affected child (%)	Affected parents having an affected child (%)
Cleft lip ± cleft palate	1–2	3:2	4	4
Club foot (talipes)	1–2	2:1	3	3
Congenital heart defects	8	1:1	1–4	2 (father affected) 6 (mother affected)
Congenital dislocation of the hip	1	1:6	6	12
Hypospadias (in males)	2	–	10	10
Manic-depressive psychosis	4	2:3	10–15	10–15
Neural tube defects				
Anencephaly	1.5	1:2	4–5	–
Spina bifida	2.5	2:3	4–5	4
Pyloric stenosis				
Male index	2.5	–	2	4
Female index	0.5	–	10	17
Schizophrenia	10	1:1	10	14

Table 20.8 Empiric recurrence risks for conditions showing causal heterogeneity

Disorder	Incidence (per 1000)	Sex ratio (M:F)	Unaffected parents having a second affected child (%)	Affected parents having an affected child (%)
Autism	0:2	3:1	2–3	–
Epilepsy (idiopathic)	5	1:1	5	5
Hydrocephalus	0.5	1:1	3	–
Mental retardation (idiopathic)	3	1:1	3–5	10
Profound childhood sensorineural deafness	1	1:1	10–15	5–10

Unfortunately empiric risks are rarely available for families in which there are several affected family members or for disorders with variable severity or different sex incidences. A computer program has been devised which allows theoretical estimates to be made in many of these more complex situations.

CONDITIONS SHOWING CAUSAL HETEROGENEITY

Many referrals to genetic clinics relate to a clinical phenotype rather than to a precise underlying diagnosis (Table 20.8). In these situations great care must be taken to ensure that all appropriate diagnostic investigations have been undertaken before resorting to the use of empiric risk data (p. 241).

It is worth emphasizing that the use of empiric risks for conditions such as sensorineural hearing loss in childhood is at best a compromise as the figure quoted to an individual family will rarely be the correct one for their particular diagnosis. Severe sensorineural hearing loss in a young child is usually caused by either single gene inheritance, most commonly autosomal recessive but occasionally autosomal dominant or sex-linked recessive, or by an environmental condition such as rubella embryopathy. Therefore, for most families the correct risk of recurrence will be either 25% or 0%. In practice it is often not possible to establish the precise cause so that the only option available is to offer the family an empiric or 'average' risk.

FURTHER READING

Bayes T 1958 An essay towards solving a problem in the doctrine of chances. Biometrika 45: 296–315
A reproduction of the Reverend Bayes' original essay on probability theory which was first published, posthumously, in 1763.
Emery A E H 1986 Methodology in medical genetics, 2nd edn. Churchill Livingstone, Edinburgh
An introduction to statistical methods of analysis in human and medical genetics.
Murphy E A, Chase G A 1975 Principles of genetic counseling. Year Book Medical Publications, Chicago
A very thorough explanation of the use of Bayes' theorem in genetic counselling.
Young I D 1999 Introduction to risk calculation in genetic counselling, 2nd edn. Oxford University Press, Oxford
A short introductory guide to all aspects of risk calculation in genetic counselling. Highly recommended!

ELEMENTS

1 Risk calculation in genetic counselling requires a knowledge and understanding of basic probability theory. Bayes' theorem enables initial background 'prior' risks to be modified by 'conditional' information to give an overall probability or risk for a particular event such as carrier status.

2 For disorders showing autosomal dominant inheritance it is often necessary to consider factors such as reduced penetrance and delayed age of onset. For disorders showing autosomal recessive inheritance, risks to offspring are determined by calculating the probability that each parent is a carrier and then multiplying the product of these probabilities by $\frac{1}{4}$.

3 In sex-linked recessive inheritance a particular problem arises if only one male in a family is affected. The results of carrier tests which show overlap between carriers and non-carriers can be incorporated in a Bayesian calculation.

4 Polymorphic DNA markers linked to the disease locus can be used in many single gene disorders for carrier detection, preclinical diagnosis and prenatal diagnosis.

5 Empiric (observed) risks are available for multifactorial disorders and for aetiologically heterogeneous conditions such as non-syndromal sensorineural hearing loss.

CHAPTER 21

Prenatal diagnosis of genetic disease

Until recently, couples at high risk of having a child with a genetic disorder had to choose between taking the risk or considering other reproductive options such as long-term contraception, sterilization and termination of all pregnancies. Other alternatives included adoption, long-term fostering and artificial insemination by donor sperm (AID).

Over the last three decades prenatal diagnosis, the ability to detect abnormalities in an unborn child, has been widely used. While it is never easy for a couple to decide to pursue prenatal diagnosis because of the possibility of subsequently having to consider termination of pregnancy, prenatal diagnosis is an option which is chosen by many couples at high risk of having a child with a serious hereditary disorder.

The ethical issues surrounding prenatal diagnosis and selective termination of pregnancy are both complex and emotive, and are considered more fully in Chapter 24 (p. 337). In this chapter we shall focus on the practical aspects of prenatal diagnosis, which can be considered under the headings of the techniques which are used and the indications for offering each of these various procedures.

TECHNIQUES USED IN PRENATAL DIAGNOSIS

There are several techniques which can be utilized for the prenatal diagnosis of hereditary disorders and structural abnormalities (Table 21.1).

AMNIOCENTESIS

Amniocentesis involves the aspiration of 10–20 ml of amniotic fluid through the abdominal wall under ultrasound guidance (Fig. 21.1). This is usually performed around the 16th week of gestation. The sample is spun down to yield a pellet of cells and supernatant fluid. The fluid can be used in the prenatal diagnosis of neural tube defects by assay of α-fetoprotein (p. 314). The cell pellet is resuspended in culture medium with fetal calf serum which stimulates cell growth. While most of these cells in the amniotic fluid which have been shed from the amnion, fetal skin and urinary tract epithelium will be non-viable, a small proportion will grow. After approximately 14 days there are usually sufficient cells for chromosome analysis, although a longer period is usually

Table 21.1 Standard techniques used in prenatal diagnosis

Technique	Optimal time (in weeks)	Disorders diagnosed
Non-invasive		
Maternal serum screening		
α-Fetoprotein	16	Neural tube defects
Triple test	16	Down's syndrome
Ultrasound	18	Structural abnormalities, e.g. CNS, heart, kidneys and limbs
Invasive		
Amniocentesis	16	
Fluid		Neural tube defects
Cells		Chromosome abnormalities, metabolic disorders, molecular defects
Chorionic villus sampling	10–12	Chromosome abnormalities, metabolic disorders, molecular defects
Fetoscopy		
Blood		Chromosome abnormalities, haematological disorders, congenital infection
Liver		Metabolic disorders, e.g. ornithine transcarbamylase deficiency
Skin		Hereditary skin disorders, e.g. epidermolysis bullosa

Fig. 21.1
A diagram of the technique of amniocentesis.

Fig. 21.2
A diagram of the technique of transvaginal chorionic villus sampling.

needed before enough cells are obtained for biochemical or DNA studies. The availability of PCR has meant that direct DNA analysis is possible without the need for culture.

When a couple is considering amniocentesis as an option they should be informed of the 0.5–1% risk of miscarriage associated with the procedure and that if the result is abnormal they will be facing the possibility of having to consider a late mid-trimester termination of pregnancy which involves an induction of labour.

Recent trials carrying out amniocentesis earlier in pregnancy, at 12–14 weeks gestation, have yielded comparable rates of success in obtaining results with a similar risk of miscarriage. Although early amniocentesis has the advantage of allowing a result to be given earlier in the pregnancy, it will usually still require a mid-trimester termination of pregnancy if the fetus is found to be affected.

CHORIONIC VILLUS SAMPLING

In contrast to amniocentesis, chorionic villus sampling, which was first developed in China, enables prenatal diagnosis to be undertaken during the first trimester. This procedure is usually carried out at 10–12 weeks gestation under ultrasound guidance by either trans-cervical or transabdominal aspiration of chorionic villi (Fig. 21.2). These are fetal in origin being derived from the outer cell layer of the blastocyst, i.e. the trophoblast. Maternal decidua, normally present in the biopsy sample, must be removed before the sample is analysed.

Placental biopsy is the term used if the procedure is carried out at later stages of pregnancy.

Chromosome analysis can be undertaken on chorionic villi either directly, looking at metaphase spreads from actively dividing cells, or following culture. Direct chromosomal analysis of chorionic villi usually allows a provisional result to be given within 24 hours. Confirmation by analysis of cultured chorionic villi is required in order to obtain good quality banded chromosomal analysis. For single gene disorders, sufficient tissue is usually obtained to allow prenatal diagnosis by biochemical assay or DNA analysis using uncultured villi.

The major advantage of chorionic villus sampling is that it offers first trimester prenatal diagnosis although it has the disadvantage that even in experienced hands this procedure conveys a 2–3% risk of causing miscarriage. There is also evidence that this technique can cause limb abnormalities in the embryo if carried out before 9 weeks gestation.

ULTRASOUND

Ultrasound offers a valuable means of prenatal diagnosis. It can be used not only for obstetric indications, such as placental localization and the diagnosis of multiple pregnancies, but also for the prenatal diagnosis of structural abnormalities which are not associated with known chromosomal, biochemical or molecular defects. Ultrasound is particularly valuable because it is non-invasive and conveys no known risk to the fetus or to the mother. It does, however, require specialized expensive equipment and a skilled and experienced operator. For example, a search can be made for polydactyly as a diagnostic feature of a multiple abnormality syndrome, such as one of the autosomal recessive short limb polydactyly syndromes which are associated with severe pulmonary hypoplasia and are invariably lethal (Fig. 21.3). Similarly, a scan can reveal that the fetus has a small jaw which can be associated with a posterior cleft palate and other more serious abnormalities in several single gene syndromes (Fig. 21.4).

Until recently, detailed ultrasound scanning for structural abnormalities was offered only to couples who had a child with a genetic disorder or syndrome for which there was no chromosomal, biochemical or molecular marker. Increasingly, however, detailed 'fetal anomaly' scanning is being offered routinely to all pregnant women around 18 weeks gestation as a screening procedure for structural abnormalities such as neural tube defects or cardiac anomalies. This technique can also identify features which suggest the presence of an underlying chromosomal abnormality (p. 315). Such a finding would lead to an offer of amniocentesis or placental biopsy for definitive chromosome analysis.

In addition, the observation that increased nuchal thickening is seen in fetuses who are subsequently born with Down's syndrome, has resulted in the introduction of measurements of nuchal pad thickness in the first trimester as a screening test for Down's syndrome. This also has the added advantage that it can also detect a number of the other common numerical chromosome abnormalities, including trisomy 18 and Turner's syndrome.

FETOSCOPY

Fetoscopy involves visualization of the fetus by means of an endoscope. Increasingly this technique is being superseded by detailed ultrasound scanning although occasionally fetoscopy is still undertaken during the second trimester to try to detect the presence of subtle structural abnormalities which would point to a serious underlying diagnosis.

Fetoscopy has also been used to obtain samples of tissue from the fetus which can be analysed as a means of achieving the prenatal diagnosis of several rare disorders. These have included inherited skin disorders such as epidermolysis bullosa and, before DNA testing became available, metabolic disorders in which the enzyme is expressed only in certain tissues or organs such as liver, e.g. ornithine transcarbamylase deficiency (p. 157), before DNA testing became available.

Unfortunately fetoscopy is associated with a 3–5% risk of miscarriage. This relatively high risk, coupled with the increasing sensitivity of ultrasound scanning and the availability of either linked DNA markers or specific mutation analysis, means that fetoscopy is used only infrequently and in highly specialized prenatal diagnostic centres.

Fig. 21.3
Ultrasound image of a transverse section of the hand of a fetus showing polydactyly.

Fig. 21.4
Longitudinal sagittal ultrasound image of the head and upper chest of a fetus showing micrognathia (small jaw) (arrowed).

CORDOCENTESIS

Although fetoscopy can also be used to obtain a small sample of fetal blood from one of the umbilical cord vessels in the procedure known as cordocentesis, improvements in ultrasound have enabled visualization of the vessels in the umbilical cord allowing transabdominal percutaneous fetal blood sampling. Fetal blood sampling is routinely used in the management of Rhesus isoimmunization (p. 187) and can be used to obtain samples for chromosome analysis to resolve problems associated with possible chromosomal mosaicism in chorionic villus or amniocentesis samples.

RADIOGRAPHY

The fetal skeleton can be visualized by radiography from 10 weeks onwards and this technique has been used in the past to diagnose inherited skeletal dysplasias. It is now rarely if ever employed because of the dangers of radiography to the fetus (p. 24) and the widespread availability of detailed ultrasound scanning.

MATERNAL SERUM SCREENING

In many centres it is now standard practice to offer screening for neural tube defects and Down's syndrome using a blood sample obtained from the mother at 16 weeks' gestation. In this way up to 75% of all cases of open neural tube defects and 60–70% of all cases of Down's syndrome can be detected. This approach is considered further in the next chapter on screening (p. 314).

NEW PRENATAL DIAGNOSTIC TECHNIQUES UNDER DEVELOPMENT

The development of non-invasive techniques which minimize the risk of pregnancy loss would offer an ideal means of prenatal diagnosis.

PREIMPLANTATION GENETIC DIAGNOSIS

A technique which is still being developed and which will almost certainly find increasing use as a reproductive option for some couples is *preimplantation genetic diagnosis* (PGD). In this procedure, an egg is removed from the female partner and fertilized in vitro using techniques developed for couples undergoing in vitro fertilization (IVF) for infertility. The fertilized oocyte is cultured in the laboratory up to the eight-cell stage of the early blastocyst. A single cell, which is known as a *blastomere*, is removed and analysed by PCR (p. 58) to see if the zygote is affected by the disorder for which the couple is at risk. If unaffected, the blastocyst is implanted into the mother's uterus. This approach has the advantage that the couple avoids having to consider the possibility of termination of pregnancy. PGD has been used diagnostically in only a very limited number of instances, e.g. to determine the sex of the zygote in the case of a couple at risk for Duchenne muscular dystrophy and for the diagnosis of cystic fibrosis and myotonic dystrophy.

PGD has found a limited use to date for a number of reasons. Despite the extreme sensitivity of PCR, even in the best centres using only a single cell as the source of DNA to amplify, there is at best only a 90–95% chance a result will be obtained and a further 90–95% chance that the result will be correct. In addition, there is a significant risk that a false-negative result will be obtained due to contamination with extraneous DNA. For example desquamated skin from the laboratory worker carrying out the procedure contaminating the reaction would contain sufficient DNA to overwhelm the signal from the single cell being analysed. For these reasons, centres developing this technique usually recommend that the mother subsequently undergoes an invasive form of prenatal diagnosis, such as chorionic villus sampling, in order to confirm the predicted result until technical developments improve its reliability.

In the small number of cases in which PGD has been carried out, the manipulation and removal of a cell from the zygote has not appeared to affect the subsequent development of the early blastocyst, embryo and fetus. A variation of this technique, which it is believed could reduce the risk of any potential harm to the developing embryo, involves the removal of the first polar body from the unfertilized oocyte, which remains adjacent to the secondary oocyte under the zona pellucida. The oocyte and first polar body divide from each other during meiosis I and therefore contain different members of each pair of homologous chromosomes. Therefore it is unlikely that a genetic defect identified in the polar body will be present in the oocyte, which can then be fertilized and implanted in the uterus.

It is important to emphasize that in most centres carrying out IVF the likelihood that a couple will have a successful pregnancy, even without the manipulation involved in preimplantation diagnosis, is still relatively low. Therefore, PGD should, for the present, be regarded as a highly specialized, largely experimental technique still under development and not a routine clinical service.

DETECTION OF FETAL CELLS IN THE MATERNAL CIRCULATION

Finally, it is possible that an entirely non-invasive means of prenatal diagnosis for chromosome and DNA abnormalities could become available. Using antibodies raised to antigens specific to the fetal trophoblast, there is evidence that cells of fetal origin are present in the maternal circulation in the first trimester. The validity of these claims has been substantiated by the use of PCR to detect the presence of paternally derived DNA markers in blood taken from women during early pregnancy. Although immunological techniques using antibodies to fetal trophoblast antigens can be used to enrich for fetal cells in the maternal circulation, problems can be encountered in excluding the possibility of significant maternal cell contamination in the sample being analysed. This technique has been used in a limited number of disorders, e.g. to predict the Rhesus status of the fetus in couples where the mother is Rh-negative and the father is heterozygous to try to determine which pregnancies need monitoring for Rhesus isoimmunization. More recently, the fact that fetal red blood cells are nucleated has been used to enrich for cells of fetal origin. Although this technique allows a couple to conceive naturally, it is important to remember that, unlike PGD, use of this approach still requires a couple to have to consider termination of pregnancy as a possible option if the fetus is found to be affected.

INDICATIONS FOR PRENATAL DIAGNOSIS

There are numerous indications for offering prenatal diagnosis. Ideally couples at high prior risk of having a baby with an abnormality should be identified and assessed before embarking upon a pregnancy so that they can be counselled and come to decisions about which options they wish to pursue at their leisure. A less satisfactory alternative is that such couples be identified early in pregnancy so that they still have an opportunity to consider all available prenatal diagnostic options as soon as possible in the pregnancy. Unfortunately many couples at an increased risk, because of their family history or previous reproductive history, are still not referred until mid-pregnancy, when it can be too late to offer the most appropriate forms of prenatal diagnosis.

ADVANCED MATERNAL AGE

This has been the most common indication for offering prenatal diagnosis. There is a well-recognized association of advanced maternal age with increased risk of having a child with Down's syndrome (Table 17.4, p. 250) and the other autosomal trisomy syndromes. No standard criterion exists for determining at what age a mother should be offered the option of an invasive prenatal diagnostic technique for fetal chromosome analysis. Most centres routinely offer amniocentesis or chorionic villus sampling to women aged 37 years or over, and the option is often discussed with women from the age of 35 years onwards. These risk figures relate to the maternal age at the expected date of delivery. The risk figures for Down's syndrome at the time of chorionic villus sampling, amniocentesis and delivery differ (Fig. 17.1, p. 250) because a proportion of pregnancies with trisomy 21 are lost spontaneously during the first and second trimesters.

PREVIOUS CHILD WITH A CHROMOSOME ABNORMALITY

Although there are a number of series with slightly different recurrence risk figures, for couples who have had a child with Down's syndrome due to non-disjunction or a de novo unbalanced Robertsonian translocation, the risk in a subsequent pregnancy is usually given as the mother's age-related risk plus approximately 0.5%. If one of the parents has been found to carry a balanced chromosomal rearrangement, such as a chromosomal translocation (p. 46) or pericentric inversion (p. 50), which has caused a previous child to be born with serious problems due to an unbalanced chromosome abnormality, then the recurrence risk is likely to be between 1–2% and 15–20%. The precise risk will depend on the nature of the parental rearrangement and the specific segments of the individual chromosomes involved (p. 51).

FAMILY HISTORY OF A CHROMOSOME ABNORMALITY

Couples are often referred for prenatal diagnosis because of a family history of a chromosome abnormality, most commonly Down's syndrome. For most couples there will usually be no increase in risk compared to the general population since most cases of trisomy 21 and other chromosomal disorders will have arisen as a result of non-disjunction rather than as a result of a familial chromosomal rearrangement. However, each situation should be carefully evaluated, either by confirming the nature of the chromosome abnormality in the affected individual or, if this is not possible, by urgent chromosome analysis of blood from the relevant parent at risk. The results of parental chromosomal analysis can usually be obtained within 3–4 days; if normal, an invasive prenatal diagnostic procedure is not then appropriate since the risk is no greater than that for the general population.

FAMILY HISTORY OF A SINGLE GENE DISORDER

If prospective parents have already had an affected child or if one of the parents is affected or has a positive family history of a single gene disorder which conveys a significant risk to offspring, then the option of prenatal diagnosis should be discussed with them. Prenatal diagnosis is available for a large and ever-increasing number of single gene disorders either by biochemical or DNA analysis.

FAMILY HISTORY OF A NEURAL TUBE DEFECT

Careful evaluation of the pedigree is necessary to determine the risk which applies to each pregnancy. Risks can be determined based on empiric data (p. 300). In high risk situations amniocentesis with assay of the chemical α-fetoprotein has been used for prenatal diagnosis in the past. Ultrasound examination of the fetus in conjunction with assay of maternal serum α-fetoprotein has proved equally reliable. Even with the best possible equipment and an experienced ultrasonographer, small closed neural tube defects can still be missed. Fortunately the latter type of neural tube defects are not usually associated with the serious problems seen with large open neural tube defects (p. 232).

FAMILY HISTORY OF OTHER CONGENITAL STRUCTURAL ABNORMALITIES

As with neural tube defects, evaluation of the family pedigree should enable the provision of a risk derived from the results of empiric studies. If the risk to a pregnancy is increased, detailed ultrasound examination looking for the specific structural abnormality can be offered at around 16–18 weeks gestation. Mid-trimester ultrasound will detect most serious cranial, cardiac, renal and limb malformations. Some couples request detailed ultrasound scanning, not because they wish to pursue the option of termination of pregnancy but because they wish to prepare themselves if the baby is found to be affected.

ABNORMALITIES IDENTIFIED IN PREGNANCY

The widespread introduction of prenatal diagnostic screening procedures, such as triple testing and fetal anomaly scanning, has meant that many couples unexpectedly present with diagnostic uncertainty during the pregnancy which can only be resolved by an invasive procedure such as amniocentesis or chorionic villus sampling. Other factors such as poor fetal growth can also be an indication for prenatal chromosome analysis, as confirmation of a serious and non-viable chromosome abnormality, such as trisomy 18 or triploidy (p. 44), can influence subsequent management of the pregnancy and mode of delivery.

OTHER HIGH RISK FACTORS

These include parental consanguinity, a poor obstetric history and certain maternal illnesses. Parental consanguinity conveys an increased risk that a child will have a hereditary disorder or congenital abnormality (p. 245). Consequently, if the parents are concerned, it is appropriate to offer detailed ultrasonography to try to exclude a serious structural abnormality. A poor obstetric history such as recurrent miscarriages or a previous unexplained stillbirth could indicate an increased risk of problems in a future pregnancy and would be an

indication for detailed ultrasound monitoring. A history of three or more unexplained miscarriages should be investigated by parental chromosome studies to exclude a chromosomal rearrangement such as a translocation or inversion (p. 264). Maternal illnesses, such as poorly controlled insulin-dependent diabetes mellitus (p. 236) or maternal epilepsy treated with anticonvulsant medications such as sodium valproate (p. 236), would also be indications for detailed ultrasonography. Both of these factors convey an increased risk of structural abnormality in a fetus.

SPECIAL PROBLEMS IN PRENATAL DIAGNOSIS

While the significance of the result of a prenatal diagnostic investigation is usually clear-cut, situations can arise which pose major problems of interpretation. Problems also occur if the diagnostic investigation is unsuccessful or if an unexpected result is obtained.

FAILURE TO OBTAIN A SAMPLE OR CULTURE FAILURE

It is important that every woman undergoing one of these invasive procedures is alerted to the possibility that, on occasion, it can prove impossible to obtain a suitable sample or the cells obtained subsequently fail to grow. Fortunately, the risk of either of these events occurring is less than 1%.

AN AMBIGUOUS CHROMOSOME RESULT

In approximately 1% of cases, chorionic villus sampling shows evidence of apparent chromosome mosaicism, i.e. the presence of two or more cell lines with different chromosome constitutions (p. 52). This can occur for several reasons:

1. The sample is contaminated by maternal cells. This is more likely to be seen using cultured cells than with direct preparations.

2. The mosaicism is a culture artefact. Usually several separate cell cultures are routinely established at the time of the procedure because of this possibility in order to rapidly help resolve this problem. If mosaicism is present in only one culture then it is probably an artefact and does not reflect the true fetal karyotype.

3. The mosaicism is limited to a portion of the placenta, or what is known as confined placental mosaicism. This arises due to an error in mitosis during the formation and development of the trophoblast and is of no consequence to the fetus.

4. There is true fetal mosaicism.

In the case of amniocentesis, in most laboratories it is routine for the sample to be split and for two or three separate cultures to be established. If a single abnormal cell is identified in only one culture this is assumed to be a culture artefact or what is termed level 1 mosaicism or *pseudomosaicism*. If the mosaicism extends to two or more cells in two or more cultures this is taken as evidence of true mosaicism or what is known as level 3 mosaicism. The most difficult situation to interpret is when mosaicism is present in two or more cells in only one culture, which is termed level 2 mosaicism. This is most likely to represent a culture artefact but there is up to a 20% chance that the mosaicism is real and will be present in the fetus.

In order to resolve the uncertainty generated by the finding of mosaicism with chromosomal analysis of chorionic villi samples it can be necessary to proceed to amniocentesis. If the latter test yields a normal chromosomal result then it is concluded that the result obtained from chorionic villi was not a true indication of the fetal karyotype.

Counselling couples in this situation is always extremely difficult. Even if true mosaicism is confirmed, it can be impossible to predict the probable phenotypic outcome for the baby. An attempt can be made to resolve ambiguous findings by proceeding to fetal blood sampling for urgent karyotype analysis. Whatever option the parents choose, it is important that tissue (blood, skin or placenta) is obtained at the time of delivery, whether the couple elect to terminate or continue with the pregnancy, in order to resolve the significance of the prenatal findings.

AN UNEXPECTED CHROMOSOME RESULT

Three different unexpected chromosome results can be given to couples, each of which usually necessitates specialized detailed genetic counselling.

A different numerical chromosomal abnormality

Although most invasive prenatal diagnostic procedures, such as chorionic villus sampling and amniocentesis, are carried out because of an increased risk of trisomy 21 through increased maternal age or as a result of increased risk through the triple test or nuchal pad screening (p. 315), a chromosomal abnormality other than trisomy 21 can be found, e.g. one of the other autosomal trisomies (trisomy 13 or 18) or one of the sex chromosome aneuploidies (45,X, 47,XXX, 47,XXY or 47,XYY). While the implication for the outcome of the pregnancy with one of the autosomal trisomies is reasonably straightforward, it is not so clear-cut with the sex chromosomal aneuploidies. Ideally all women undergoing amniocentesis should be alerted to this possibility before the test is carried out, although in practice this is rarely done. When a diagnosis

such as Turner's syndrome (45,X) or Klinefelter's syndrome (47,XXY) is obtained it is essential that the parents be given full details of the nature and consequences of the diagnosis. Recent studies have shown that when objective and informed counselling is available, less than 50% of the parents of a fetus with an 'incidental' diagnosis of a sex chromosome abnormality opt for termination of pregnancy.

A structural chromosomal rearrangement

A second difficult situation not infrequently encountered when providing prenatal diagnosis by amniocentesis or chorionic villus biopsy is the discovery of an apparently balanced chromosome rearrangement in the fetus, such as an inversion or translocation. If analysis of parental chromosomes shows that one of the parents has the same structural chromosomal rearrangement, then the parents can be reassured that it is very unlikely that this will cause any problems in the fetus. If, however, the apparently balanced chromosomal rearrangement has occurred as a de novo event in the fetus, then there is between a 5% and 10% chance that the fetus will have physical abnormalities and/or subsequently show developmental delay. This is likely to reflect a subtle chromosomal imbalance which cannot be detected using conventional cytogenetic techniques, or damage to a critical gene at one or both of the rearrangement break-points. It is not surprising that couples in this situation can have great difficulty in deciding what to do. Detailed ultrasonography, if normal, can provide some, but not complete, reassurance. The opportunity should, in due course, be taken to investigate the extended family if the rearrangement is found to be present in one of the parents.

The presence of a marker chromosome

A third situation which presents difficulty in counselling is the discovery in the amniocentesis or CVS sample of a small additional chromosome known as a *marker chromosome*, i.e. a small chromosomal fragment the specific identity of which cannot be determined by conventional cytogenetic techniques (p. 31). If this is found to be present in one of the parents, then it is unlikely that it will be of any significance to the fetus. If, on the other hand, it is a de novo finding, there is up to a 15% chance that the fetus will be phenotypically abnormal. The risk is lower if the marker chromosome contains satellite material (p. 30), or is largely made up of heterochromatin (p. 30), than if it does not have satellites and is mostly made up of euchromatin (p. 30). The availability of fluorescent in situ hybridization (p. 34) means that the origin of the marker chromosome can often be more specifically determined so that it is often possible to give more precise prognostic information.

ULTRASOUND 'SOFT' MARKERS

The increasing sophistication of mid-trimester ultrasonography has resulted in the identification of subtle anomalies in the fetus, the significance of which is not always clear. For example, choroid plexus cysts are sometimes seen in the developing cerebral ventricles in mid-trimester (Fig. 21.5). Initially it was thought that these were invariably associated with the fetus having trisomy 18. It is now known that choroid plexus cysts occur frequently in normal fetuses, although if they are very large and do not disappear spontaneously they can be indicative of a chromosome abnormality.

More recently, increased echogenicity of the fetal bowel has been reported as being associated with the baby subsequently having cystic fibrosis. It is presumed that this is the prenatal equivalent of meconium ileus (p. 276). Although initial reports suggested that the finding of 'echogenic bowel' could convey a risk as high as 10% for the fetus having cystic fibrosis, it is now clear that this risk is probably no greater than 1–2%. These types of novel ultrasound findings associated with possible fetal abnormalities are often called *soft markers*.

The difficulty in distinguishing normal from abnormal variation, coupled with lack of knowledge of the natural history of other commonly observed findings, emphasizes the importance of viewing reports of ultrasound soft markers and their possible association with abnormality in the fetus with great caution!

Fig. 21.5
Ultrasound scan of a fetal brain showing bilateral choroid plexus cysts (arrowed).

TERMINATION OF PREGNANCY

The presence of a serious abnormality in a fetus in the majority of developed countries is an acceptable legal indication for termination of pregnancy. This does not mean, however, that this is an easy choice for a couple to make. It is essential that all couples undergoing any form of prenatal diagnostic investigation, whether invasive or non-invasive, be provided with information about the practical aspects of termination of pregnancy before the prenatal diagnostic procedure is carried out. This should include a practical explanation that termination in the first trimester is carried out by surgical means under general anaesthetic, whereas a woman undergoing a mid-trimester termination will have to experience labour and delivery.

PRENATAL TREATMENT

So far in this chapter attention has focused on the prenatal diagnosis of abnormalities with the subsequent option of termination of pregnancy. While this is the only option in most situations, there is cautious optimism that prenatal diagnosis will, in time, lead to the possibility of effective treatment in utero.

A possible model for successful prenatal treatment is provided by the autosomal recessive disorder congenital adrenal hyperplasia (CAH) (pp. 158, 261). Affected female infants are born with virilization of the external genitalia. There is evidence that in a proportion of cases the virilization can be prevented if the mother takes a powerful steroid known as dexamethasone in a very small dose from 4–5 weeks gestation onwards. Specific prenatal diagnosis of CAH can be achieved by DNA analysis of chorionic villi. If this procedure confirms that the fetus is both female and affected, then the mother continues to take low doses of dexamethasone throughout pregnancy which suppresses the fetal pituitary–adrenal axis and can prevent virilization of the female fetus. If the fetus is male and affected or unaffected, the mother ceases to take dexamethasone and the pregnancy can proceed uneventfully.

More recently, in utero treatment of a fetus affected with severe combined immunodeficiency (p. 184) has been reported. The immunological tolerance of the fetus to foreign antigens introduced in utero means that the transfused stem cells are recognized as 'self', with the prospect of good long-term results.

When gene therapy (p. 327) has been proved to be both safe and effective, the immunological tolerance of the fetus should make it easier to commence such therapy before birth rather than afterwards. This will have the added advantage of reducing the period in which irreversible damage can occur in organs such as the central nervous system, which can be affected by progressive neuro-degenerative disorders (p. 163).

FURTHER READING

Brock D J H, Rodeck C H, Ferguson Smith M A (eds) 1992 Prenatal diagnosis and screening. Churchill Livingstone, Edinburgh
A very comprehensive multiauthor textbook covering all aspects of prenatal diagnosis.
Drife J O, Donnai D (eds) 1991 Antenatal diagnosis of fetal abnormalities. Springer-Verlag, London

The proceedings of a workshop on the practical aspects of prenatal diagnosis.
Lilford R J (ed) 1990 Prenatal diagnosis and prognosis. Butterworth, London
Provides useful information on recurrence risks for Down's syndrome, the prognosis for abnormalities detected by ultrasound, and decision analysis.
Stranc L C, Evans J A, Hamerton J L 1997 Chorionic villus sampling and amniocentesis for prenatal diagnosis. Lancet 349: 711–714
A good review of the practical and ethical aspects of the two main prenatal invasive diagnostic techniques.
Whittle M J, Connor J M (eds) 1989 Prenatal diagnosis in obstetric practice. Blackwell, Oxford
Describes prenatal diagnostic techniques and the types of abnormalities identified.

ELEMENTS

1 Prenatal diagnosis can be carried out by non-invasive procedures such as maternal serum α-fetoprotein screening for neural tube defects, the triple test and nuchal pad screening for Down's syndrome and ultrasonography for structural abnormalities.

2 Specific prenatal diagnosis of chromosome and single gene disorders usually requires an invasive technique such as amniocentesis or chorionic villus sampling by which material of fetal origin can be obtained for analysis.

3 Invasive prenatal diagnostic procedures convey small risks for causing miscarriage, e.g. amniocentesis 0.5–1%, cordocentesis 1–2%, chorionic villus sampling 2–3%, fetoscopy 3–5%.

4 The commonest indication for prenatal diagnosis is advanced maternal age. Other indications include a family history of a chromosome, single gene or structural abnormality or an increased risk predicted on the result of a screening test.

5 While the significance of most prenatal diagnostic findings is clear, situations can arise in which the implications for the fetus are very difficult to predict. When this occurs the parents should be offered specialized genetic counselling.

CHAPTER 22

Population screening and community genetics

Increasing awareness of the role of genetics in the aetiology of disease and its overall impact on the burden imposed on individuals, families and society has led to the introduction of several population genetic screening programmes. The branch of medical genetics which is concerned with screening and the prevention of genetic disease on a population basis is known as *community genetics*.

Population screening involves the offer of genetic testing on an equitable basis to all relevant individuals in a defined population. Its primary objective is to enhance autonomy by enabling individuals to be better informed about genetic risks and reproductive options. A secondary goal is the prevention of morbidity due to genetic disease and alleviation of the suffering that this would impose.

CRITERIA FOR A SCREENING PROGRAMME

These can be considered under the headings of the disease, the test and the practical aspects of the programme (Table 22.1).

THE DISEASE

The disease should be relatively common and have potentially serious effects which are amenable to prevention or amelioration. This can involve the early introduction of treatment, as in the case of neonatally diagnosed phenylketonuria (p. 151), or the offer of termination of pregnancy for disorders which cannot be treated effectively and which are associated with serious morbidity and/or mortality.

THE TEST

The test should be accurate and reliable with high sensitivity and specificity. *Sensitivity* refers to the proportion of cases which are detected. A measure of sensitivity can

Table 22.1 Criteria for a screening programme

Disease	— high incidence in target population
	— serious effect on health
	— treatable or preventable
Test	— non-invasive and easily carried out
	— accurate and reliable
	— inexpensive
Programme	— widespread and equitable availability
	— voluntary participation
	— acceptable to the target population
	— full information and counselling provided

be made by determining the proportion of *false-negative* results, i.e. how many cases are missed. Thus if a test detects only 70 out of 100 cases then it shows a sensitivity of 70%. *Specificity* refers to the extent to which the test detects only affected individuals. If unaffected persons test positive, these are referred to as *false-positives*. Thus if 10 out of 100 unaffected individuals give a false-positive test result, then the test shows a specificity of 90%.

THE PROGRAMME

The programme should be offered in a fair and equitable manner and should be widely available. It must also be morally acceptable to a substantial proportion of the population to which it is offered. Participation must be entirely voluntary. Easily understood information and well-informed counselling should both be readily available.

It is often stated that the cost of a screening programme should be reasonable and affordable. This does not mean that the potential savings gained through a reduction in the number of affected cases requiring treatment should exceed or even balance the cost of screening, although this is an argument which is popular with health administrators and planners who have to fund the programme. It is reasonable to point out that cost–benefit analyses also have to take into account non-tangible factors such as the emotional costs of human suffering borne by both the affected individuals and those who care for them.

PRENATAL SCREENING

NEURAL TUBE DEFECTS

In 1972 it was recognized that many pregnancies in which the baby had an open neural tube defect (NTD) (p. 232) could be detected at 16 weeks' gestation by assay of a protein in maternal serum known as α-fetoprotein (αFP). αFP is the fetal equivalent of albumin and is the major protein in fetal blood. If the fetus has an open NTD, the level of αFP is elevated in both the amniotic fluid and maternal serum as a result of leakage from the open defect. Open NTDs fulfil the criterion of being serious disorders, as anencephaly is invariably fatal and between 80% and 90% of the small proportion of babies who survive with an open lumbo-sacral lesion are severely handicapped.

Unfortunately maternal serum αFP screening for NTDs is neither 100% sensitive nor 100% specific. The curves for the levels of maternal serum αFP in normal and affected pregnancies overlap (Fig. 22.1), so that in practice an arbitrary cut-off level has to be introduced below which no further action is taken. This is usually either the 95th centile or 2.5 multiples of the median, and as a result around 75% of screened open spina bifida cases are detected. Those pregnant women with results which lie above this arbitrary cut-off level are offered further investigations such as detailed ultrasonography and possibly also amniocentesis, which gives a clearer distinction between the levels of αFP in normal and affected pregnancies.

Lack of specificity results from the elevation in maternal serum αFP which can occur for reasons other than an open NTD (Table 22.2) such as a threatened miscarriage,

a twin pregnancy, or a fetal abnormality such as exomphalos, in which there is a protrusion of abdominal contents through the umbilicus.

Despite these limitations prenatal maternal serum αFP screening has been implemented widely and is one of the main factors which have led to a striking decline in the incidence of open NTDs in liveborn and stillborn babies. Other contributory factors are a general improvement in diet and the introduction of periconceptional folic acid supplementation (p. 233). In England and Wales the combined incidence of anencephaly and spina bifida in liveborn and stillborn babies fell from 1 in 250 in 1973 to 1 in 6250 in 1993.

DOWN'S SYNDROME AND OTHER CHROMOSOME ABNORMALITIES

The triple test

Confirmation of a chromosome abnormality in an unborn baby requires cytogenetic studies using material obtained by an invasive procedure such as chorionic villus sampling or amniocentesis (p. 303). However, chromosome abnormalities, and in particular Down's syndrome, can be screened for in pregnancy by taking into account risk factors such as maternal age and the levels of three biochemical markers in maternal serum (Table 22.3).

This latter approach is based on the discovery that, at 16 weeks' gestation, maternal serum αFP and unconjugated oestriol levels tend to be reduced in Down's syndrome pregnancies as compared with normal pregnancies,

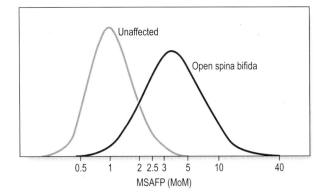

Fig. 22.1
Maternal serum αFP levels at 16 weeks gestation plotted on a logarithmic scale as multiples of the median (MoMs). Women with a value on or above 2.5 multiples of the median are offered further investigations. (Adapted from Brock D J H, Rodeck C H, Ferguson-Smith M A (eds) 1992 Prenatal diagnosis and screening. Churchill Livingstone, Edinburgh.)

Table 22.2 Causes of elevated maternal serum αFP

Anencephaly
Open spina bifida
Incorrect gestational age
Intra-uterine fetal bleed
Threatened miscarriage
Multiple pregnancy
Congenital nephrotic syndrome
Abdominal wall defect

Table 22.3 Maternal risk factors for Down's syndrome

Advanced age (35 years or over)	
Maternal serum	*MoM**
α-Fetoprotein (αFP)	(0.75)
Unconjugated oestriol (μE3)	(0.73)
Human chorionic gonadotrophin (hCG)	(2.05)
Inhibin-A	(2.10)

*Numbers in brackets refer to the mean values in affected pregnancies expressed as multiples of the median (MoMs) in normal pregnancies

whereas the level of maternal serum human chorionic gonadotrophin is usually elevated. None of these parameters gives absolute discrimination, but taken together they provide a means of modifying a woman's prior age-related risk to give an overall probability that the unborn baby is affected. When this probability exceeds 1 in 250, invasive testing in the form of amniocentesis or placental biopsy is offered.

Using age alone as a screening parameter, if all pregnant women aged 35 years and over opt for fetal chromosome analysis approximately 35% of all Down's syndrome pregnancies will be detected (Table 22.4). If the aforementioned three biochemical markers are also included, this being the so-called *triple test*, 60% of all Down's syndrome pregnancies will be detected using a risk of 1 in 250 or greater as the criterion for offering amniocentesis. This approach will also result in the detection of approximately 50% of all cases of trisomy 18 (p. 252).

It has recently been shown that another biochemical marker, inhibin-A, is also increased in maternal serum in Down's syndrome pregnancies. If this fourth marker is used as part of a 'quadruple' serum screening test, the proportion of Down's syndrome pregnancies detected rises from 60% to 75% if amniocentesis is offered to the 5% of mothers tested who have the highest risk.

Recently published results from California provide a useful indication of the outcome of a triple test prenatal screening programme. California has a population of 32 million and all pregnant women are offered triple test screening. This was accepted by 67% of all eligible women, of whom 2.6% went on to have amniocentesis resulting in the detection of 41% of all cases of Down's syndrome. These figures are similar to those observed in other studies and serve to illustrate the discrepancy between what is possible in theory (i.e. a detection rate of 60%) and what actually happens in practice.

Ultrasonography

Almost all pregnant women are routinely offered a 'dating' scan at around 12 weeks' gestation. It has recently been shown that at around this time there is a strong association between chromosome abnormalities and abnormal accumulation of fluid behind the baby's neck, a finding referred to as increased 'fetal nuchal translucency'. This applies both to Down's syndrome and to the other autosomal trisomy syndromes, i.e. trisomy 13 and trisomy 18 (p. 252). By combining information on maternal age with the results of fetal nuchal translucency and thickness measurements, it is possible to detect approximately 80% of fetuses with trisomy 21 if invasive testing is offered to the 5% of pregnant women with the highest risk.

In many centres it is also standard practice to offer a detailed 'fetal anomaly' scan to all pregnant women at 18

Table 22.4 Detection rates using different Down's syndrome screening strategies

Screening procedure	% of all pregnancies tested	% of Down's syndrome cases detected
Age alone		
40 years and over	1.5	15
35 years and over	7	35
Age + αFP	5	34
Age + αFP, μE3 + hCG	5	61
Age + αFP, μE3, hCG + inhibin-A	5	75

Fig. 22.2
Ultrasound scan at 18 weeks showing exomphalos. (Courtesy of Dr D Rose, City Hospital, Nottingham.)

Table 22.5 Prenatal ultrasound findings suggestive of a chromosome abnormality

Feature	Chromosome abnormality
Cardiac defect (especially common atrio-ventricular canal)	Trisomy 13, 18, 21
Clenched overlapping fingers	Trisomy 18
Cystic hygroma or fetal hydrops	Trisomy 13, 18, 21, Turner's syndrome
Duodenal atresia	Trisomy 21
Exomphalos	Trisomy 13, 18
Rocker bottom foot	Trisomy 18

weeks. Although chromosome abnormalities cannot be diagnosed directly, their presence can be suspected by the detection of an abnormality such as exomphalos (Fig. 22.2) or a rocker-bottom foot (Fig. 22.3) (Table 22.5). A chromosome abnormality is found in 50% of fetuses with an exomphalos identified at 18 weeks, and a rocker-

A   B

Fig. 22.3
(A) Ultrasound scan at 18 weeks showing a rocker-bottom foot in a fetus subsequently found to have trisomy 18, together with (B) a photograph of the feet of a newborn with trisomy 18. (Courtesy of Dr D Rose, City Hospital, Nottingham.)

bottom foot is a very characteristic finding in babies with trisomy 18 (p. 252). The use of other ultrasound 'soft markers' in identifying chromosome abnormalities in pregnancy is discussed in Chapter 21 (p. 310).

NEONATAL SCREENING

Newborn screening programmes have been introduced on a widespread basis for phenylketonuria, galactosaemia and congenital hypothyroidism. In all of these disorders early treatment can prevent the development of mental retardation. Screening for several other disorders is carried out more selectively in different centres (Table 22.6). For most of these conditions the rationale is to try to prevent subsequent morbidity. However in the case of Duchenne muscular dystrophy (p. 280) there is no effective treatment. In this situation the indication is to try to identify families to whom genetic counselling could be offered with a view to alerting relevant females to their possible carrier status.

PHENYLKETONURIA

Routine biochemical screening of newborn infants for phenylketonuria was recommended by the Ministry of Health in the United Kingdom in 1969 after it had been shown that a low phenylalanine diet could prevent the severe mental retardation which previously had been a hallmark of this condition (p. 151). The screening test,

which is sometimes known as the Guthrie test, is carried out on a small sample of blood obtained by heel-prick at age 7 days. An abnormal test result is further investigated by repeat analysis of phenylalanine levels in a venous blood sample. A low phenylalanine diet is extremely effective in preventing mental retardation, and, although it is not particularly palatable, most affected children can be persuaded to adhere to it until early adult life when it

Table 22.6   Conditions for which neonatal screening can be undertaken

Disorder	Test/method
Widely applied	
Phenylketonuria	Guthrie* or automated fluorometric assay
Congenital hypothyroidism	Thyroxine or thyroid stimulating hormone
Other inborn errors	
Biotinidase deficiency	Specific enzyme assay
Galactosaemia	Modified Guthrie
Homocystinuria	Modified Guthrie
Maple syrup urine disease	Modified Guthrie
Tyrosinaemia	Modified Guthrie
Miscellaneous	
Congenital adrenal hyperplasia	17-Hydroxyprogesterone assay
Cystic fibrosis	Immunoreactive trypsin and DNA analysis
Duchenne muscular dystrophy	Creatine kinase
Sickle-cell disease	Haemoglobin electrophoresis

*The Guthrie test is based on reversal of bacterial growth inhibition by a high level of phenylalanine

can be relaxed. Any woman with phenylketonuria who is contemplating pregnancy should adhere to a strict low phenylalanine diet both before and during pregnancy to minimize the risk of brain damage to her unborn child (pp. 155, 236). Without strict dietary control this risk is very high.

GALACTOSAEMIA

Classical galactosaemia affects approximately 1 in 50 000 newborn infants and usually presents with vomiting, lethargy and severe metabolic collapse within the first 2 or 3 weeks of life. Newborn screening is based on a modification of the Guthrie test with subsequent confirmation by specific enzyme assay. The early introduction of appropriate dietary restriction can prevent the development of serious complications such as cataracts, liver failure and mental retardation.

CONGENITAL HYPOTHYROIDISM

Screening for congenital hypothyroidism was first introduced in the United States in 1974 and is now undertaken in most parts of the developed world. The test is based on assay of either thyroxine or thyroid stimulating hormone. This disorder is particularly suitable for screening as it is relatively common with an incidence of approximately 1 in 4000 and treatment with life-long thyroxine replacement is extremely effective in preventing the severe developmental problems associated with the classical picture of 'cretinism'. The most common cause of congenital hypothyroidism is absence of the thyroid gland rather than an inborn error of metabolism (p. 154). Congenital absence of the thyroid gland is usually not caused by genetic factors.

CYSTIC FIBROSIS

Newborn screening for cystic fibrosis has been introduced in several countries with a significant population of northern European origin. It is based on the detection of an elevated blood level of immunoreactive trypsin, which is a consequence of blockage of pancreatic ducts in utero, supplemented by DNA analysis (p. 277). The rationale for screening is that it is hoped that early treatment with physiotherapy and antibiotics will improve the long-term prognosis. Initial results are encouraging but absolute confirmation of long-term benefit has not yet been forthcoming.

SICKLE-CELL DISEASE

Newborn screening based on haemoglobin electrophoresis is undertaken in many countries with a significant Afro-Caribbean community. As with cystic fibrosis, it is hoped that early prophylaxis will reduce morbidity and mortality, thereby improving the long-term outlook. In the case of sickle-cell disease treatment involves the use of oral penicillin to reduce the risk of pneumococcal infection resulting from immune deficiency secondary to splenic infarction (p. 144). Even in Western countries with good medical facilities, a significant proportion of sickle-cell homozygotes, possibly as many as 15%, die as a result of infection in early childhood.

POPULATION CARRIER SCREENING

Widespread screening for carriers of autosomal recessive disorders in high incidence populations was first introduced for the haemoglobinopathies (p. 142) and has been extended to several other disorders (Table 22.7). The rationale behind these programmes is that carrier detection can be supported by genetic counselling so that carrier couples can be forewarned of the 1 in 4 risk that each of their children could be affected.

Experience with the two common haemoglobinopathies, thalassaemia and sickle-cell disease, illustrates the extremes of success and failure which can result from well- or poorly-planned screening programmes.

Table 22.7 Autosomal recessive disorders suitable for population carrier screening

Disorder	Ethnic group or community	Test
α Thalassaemia	China and eastern Asia	Mean corpuscular haemoglobin and haemoglobin electrophoresis
β Thalassaemia	Indian subcontinent and Mediterranean countries	Mean corpuscular haemoglobin and haemoglobin electrophoresis
Sickle-cell disease	Afro-Caribbeans	Sickle test and haemoglobin electrophoresis
Cystic fibrosis	Western European caucasians	Common mutation analysis
Tay–Sachs disease	Ashkenazi Jews	Hexosaminidase A

THALASSAEMIA

α and β thalassaemia are caused by abnormal globin chain synthesis due to mutations involving the α- and β-globin genes or their promotor regions (p. 145). Both disorders show autosomal recessive inheritance, and both are extremely common in certain parts of the world, notably China (α thalassaemia) and Cyprus, Italy and the Indian subcontinent (β thalassaemia).

In Cyprus in 1974 the birth incidence of β thalassaemia was 1 in 250. Following the introduction of a comprehensive screening programme to determine the carrier status of young adults, the incidence of affected babies declined by over 95% within 10 years. Similar programmes in Greece and Italy have seen a drop in the incidence of affected homozygotes of over 50%.

If it is acceptable to judge the outcome of these screening programmes on the basis of a reduction in the births of affected babies, then they have been very successful, due largely to the efforts of highly motivated staff interacting with a well-informed target population which has usually opted not to have affected children.

SICKLE-CELL DISEASE

In contrast to the Cypriot response to β thalassaemia screening, early attempts to introduce sickle-cell carrier detection in the black population of North America were disastrous. Information pamphlets tended to confuse the sickle-cell carrier state, or trait, which is usually harmless, with the homozygous disease which conveys significant morbidity (p. 144). Several US states passed legislation making sickle-cell screening in black people mandatory, and sickle-cell carriers began to be discriminated against by employers and insurance companies. It is not surprising that public criticism was aroused leading to abandonment of the screening programmes and amendment of the ill-conceived legislation.

This experience with sickle-cell carrier screening emphasizes the importance of ensuring voluntary participation and providing adequate and appropriate information and counselling. More recent pilot studies in the United States and in Cuba have shown that individuals of Afro-Caribbean origin are perfectly receptive to well-planned non-directive sickle-cell screening programmes.

CYSTIC FIBROSIS

The discovery in 1989 that the ΔF508 deletion/mutation accounts for a high proportion of all cystic fibrosis heterozygotes soon led to the suggestion that screening programmes could be implemented for carrier detection on a population basis. In the white population of the United Kingdom, the cystic fibrosis carrier frequency is approximately 1 in 22 and the ΔF508 mutation accounts for 75–80% of all heterozygotes. A further 10% of carriers can be detected relatively easily and cheaply using a multiplex PCR analytical procedure.

Initial studies of attitudes to cystic fibrosis carrier detection yielded quite divergent results. A casual written invitation generates a poor take-up response of around 10%, whereas personal contact during early pregnancy, whether mediated through general practice or the antenatal clinic, results in uptake rates of over 80%. Further studies are underway to explore attitudes to cystic fibrosis screening among specific groups such as school leavers and women in early pregnancy.

Two approaches for screening pregnant women have been considered. The first is referred to as 'two-step' and involves testing pregnant mothers at the antenatal clinic. Those who test positive for a common mutation, i.e. approximately 85% of all cystic fibrosis carriers, are informed of the result and invited to bring their partners for testing — hence 'two-step' testing. If both partners are found to be carriers then an offer of prenatal diagnosis is made. This approach has the advantage that all carriers detected are informed of their result and further family studies ('cascade screening') can be initiated. The disadvantages are that those women whose partners are subsequently found to have a normal result experience considerable unnecessary anxiety which creates a need for counselling and support.

The second approach is referred to as 'couple screening'. This involves testing both partners simultaneously and only disclosing positive results if both partners are found to be carriers. In this way much less anxiety is generated but the opportunity for offering tests to the extended family when only one partner is a carrier is lost. At present it is not clear which, if either, of these approaches will be recommended for widespread implementation. The results of pilot studies indicate that these 'two-step' and 'couple screening' approaches are equally acceptable to pregnant mothers with take-up rates of approximately 70%.

POSITIVE AND NEGATIVE ASPECTS OF POPULATION SCREENING

Well-planned population screening enhances informed choice and offers the prospect of a significant reduction in the incidence of disabling genetic disorders. These potential advantages have to be weighed against the potential disadvantages which can arise from the over-enthusiastic pursuit of a poorly planned or ill-judged screening programme (Table 22.8). Experience to date indicates that in relatively small well-informed groups, such as the Greek Cypriots and American Ashkenazi Jews, community screening is welcomed. When screening is offered to larger populations the outcome is less certain.

Table 22.8 Potential advantages and disadvantages of genetic screening

Advantages
Informed choice
Improved understanding
Early treatment when available
Reduction in births of affected homozygotes

Disadvantages and hazards
Pressure to participate causing mistrust and suspicion
Stigmatization of carriers (social, insurance and employment)
Inappropriate anxiety in carriers
Inappropriate reassurance if test is not 100% sensitive

Table 22.9 Roles of a genetic register

To maintain an informal two-way communication process between the family and the genetics unit

To offer carrier detection to relevant family members as they reach adult life

To coordinate presymptomatic and prenatal diagnosis when requested

To coordinate multidisciplinary management of patients with complex hereditary conditions such as the familial cancer syndromes

To ensure effective implementation of new technology and treatment

To provide a long term source of information and support

A 3-year follow-up of almost 750 individuals screened for the cystic fibrosis carrier status in the United Kingdom revealed that a positive test result had not caused undue anxiety, although some carriers did have a relatively poor perception of their own general health. A more worrying outcome was that almost 50% of the individuals tested could not accurately recall or interpret their results. This emphasizes the importance of pretest counselling and the provision of accurate information which can be easily processed and fully understood.

GENETIC REGISTERS

Most clinical genetic units maintain what is known as a *genetic register* of families and individuals who are either affected by or at risk of developing a serious hereditary disorder. The primary purpose of a genetic register is to maintain two-way contact between a genetics unit and relevant family members (Table 22.9). This permits investigations to be offered as appropriate and ensures that families do not feel abandoned or excluded from a source of information and support.

Entry on to a genetic register should be entirely voluntary and it is essential that confidentiality is not breached. Information is never revealed to outside agencies without the consent of the relevant individual.

Genetic registers are most appropriate for conditions which are relatively common, have potentially serious effects, convey high risks to other family members and in which complications can be treated or prevented (Table 22.10). They are particularly valuable for conditions which show a delayed age of onset or for which unaffected carriers could be at high risk of having seriously affected children.

Well-organized genetic registers can also play a key role in coordinating a multidisciplinary approach to the management of patients with conditions such as the familial cancer-predisposing syndromes (p. 202). The management

Table 22.10 Disorders suitable for a genetics register

Disorder	Chromosome location
Autosomal dominant	
Adult onset polycystic kidney disease	16
Familial adenomatous polyposis	5
Familial hypercholesterolaemia	19
Huntington's disease	4
Multiple endocrine neoplasia types 1 and 2	10, 11
Myotonic dystrophy	19
Neurofibromatosis types I and II	17, 22
Retinoblastoma	13
Von Hippel–Lindau syndrome	3
Autosomal recessive	
Cystic fibrosis	7
Sickle-cell disease	11
Thalassaemia	11, 16
X-linked	
Duchenne/Becker muscular dystrophy	
Fragile X syndrome	
Haemophilia	
Retinitis pigmentosa	
Chromosomal	
Deletions/insertions	
Inversions	
Translocations	

of such patients often involves the interpretation of molecular investigations and the organization of regular visits to other hospital departments where screening for early signs of malignancy can be undertaken (p. 204). Programmes of this nature are much appreciated by family members and can make a major contribution to improving the quality of life for individuals and families at risk of developing serious genetic disease. Genetic registers will prove to be particularly valuable when effective methods of gene therapy have been developed for the common single gene disorders.

ELEMENTS

1 Population screening involves the offer of genetic testing to all members of a particular population, with the primary objective being the enhancement of informed personal choice.

2 Participation should be voluntary and each programme should be widely available, equitably distributed, acceptable to the target population and supported by full information and counselling.

3 Prenatal screening is now offered routinely for neural tube defects, by assay of maternal serum α-fetoprotein, and for chromosome abnormalities by assay of three or four biochemical markers constituting either the 'triple' or the 'quadruple' test.

4 Neonatal screening is widely available for phenylketonuria, galactosaemia and congenital hypothyroidism. Other conditions are screened for in specific populations.

5 Population screening programmes for carriers of β thalassaemia have resulted in a major fall in the births of affected homozygotes. Similar programmes could be equally effective for sickle-cell disease and cystic fibrosis if care is taken to ensure that they are acceptable to their target populations.

6 Well-organized genetic registers provide an effective means of maintaining two-way contact between genetics centres and families with hereditary disease.

FURTHER READING

Axworthy D, Brock D J H, Bobrow M, Marteau T M 1996 Psychological impact of population-based carrier testing for cystic fibrosis: 3-year follow-up. Lancet 347: 1443–1446
A review of the impact of carrier testing for cystic fibrosis on over 700 individuals.
Brock D J H, Rodeck C H, Ferguson Smith M A (eds) 1992 Prenatal diagnosis and screening. Churchill Livingstone, Edinburgh
A huge multiauthor textbook with excellent chapters on all aspects of genetic screening.
Cunningham G C, Tompkinson D G 1999 Cost and effectiveness of the California triple marker prenatal screening program. Genet Med 1: 199–206
A detailed review of the impact of triple test screening over a 10-year period in California.
Genetic screening ethical issues 1993 Nuffield Council on Bioethics, London
The report of a working party on genetic screening on the associated ethical and societal issues.
Modell B, Modell M 1992 Towards a healthy baby. Oxford University Press, Oxford
A clearly written and easily understood guide to genetic counselling and community genetics.

The human genome project, treatment of genetic disease and gene therapy

BEGINNING AND ORGANIZATION OF THE HUMAN GENOME PROJECT

The concept of a map of the human genome was proposed as long ago as 1969 by Victor McKusick, one of the founding fathers of medical genetics. Human gene mapping workshops were held regularly from 1973 to collate the mapping data. The human genome project as an entity in its own right had its beginnings in a workshop held in Alta, Utah under the auspices of the US Department of Energy (DOE) in 1984. The involvement of the DOE might at first appearance seem odd but they had historically been interested in the detection of mutations in DNA to assess the effects of exposure to radiation and chemicals. A subsequent report on the technologies involved in detecting mutations in DNA and a further international meeting organized by the DOE held in 1986 at Sante Fe, New Mexico, led to the idea of a dedicated human genome project. The DOE in the following year produced a report on the Human Genome Initiative outlining the major objectives.

In the subsequent year the United States Congress approved a 15-year US human genome project which started in 1991 with an estimated budget of $200 000 000 per annum. Other nations, notably France, the United Kingdom and Japan, soon followed with their own major national human genome programmes and have subsequently been joined by a number of other countries. These individual national projects are all coordinated by the Human Genome Organization (HUGO) which has three centres, one for the Americas based in Bethesda, Maryland, one for Europe located in London and one for the Pacific in Tokyo.

The US Human Genome Project (HGP) is run jointly under the auspices of the National Institute of Health's National Center for Human Genome Research (NCHGR), initially headed by James Watson who was succeeded by

Francis Collins, and the DOE through the National Laboratories at Lawrence Livermore, Lawrence Berkeley and Los Alamos.

OBJECTIVES OF THE HUMAN GENOME PROJECT

Many persons, particularly the general public, have the impression that the only objective of the human genome project is to sequence all 3×10^9 base pairs of the human genome. This is, however, only one of the six main objectives/areas of work of the human genome project.

Human gene maps and mapping of human inherited diseases

Designated genome mapping centres with earmarked funding were involved in the coordination and production of genetic or recombination and physical maps of the human genome. The genetic maps initially involved the production of fairly low level resolution index, skeleton or framework maps, which were based on polymorphic variable number di-, tri- and tetranucleotide tandem repeats (p. 16) spaced at approximately 10 cM intervals throughout the genome. The most recent high level resolution maps have polymorphic markers which are, on average, spaced at intervals of less than 1 cM.

The mapping information from these genetic maps has been integrated with high resolution physical maps (Fig. 23.1). The information for the latter maps comes from a variety of sources using a number of different technologies which include fluorescent in situ hybridization (FISH) (p. 34), somatic cell and radiation hybrids (p. 57), and YAC or cosmid contigs (p. 71). Access to the detailed information from these high resolution genetic and physical maps allows individual research groups, often interested in a specific or particular inherited disease or group of diseases, to rapidly and precisely localize or map a disease gene to a specific region of a chromosome.

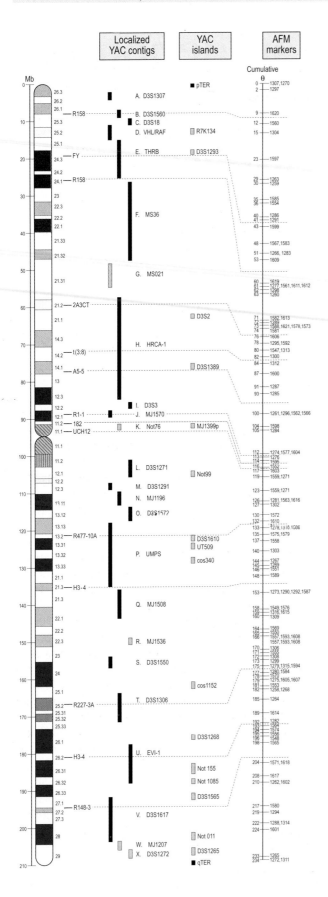

The presence of CpG islands (p. 73), exon trapping (p. 73) and/or expressed sequence tags (ESTs) (p. 73) can be used to identify coding sequences in the region involved. Along with the known genes or ESTs which map to the region, these can then serve as positional candidate genes (p. 74) for analysis to determine whether they are responsible for an inherited disorder.

Development of new DNA technologies

A second major objective is the development of new DNA technologies for human genome research. For example, at the outset of the human genome project, the technology involved in DNA sequencing was very time consuming, laborious and relatively expensive. The development of automated genome sequencing technology, along with the use of fluorescent labelling, has helped transform the ease and cost of large-scale DNA sequencing projects. Future developments in the use of DNA microchip technology are likely to further revolutionize analytical applications of the information from the human genome sequence project.

Sequencing of the human genome

While sequencing the entire human genome would have been seen to be the obvious main focus of the human genome project, it was not initially the straightforward proposal it seemed. The human genome contains large sections of repetitive DNA (p. 16) which are often technically difficult to clone and sequence. In addition, it would seem a waste of time to collect sequence data on the entire genome when only a small proportion is made up of expressed sequences or genes, the latter being most likely to be the regions of greatest medical and biological importance. Furthermore, the sheer magnitude of the prospect of sequencing all 3×10^9 base pairs of the human genome seemed overwhelming. With conventional sequencing technology, as was carried out in the early 1990s, it was estimated that a single laboratory worker could sequence up to approximately 2000 base pairs per day. This would mean that it would have taken 1.5×10^6 person-days to sequence the whole of the human genome!

Fig. 23.1

A summary map of human chromosome 3, estimated to be 210 Mb in size, which integrates physical mapping data covered by 24 YAC contigs and the Genethon genetic map with cumulative map distances. (From Gemmill R M, Chumakov I, Scott P et al 1995 A second-generation YAC contig map of human chromosome 3. Nature 377: 299–319, with permission.)

Projects involving sequencing of other organisms with smaller genomes have shown how much work is involved as well as how the rate of producing sequence data has increased with the development of new DNA technologies. For example, initial efforts at producing genome sequence data for yeast took an international collaboration involving 35 laboratories in 17 countries from when it was started in 1989 until 1995 to sequence just 315 000 base pairs of chromosome 3, one of the 16 chromosomes which make up the 14 000 000 base pairs of the yeast genome. Advances in the DNA technologies meant, however, that by the middle of 1995 more than one-half of the yeast genome had been sequenced, with the complete genomic sequence being reported the following year.

Further advances in DNA sequencing technology have resulted in the reporting of the full sequence of the nematode *C. elegans* in 1998, the 50 million base pairs of the DNA sequence of human chromosome 22 at the end of 1999 and the sequence of the 125 million base pairs of the fruit fly in early 2000, the latter some 3 years ahead of schedule. As a consequence of these technical developments, the 'draft' sequence of the human genome was reported in the spring of 2000 with the expectation of the complete sequence in 2003.

This portion of the human genome project has been associated with much controversy. Substantial sums of public money have been dedicated to the sequencing of the human genome project with involvement of a number of centres with the sequence information generated being freely available to the scientific community. The strategy being used was to carry out the DNA sequencing on an ordered modular basis, i.e. different groups concentrating on specific chromosomes with the sequencing being carried on a clone-by-clone basis using the mapping information previously generated.

The approach of the commercial sector to the sequencing of the human genome has been, perhaps not surprisingly, different. Rather than the modular approach they suggested it was simpler and more efficient just to 'shotgun' sequence the whole of the human genome at random and then to take the sequence information generated and assemble it by means of a computer program which recognizes overlapping DNA sequences. Although many members of the scientific community were sceptical at the time it was proposed about the likelihood of this approach succeeding, a combination of this method with the existing genome maps led to the complete sequence becoming available well ahead of the planned schedule.

In addition, although the commercial sector originally indicated that they would release the DNA sequence information they generated into the public domain (appendix: GenBank), they have maintained that they have the right to release this information on a 'non-redistribution' basis, i.e. that they should have the right to sell the human genome sequence information they generated. They argue that it is reasonable for them to expect commercial returns on their investment which would be likely to result from the identification of novel genes which would allow elucidation of the role of their gene products in biological pathways involved in health and disease with the potential for the development of diagnostic tools and pharmacological therapeutic interventions. This is an area of controversy which also involves ethical and social aspects and will not easily be resolved. It is clear, however, that public–private partnerships give added value, if the various potentially conflicting interests can be accommodated.

Development of bioinformatics

Essential to the overall success of the human genome project, is what is known as bioinformatics — the establishment of facilities for collecting, storing, organizing, interpreting, analysing and communicating the data from the project which can be widely shared by the scientific community at large. It is vital for anyone involved in any aspect of the human genome project to have rapid and easy access to the data/information arising from it. This dissemination of information has been met by the establishment of a large number of electronic databases available on the World Wide Web (WWW) on the Internet (appendix). These include protein and DNA sequence databases (for example GenBank and EMBL), databases of genetic maps for humans (such as the GDB, Genethon, CEPH, CHLC and the Whitehead Institute sites) and other species (the Mouse Genome Database and the *Caenorhabditis elegans* database), linkage analysis programs (e.g. the Rockefeller University Web site) and the catalogue of inherited diseases in humans (Online Mendelian Inheritance in Man or OMIM). The latter was first set up as a computer-based information system by Victor McKusick more than 30 years ago.

These developments in bioinformatics now allow the prospect of identifying coding sequences and determining their likely function(s) from homologies to known genes, leading to the prospect of identifying a new gene without the need for any laboratory experimental work, or what has been called 'cloning in silico'.

Comparative genomics

In addition to the human genome project, there are separate genome projects for a number of other species, for what are known as 'model organisms'. These include various prokaryotic organisms such as the bacteria

Escherichia coli and *Haemophilus influenzae* as well as eukaryotic organisms such as *Saccharomyces cerevisiae* (yeast), *Caenorhabditis elegans* (flatworm), *Drosophila melanogaster* (fruit fly), *Mus musculus* (mouse), *Rattus norvegicus* (rat) and *Fugu rubripes rupripes* (puffer fish). While the impact of what is called *comparative genomics* is not necessarily immediately obvious, it is of vital importance in the human genome project.

For example, the availability of the total genome sequence of yeast revealed it to contain a total of approximately 6000 genes, only some 2300 of which had been previously identified from traditional genetic studies in yeast. In addition, of the 3700 new genes identified by the sequencing project, only approximately 2300 shared significant sequence homology with any known genes from any other organism, i.e. they are novel genes whose functions are unknown. The sequencing of the fruit fly has also revealed so far some 13 000 genes half of whose functions are unknown. Mapping of the human homologues of these newly identified genes from other species provides new 'candidate' genes for inherited diseases in humans.

Functional genomics

The second major way in which model organisms are proving to be invaluable in the human genome project is to provide the means to follow the expression of genes and the function of their protein products in normal development as well as their dysfunction in inherited disorders. This is referred to as *functional genomics* or what has also been called *post-genomic genetics*.

The ability to introduce targeted mutations in specific genes (p. 64), along with the production of transgenic animals (p. 69), for example in the mouse, allows the production of animal models to study the pathodevelopmental basis for inherited human disorders as well as serve as a test system for the safety and efficacy of gene therapy and other treatment modalities (p. 327). Strategies using different model organisms in a complementary fashion, taking into account factors, such as the ease/complexity of producing transgenic organisms and the generation times of different species, allow the possibility of relatively rapid analysis of gene expression, function and interactions in providing an understanding of the complex pathobiology of inherited diseases in humans.

In addition, in the last few years the development of *microarrays* provides a useful tool for the analysis of the pattern of gene expression in health and disease. This technique which has come out of the developments in DNA microchip technology (p. 64), involves use of robotic automated miniaturized microscopic spots of aliquots of cDNAs or oligonucleotides from specific genes in a standardized high density gridded arrangement on glass (Fig. 23.2). This allows large-scale analysis

Fig. 23.2

Diagrammatic representation of a cDNA microarray. Aliquots of cDNAs of interest are gridded on a glass template using a computer controlled robot. The test and reference RNA samples which are labelled with different coloured fluorochromes by reverse transcription are mixed and allowed to hybridize with the cDNAs on the microarray. The templates are exposed to laser light and the excitation pattern generated is compared identifying genes which show differences in expression between the reference and test samples.

of the pattern of gene expression by analysis of RNA species looking at differences between tissues, at different times of development and differentiation, as well as under a variety of different conditions, e.g. exposure to hormones, drugs, and so on.

Microarray gene expression analysis has an enormous potential, allowing whole genome expression screening, offering the prospect of being able to move from the 'anatomy' of the genes of the human genome in the form of DNA sequence information to its 'function', through what has been termed *proteomics*. This is the identification of the respective proteins and the elucidation of their involvement in the biological pathways and interactions in development, differentiation, health and disease.

ETHICAL, LEGAL AND SOCIAL ISSUES OF THE HUMAN GENOME PROJECT

The rapid advances in the science and application of developments from the human genome project present complex ethical issues for both the individual and society. Five per cent of the budget from the Department of Energy and the National Institutes of Health in the United States for the human genome project is devoted to the study of the ethical, legal and social issues (ELSI) surrounding the availability of genetic information. These issues include ones of immediate practical relevance such as who owns and should control genetic information with respect to privacy and confidentiality: who is entitled to access to it and how, whether it should be used by employers, schools, etc., the psychological impact and potential stigmatization of persons positive for genetic testing and the use of genetic testing in reproductive decision making. Other issues which will be increasingly important in future as developments from the human genome project become more widespread are the concept of disability/differences which have a genetic basis in relation to the treatment of genetic disorders/ diseases by gene therapy and the possibility of genetic enhancement, i.e. using gene therapy to supply certain characteristics such as height. Lastly, issues need to be resolved with regard to the appropriateness and fairness of the use of the genetic technologies which come out of the human genome project with prioritization of the use of public resources and commercial involvement and property rights, especially with regard to patenting. It is probably fair to say that although the public debate is appropriate and much overdue, a quick and simple resolution of many of these complex issues is unlikely.

PROS AND CONS OF THE HUMAN GENOME PROJECT

Opponents of the human genome project argue that an expenditure likely to exceed the planned total of $3 billion over the 15 years of the project could be better used in other medical and scientific research. Many such critics have often mistakenly viewed the human genome project as a mindless sequencing exercise which will be devoid of any intrinsic biological interest. Others, through a misunderstanding of the normal interaction which takes place between the genetic make-up and environ-

mental factors in development of the characteristics and health of an individual, cite the danger of what is commonly called *biological* or *genetic determinism*, i.e. that we will be able to precisely predict the intelligence or characteristics of a person or when and what they will die of. Persons with such concerns often feel it is a short step to raise the potential dangers of the misuse of this information in the form of positive or negative eugenics.

Supporters of the human genome project maintain that it will be of major benefit to humankind by improving our understanding and development of new strategies for the prevention and treatment of inherited disease. It is clear, however, from the progress of the human genome project to date, that while many of the developments and findings have occurred as were planned and predicted, a large number have been unplanned and unexpected. In addition, the rate of progress of the project is likely to accelerate with the development of new technologies and the convergence of findings from various component parts of the project. While it is obvious that the information and understanding which will come from the human genome project will be of enormous benefit and importance to those individuals and families with or at risk of inherited diseases, there should be genuine and real concern that the same developments could be misused, for example by employers or insurance companies, to discriminate against the same such individuals. The right of ownership of this information and its confidentiality are vital concerns for any developed and caring society (p. 337).

TREATMENT OF GENETIC DISEASE

Many genetic disorders are characterized by progressive disability or chronic ill-health for which there is, at present, no effective treatment. Consequently one of the most exciting aspects of the developments in biotechnology is the prospect of successful gene therapy. It is important, however, to keep a perspective on the limitations of gene therapy for the immediate future and to consider, in the first instance, conventional approaches to the treatment of genetic disease.

CONVENTIONAL APPROACHES TO TREATMENT OF GENETIC DISEASE

Most genetic disorders cannot be cured or even ameliorated using conventional methods of treatment. Often this is because the underlying gene and gene product have not been identified so that there is little, if any, understanding of the basic metabolic or molecular defect. If, however, this is understood then dietary restriction, as in phenylketonuria (p. 151), or hormone replacement, as in congenital adrenal hyperplasia (p. 158), can be used very successfully in the treatment of the disorder. In a few disorders, such as homocystinuria (p. 156) and some of the organic acidurias (p. 166), supplementation with a vitamin or coenzyme can increase the activity of the defective enzyme with beneficial effect (Table 23.1).

Protein/enzyme replacement

If a genetic disorder is found to be the result of a deficiency of or an abnormality in a specific enzyme or protein then, in theory, treatment could involve replacement of the deficient or defective enzyme or protein. An obviously successful example of this is the use of factor VIII concentrate in the treatment of haemophilia A (p. 282).

In most of the inborn errors of metabolism in which an enzyme deficiency has been identified, simple enzyme replacement is not possible because, until recently, sufficient quantities of the enzyme or protein have not been available. In addition, even if recombinant DNA techniques are used to biosynthesize the missing or defective gene product, injection of the enzyme or protein could be predicted to be unsuccessful as the metabolic processes involved are carried out within cells and the protein or enzyme is not normally transported into the cell. Artificial delivery systems, such as liposomes, allow proteins to cross the cell membrane. Liposomes are artificially prepared cell-like structures in which one or more bimolecular layers of phospholipid enclose one or more aqueous compartments, which can include specific proteins. Although, in theory, it was thought liposomes would work, they have met with little success in the treatment of genetic disorders such as the mucopolysaccharidoses, in which it was hoped that such a therapy could be effective. In some instances, however, biochemical modification of the protein or enzyme allows utilization of normal cellular transport mechanisms to target the enzyme to its normal location within the cell. For example, modifications in β-glucosidase as used in the treatment of Gaucher's disease enable it to enter the lysosomes, resulting in an effective form of treatment (p. 164).

Drug treatment

In some genetic disorders drug therapy is possible, e.g. certain drugs can help lower cholesterol levels in familial hypercholesterolaemia (p. 160). In others, avoidance of certain drugs or foods can prevent the manifestation of the disorder, e.g. sulphonamides and fava beans in glucose-6-phosphate dehydrogenase (G6PD) deficiency (p. 171).

Table 23.1 Examples of various methods for treating genetic disease

Treatment	Disorder
Enzyme induction by drugs	
Phenobarbitone	Congenital non-haemolytic jaundice
Replacement of deficient enzyme/protein	
Blood transfusion	SCID due to adenosine deaminase deficiency
Bone marrow transplantation	Mucopolysaccharidoses
Enzyme/protein preparations	
Trypsin	Trypsinogen deficiency
α_1-Antitrypsin	α_1-Antitrypsin deficiency
Cryoprecipitate/factor VIII	Haemophilia A
β-Glucosidase	Gaucher's disease
Replacement of deficient vitamin or coenzyme	
B_6	Homocystinuria
B_{12}	Methylmalonic acidaemia
Biotin	Propionic acidaemia
D	Vitamin D-resistant rickets
Replacement of deficient product	
Cortisone	Congenital adrenal hyperplasia
Thyroxine	Congenital hypothyroidism
Substrate restriction in diet	
Amino acids	
Phenylalanine	Phenylketonuria
Leucine, isoleucine, valine	Maple syrup urine disease
Carbohydrate	
Galactose	Galactosaemia
Lipid	
Cholesterol	Familial hypercholesterolaemia
Protein	Urea cycle disorders
Drug therapy	
Aminocaproic acid	Angioneurotic oedema
Dantrolene	Malignant hyperthermia
Cholestyramine	Familial hypercholesterolaemia
Pancreatic enzymes	Cystic fibrosis
Penicillamine	Wilson's disease, cystinuria
Drug/dietary avoidance	
Sulphonamides	G6PD deficiency
Barbiturates	Porphyria
Replacement of diseased tissue	
Kidney transplantation	Adult onset polycystic kidney disease, Fabry's disease
Bone marrow transplantation	X-linked SCID, Wiskott–Aldrich syndrome
Removal of diseased tissue	
Colectomy	Familial adenomatous polyposis
Splenectomy	Hereditary spherocytosis

Tissue removal/transplant

Replacement of defective tissue is another option which became available with the advent of tissue typing (p. 182), e.g. renal transplantation in adult polycystic kidney disease. Removal of diseased tissue to prevent complications is a prophylactic or therapeutic option in many of the familial cancer-predisposing syndromes, e.g. colectomy in persons with familial adenomatous polyposis (p. 200).

Experimental methods of treatment

For a number of serious genetic disorders it is necessary to consider less frequently used and, on occasion, drastic and/or unproven therapeutic options. These include bone marrow transplantation for some of the neuro-degenerative storage disorders, such as the more severe mucopolysaccharidoses, e.g. Hurler's and Hunter's syndromes (p. 162), which has met with limited success.

THERAPEUTIC APPLICATIONS OF RECOMBINANT DNA TECHNOLOGY

The advent of recombinant DNA technology has also led to rapid progress in the availability of biosynthetic gene products for the treatment of certain inherited diseases.

Biosynthesis of gene products

Insulin used in the treatment of diabetes mellitus was, until recently, obtained from pig pancreases. This had to be very carefully purified for use and even then it occasionally produced sensitivity reactions in patients. However, with recombinant DNA technology, microorganisms can be used to synthesize insulin from the human insulin gene. This is inserted, along with appropriate sequences to ensure efficient transcription and translation, into a recombinant DNA vector such as a plasmid and cloned in a microorganism, such as *E. coli*. In this way large quantities of insulin can be made. An artificial gene which is not identical with the natural gene needs to be constructed for this purpose, however, because synthetically produced genes cannot contain the non-coding intervening sequences, or introns (p. 15), found in the majority of structural genes in eukaryotic organisms, since microorganisms such as *E. coli* do not possess a means for splicing of the mRNA after transcription.

Recombinant DNA technology is being employed in the production of a number of other biosynthetic products (Table 23.2). The biosynthesis of medically important peptides in this way is usually more expensive than obtaining the product from conventional sources because of the research and development involved. However, biosynthetically derived products have the dual advantages of providing a pure product which is unlikely to induce a sensitivity reaction and one which is free of the risk of chemical or biological contamination. In the past, the use of growth hormone

Table 23.2   Proteins produced biosynthetically using recombinant DNA technology

Protein	Disease
Insulin	Insulin-dependent diabetes mellitus
Growth hormone	Short stature due to growth hormone deficiency
Factor VIII	Haemophilia A
Factor IX	Haemophilia B
Interferon	Infections, cancer (?)
α_1-Antitrypsin	Emphysema due to α_1-antitrypsin deficiency (?)
Somatostatin	Excess growth
Vaccines	Hepatitis B, malaria and other tropical diseases (?)

? = effectiveness not yet proven.

from human cadaver pituitaries has been associated with the transmission of Creutzfeldt-Jakob disease, and the human immunodeficiency virus (HIV) has been a contaminant in cryoprecipitate containing factor VIII used in the treatment of haemophilia A (p. 282).

GENE THERAPY

Gene therapy can be defined as the replacement of a deficient gene product or correction of an abnormal gene. Gene therapy can be carried out either in vitro (or ex vivo) by treatment of cells or tissue from an affected individual in culture, with reintroduction into the affected individual, or in vivo if cells cannot be cultured or be replaced in the affected individual.

The possibility of successful gene therapy belonged to the realms of science fiction until the very recent past. However, advances in molecular biology leading to the identification of many important human disease genes and their protein products have raised the prospect of gene therapy for many genetic and non-genetic disorders. It is important to emphasize that although gene therapy is often presented as the new panacea in medicine, it will have a limited impact in the short term and its application will be fraught with many practical difficulties for the near future.

REGULATORY REQUIREMENTS

There has been much publicity about the potential uses and abuses of gene therapy. Regulatory bodies have been established in several countries to oversee the technical, therapeutic and safety aspects of gene therapy programmes (p. 342). There is universal agreement that *germ line gene therapy*, in which genetic changes could be distributed to both somatic and germ cells and therefore be transmitted to future generations, is morally and ethically unacceptable. Therefore all programmes are focusing only on *somatic cell gene therapy*, in which the alteration in genetic information is targeted to specific cells, tissues or organs in which the disorder is manifest.

In the United States the Human Gene Therapy Subcommittee of the National Institutes of Health has produced guidelines for protocols of trials of gene therapy which must be submitted for approval to both the Food and Drug Administration and the Recombinant DNA Advisory Committee, along with their institutional review boards (IRBs). In the United Kingdom the Gene Therapy Advisory Committee (GTAC) has recommended that all gene therapy programmes must be approved by hospital research ethical committees.

Over 300 clinical trials of gene therapy have been approved for children and adults for a variety of genetic and non-genetic disorders. For the most part these appear to be proceeding without event, but the unexpected death of a patient in one trial has highlighted the need to consider whether external monitoring of the clinical trials in gene therapy is appropriate. Exaggerated expectations and fierce competition to succeed could lead to potential conflicts of interest.

TECHNICAL ASPECTS

Before a gene therapy trial is possible, there are a number of technical aspects which must be addressed.

Gene characterization

One of the basic prerequisites of gene therapy is that the gene involved should have been cloned. This should include not only the structural gene but also the DNA sequences involved in the control and regulation of expression of that gene. This prerequisite would seem obvious, but some of the early attempts at gene therapy were carried out in the early 1980s when little was known about the regulatory or control regions needed for normal gene expression. In retrospect, it is clear that these early attempts at gene therapy were both premature and naive in their expectation of achieving success.

Target cells/tissue/organ

The specific cells, tissue or organ affected which is to be treated must be identified and accessible. Again this seems obvious. Some of the early attempts at treating the inherited disorders of haemoglobin, such as β thalassaemia, involved removing bone marrow from affected individuals, treating it in vitro, and then returning it to the patient by transfusion. While in principle this could have worked, in order to have any likelihood of success the particular cells which needed to be targeted were the small number of bone marrow stem cells from which the immature red blood cells, or reticulocytes, develop.

Vector system

The means by which a foreign gene is introduced needs to be both efficient and safe. If gene therapy is to be considered as a realistic alternative to conventional treatments, there should be unequivocal evidence from trials of gene therapy carried out in animal models that the inserted gene functions adequately with appropriate regulatory, promoter and enhancer sequences. In addition, it needs to be shown that the treated tissue or cell population has a reasonable life span, that the gene product continues to be expressed and that the body does not react adversely to the gene product, e.g. by producing antibodies to the protein product. Lastly, it is essential to demonstrate that introduction of the foreign gene or DNA sequence has no deleterious effects, such as inadvertently leading to a malignancy or a mutagenic effect on either the somatic or the germ cell lines, e.g. through mistakes arising as a result of the insertion of the gene or DNA sequence into the host DNA or what is known as *insertional mutagenesis*. The possibility of affecting the germ cells needs to be considered even if the treatment is directed at somatic tissues.

METHODS OF GENE THERAPY

These can be divided into two main types, viral and non-viral methods.

Viral agents

A number of different viruses can be used to transport foreign genetic material into cells. Each of these has its own particular advantages and disadvantages.

Retroviruses

These are derived from a family of viruses which includes the human immunodeficiency virus and viruses which can cause cancer in certain species. Retroviruses integrate into the host DNA by making a copy of their RNA molecule using the enzyme reverse transcriptase (p. 190). The provirus so formed is the template for the production of the mRNAs for the various viral gene products and the new genomic RNA of the virus. If the provirus is stably integrated into dividing stem cells, all subsequent progeny cells will inherit a copy of the viral genome.

Retroviruses used in gene therapy are rendered incapable of independent replication so as not to produce the side-effects associated with infectivity. For this to be achieved, retroviruses used in gene therapy require two elements, a *packaging cell line* and a *vector* or *helper virus*.

Packaging cell line

The packaging cell line is a cell line which has been infected with a retrovirus in which the provirus is genetically engineered to lack the region of the proviral DNA called the packaging sequence. This means that the cells will produce all of the normal viral proteins but the provirus cannot be packaged into infectious virus particles.

Vector or helper virus

Another retroviral provirus is engineered with more than 90% of the viral genetic material removed, leaving only the minimal DNA sequences necessary to produce copies of the viral RNA sequences along with the sequences necessary for packaging of the viral genomic RNA. This is the vector backbone into which the foreign DNA or gene can be inserted. If this vector, or helper virus, is introduced into the packaging cell line which contains the provirus missing the packaging sequences, the RNA produced by the vector provirus can be packaged into viruses. These virions can be used to infect, or what is commonly termed *transfect*, the particular target cells or tissue. The virions do not replicate to produce further infective virions since the retrovirus vector cannot replicate because it lacks the sequences necessary for this to occur (Fig. 23.3).

Disadvantages of the use of retroviruses

One of the disadvantages associated with the use of retroviruses as a vector system in gene therapy is that only a relatively small DNA sequence can be introduced into the target cells, usually less than 7 kb, limiting their use in gene therapy. For example, even if all of the introns were removed from the dystrophin gene (p. 281) for use in gene therapy of Duchenne muscular dystrophy, the gene would still be much too large to be incorporated into a retroviral vector. Attempts have been made to overcome this by inserting a modified dystrophin gene in which a large amount of the gene has been deleted but which still has relatively normal function. This is known as a *minidystrophin* gene (p. 282).

A second disadvantage of using retroviruses as vectors in gene therapy is that they can only infect dividing cells. This means that genetic disorders which involve, for example, the central nervous system cannot be treated using retroviruses. In addition, at present, retroviruses can only be used to treat cells or tissues in vitro. In theory, with identification of the receptors on cells for

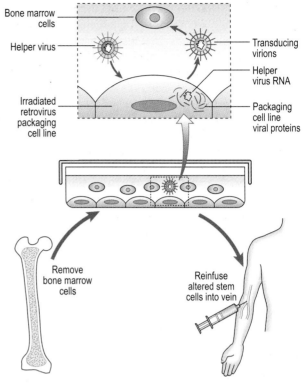

Fig. 23.3
Diagrammatic representation of retrovirus gene therapy using bone marrow cells.

retroviruses, they could also be used to target specific cell types or tissues in vivo.

A further disadvantage of retroviruses is that they are unstable and cannot be purified for use in gene therapy without reducing their ability to transduce their target cells. As a consequence, retrovirus preparations from cultured cells cannot be fully characterized. This means that it is not possible to completely exclude the possibility of contamination with replication competent retroviruses or packaging of cellular RNAs which could have oncogenic potential (p. 191). These are not simply theoretical risks since there has been a report of lymphoma occurring in rhesus monkeys subjected to trials of retroviral gene therapy.

Difficulties in controlling the level of expression of the introduced gene or DNA sequence have been encountered in animal trials of retrovirus-mediated gene therapy. Improvements in the techniques used in retrovirus-mediated gene therapy are likely with targeting of specific cells, e.g. stem cells in bone marrow, including the appropriate control or regulatory sequences.

Adenoviruses

Adenoviruses can be used as vectors in gene therapy since they infect a wide variety of cell types. They have advantages over retroviruses in that they are stable and can be easily purified to produce high titres for infection. In addition, they are suitable for targeted treatment of specific tissues such as the respiratory tract. Unlike retroviruses, they can infect non-dividing cells and carry up to 36 kb of foreign DNA.

Adenoviruses do not integrate into the host genome which avoids the possibility of insertional mutagenesis but has the disadvantage that expression of the introduced gene is usually unstable and often transient. In addition, by virtue of their infectivity, they can produce adverse effects secondary to infection and by stimulating the host immune response. Lastly, adenoviruses contain genes known to be involved in the process of malignant transformation so that there is a potential risk that they could inadvertently induce malignancy.

Adeno-associated viruses

Adeno-associated viruses are non-pathogenic parvo-viruses in humans which require coinfection with helper adenoviruses or certain members of the herpes virus family to achieve infection. In the absence of the helper virus the adeno-associated virus DNA integrates into chromosomal DNA at a specific site on the long arm of chromosome 19 (19q13.3–qter). Subsequent infection with an adenovirus activates the integrated adeno-associated viral DNA producing virions. They have the advantages of being able to infect a wide variety of cell types, exhibiting long term gene expression and lack of generation of an immune response to transduced cells. The safety of adeno-associated viruses as vectors occurs by virtue of their site-specific integration but, unfortunately, this is often impaired with the inclusion of foreign DNA in the virus. The disadvantages of adeno-associated viruses include the fact that they can be activated by any adenovirus infection and that, although 95% of the vector genome is removed, they can only take inserts of foreign DNA up to 5 kb in size.

Some of the more recent developments of the adeno-associated viruses as vectors for gene therapy allow the prospect of the introduction of pharmacologically controlled induction of the expression of transduced genes.

Herpes virus

Herpes viruses are neurotropic, i.e. infect nervous tissue, and, if suitably modified, could be used to target gene therapy to the central nervous system. An immediate disadvantage of using herpes viruses as a vector system is their direct toxic effects on nerve cells as well as the consequent immune response, although recent modifications of this potential neurotropic vector have been produced which are devoid of viral expression and neurotoxicity. Herpes viruses, however, do not integrate

into the host genome and therefore it is likely that the expression of introduced genes would be temporary and unstable.

Other viruses

Other viruses, including the influenza, vaccinia and a number of other RNA viruses, could be used as vectors in gene therapy since they produce large quantities of gene product. However, they are likely to have problems similar to those seen with other vector systems. Many, like adenoviruses, will elicit an immune response, thereby limiting their potential for repeated use.

Non-viral agents

There are a number of different non-viral methods of gene therapy. These have the theoretical advantage of not eliciting an immune response and being safer and simpler to use, as well as allowing large-scale production, but differ in their efficacy.

Naked DNA

Direct injection of DNA into cells has been used in gene therapy, e.g. the minidystrophin gene into myoblasts in the mouse model for Duchenne muscular dystrophy (p. 291). While success has been reported in terms of evidence of localized gene expression, clearly this approach has a limited place except for the possibility of the expression of hormones or proteins for which small amounts will result in a significant clinical effect, e.g. erythropoietin or factor VIII.

Liposome-mediated DNA transfer

Liposomes are lipid bilayers surrounding an aqueous vesicle (p. 326) which can facilitate the introduction of foreign DNA into a target cell (Fig. 23.4). A disadvantage of liposomes is that they are not very efficient in gene transfer and the expression of the foreign gene is transient, so that the treatment has to be repeated. An advantage of liposome-mediated gene transfer is that a much larger DNA sequence can be introduced into the target cells or tissues than with viral vector systems. This can be as large as an artificially constructed mini-chromosome which, in addition to a specific structural gene, can include elements involved in the regulation of gene expression in a physiologically controlled fashion, as well as centromeric and telomeric sequences which will allow replication of the foreign DNA in mitotic divisions. Recent modifications of cationic lipid/DNA complexes have been developed which enhance the efficacy of gene transduction.

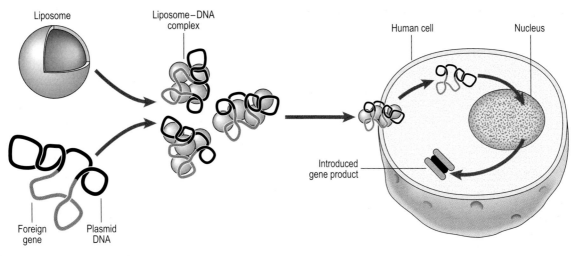

Fig. 23.4
Diagrammatic representation of liposome-mediated gene therapy.

Receptor-mediated endocytosis

A variation of liposome-mediated gene transfer is to target the DNA to specific receptors on the surfaces of cells. A complex is made between plasmid DNA containing the foreign gene or DNA sequence and specific polypeptide ligands for which the cell has a receptor on its surface. For example, DNA complexed to a glycoprotein containing galactose will be recognized by receptors on the surface of liver cells which are specific to glycoproteins with a terminal galactose. This results in internalization of the complex into endocytic vesicles, which are then transported to the lysosomes where the complex is degraded. In order for the foreign gene to then be expressed, it has to escape from the lysosome. The rate at which it escapes from the lysosomes can be increased by inclusion of adenovirus or influenza gene products.

Oligonucleotides

It is possible to synthesize what are known as antisense oligonucleotides, which bind to specific mRNA sequences, or specifically engineered RNA molecules known as ribozymes, which have intrinsic RNA catalytic properties resulting in cleavage of RNA transcripts. This can result in blocking of mRNA processing and subsequent translation of a particular mRNA species. Difficulties arise both in the stability of the oligonucleotides and their entry into the relevant target cells. Alternatively, an oligonucleotide can be synthesized to a sequence in a gene which will form a triple helical structure with double stranded genomic DNA. If the stretch of triple helix is then alkylated, then that gene can be disabled permanently. This latter approach is also of limited value as the oligonucleotide must be up to 15–18 bp in length

and composed primarily of the purine nucleotides adenine and guanine, a combination which occurs only rarely in the coding sequences of most genes. Recently, it has been proposed that RNA/DNA chimeras which utilize the normal mismatch repair system (p. 200) could be used for targeted gene repair.

Future methods of gene therapy

It is likely that the development of vector systems for gene therapy in the future will involve a convergence of viral and non-viral technologies, such as virus-targeted integration into a specific region of DNA in certain limited cell types or tissues through specific receptor-mediated endocytosis, along with removal of sequences involved in interactions with native receptors which lead to toxicity by generation of an immune response.

In addition, the extension of the treatment of genetic diseases to the antenatal period in utero may offer the prospect of another option for couples at risk for having children with certain serious genetic disorders.

Stem cell transplantation

Transplantation of the relevant stem cells, e.g. pluripotent haematopoietic stem cells, in utero offers the prospect of a novel mode of treatment of genetic disorders with a congenital onset. The immaturity of the fetal immune system means that the fetus will be tolerant of foreign cells so that there is no need to match the donor cells with those of the fetus. Trials of in utero stem cell transplantation are under way for a number of disorders which include severe combined immunodeficiency (SCID), α and β thalassaemia and sickle-cell disease.

Stem cell gene therapy

The ability to identify the process and factors involved in the differentiation of committed stem and progenitor cells in various tissues, e.g. haematopoietic tissues, offers the prospect of gene therapy targeted to cells committed to a particular tissue or organ.

In utero fetal gene therapy

The report of successful in utero gene therapy in a cystic fibrosis mouse model means that fetal gene therapy in utero is possible in humans, but it is considered unacceptable at present because of the possibility of inadvertent germ cell gene therapy. The possibility of somatic cells being treated by gene therapy in vitro and then transplanted back in utero however, is likely to have a place for some of the more serious neurodegenerative disorders with a very early onset, such as Krabbe's disease or Hurler's syndrome (p. 162).

Animal models

One of the basic prerequisites for assessing the suitability of gene therapy trials in humans is the existence of an animal model. While there are naturally occurring animal models for some inherited human diseases, for most there is no animal counterpart. Site-directed DNA mutagenesis allows the targeted introduction of mutations into a gene (p. 64). If carried out in the embryonic cells of an inbred species, the subsequent offspring will be mosaics for the normal and mutated gene. These animals can then be interbred to produce animals which will be homozygous for the introduced mutation in that particular gene. Several groups, using homologous recombination (p. 64), have been able to knock out the *CFTR* gene (p. 276) in mouse embryonic cells to produce a mouse model for cystic fibrosis. These mice have been confirmed as transgenic animal models for cystic fibrosis by having findings similar to those seen in humans with the disease. This animal model has been used to evaluate several types of gene therapy before trials in humans.

Target organs

In most instances gene therapy will need to be and should be directed or limited to a particular organ, tissue or body system.

Liver

Viral vectors for gene therapy of inherited hepatic disorders have been of limited use due to the lack of vectors which specifically target hepatocytes. Although liver cells are refractory to retroviruses in vivo, they are, somewhat surprisingly, susceptible to transfection by retroviruses in vitro. Cells removed from the liver by partial hepatectomy can be treated in vitro and then reinjected via the portal venous system from which they seed in the liver. The effectiveness of this approach has been demonstrated by the lowering of cholesterol levels in a rabbit animal model with a defect in the low density lipoprotein (LDL) receptor. The injection of the hepatocytes into the portal venous system is, however, associated with a significant risk of thrombosis of the portal venous system which can lead to the complication of portal hypertension. Nevertheless, because of the serious outlook for homozygotes with mutations in the LDL receptor (p. 160), gene therapy by this means has been attempted in a woman homozygous for an LDL receptor defect. This has led, in the short term, to a reduction of LDL levels, although the long term benefit is, as yet, undetermined. Other disorders affecting or involving the liver in which a similar approach could be considered are phenylketonuria, α_1-antitrypsin deficiency and haemophilia A.

CNS

CNS directed vector systems are being developed in which replication-defective neurotropic adenoviruses lacking the so-called E1 region can be produced and then be made infective by growing them in cells engineered to express the E1 genes. In addition, it has been suggested that slow viruses, or what are known as lentiviruses, could be used for the treatment of central nervous system disorders, such as Parkinson's and Alzheimer's diseases, because they integrate into the host genome of non-dividing cells and could therefore act as a delivery system for stable expression.

Another approach which has been suggested in genetic disorders affecting the CNS is to transplant cells which have been genetically modified in vitro into specific regions of the brain, such as the caudate nucleus in persons with or at risk of Huntington's disease.

Muscle

Unlike other tissues, direct injection of foreign DNA into muscle has met with some success in terms of retention and expression of the foreign gene in the treated muscle. Alternatively, injection of myoblasts into muscle results in their incorporation into recipient muscle bundles. Although animal model work showed some promise of efficacy, this approach has met with difficulties in humans. Direct DNA injection has, however, been used to express the protein products of genes, transferred in vitro into myoblasts, which are unrelated to muscle function, such as human growth hormone and factor VIII. Other primary cell types, such as fibroblasts treated in vitro, could also be transplanted back as skin grafts to deliver circulating gene products.

Bone marrow

In the treatment of disorders affecting the bone marrow, problems arise due to the small numbers of stem cells, which need to be transduced if there is to be more than a transient response with gene therapy. Stem cells often constitute less than 1% of the total cells present. Pretreatment of the bone marrow to expand the number of stem cells has been tried for certain inherited immunological disorders by the use of growth factors such as the granulocyte colony stimulating factor (G-CSF) and the cytotoxic agent 5-fluorouracil. Reliable identification of specific stem cell types would enable them to be enriched for, thereby increasing the likelihood of success.

DISEASES AMENABLE TO GENE THERAPY

The disorders which are possible candidates for gene therapy include both genetic and non-genetic diseases (Table 23.3).

Genetic disorders

There are a number of single gene diseases which are obvious candidates for gene therapy. One of the first diseases for which gene therapy has been attempted in humans is the inherited immunodeficiency disorder caused by adenosine deaminase (ADA) deficiency (p. 165). Somewhat surprisingly, it has been found that persons with this disorder respond to simple blood transfusions. The ADA activity present in the red blood cells of the transfused blood transiently corrects the immunodeficiency in the lymphocytes of the affected patients. Treatment with polyethylene-conjugated ADA increases the half-life of the enzyme in the circulation. Trials of treatment of lymphocytes or bone marrow from patients with ADA deficiency transduced with a retroviral vector with the ADA gene are under way at present.

Attempts at treating β thalassaemia and sickle-cell disease by gene therapy have not been effective as yet, primarily because of difficulties in the identification of sequences involved in the normal control of the expression of the globin genes (p. 139).

Double blind trials are being carried out in the United Kingdom and the United States treating cystic fibrosis patients using either a liposome–gene complex or an adenovirus vector sprayed into the nasal passages. Studies of their efficacy and safety involve looking for

Table 23.3 Genetic and non-genetic diseases which can potentially be treated by gene therapy

Genetic disorder	Defect
Immune deficiency	Adenosine deaminase deficiency Purine nucleoside phosphorylase deficiency Chronic granulomatous disease
Hypercholesterolaemia	Low density lipoprotein receptor abnormalities
Haemophilia	Factor VIII deficiency (A) Factor IX deficiency (B)
Gaucher's disease	Glucocerebrosidase deficiency
Mucopolysaccharidosis VII	β-Glucuronidase deficiency
Emphysema	α_1-Antitrypsin deficiency
Cystic fibrosis	CFTR mutations
Phenylketonuria	Phenylalanine hydroxylase deficiency
Urea cycle abnormalities	
Hyperammonaemia	Ornithine transcarbamylase deficiency
Citrullinaemia	Argininosuccinate synthetase deficiency
Muscular dystrophy	Dystrophin mutations
Thalassaemia/sickle-cell disease	α- and β-globin mutations
Cancer Malignant melanoma Ovarian cancer Brain tumours Neuroblastoma Renal cancer Lung cancer	
Acquired immune deficiency syndrome (AIDS)	
Cardiovascular diseases	
Rheumatoid arthritis	

the presence of the introduced *CFTR* gene in biopsies of the nasal epithelium and measurement of ion transport in nasal epithelial cells. Reports to date of trials of gene therapy in cystic fibrosis have shown that it is not obviously harmful, although there is very limited evidence of efficacy.

Common multifactorial diseases

In the majority of human diseases in which there is a genetic aetiology, both genes and environmental factors are involved (pp. 127, 209). Gene therapy will have a much more widespread impact in medicine if it can be used in this group of disorders. It is important, however, to remember that for most of the common multifactorial diseases in humans, the identification and subsequent avoidance of causative environmental factors is likely to be much more effective than gene therapy at present or in the near future.

Cancer

Gene therapy for cancer involves the introduction of toxic genetic elements to selectively kill off cancer cells.

Supply tumour suppressor genes

It has been proposed that the targeted introduction of recognized tumour suppressor genes (p. 195), such as *Tp53*, to cancer cells could result in control of their growth. More detailed knowledge of the biology of cancer will be needed before this approach can be reliable and safe.

Target immunological mitogen genes into tumour cells

Mitogens, such as interleukin-2, introduced in vitro into melanosomes, which have been removed from patients with malignant melanoma and then reintroduced into the patient, could be used to activate the patient's immune response. The use of liposome-bound plasmid DNA containing foreign histocompatibility genes to transduce tumour cells to enhance the immune response has also been proposed as a possible form of gene therapy in cancer. Again, a better understanding of the malignant process and the body's immune response to malignancy will be necessary before this form of gene therapy can be effective.

Introduce genes which selectively damage cancer cells

The introduction of the tumour necrosis factor gene into tumour-infiltrating lymphocytes, which can then be returned to the patient, has been promoted as another approach for gene therapy in cancer. More recently, a proposal has been made to introduce what have been called *conditionally toxic* or *suicide genes* into cancer cells. An example is the thymidine kinase gene of the herpes simplex virus which allows the metabolism of the substance gancyclovir by cellular kinases into the triphosphate form which inhibits DNA polymerase, resulting in the death of the cancer cells as well as surrounding cells through a 'bystander' effect. It has also been proposed that 'antiangiogenic' genes could be used to compromise the circulatory supply of tumours.

Other modalities

These include the use of antisense oligonucleotides to block the gene products of oncogenes, as well as the introduction of genes into bone marrow cells to render them resistant to chemotherapeutic agents.

Coronary artery disease

It has been proposed that gene therapy could be used to introduce the LDL receptor into persons with a family history of early coronary artery disease even if they do not have familial hypercholesterolaemia.

Peripheral vascular disease

A number of different trials of gene therapy in persons with peripheral arterial vascular disease are under way, involving introduction of genes which lead to proliferation of new vessels and the production of anticlotting agents.

Autoimmune disorders

The use of gene therapy in autoimmune disorders to restore immune homeostasis has been suggested. Interleukin-1 (IL-1) is an immune system signal which triggers inflammation. For example, it has been proposed that gene therapy could be used to introduce genes for the IL-1 receptor antagonist protein into synovial cells in persons with rheumatoid arthritis, in which the inflammatory process is believed to play a key aetiological role.

Gene therapy in transplantation

It has been suggested that gene therapy be used to reduce the immune response in order to increase the success rate of tranplants and reduce the immunotoxicity associated with immunosuppressants used to prevent rejection could involve the introduction of genes which lead to the inhibition of T cell stimulation, immunosuppressive cytokines or the major histocompatibility genes.

FURTHER READING

Adams M D, Celniker S E, Holt R A et al 2000 The genome sequence of the *Drosophia melanogaster*. Science 287: 2185–2195
The sequence of the fruit fly, one of the first 'model' organisms in genetics.
Anderson W F 1992 Human gene therapy. Science 256: 808–813
A consideration of gene therapy by one of its main proponents.
Cappecchi M R 1994 Targeted gene replacement. Sci Am 270: 34–41
Review of the techniques to produce transgenic animal models for inherited diseases in humans.
Dunham I, Shimizu N, Roe B A et al 1999 The DNA sequence of chromosome 22. Nature 402: 489–95
The first report of the DNA sequence of a human chromosome.
Müller-Hill B 1993 The shadow of genetic injustice. Nature 362: 491–492
A brief commentary urging caution against being caught up in the enthusiasm for the human genome project.
Mulligan R C 1993 The basic science of gene therapy. Science 260: 926–936
A considered review of the problems and approaches to gene therapy.

ELEMENTS

1 The human genome project is an international research effort, the purpose of which is to track down the genes responsible for inherited disease in humans and determine the sequence of the human genome. Although justification of the planned expenditure is controversial, this research is likely to pay dividends in our understanding of both genetic and non-genetic diseases.

2 Treatment of genetic disease by conventional means requires identification of the gene product and an understanding of the pathophysiology of the disease process. Therapeutic options can include dietary restriction or supplementation, drug therapy, replacement of an abnormal or deficient protein or enzyme and replacement or removal of an abnormal tissue.

3 Recombinant DNA technology has enabled human-derived biosynthetic gene products such as human insulin and growth hormone to be produced for the treatment of human disease.

4 Before a trial of gene therapy is carried out in humans, the gene involved must be characterized, the particular cell type or tissue to be targeted must be identified, an efficient, reliable and safe vector system which results in stable continued expression of the introduced gene has to be developed, and the safety and effectiveness of the particular modality of gene therapy has to be demonstrated in an animal model.

5 Germ line gene therapy is universally viewed as ethically unacceptable, while somatic cell gene therapy is generally viewed as being acceptable, as this is seen as similar to existing treatments such as organ transplantation.

CHAPTER

24

Ethical issues in medical genetics

Ethical issues can be defined as those which involve moral questions and dilemmas. Traditionally they are approached by applying a set of moral principles, usually based on a synthesis of the philosophical and religious views of well-informed, respected, thinking members of society. In this way a code of practice evolves which is seen as reasonable and acceptable by a majority and which often forms the basis for professional guidelines or regulations.

Ethical issues arise in all branches of medicine but are particularly contentious in genetics because of the way this subject impinges not just on an individual but also on the extended family and on society in general. In the minds of the general public, clinical genetics and genetic counselling can easily be confused with *eugenics*, which can be defined as the science of 'improving' a species through breeding. It is important to stress that the modern specialty of clinical genetics has absolutely nothing in common with the totally unacceptable eugenic phil-osophies which were practised in Nazi Germany and, to a much lesser extent, elsewhere in Europe and in the United States between the two World Wars. Emphasis has already been made on the fundamental principle that genetic counselling is a **non-directive** and **non-judgemental** communication process whereby factual knowledge is imparted to facilitate informed personal choice (ch.15). Coercion and eugenics have no place in modern medical genetics.

Nevertheless this is a subject which lends itself to ethical debate, not least because of the new opportunities provided by discoveries in molecular genetics. In this chapter some of the more controversial and difficult areas will be considered. It will soon become apparent that for many of these issues there is no clear right or wrong approach and individual views will vary widely. Sometimes in a clinical setting the best that can be hoped for is to arrive at a mutually acceptable compromise with an explicit agreement that opposing views are respected and, personal conscience permitting, a patient's expressed wishes are carried out.

GENERAL PRINCIPLES

When undertaking any patient contact there are a number of important general principles to keep in mind.

INFORMED CONSENT

A patient is entitled to an honest and full explanation before any procedure or test is undertaken. Information should include details of the risks, limitations, implica-tions and possible outcomes of each procedure.

INFORMED CHOICE

A patient is entitled to full information about all options available including the option of not participating. Potential consequences should be discussed. No duress should be applied and the doctor or nurse should not have a vested interest in the patient pursuing any particular course of action.

AUTONOMY

The patient is in charge. At any stage he or she can decide to proceed no further. In genetics this is particularly relevant in the context of predictive testing when, for example, a patient is fully entitled to opt out at any stage in the pre-test counselling process.

CONFIDENTIALITY

A patient has a right to complete confidentiality which can only be breached under extreme circumstances, such as when it is deemed that an individual's behaviour could convey a high risk of harm to him- or herself or to others.

ETHICAL DILEMMAS IN CLINICAL GENETICS

Everyone involved in the discipline of clinical genetics is confronted by complex and challenging ethical situations on an all too frequent basis. Some of those areas which pose particularly difficult problems shall be considered. In dealing with these the clinician/counsellor, who sometimes faces an almost impossible task, has to keep in mind the basic ethical principles which form the cornerstone of all good medical practice (Table 24.1). On occasions some of the dilemmas which arise in clinical genetics would tax even the wisdom of Solomon!

PRENATAL DIAGNOSIS

Many methods are now widely available for diagnosing structural abnormalities and genetic disorders during the first and second trimesters (ch. 21). The issue of prenatal diagnosis and subsequent offer of termination of pregnancy raises many difficult issues for individuals and families and raises serious questions about the way in which society views and cares for both children and adults with disability. In the United Kingdom termination of pregnancy is permitted up to and beyond 24 weeks gestation if the fetus has a lethal condition such as anencephaly, or if there is a serious risk of major physical or mental handicap. Terms such as 'serious' are not defined in the relevant legislation.

The difficulties surrounding prenatal diagnosis can be illustrated by considering some of the general principles which have already been discussed. At the top of the list comes informed consent. In the United Kingdom approximately 70% of all pregnancies are monitored for the presence of a neural tube defect by measurement of α-fetoprotein in maternal serum at approximately 16 weeks' gestation (p. 314). In theory all women undertaking this test should have a full understanding of its potential implications. This also applies to every woman who is offered a detailed ultrasound scan to assess fetal anatomy at around 18 weeks' gestation (p. 304). For fully informed consent to be obtained in these situations it is essential that pregnant women should have access to detailed counselling by unhurried staff who are well informed, experienced and sympathetic. In practice it is unlikely that this always applies.

The most difficult problems in prenatal diagnosis are those involving autonomy and individual choice. This relates particularly to severity and to who should be able to decide when termination is justified. This can be illustrated by considering the following situations. First of all a mother presents with a request that the sex of her unborn baby be determined; she already has five healthy daughters and states that she will only continue with the pregnancy if tests show that the unborn baby is male. There is general agreement in the medical genetics community that being of the 'wrong' sex is not an abnormality and does not provide grounds for termination of pregnancy. Yet for this woman the prospect of another daughter is unacceptable. Faced with this impossible situation how should the genetic counsellor proceed?

Next consider the unusual but not unprecedented dilemma which arises when parents with an inherited condition indicate that they only wish to continue with a pregnancy if tests show that their unborn baby is also affected. Examples of conditions which could generate a request of this nature include achondroplasia and congenital sensorineural hearing loss. If the family's autonomy and right to choose is to be respected then their request should be granted. Many readers of this chapter will be very uncomfortable with the suggestion that an unaffected pregnancy should be terminated. This particular scenario illustrates the difficulty of defining what is normal.

The issue of autonomy and individual choice can also arise when a fetus is found to have a relatively mild abnormality, such as a non-syndromal cleft lip and palate, for which surgical correction usually achieves an excellent outcome. For some parents, particularly those who themselves have had an unhappy childhood because of being stigmatized for a similar problem, the prospect of having a similarly affected child can be unacceptable. Understandably medical and nursing staff may feel very uneasy about complying with a request for termination of pregnancy in this situation.

It is inevitable that a subject as emotive as termination of pregnancy will generate controversy and the ethical dilemmas which arise are not easily resolved. Proponents of choice argue that selective termination should be available, particularly if the alternative involves a lifetime of pain and suffering. More often than not prenatal diagnostic techniques provide reassurance and their availability allows many couples to embark upon a pregnancy who would otherwise have been deterred. When viewed in the context of abortion in general, termination on the grounds of fetal abnormality constitutes less than 2% of the total of well over 100 000 abortions carried out each year in the United Kingdom.

Table 24.1   Fundamental ethical principles
Informed consent
Respect for individual autonomy
Fairness and justice
Do good and do not harm
Equity of access and opportunity
Privacy and confidentiality

Those who hold opposing views argue on religious, moral or ethical grounds that selective termination is little less than legalized infanticide. There is also concern that prenatal diagnostic screening programmes could lead to a devaluing of handicapped individuals in society with a possible shift of resources away from their care to the funding of programmes aimed at 'preventing' their birth. The debate about the ethics of prenatal diagnosis is a fierce one which will become even more difficult when genes are identified for common multifactorial disorders such as depression and schizophrenia.

PREDICTIVE TESTING IN CHILDHOOD

Understandably, parents sometimes wish to know whether or not a child has inherited the gene for an adult onset autosomal dominant disorder which runs in the family. It could be argued that this knowledge will help the parents guide their child towards the most appropriate educational and career opportunities and that to refuse their request is a denial of their rights as parents. Similarly parents sometimes request information about the carrier status of young healthy siblings of a child with a recessive disorder such as cystic fibrosis. Sometimes this information will have become available as a result of prenatal diagnostic testing for the homozygous affected state.

The problem with agreeing to this type of request is that it is a clear infringement of the child's own future autonomy. Increasingly, it is felt that testing should be delayed until the child reaches an age when he or she can make his or her own informed decision. There is also concern about the possible deleterious effects on a child of growing up with the certain knowledge of developing a serious adult onset hereditary disorder or being a carrier of a recessive disorder, particularly if the tests have proved negative in that child's other siblings. Such a situation could raise a very real possibility of stigmatization.

The situation is very different if predictive testing could be of direct medical benefit to the child. This applies to conditions such as familial hypercholesterolaemia (p. 160) for which early dietary management can be introduced and also to some of the familial cancer-predisposing syndromes (p. 202) for which early screening is indicated. Generally it is felt that in these situations genetic testing is acceptable at around the time when other screening tests or preventive measures would be initiated.

IMPLICATIONS FOR THE IMMEDIATE FAMILY (INADVERTENT TESTING OR TESTING BY 'PROXY')

A positive test result in an individual can have major implications for close antecedent relatives who themselves do not wish to be informed of their disease status. For example, consider Huntington's disease (HD) for which direct mutational analysis is now available (p. 267). A young man aged 20 years requests predictive testing prior to starting his family; his fears are based on a confirmed diagnosis in his 65-year-old paternal grandfather. Predictive testing would be relatively straightforward were it not for the fact that his father, who is obviously at a prior risk of 1 in 2, specifically does not wish to know whether he will develop the disease.

Thus the young man has raised the difficult question of how to comply with his request without inadvertently carrying out a predictive test on his father. A negative result in the young man leaves scope for doubt; in principle no harm would be done. A positive result in the son, however, would be difficult to conceal from an observant father who will be alert to his son's subsequent behaviour. Clearly a positive result in the son would indicate that the father must be heterozygous for the HD gene.

There is no easy solution to this particular problem. In the guidelines drawn up in 1994 for predictive testing in Huntington's disease it was concluded that 'every effort should be made by the counsellors and the persons concerned to come to a satisfactory solution' with the rider that 'if no consensus can be reached the right of the adult child to know should have priority over the right of the parent not to know'.

IMPLICATIONS FOR THE EXTENDED FAMILY

It is widely agreed that the identification of a condition which could have implications for other family members should lead to the offer of tests for the extended family. This applies particularly to balanced translocations and serious X-linked recessive disorders. In the case of translocations this is sometimes referred to as translocation 'chasing'. For an autosomal recessive disorder such as cystic fibrosis the term 'cascade screening' is applied (p. 318).

The main ethical problem which arises here is that of confidentiality. A carrier of a translocation or serious X-linked recessive disorder is usually urged to alert close family relatives to the possibility that they could also be carriers and therefore be at risk of having affected children. Alternatively, permission can be sought for members of the genetics team to make these approaches. Occasionally a patient, for whatever reason, will refuse to allow this information to be disseminated.

Faced with this situation what should the clinical geneticist do? In practice most clinical geneticists would try to convince their patient of the importance of offering tests to relatives, possibly by providing an explanation of the consequences and ill-feeling which could arise in the future if a relative was to have an affected child whose birth could have been predicted and perhaps avoided. Often skilled and sensitive counselling will lead to a satisfactory solution. Ultimately, however, most clinical geneticists would opt to respect their patient's confidentiality rather than break the trust which forms a cornerstone of the traditional doctor–patient relationship.

INFORMED CONSENT IN GENETIC RESEARCH

All individuals who agree to undergo genetic testing in a service context are obviously entitled to a full and clear explanation of what the test involves and how the results could have implications for both themselves and other family members. Vigorous efforts are usually made to ensure that these basic principles are adhered to, particularly when predictive testing for serious late onset genetic disorders is being undertaken.

The issues relating to informed consent when participating in genetic research are just as complex. Many people are perfectly willing to hold out their arm for a blood test 'which might help others', particularly if they have personal experience of a serious disorder in their own family. However, few will have given any serious thought to the possible ramifications of their simple act of altruism. For example, it is unlikely that they will ever have considered whether their sample will be tested anonymously, who will be informed of the result or whether other tests will be carried out on stored DNA in the future as new techniques are developed. These concerns among others (Table 24.2) have prompted the NIH Office of Protection from Research Risks to draw up proposals on the steps which should be taken to try to ensure that all aspects of informed consent are addressed when samples are collected for genetic research.

ETHICAL DILEMMAS IN A WIDER CONTEXT

Recent progress in genetics, most notably in the area of molecular testing, has brought the ethical debate into a much wider public arena. Topics such as insurance, patenting, gene therapy and population screening are now rightly viewed as being of major societal, commercial and political importance, and perhaps not surprisingly they feature prominently in media discussion. All of these subjects impact on the specialty of medical genetics and each of these shall now be considered in turn.

GENETICS AND INSURANCE

The availability of predictive tests for disorders of adult onset which convey a risk for chronic ill health with the possibility of a reduction in life expectancy has generated widespread concern about the extent to which the

---

Table 24.2 **Issues of disclosure and consent in genetic research**
The nature of the study
Who is doing the study and where is it being carried out?
Availability of results and their implications for the individual and extended family regarding health, employment and insurance
Anonymity of testing and confidentiality of results
Long term storage of DNA and its possible use in other research projects
Potential commercial applications and profit

---

results of these tests should be revealed to outside agencies. Chief among these are the life insurance companies. In countries with only limited welfare medical services, this is also an issue for private health care insurance, including critical illness and disability income. In addition, if either life or health insurance is arranged through an employer, then in theory there could also be implications for long term career prospects as a positive predictive genetic test could lead to withdrawal of an offer of employment.

The life insurance industry is competitive and profit driven. Private insurance is based on the concept of 'mutuality', whereby risks are pooled for individuals in similar circumstances. In contrast public health services are based on the principle of 'solidarity' whereby health provision for everyone is funded from general taxation. It is understandable that the life insurance industry is concerned that individuals who receive a positive result from a predictive test will take out large policies without revealing their true risk status. This is referred to as 'antiselection' or 'adverse selection'. On the other hand there is a very real fear among the genetics community that individuals who test positive will find themselves victims of discrimination, possibly to the extent that they become uninsurable. This concern also extends to those who have a family history of a late onset disorder who might be refused insurance unless they undergo predictive testing.

Concerns about this very real possibility that DNA testing will create an uninsurable 'genetic underclass' have led to the introduction of legislation in many parts of the United States aimed at limiting the use of genetic information by health insurers. This culminated in 1996 in President Clinton signing 'The Health Insurance Portability and Accountability Act', which expressly prevents employer-based health plans refusing coverage on genetic grounds when a person changes employment. In the United Kingdom this whole area was considered in 1995 by the House of Commons Science and Technology Committee, which recommended that a Human Genetics Advisory Commission be established to overview developments in human genetics. In 1997 this

Advisory Commission recommended that applicants for life insurance should not have to disclose the results of any genetic test to a prospective insurer and that a moratorium on disclosure of genetic test results should last for at least 2 years until genetic testing had been carefully evaluated.

To the disappointment of the genetics community, the UK government opted not to accept the recommendation of this advisory body, preferring instead to allow the recommendations of the Association of British Insurers (ABI) to prevail. Some of the key points in these recommendations are listed in Table 24.3. In the 1999 revision of its Code of Practice, the ABI reiterated its view that applicants should not be asked to undergo genetic testing and that existing genetic test results need not be disclosed in applications for mortgage related life assurance up to a total of £100 000.

In the UK the Genetics and Insurance Committee has been established with a broad membership drawn from the insurance industry, the medical community and interested public bodies. One of the chief remits of this committee is to evaluate genetic tests as they are developed, and the ABI has stated in its code of practice that genetic test results should not be taken into account until each specific test is fully validated.

The issues involved in genetic testing and the insurance industry are not going to be easily resolved. If 'polygenes' conveying susceptibility to common disorders of adult life are identified, then almost the entire population could find itself at the mercy of a profit driven commercially focused insurance industry. Among the genetics community there is a strong view that legislation is needed urgently to ensure that those who are genetically disadvantaged, through no fault of their own, do not face discrimination when seeking health care or long term life insurance.

GENE PATENTING AND THE HUMAN GENOME PROJECT

The controversy surrounding the patenting of naturally occurring human DNA sequences, be they complete genes or ESTs, neatly encapsulates the conflict between harsh commercial realism and altruistic academic idealism. On the one hand biotechnology companies which have invested heavily in molecular research can argue with conviction that both they and their shareholders are entitled to benefit from the fruits of their labours. Biotechnology research is indeed expensive and it can reasonably be argued that any commercial company is entitled to a fair return on its investments. Those who embrace a more idealistic view have argued that the human genome represents mankind's 'common heritage' and that information gained through the Human Genome Project, or other molecular research, should be freely available for the benefit of everyone. Proponents of this latter view frequently cite alleged exploitation of patients and communities who have donated their blood samples for research, little realizing that their generosity could be exploited for financial gain. This is amply illustrated by the furore surrounding the proposed use (or abuse) of a centralized medical database of the entire Icelandic population to help identify 'polygenes' for potential commercial gain (p. 132).

Given the complexity of the legal issues involved it is not surprising that the international community has struggled to identify satisfactory solutions. With the exception of the United States, most international regulatory bodies prohibit payment for the procurement of human genetic material, but their views on patenting are much less well defined. As the new millennium dawns, the reality is that many important human genes have been patented and companies such as Myriad Genetics in the United States have clearly indicated that they intend to exercise their exclusive license for genetic testing for *BRCA1* and *BRCA2* (p. 201). In the short term the impact of gene patents will be mainly on single gene disorders and clearly if excessive costs are imposed this will raise a direct challenge to the fundamental ethical principle of equity of access. In the longer term gene patenting could impinge directly on testing for common polygenic disorders and for treating both genetic and non-genetic problems, such as baldness and obesity, using gene therapy. As illustrations of the prevailing levels of investment it is worth noting that the rights to one gene associated with obesity were sold in 1995 for $70 million, while in 1997 DeCODE, the Icelandic genomics company at the centre of the controversy regarding national assent, sold the potential rights to 12 genes possibly associated

---

Table 24.3 Key points in the Association of British Insurers (ABI) Code of Practice for genetic testing (1999)

- Applicants must not be asked to undergo genetic testing*
- Results of genetic tests which have been undertaken should be disclosed
- Only test results which have been validated should be taken into account
- Existing genetic test results need not be disclosed in applications for mortgage related life assurance up to a total of £100 000.
- The results of genetic tests undertaken by an applicant will not be taken into account when assessing an application from another individual and vice versa

---

*A genetic test is defined as 'an examination of the chromosome, DNA or RNA to find out if there is an otherwise undetectable related genotype, which may indicate an increased chance of that individual developing a specific disease in the future' with common complex diseases to Hoffman-La Roche for $200 million.

GENE THERAPY

One of the most exciting aspects of recent progress in molecular biology is the prospect of successful gene therapy (p. 327), although it is obviously disappointing that this potential has not as yet been realized. It is understandable that both the general public and the health care professions should be concerned about the possible side-effects and its abuse. Frequent reference has been made to the 'slippery slope' argument whereby it is claimed that one innocent concession will lead inevitably to uncontrolled experimentation. To address these anxieties, advisory or regulatory committees have been established in several countries to assess the practical and ethical aspects of gene therapy research programmes.

Concern centres around two fundamental issues. The first relates to the practical aspects of ensuring informed consent on the part of patients who wish to participate in gene therapy research. Adult patients and parents of affected children could well be desperate to participate in gene therapy research particularly if their disease is otherwise incurable. Consequently they could be tempted to disregard the possible hazards of what is essentially a new, untried and unproven therapeutic approach. In the United Kingdom, the Committee on the Ethics of Gene Therapy has recommended that until this is shown to be safe, all gene therapy programmes should be subjected to careful scrutiny by local hospital research ethical committees. In addition, a national supervisory body, the Gene Therapy Advisory Committee, has been established to review all proposals to conduct gene therapy in humans and to monitor and record complications in ongoing gene therapy trials. In this way it is anticipated that the rights of individual patients in terms of both consent and confidentiality will be safeguarded.

The second aspect of gene therapy which generates concern is the possibility that it could be used for eugenic purposes. On this point the British committee has recommended that genetic modification involving the germ line (p. 328) should not be attempted. Therefore by limiting gene therapy to somatic cells it should not be possible for newly modified genes to be transmitted to future generations. This committee has also recommended that somatic cell gene therapy should only be used to try to treat serious diseases and not to alter human characteristics such as intelligence or athletic prowess.

The potential benefits of gene therapy are enormous and, although it is disappointing that initial success has been very limited, it is inevitable that both somatic and germ line gene therapy will continue to be the focus of intense research activity. The degree of caution exercised by national committees overseeing the ethics of gene therapy illustrates the care which is being taken by medical and governing bodies to ensure that human gene manipulation will not be abused. This is demonstrated by the recent halting of gene therapy trials at an American institute following the death of a young man who was being treated for ornithine decarboxylase deficiency. The US Food and Drug Administration promptly suspended this particular study and halted all others pending further investigations.

POPULATION SCREENING

Population screening programmes offering carrier detection for common autosomal recessive disorders have been in operation for many years (p. 317). These have been well received for thalassaemia and Tay–Sachs disease, for which screening has been carefully planned with well-informed and highly motivated target populations. In contrast, early efforts to introduce sickle-cell carrier detection in North America were largely unsuccessful because of misinformation, discrimination and stigmatization. Pilot studies assessing the responses to cystic fibrosis carrier screening in Caucasian populations have yielded conflicting results (p. 318).

The differing receptions to these various screening programmes illustrate the importance of informed consent and the difficulties of ensuring both autonomy and informed choice. For example, it has been suggested that screening for the cystic fibrosis carrier status could be included in the neonatal screening programme or be introduced as an option for all school children at age 16 years. Clearly newborn infants cannot make an informed choice and it is doubtful whether all 16-year-olds are sufficiently mature to make a fully reasoned decision for themselves.

Consequently many pilot studies have focused on adults and their responses to the offer of carrier testing from either their general practitioner or at the antenatal clinic. This has raised the vexed question of whether an offer from a respected family doctor could be interpreted as an implicit recommendation to participate which cannot be easily refused. A personal 'opportunistic' invitation to participate from a general practitioner yields a much higher acceptance rate than a casual written invitation to attend for screening at a future date. This difference in rates of uptake could simply be a reflection of inertia but could also indicate that individuals feel pressurized to agree to a test which they do not necessarily want.

It is therefore important that even the most well-intended offer of carrier detection should be worded carefully so as to ensure that participation is entirely voluntary. Full counselling in the event of a positive result is also essential to minimize the risk of any feeling of stigmatization or genetic inferiority.

In population screening confidentiality is also important. Many will not wish their carrier status to be known among classmates or colleagues at work. The issue of confidentiality will become particularly difficult for individuals who are found to be genetically susceptible to a potential industrial hazard such as smoke or dust. There is concern that such individuals will be discriminated against by potential employers (p. 175) and doctors could find themselves in the invidious position of having to provide information which jeopardizes their patient's employment prospects.

These anxieties led in 1995 to the Equal Employment Opportunity Commission in the United States issuing a guideline that allows for anyone denied employment because of a disease susceptibility to claim protection under the 'Americans with Disabilities Act'.

CONCLUSION

It is clear that ethical issues are of major importance in medical genetics. Each new discovery brings new challenges and raises new dilemmas for which there are usually no easy answers. On a global scale the computerization of medical records together with the widespread introduction of genetic testing make it essential that safeguards are introduced to ensure that fundamental principles such as privacy and confidentiality are maintained. Members of the medical genetics community shall continue to play a pivotal role in trying to balance the needs of their patients and families with the demands of an increasingly cost conscious society and a commercially driven biotechnology industry. Cost–benefit arguments can be persuasive in cold financial terms but take no account of the fundamental human and social issues which are often involved. Increasingly it will fall upon the shoulders of the medical genetics community to try to ensure that the interests of their patients and families take precedence and towards that end it is hoped that this chapter, and indeed the rest of this textbook, can make a positive contribution.

FURTHER READING

American Society of Human Genetics Report 1996 Statement on informed consent for genetic research. Am J Hum Genet 59: 471–474
The statement of the American Society of Human Genetics Board of Directors on the issues relating to informed consent in genetic research.

Association of British Insurers 1999 Genetic testing. ABI code of practice. ABI, London.
A formal statement of the principles and practice adopted by the British insurance industry with regard to genetic testing.

British Medical Association 1998 Human genetics. Choice and responsibility. Oxford University Press, Oxford
A comprehensive wide ranging report produced by a BMA medical ethics committee steering group on the ethical issues raised by genetics in clinical practice.

Collins F S 1999 Shattuck lecture — medical and societal consequences of the human genome project. New Engl J Med 341: 28–37
A contemporary overview of the human genome project with due emphasis on its possible ethical and social implications.

Harper P S, Clarke A J 1997 Genetics society and clinical practice. βios Scientific, Oxford.
A thoughtful account of the important ethical and social aspects of recent developments in clinical genetics.

Knoppers B M 1999 Status, sale and patenting of human genetic material: an international survey. Nat Genet 22: 23–26
An overview of current international policies on gene patenting.

McInnis M G 1999 The assent of a nation: genethics and Iceland. Clin Genet 55: 234–239
A critical review of the complex ethical issues raised by the decision of the Icelandic government to collaborate in genetic research with a biotechnology company.

Pokorski R J 1997 Insurance underwriting in the genetic era. Am J Hum Genet 60: 205–216
A detailed account of the issues surrounding the use of genetic tests by the insurance industry.

Report of the Committee on the Ethics of Gene Therapy 1992 HMSO, London
The recommendations of the committee chaired by Sir Cecil Clothier on the ethical aspects of somatic cell and germ line gene therapy.

ELEMENTS

1 Ethical considerations impinge on almost every aspect of clinical genetics. In a wider context developments in molecular biology have important ethical implications for society at large.

2 Subjects which can generate particularly difficult problems in clinical genetics include prenatal diagnosis, predictive testing in childhood and genetic testing in the extended family.

3 Possible applications of molecular genetics of importance on a wider scale include the use of genetic test results by the insurance industry, gene patenting, gene therapy and population screening.

4 There are no easy or correct solutions for many of the difficult ethical problems which arise in clinical genetics. It is important that guidelines and regulations are established which recognize each individual's fundamental entitlement to respect for autonomy, informed choice and consent, privacy and confidentiality.

Appendix

The rate of generation of information about human, medical and clinical genetics and the human genome project means that access to current information is vital to both the student and the doctor, particularly since patients and families often come to the clinic armed with the same information!

There are a number of general Web sites which students will find useful as entry points with a wealth of links to other sites for 'surfing'. Other specialized Web sites may be of interest, in relation to specific interests.

Clinical geneticists regularly use a number of expert databases to assist in the diagnosis of genetic disorders and diseases, some of which are listed. Some clinical genetics services have Web sites describing their service, as well as education aspects and other useful links.

Lastly, students may find it of interest and value to see the range of material available for teaching and learning medical genetics in medical schools throughout the world.

GENERAL GENETIC INTERNET WEB SITES

Online Mendelian Inheritance in Man (OMIM)
http://www3.ncbi.nlm.nih.gov/omim/
Online access to McKusick's catalogue, an invaluable resource for clinical genetic information with a wealth of links to many other resources.

Genome Database
http://gdbwww.gdb.org/
An encyclopedia of the current state of knowledge of the human genome.

Public Human Diseases Menu
http://www.hgmp.mrc.ac.uk/Public/diseases.html
Site available to the public for information about inherited human diseases and their support groups.

Human Genome Organization
http://www.gene.ucl.ac.uk/hugo/
The Web site of the international organization of scientists involved in the Human Genome Project.

Science's Human Gene Map
http://www.ncbi.nlm.nih.gov./genemap99/
A map of the human genome with information about important genes.

SPECIALIZED WEB SITES

GenBank
http://www.ncbi.nlm.nih.gov/Genbank/index.html
GenBank is an annotated genetic sequence database.

Human Gene Mutation Database
http://www.uwcm.ac.uk/uwcm/mg/hgmd0.html
A database of the reported mutations in human genes.

Whitehead Institute for Biomedical Research/MIT Center for Genome Research
http://www-genome.wi.mit.edu/
Human gene map, sequencing and software programs.

The Cooperative Human Linkage Center
http://lpg.nci.nih.gov/CHLC/
Human gene maps and markers.

Genelink
http://www.genlink.wustl.edu/
Genetic maps and databases.

The Rockefeller University Genetic Linkage Analysis Resources
http://linkage.rockefeller.edu/
Linkage analysis and marker mapping programs.

Research Program on Ethical, Legal and Social Implications of Human Genome Project
http://www.nhgri.nih.gov./About_NHGRI/Der/Elsi/index.html
Site about ethical, legal and social implications of the human genome project.

Mammalian Genetics Unit and Mouse Genome Centre
http://www.mgu.har.mrc.ac.uk/MGU-welcome.html
Mouse genome site.

Drosophila melanogaster Genome Database
http://flybase.bio.indiana.edu:82/
A comprehensive database for information on the genetics and molecular biology of D. melanogaster including the genome sequence.

Caenorhabditis elegans Genetics and Genomics
http://elegans.swmed.edu/genome.shtml
C. elegans genome project information.

Yeast Genome Project
http://www.mips.biochem.mpg.de/project/yeast/
Yeast genome project information.

UNIVERSITY AND MEDICAL SCHOOL HUMAN/MEDICAL GENETICS WEB SITES

Yale University School of Medicine
http://info.med.yale.edu/genetics/clinical/HG500/
First year medical school course

University of Michigan Medical School
http://www.med.umich.edu/lrc/coursepages/M1/
humangenetics/humangenetics.html
Course information, practice quizzes

Louisiana State University
http://www.sh.lsumc.edu/pediatrics/genetics/tableof.htm
Course material, assignments and answers, case studies

University of California, San Diego
http://www.biology.ucsd.edu/classes/CBB-
Genetics/CBB1997A.html
Syllabus, lecture outline and links

Robert Wood Johnson Medical School of the University of Medicine and Dentistry, NJ
http://www2.umdnj.edu/~genetics/hg-1.htm
Course outline, syllabus

University of Leeds
http://www.leeds.ac.uk/medicine/admin/taught/bm/medgen/index.htm
Lecture notes and slides, sample questions

CLINICAL GENETICS SERVICES WEB SITES

University of South Dakota School of Medicine
http://www.kumc.edu/gec/prof/guide_sd.html
Clinical Genetics: A Self-Study Guide

Tulane University
http://www.tmc.tulane.edu/departments/human_genetics/main.htm
Clinical genetics services

Vanderbilt University Medical School
http://peds.mc.vanderbilt.edu/VCHWEB_1/Medical-Genetics.html
Links to teaching resources

Yorkshire Regional Genetics Service
http://www.yorkshireclingen.demon.co.uk/
Regional genetics service in the United Kingdom

CLINICAL DATABASES

London Dysmorphology Database (LDDB) Winter R M, Baraitser M. Oxford Medical, Oxford University Press, Oxford
A diagnostic database which contains a detailed list of clinical features and references for each of the syndrome entries along with an abstract.

Pictures of Standard Syndromes and Undiagnosed Malformations (POSSUM) Bankier A. The Murdoch Institute for Research into Birth Defects, PO Box 1100, Parkville 3052, Melbourne, Australia
A database for the diagnosis of dysmorphic syndromes with description of the syndrome, clinical features, references, photographs and video sequences.

The Human Cytogenetic Database (HCDB) Schinzel A. Oxford Medical, Oxford University Press, Oxford
A diagnostic database with features and references on 1200 chromosomal abnormalities.

London Neurological Database (LNDB) Winter R M, Baraitser M. Oxford Medical, Oxford University Press, Oxford
A database for the diagnosis of neurogenetic syndromes or disorders containing an abstract and information about clinical features and references.

A Radiological Electronic Atlas of Malformation Syndromes and Skeletal Dysplasias (REAMS). Hall C, Washbrook J Oxford University Press, Oxford
A database for the diagnosis of skeletal dysplasias and malformation syndromes to assist with diagnosis.

Program Listing Abnormalities in Prenatal Ultrasound (Platypus) Benzie R J (ed) Toikinnoin, Inc., Ottawa, Canada
A reference source demonstrating real time images of 337 fetal anomalies with a diagnostic search facility and information and references on 3500 associated syndromes.

Glossary

A. Abbreviation for adenine.

Acentric. Lacking a centromere.

Acetylation. The introduction of an acetyl group into a molecule; often used by the body to help eliminate substances by the liver.

Acrocentric. Term used to describe a chromosome where the centromere is near one end and the short arm usually consists of satellite material.

Acute phase proteins. A number of proteins involved in innate immunity produced in reaction to infection which include C-reactive protein, mannose binding protein and serum amyloid P component.

Adenine. A purine base in DNA and RNA.

Adenomatous polyposis coli (APC). See *Familial adenomatous polyposis*.

AIDS. Acquired immunodeficiency syndrome.

Allele (= allelomorph). Alternative form of a gene found at the same locus on homologous chromosomes.

Allograft. A tissue graft between non-identical individuals.

Allotypes. Genetically determined variants of antibodies.

Alpha (α) thalassaemia. Inherited disorder of haemoglobin involving underproduction of the α-globin chains occurring most commonly in persons from South-East Asia.

Alternative pathway. One of the two pathways of the activation of complement which, in this instance, involves cell membranes of microorganisms.

Alu repeat. Short repeated DNA sequences which appear to have homology with transposable elements in other organisms.

Am. The group of genetic variants associated with the IgA heavy chain.

Amino acid. An organic compound containing both carboxyl ($-COOH$) and amino groups ($-NH_2$).

Amniocentesis. Procedure for obtaining amniotic fluid and cells for prenatal diagnosis.

Amorph. A mutation which leads to complete loss of function.

Anaphase. The stage of cell division when the chromosomes leave the equatorial plate and migrate to opposite poles of the spindle.

Anaphase lag. Loss of a chromosome as it moves to the pole of the cell during anaphase which can lead to monosomy.

Aneuploid. A chromosome number which is not an exact multiple of the haploid number, i.e. $2N - 1$ or $2N + 1$ where N is the haploid number of chromosomes.

Anterior information. Information previously known which leads to the *prior probability*.

Antibody (= immunoglobulin). A serum protein which is formed in response to an antigenic stimulus and reacts specifically with that antigen.

Anticipation. The tendency for some autosomal dominant diseases to manifest at an earlier age and/or to increase in severity with each succeeding generation.

Anticodon. The complementary triplet of the tRNA molecule which binds to it with a particular amino acid.

Antigen. A substance which elicits the synthesis of antibody with which it specifically reacts.

Antigen binding fragment (Fab). The fragment of the antibody molecule produced by papain digestion responsible for antigen binding.

Antiparallel. Opposite orientation of the two strands of a DNA duplex, one runs in the 3′ to 5′ direction, the other in the 5′ to 3′ direction.

Antisense oligonucleotide. A short oligonucleotide synthesized to bind to a particular RNA or DNA sequence to block its expression.

Antisense strand. The template strand of DNA.

Apical ectodermal ridge. Area of ectoderm in the developing limb bud which produces growth factors.

Apolipoproteins. A number of different proteins which are involved in lipid transportation in the circulation.

Apoptosis. Programmed involution or cell death of a developing tissue or organ of the body.

Artificial insemination by donor (AID). Use of semen from a male donor as a reproductive option for couples at high risk of transmitting a genetic disorder.

Ascertainment. The finding and selection of families with a hereditary disorder.

Association. The occurrence of a particular allele in a group of patients more often than can be accounted for by chance.

Assortative mating (= non-random mating). The preferential selection of a spouse with a particular phenotype.

Atherosclerosis. The fatty degenerative plaque which accumulates in the intimal wall of blood vessels.

Autoimmune diseases. Diseases which are thought to be caused by the body not recognizing its own antigens.

Autonomous replication sequences. DNA sequences which are necessary for accurate replication within yeast.

Autoradiography. Detection of radioactively labelled molecules on an X-ray film.

Autosomal dominant. A gene on one of the non-sex chromosomes which manifests in the heterozygous state.

Autosomal inheritance. The pattern of inheritance shown by a disorder or trait determined by a gene on one of the non-sex chromosomes.

Autosomal recessive. A gene located on one of the non-sex chromosomes which manifests in the homozygous state.

Autosome. Any of the 22 non-sex chromosomes.

Autozygosity. Homozygosity as a result of identity by descent from a common ancestor.

Azoospermia. Absence of sperm in semen.

B lymphocytes. Antibody-producing lymphocytes involved in humoral immunity.

Bacterial artificial chromosome (BAC). An artificial chromosome created from modification of the fertility factor of plasmids which allows incorporation of up to 330 kb of foreign DNA.

Bacteriophage (= phage). A virus which infects bacteria.

Balanced polymorphism. Two different genetic variants which are stably present in a population, i.e. selective advantages and disadvantages cancel each other out.

Balanced translocation. See *Reciprocal translocation*.

Bare lymphocyte syndrome. A rare autosomal recessive form of severe combined immunodeficiency due to absence of the class II molecules of the major histocompatibility complex.

Barr body. The condensation of the inactive X chromosome seen in the nucleus of certain types of cells from females. See *Sex chromatin*.

Base. Short for the nitrogenous bases in nucleic acid molecules (A = adenine; T = thymine; U = uracil; C = cytosine, G = guanine).

Base pair (bp). A pair of complementary bases in DNA (A with T, G with C).

Bayes' theorem. Combining the prior and conditional probabilities of certain events or the results of specific tests to give a joint probability to derive the posterior or relative probability.

Bence Jones protein. The antibody of a single species produced in large amounts by a person with multiple myeloma, a tumour of antibody producing plasma cells.

Beta (β) thalassaemia. Inherited disorder of haemoglobin involving underproduction of the β-globin chain occurring most commonly in persons from the Mediterranean region and Indian subcontinent.

Bias of ascertainment. An artefact, which must be taken into account in family studies when looking at segregation ratios, caused by families coming to attention because they have affected individual(s).

Biochemical disorder. An inherited disorder involving a metabolic pathway, i.e. an inborn error of metabolism.

Biological or genetic determinisim. The premise that our genetic make-up is the only factor determining all aspects of our health and disease.

Biosynthesis. Use of recombinant DNA techniques to produce molecules of biological and medical importance in the laboratory or commercially.

Bipolar illness. Affective manic-depressive illness.

Bivalent. A pair of synapsed homologous chromosomes.

Blastocyst. Early embryo consisting of embryoblast and trophoblast.

Blastomere. A single cell of the early fertilized conceptus.

Blood chimera. A mixture of cells of different genetic origin present in twins as a result of an exchange of cells via the placenta between non-identical twins in utero.

Boundary elements. Short sequences of DNA, usually 500 bp to 3 kb in size, which block or inhibit the influence of regulatory elements of adjacent genes.

Break-point cluster (bcr). Region of chromosome 22 involved in the translocation seen in the majority of persons with chronic myeloid leukaemia.

C. Abbreviation for cytosine.

CAAT box. A conserved, non-coding, so-called 'promoter' sequence about 80 bp upstream from the start of transcription.

Cancer family syndrome. A term used to describe the clustering in certain families of particular types of cancers, in which it has been proposed that the different types of malignancy could be due to a single dominant gene, specifically Lynch type II.

Cancer genetics. The study of the genetic causes of cancer.

Candidate gene. A gene whose function or location suggests that it is likely to be responsible for a particular genetic disease or disorder.

5′ Cap. Modification of the nascent mRNA by the addition of a methylated guanine nucleotide to the 5′ end of the molecule by an unusual 5′ to 5′ triphosphate linkage.

CA repeat. A short dinucleotide sequence present as tandem repeats at multiple sites in the human genome producing microsatellite polymorphisms.

Carrier. Person heterozygous for a recessive gene, male or female for autosomal genes or female for X-linked genes.

Cascade screening. Identification within a family of carriers for an autosomal recessive disorder or persons with an autosomal dominant gene following ascertainment of an index case.

Cell-mediated immunity. Immunity which involves the T lymphocytes to fight intracellular infection and is involved in transplantation rejection and delayed hypersensitivity.

Cellular oncogene. See *Proto-oncogene*.

CentiMorgan (cM). Unit used to measure map distances, equivalent to a 1% chance of recombination (crossing over).

Central dogma. The concept that genetic information is usually only transmitted from DNA to RNA to protein.

Centric fusion. The fusion of the centromeres of two acrocentric chromosomes to form a Robertsonian translocation.

Centriole. The cellular structure from which microtubules radiate in the mitotic spindle involved in the separation of chromosomes in mitosis.

Centromere (= kinetochore). The point at which the two chromatids of a chromosome are joined, and the region of the chromosome which becomes attached to the spindle during cell division.

Chemical cleavage mismatch. A DNA mutation detection system which involves the addition of the chemicals hydroxylamine and osmium tetroxide which react with free cytosine and thymine nucleotides respectively. By denaturing the double stranded DNA being screened and allowing it to hybridize with a single stranded radiolabelled DNA probe, any mismatched cytosine or thymine nucleotides will be exposed and therefore be susceptible to reaction with the hydroxylamine and osmium tetroxide. The addition of piperidine results in cleavage of the DNA being screened at any such sites allowing identification of mutations.

Chemotaxis. The attraction of phagocytes to the site of infection by components of complement.

Chiasmata. Cross-overs between chromosomes in meiosis.

Chimera. An individual composed of two populations of cells with different genotypes.

Chorion. Layer of cells covering a fertilized ovum some of which, the chorion frondosum, will later form the placenta.

Chorionic villus sampling. Procedure using ultrasound guidance to obtain chorionic villi from the chorion frondosum for prenatal diagnosis.

Chromatid. During cell division each chromosome divides longitudinally into two strands, or chromatids, which are held together by the centromere.

Chromatin. The tertiary coiling of the nucleosomes of the chromosomes with associated proteins.

Chromatin fibre FISH. Use of extended chromatin or DNA fibres with fluorescent in situ hybridization to physically order DNA clones or sequences.

Chromosomal analysis. The process of counting and analysing the banding pattern of the chromosomes of an individual.

Chromosomal fragments. Acentric chromosomes which can arise as a result of segregation of a paracentric inversion and which are usually incapable of replication.

Chromosome instability. The presence of breaks and gaps in the chromosomes from persons with a number of disorders associated with an increased risk of neoplasia.

Chromosome mapping. Assigning a gene or DNA sequence to a specific chromosome or a particular region of a chromosome.

Chromosome-mediated gene transfer. The technique of transferring chromosomes or parts of chromosomes to somatic cell hybrids to enable more detailed chromosome mapping.

Chromosome painting. The hybridization in situ of fluorescent labelled probes to a chromosome preparation to allow identification of a particular chromosome(s).

Chromosome walking. Using an ordered assembly of clones to extend from a known start point.

Chromosomes. Thread-like, darkly staining bodies within the nucleus, composed of DNA and chromatin which carry the genetic information.

Cis-acting. Regulatory elements in the promoter region which act on genes on the same chromosome.

Class switching. Term used for the normal change in antibody class from IgM to IgG in the immune response.

Classical gene families. Multigene families which show a high degree of sequence homology.

Classical pathway. One of the two ways of activation of complement, in this instance, involving antigen–antibody complexes.

Clone. A group of cells, all of which are derived from a single cell by repeated mitoses, all having the same genetic information.

Clone contigs. Assembly of clones which have been mapped and ordered to produce an overlapping array.

Cloning in silico. The use of a number of computer programs which can search genomic DNA sequence databases for sequence homology to known genes, as well as DNA sequences specific to all genes such as the conserved intron/exon splice junctions, promoter sequences, polyadenylation sites and stretches of open-reading frames (ORFs) to identify novel genes.

cM. Abbreviation for centiMorgan.

Codominance. When both alleles are expressed in the heterozygote.

Codon. A sequence of three adjacent nucleotides which codes for one amino acid or chain termination.

Common cancers. The cancers which occur commonly in humans, such as bowel and breast cancer.

Common diseases. The diseases which occur commonly in humans, e.g. cancer, coronary artery disease, diabetes, etc.

Community genetics. The branch of medical genetics concerned with screening and the prevention of genetic diseases on a population basis.

Comparative genomics. The identification of orthologous genes in different species.

Competent. Making bacterial cell membrane permeable to DNA by a variety of different methods including exposure to certain salts or high voltage.

Complement. A series of at least 10 serum proteins in humans (and other vertebrates) that can be activated by either the 'classical' or the 'alternative' pathways and which interact in sequence to bring about the destruction of cellular antigens.

Complementary DNA (cDNA). DNA synthesized from mRNA by the enzyme reverse transcriptase.

Complementary strands. The specific pairing of the bases in the DNA of the purines adenine and guanine with thymine and cytosine.

Complete ascertainment. A term used in segregation analysis for a type of study which identifies all affected individuals in a population.

Compound heterozygote. An individual who is affected with an autosomal recessive disorder having two different mutations in homologous genes.

Concordance. When both members of a pair of twins exhibit the same trait they are said to be concordant. If only one twin has the trait they are said to be discordant.

Conditional knockout. A mutation that is only expressed under certain conditions, e.g. raised temperature.

Conditional probability. Observations or tests which can be used to modify prior probabilities using Bayesian calculation in risk estimations.

Conditionally toxic or **suicide gene.** Genes that are introduced in gene therapy and which, under certain conditions or after the introduction of a certain substance, will kill the cell.

Confined placental mosaicism. The occurrence of a chromosomal abnormality in chorionic villus samples obtained for first trimester prenatal diagnosis in which the fetus has a normal chromosomal complement.

Congenital. Any abnormality, whether genetic or not, which is present at birth.

Congenital hypertrophy of the retinal pigment epithelium (CHRPE). Abnormal retinal pigmentation which, when present in persons at risk for familial adenomatous polyposis, is evidence of the heterozygous state.

Conjugation. A chemical process in which two molecules are joined, often used to describe the process by which certain drugs or chemicals can then be excreted by the body, e.g. acetylation of isoniazid by the liver.

Consanguineous marriage. A marriage between 'blood relatives', that is between persons who have one or more ancestors in common, most frequently between first cousins.

Consanguinity. Relationship between blood relatives.

Consensus sequence. A GGGCGGG sequence promoter element to the 5' side of genes in eukaryotes involved in the control of gene expression.

Conservative substitution. Single base pair substitution which, although resulting in the replacement by a different amino acid, if chemically similar, has no functional effect.

Constant region. The portion of the light and heavy chains of antibodies in which the amino acid sequence is relatively constant from molecule to molecule.

Constitutional. Present in the fertilized gamete.

Constitutional heterozygosity. The presence in an individual at the time of conception of obligate heterozygosity at a locus when the parents are homozygous at that locus for different alleles.

Consultand. The person presenting for genetic advice.

Contigs. Contiguous or overlapping DNA clones.

Contiguous gene syndrome. Disorder resulting from deletion of adjacent genes.

Continuous trait. A trait, such as height, for which there is a range of observations or findings, in contrast to traits which are all or none, cf. *discontinuous*, such as cleft lip and palate.

Control gene. A gene which can turn other genes on or off, i.e. regulate.

Cordocentesis. The procedure of obtaining fetal blood samples for prenatal diagnosis.

Corona radiata. Cellular layer surrounding the mature oocyte.

Cor pulmonale. Right-sided heart failure which can occur after serious lung disease, such as in persons with cystic fibrosis.

Correlation. Statistical measure of the degree of association or resemblance between two parameters.

Cosmid. A plasmid which has had the maximum DNA removed to allow the largest possible insert for cloning but still has the DNA sequences necessary for in vitro packaging into an infective phage particle.

Co-twins. Both members of a twin pair, whether dizygotic or monozygotic.

Counsellee. Person receiving genetic counselling.

Coupling. When a certain allele at a particular locus is on the same chromosome with a specific allele at a closely-linked locus.

CpG dinucleotides. The occurrence of the nucleotides cytosine and guanine together in genomic DNA which is frequently methylated and which is associated with spontaneous deamination of cytosine converting it to thymine as a mechanism of mutation.

CpG islands. Clusters of unmethylated CpGs occur near the transcription sites of many genes.

Cross-over (= **recombination**). The exchange of genetic material between homologous chromosomes in meiosis.

Cross-reacting material (CRM). Immunologically detected protein or enzyme which is functionally inactive.

Cryptic splice site. A mutation in a gene leading to the creation of the sequence of a splice site which results in abnormal splicing of the mRNA.

Cystic fibrosis transmembrane conductance regulator (CFTR). The gene product of the cystic fibrosis gene responsible for chloride transport and mucin secretion.

Cytogenetics. The branch of genetics concerned principally with the study of chromosomes.

Cytokinesis. Division of the cytoplasm to form two daughter cells in meiosis and mitosis.

Cytoplasm. The ground substance of the cell in which are situated the nucleus, endoplasmic reticulum and mitochondria, etc.

Cytoplasmic inheritance. See *Mitochondrial inheritance.*

Cytosine. A pyrimidine base in DNA and RNA.

Cytosol. The semi-soluble contents of the cytoplasm.

Cytotoxic T cells. A subclass of T lymphocytes sensitized to destroy cells bearing certain antigens.

Cytotoxic T lymphocytes (= killer). A group of T cells which specifically kill foreign or virus infected vertebrate cells.

Daltonism. A term given in the past to X-linked inheritance after John Dalton who noted this pattern of inheritance in colour blindness.

Deformation. A birth defect which results from an abnormal mechanical force which distorts an otherwise normal structure.

Degeneracy. Certain amino acids being coded for by more than one triplet codon of the genetic code.

Deleted in colorectal carcinoma (DCC). A region on the long arm of chromosome 18 often found to be deleted in colorectal carcinomas.

Deletion. A type of chromosomal aberration or mutation at the DNA level in which there is loss of part of a chromosome or one or more nucleotides.

Delta-beta (δβ) thalassaemia. A form of thalassaemia in which there is reduced production of both the δ- and β-globin chains.

Denaturing gradient gel electrophoresis. A mutation detection system which involves mixing a radiolabelled single stranded DNA probe with the double stranded DNA being screened, which is heated to make it single stranded. This mixture is electrophoresed on a denaturing gradient gel. DNA which is identical with the sequence of the DNA probe will form a homoduplex, which under the denaturing conditions of the gel will remain hybridized. Any mismatches of the DNA being screened with the DNA probe will result in the formation of a heteroduplex, which, as it is run down the denaturing gradient of the gel, will become single stranded at a certain point, resulting in a branched structure which has decreased mobility. This results in an altered position compared to the homoduplex which can be detected on an autoradiograph.

De novo. Literally 'from new', as opposed to inherited.

Deoxyribonucleic acid. See *DNA*

Desert hedgehog. One of three mammalian homologues of the segment polarity hedgehog genes.

Dicentric. Possessing two centromeres.

Dictyotene. The stage in meiosis I in which primary oocytes are arrested in females until the time of ovulation.

Digenic inheritance. An inheritance mechanism resulting from the interaction of two non-homologous genes.

Diploid. The condition in which the cell contains two sets of chromosomes. Normal state of somatic cells in humans where the diploid number (2N) is 46.

Discontinuous trait. A trait which is all or none, e.g. cleft lip and palate, in contrast to *continuous* traits such as height.

Discordant. Differing phenotypic features between individuals, classically used in twin pairs.

Disomy. The normal state of an individual having two homologous chromosomes.

Dispermic chimera. Two separate sperm fertilize two separate ova and the resulting two zygotes fuse to form one embryo.

Dispermy. Fertilization of an oocyte by two sperm.

Disruption. An abnormal structure of an organ or tissue as a result of external factors disturbing the normal developmental process.

Diversity region. DNA sequences coding for the segments of the hypervariable regions of antibodies.

Dizygotic twins (= fraternal). Type of twins produced by fertilization of two ova by two sperm.

DNA (= deoxyribonucleic acid). The nucleic acid in chromosomes in which genetic information is coded.

DNA chip. DNA microarrays which, with the appropriate computerised software allow rapid, automated high throughput DNA sequencing and mutation detection.

DNA fingerprint. Pattern of hypervariable tandem DNA repeats of a core sequence which is unique to an individual.

DNA haplotype. The pattern of DNA sequence polymorphisms flanking a DNA sequence or gene of interest.

DNA library. A collection of recombinant DNA molecules from a particular source, e.g. genomic or cDNA.

DNA ligase. An enzyme which catalyses the formation of a phosphodiester bond between a 3'-hydroxyl and a 5'-phosphate group in DNA thereby joining two DNA fragments.

DNA mapping. The physical relationships of flanking DNA sequence polymorphisms and the detailed structure of a gene.

DNA polymorphisms. Inherited variation in the nucleotide sequence usually of non-coding DNA.

DNA probes. A DNA sequence which is labelled, usually either radioactively or fluorescently, and used to identify a gene or DNA sequence, e.g. a cDNA or genomic probe.

DNA repair. DNA damaged through a variety of mechanisms can be removed and repaired by a complex set of processes.

DNA replication. The process of copying the nucleotide sequence of the genome from one generation to the next.

DNA sequence amplification. See *Polymerase chain reaction.*

DNA sequence variants. See *DNA polymorphisms.*

DNA sequencing. Analysis of the nucleotide sequence of a gene or DNA fragment.

Dominant. A trait which is expressed in individuals who are heterozygous for a particular allele.

Dominant-negative mutation. A mutant allele in the heterozygous state which results in the loss of activity/function of its mutant gene product as well as interfering with the function of the normal gene product of the corresponding allele.

Dosage compensation. The phenomenon in women who have two copies of genes on the X chromosome having the same level of the products of those genes as males who have a single X chromosome.

Dosimetry. The measurement of radiation exposure.

Double heterozygote. An individual who is heterozygous at two different loci.

Double-minute chromosomes. Amplified sequences of DNA in tumour cells which can occur as small extra chromosomes, as in neuroblastoma.

Drift (= random genetic drift). Fluctuations in gene frequencies which tend to occur in small isolated populations.

Dynamic mutation. See *Unstable mutation.*

Dysmorphology. The study of the definition, recognition and aetiology of multiple malformation syndromes.

Dysplasia. An abnormal organization of cells into tissue.

Dystrophin. The product of the Duchenne muscular dystrophy gene.

Ecogenetics. The study of genetically determined differences in susceptibility to the action of physical, chemical and infectious agents in the environment.

Em. The group of genetic variants of the IgE heavy chain of immunoglobulins.

Embryoblast. Cell layer of the blastocyst which forms the embryo.

Embryonic stem cells. A cell in the early embryo which is totipotent in terms of cellular fate.

Empiric risks. Advice given in recurrence risk counselling for multifactorially determined disorders based on observation and experience, in which the inherited contribution is due to a number of genes, i.e. polygenic.

Endoplasmic reticulum. A system of minute tubules within the cell involved in the biosynthesis of macromolecules.

Endoreduplication. Duplication of a haploid sperm chromosome set.

Enhancer. DNA sequence which increases transcription of a related gene.

Enzyme. A protein which acts as a catalyst in biological systems.

Epidermal growth factor (EGF). A growth factor which stimulates a variety of cell types including epidermal cells.

Epistasis. Interaction between non-allelic genes.

Erythroblastosis fetalis. See *Haemolytic disease of the newborn.*

Essential hypertension. Increased blood pressure for which there is no recognized primary cause.

Euchromatin. Genetically active regions of the chromosomes.

Eugenics. The 'science' which promotes the improvement of the hereditary qualities of a race or a species.

Eukaryote. Higher organism with a well-defined nucleus.

Exon (= expressed sequence). Region of a gene which is not excised during transcription forming part of the mature mRNA and therefore specifying part of the primary structure of the gene product.

Exon trapping. A process by which a recombinant DNA vector which contains the DNA sequences of the splice site junctions is used to clone coding sequences or exons.

Expansion. Refers to the increase in the number of triplet repeat sequences in the various disorders due to dynamic or unstable mutations.

Expressed sequence tags. Sequence-specific primers from cDNA clones designed to identify sequences of expressed genes in the genome.

Expressivity. Variation in the severity of the phenotypic features of a particular gene.

Extinguished. Loss of one allelic variant at a locus due to random genetic drift.

Extrinsic malformation. Term previously used for *disruption.*

Fab. The two antigen binding fragments of an antibody molecule produced by digestion with the proteolytic enzyme papain.

False-negative. Affected cases missed by a diagnostic or screening test.

False-positive. Unaffected cases incorrectly diagnosed as affected by a screening or diagnostic test.

Familial adenomatous polyposis. A dominantly inherited cancer-predisposing syndrome characterized by the presence of a large number of polyps of the large bowel with a high risk of developing malignant changes.

Familial cancer-predisposing syndrome. One of a number of syndromes in which persons are at risk of developing one or more types of cancer.

Favism. A haemolytic crisis due to G6PD deficiency occurring after eating fava beans.

Fc. The complement binding fragment of an antibody molecule produced by digestion with the proteolytic enzyme papain.

Fetoscopy. Procedure used to visualize the fetus and often to take skin and/or blood samples from the fetus for prenatal diagnosis.

Fetus. The name given to the unborn infant during the final stage of in utero development, usually from 12 weeks gestation to term.

Filial. Offspring.

First-degree relatives. Closest relatives, that is, parents, offspring, sibs, sharing on average 50% of their genes.

Fitness (= biological fitness). The number of offspring who reach reproductive age.

Five-prime (5′) end. The end of a DNA or RNA strand with a free 5′ phosphate group.

Fixed. The establishment of a single allelic variant at a locus due to random genetic drift.

Fixed mutation. See *Stable mutation*.

Flanking DNA. Nucleotide sequence adjacent to the DNA sequence being considered.

Flanking markers. Polymorphic markers which are located adjacent to a gene or DNA sequence of interest.

Flow cytometry. See *Fluorescent activated cell sorting*.

Flow karyotype. A distribution histogram of chromosome size obtained using a fluorescent activated cell sorter.

Fluorescent activated cell sorting (FACS). A technique in which chromosomes are stained with a fluorescent dye which selectively binds to DNA; the differences in fluorescence of the various chromosomes allows them to be physically separated by a special laser.

Fluorescent in situ hybridization (FISH). Use of a single stranded DNA sequence with a fluorescent label to hybridize with its complementary target sequence in the chromosomes, allowing it to be visualized under ultraviolet light.

Foreign DNA. A source of DNA incorporated into a vector in producing recombinant DNA molecules.

Founder effect. Certain genetic disorders can be relatively common in particular populations through all individuals being descended from a relatively small number of ancestors, one or a few of whom had a particular disorder.

Fragile site. A non-staining gap in a chromatid where breakage is liable to occur.

Frameshift mutations. Mutations, such as insertions or deletions, which change the reading frame of the codon triplets.

Framework map. A set of markers distributed at defined approximately evenly spaced intervals along the chromosomes in the human genome.

Framework region. Parts of the variable regions of antibodies which are not hypervariable.

Fraternal twins. Non-identical twins.

Freemartin. A chromosomal female twin calf with ambiguous genitalia due to gonadal chimerism.

Frequency. The number of times an event occurs in a period of time, e.g. 1000 cases per year.

Full ascertainment. See *Complete ascertainment*.

Functional cloning. Identification of a gene through its function, e.g. isolation of cDNAs expressed in a particular tissue in which a disease or disorder is manifest.

Functional genomics. The normal pattern of expression of genes in development and differentiation and the function of their protein products in normal development as well as their dysfunction in inherited disorders.

Fusion polypeptide. Genes which are physically near to each other and have DNA sequence homology can undergo a cross-over, leading to formation of a protein that has an amino acid sequence which is derived from both of the genes involved.

G. Abbreviation for the nucleotide guanine.

Gain-of-function. Mutations which in the heterozygote result in new functions.

Gap mutant. Developmental genes identified in *Drosophila* which delete groups of adjacent segments.

Gastrulation. The formation of the bi- then tri-laminar disc of the inner cell mass which becomes the early embryo.

Gene. A part of the DNA molecule of a chromosome which directs the synthesis of a specific polypeptide chain.

Gene amplification. Process in tumour cells of the production of multiple copies of certain genes, the visible evidence of which are *homogeneously staining regions* and *double-minute chromosomes*.

Gene flow. A term used to describe differences in allele frequencies between populations which reflect migration or contact between them.

Gene superfamilies. Multigene families which have limited sequence homology but are functionally related.

Gene targeting. The introduction of specific mutations into genes by homologous recombination in embryonic stem cells.

Gene therapy. Treatment of inherited disease by addition, insertion or replacement of a normal gene or genes.

Genetic code. The triplets of DNA nucleotides which code for the various amino acids of proteins.

Genetic counselling. The process of providing information about a genetic disorder which includes details about the diagnosis, its cause, the risk of recurrence and options available for prevention.

Genetic heterogeneity. The phenomenon that a disorder can be caused by different allelic or non-allelic mutations.

Genetic isolates. Groups which are isolated for geographical, religious or ethnic reasons that often show differences in allele frequencies.

Genetic load. The total of all kinds of harmful alleles in a population.

Genetic register. A list of families and individuals who are either affected by or at risk of developing a serious hereditary disorder.

Genetic susceptibility. An inherited predisposition to a disease or disorder which is not due to a single gene cause and is usually the result of a complex interaction of the effects of multiple different genes, i.e. *polygenic inheritance*.

Genocopy. The same phenotype due to different genetic causes.

Genome. All the genes carried by a cell.

Genomic DNA. The total DNA content of the chromosomes.

Genomic imprinting. Differing expression of genetic material dependent on the sex of the transmitting parent.

Genotype. The genetic constitution of an individual.

Genotype–phenotype correlation. Correlation of certain mutations with particular phenotypic features.

Germ cells. The cells of the body which transmit genetic information to the next generation.

Germ line gene therapy. The alteration or insertion of genetic material in the gametes.

Germ line mosaicism. The presence in the germ line or gonadal tissue of two populations of cells which differ genetically.

Germ line mutation. A mutation in a gamete.

Gestational diabetes. Onset of an abnormal glucose tolerance in pregnancy which usually reverts to normal after delivery.

Gm. Genetic variants of the heavy chain of IgG immunoglobulins.

Goldberg–Hogness box. See *CAAT box*.

Gonad dose. Term used in radiation dosimetry to describe the radiation exposure of an individual to a particular radiological investigation or exposure.

Gonadal mosaicism. See *Germ line mosaicism*.

Gray (Gy). Equivalent to 100 rad.

Growth factors. A substance which must be present in culture medium to permit cell multiplication, or substances involved in promoting growth of certain cell types, tissues or parts of the body in development, e.g. fibroblast growth factor.

Growth factor receptors. Receptors on the surfaces of cells for a growth factor.

Guanine. A purine base in DNA and RNA.

Haem. The iron-containing group of haemoglobin.

Haemoglobinopathy. An inherited disorder of haemoglobin.

Haemolytic disease of the newborn. Anaemia due to antibody produced by an Rh-negative mother to the Rh-positive blood group of the fetus crossing the placenta and causing haemolysis. If this haemolytic process is severe, it can cause death of the fetus

351

due to heart failure because of the anaemia or what is known as *haemolytic disease of the newborn*.

Haploid. The condition in which the cell contains one set of chromosomes, i.e. 23. This is the chromosome number in a normal gamete.

Haploinsufficiency. Mutations in the heterozygous state which result in half normal levels of the gene product leading to phenotypic effects, i.e. are sensitive to gene dosage.

Haplotype. Conventionally used to refer to the particular alleles present at the four genes of the HLA complex on chromosome 6. The term is also used to describe DNA sequence variants on a particular chromosome adjacent to or closely flanking a locus of interest.

Hardy–Weinberg equilibrium. The maintenance of allele frequencies in a population with random mating and absence of selection.

Hardy–Weinberg formula. A simple binomial equation in population genetics which can be used to determine the frequency of the different genotypes from one of the phenotypes.

Hardy–Weinberg principle. The relative proportions of the different genotypes remain constant from one generation to the next.

Hb Barts. The tetramer of γ-globin chains found in the severe form of α thalassaemia, which causes hydrops fetalis.

Hb H. Tetramer of the β-globin chains found in the less severe form of thalassaemia.

Hedgehog. A group of morphogens produced by segment polarity genes.

Helix-loop-helix. DNA binding motif controlling gene expression.

Helix-turn-helix proteins. Proteins made up of two alpha helices connected by a short chain of amnio acids which make up a 'turn'.

Helper lymphocytes. A subclass of T lymphocytes necessary for the production of antibodies by B lymphocytes.

Helper virus. A retroviral provirus engineered to remove all but the sequences necessary to produce copies of the viral RNA sequences along with the sequences necessary for packaging of the viral genomic RNA in retroviral-mediated gene therapy.

Hemizygous. A term used when describing the genotype of a male with regard to an X-linked trait, since males have only one set of X-linked genes.

Hereditary non-polyposis colorectal cancer (HNPCC). A form of familial cancer in which persons are at risk of developing bowel cancer, not associated with a large number of polyps as in familial polyposis coli, in which the bowel cancer is usually proximal and right-sided.

Hereditary persistence of fetal Hb (HPFH). Persistence of the production of fetal haemoglobin into childhood and adult life.

Heritability. The proportion of the total variation of a character attributable to genetic as opposed to environmental factors.

Hermaphrodite. An individual with both male and female gonads often in association with ambiguous external genitalia.

Heterochromatin. Genetically inert or inactive regions of the chromosomes.

Heterogeneity. The phenomenon of there being more than a single cause for what appears to be a single entity. See *Genetic heterogeneity*.

Heteromorphism. An inherited structural polymorphism of a chromosome.

Heteroplasmy. The mitochondria of an individual consisting of more than one population.

Heteropyknotic. Condensed darkly staining chromosomal material, e.g. the inactivated X chromosome in females.

Heterozygote (= carrier). An individual who possesses two different alleles at one particular locus on a pair of homologous chromosomes.

Heterozygote advantage. An increase in biological fitness seen in unaffected heterozygotes compared to unaffected homozygotes, e.g. sickle-cell trait and resistance to infection by the malarial parasite.

Heterozygous. The state of having different alleles at a locus on homologous chromosomes.

High resolution DNA mapping. Detailed physical mapping at the level of restriction site polymorphisms, expressed sequence tags, etc.

Histocompatibility. Antigenic similarity of donor and recipient in organ transplantation.

Histone. Type of protein rich in lysine and arginine found in association with DNA in chromosomes.

HIV. Human immunodeficiency virus.

HLA (human leucocyte antigen). Antigens present on the cell surfaces of various tissues, including leucocytes.

HLA complex. The genes on chromosome 6 responsible for determining the cell-surface antigens important in organ transplantation.

Hogness box (= TATA box). A conserved, non-coding, so-called 'promoter' sequence about 30 bp upstream from the start of transcription.

Holandric inheritance. The pattern of inheritance of genes on the Y chromosome: only males are affected and the trait is transmitted by affected males to their sons but to none of their daughters.

Homeobox. A stretch of approximately 180 bp conserved in different homeotic genes.

Homeotic gene. Genes which are involved in controlling the development of a region or compartment of an organism producing proteins or factors which regulate gene expression by binding particular DNA sequences.

Homogeneously staining regions (HSR). Amplification of DNA sequences in tumour cells which can appear as extra or expanded areas of the chromosomes which stain evenly.

Homograft. Graft between individuals of the same species but with different genotypes.

Homologous chromosomes. Chromosomes which pair during meiosis and contain identical loci.

Homologous recombination. The process by which a DNA sequence can be replaced by one with a similar sequence to determine the effect of changes in DNA sequence in the process of site-directed mutagenesis.

Homoplasmy. The mitochondria of an individual consisting of a single population.

Homozygote. An individual who possesses two identical alleles at one particular locus on a pair of homologous chromosomes.

Homozygous. The presence of two identical alleles at a particular locus on a pair of homologous chromosomes.

Hormone nuclear receptors. Intracellular receptors involved in the control of transcription.

Housekeeping genes. Genes which express proteins common to all cells, e.g. ribosomal, chromosomal and cytoskeletal proteins.

HTF islands. Methylation-free clusters of CpG dinucleotides found near transcription initiation sites at the 5' end of many eukaryotic genes which can be detected by cutting with the restriction enzyme *Hpa*II producing tiny DNA fragments.

Human genome project. A major international collaborative effort to map and sequence the entire human genome.

Humoral immunity. Immunity which is due to circulating antibodies in the blood and other bodily fluids.

Huntingtin. The protein product of the Huntington's disease gene.

H–Y antigen. A histocompatibility antigen originally detected in the mouse and thought to be located on the Y chromosome.

Hydatidiform mole. An abnormal conceptus which consists of abnormal tissues: a complete mole contains no fetus but can undergo malignant change and receives both sets of chromosomes from the father; a partial mole contains a chromosomally abnormal fetus with triploidy.

Hydrops fetalis. The most severe form of α thalassaemia resulting in death of the fetus in utero due to heart failure secondary to the severe anaemia caused by haemolysis of the red cells.

Hypervariable DNA length polymorphisms. A number of different types of variation in DNA sequence which are highly polymorphic, e.g. variable number tandem repeats, mini- and microsatellites.

Hypervariable minisatellite DNA. Highly polymorphic DNA consisting of a 9–24 bp sequence often located near the telomeres.

Hypervariable region. A number of small regions present in the variable regions of the light and heavy chains of antibodies in which the majority of the variability in antibody sequence occurs.

Hypomorph. Loss-of-function mutations which result in either reduced activity or complete loss of the gene product due to either reduced activity or to decreased stability of the gene product.

Identical twins. See *Monozygotic twins.*

Idiogram. An idealized representation of an object, e.g. an idiogram of a karyotype.

Immunoglobulin. See *Antibody.*

Immunoglobulin allotypes. Genetically determined variants of the various antibody classes, e.g. the Gm system associated with the heavy chain of IgG.

Immunoglobulin superfamily. The multigene families primarily involved in the immune response with structural and DNA sequence homology.

Immunological memory. The ability of the immune system to 'remember' previous exposure to a foreign antigen or infectious agents, leading to the enhanced secondary immune response upon re-exposure.

Imprinting. The phenomenon of a gene or region of a chromosome showing different expression depending on the parent of origin.

Inborn error of metabolism. An inherited metabolic defect which results in deficient production or synthesis of an abnormal enzyme.

Incest. Union between first-degree relatives.

Incestuous. Description of a relationship between first-degree relatives.

Incidence. The rate at which new cases occur, e.g. 2 in 1000 births are affected by neural tube defects.

Incompatibility. A donor and host are incompatible if the latter rejects a graft from the former.

Incomplete ascertainment. A term used in segregation analysis to describe family studies in which complete ascertainment is not possible.

Index case. See *Proband.*

Index map. See *Framework map.*

Indian hedgehog. One of three mammalian homologues of the segment polarity hedgehog genes.

Inducer. Small molecule which interacts with a regulator protein and triggers gene transcription.

Informative. Variation in a marker system in a family which enables a gene or inherited disease to be followed in that family.

Innate immunity. A number of non-specific systems involved in immunity which don't require or involve prior contact with the infectious agent.

Insertion. Addition of chromosomal material or DNA sequence of one or more nucleotides within the genome.

Insertional mutagenesis. The introduction of mutations at specific sites to determine the effects of these changes.

In situ hybridization. Hybridization with a DNA probe carried out directly on a chromosome preparation or histological section.

Insulin-dependent diabetes mellitus. Diabetes requiring the use of insulin, usually of juvenile onset, also known as type 1 diabetes.

Intermediate inheritance. See *Codominance.*

Interphase. The stage between two successive cell divisions during which DNA replication occurs.

Interphase cytogenetics. The study of chromosomes during interphase, usually by FISH.

Intersex. An individual with external genitalia not clearly male or female.

Interval cancer. Developing cancer in the interval between repeated screening procedures.

Intra-cytoplasmic sperm injection (ICSI). A technique whereby a secondary spermatocyte or spermatozoon is removed from the testis and used to fertilize an egg.

Intrinsic malformation. A malformation due to an inherent abnormality in development.

Intron (= intervening sequence). Region of DNA which generates that part of precursor RNA which is spliced out during transcription and does not form mature mRNA and therefore does not specify the primary structure of the gene product.

Inv. The group of genetic variants of the κ light chains of immunoglobulins.

Inversion. A type of chromosomal aberration or mutation in which part of a chromosome or sequence of DNA is reversed in its order.

Inversion loop. The structure formed in meiosis I by a chromosome with either a para- or pericentric inversion.

In vitro. In the laboratory, literally 'in glass'.

In vivo. In the normal cell, literally 'in the living organism'.

Ionizing radiation. Electromagnetic waves of very short wavelength (X-rays and γ rays), and high energy particles (α particles, β particles and neutrons).

Isochromosome. A type of chromosomal aberration in which one of the arms of a particular chromosome is duplicated because the centromere divides transversely and not longitudinally as normal during cell division. The two arms of an isochromosome are therefore of equal length and contain the same set of genes.

Isolate. A term used to describe a population or group of individuals who for religious, cultural or geographical reasons have remained separate from other groups of persons.

Isozymes. Enzymes that exist in multiple molecular forms which can be distinguished by biochemical methods.

Joining region. Short conserved sequence of nucleotides involved in somatic recombinational events in the production of antibody diversity.

Joint probability. The product of the prior and conditional probability for two events.

Karyogram. Photomicrograph of chromosomes arranged in descending order of size.

Karyotype. The number, size and shape of the chromosomes of an individual. Also used for the photomicrograph of an individual's chromosomes arranged in a standard manner.

Kb. Abbreviation for kilobase.

Killer lymphocytes. See *Cytotoxic T lymphocytes.*

Kilobase. 1000 base pairs (bp).

Km. Genetic variants of the κ light chain of immunoglobulins.

Knockout mutation. Complete loss of function of a gene.

Lagging strand. One of the two strands created in DNA replication which is synthesized in the 3′ to 5′ direction made up of pieces synthesized in the 5′ to 3′ direction which are then joined together as a continuous strand by the enzyme DNA ligase.

Law of addition. If two or more events are mutually exclusive then the probability that *either* one *or* the other will occur equals the *sum* of their individual probabilities.

Law of independent assortment. Members of different gene pairs segregate to offspring independently of one another.

Law of multiplication. If two or more events or outcomes are independent, then the probability that *both* the first *and* the second will occur equals the *product* of their individual probabilities.

Law of segregation. Each individual possesses two genes for a particular characteristic, only one of which can be transmitted at any one time.

Law of uniformity. When two homozygotes with different alleles are crossed, all the offspring in the F1 generation are identical and heterozygous, i.e. the characteristics do not blend and can reappear in later generations.

Leading strand. The synthesis of one of the DNA strands created in DNA replication which occurs in the 5′ to 3′ direction synthesized as a continuous process.

Lethal mutation. A mutation which leads to the premature death of an individual or organism.

Leucine zipper. A DNA binding motif controlling gene expression.

Liability. A concept used in disorders which are multifactorially determined to take into account all possible causative factors.

Library. Set of cloned DNA fragments derived from a particular DNA source, e.g. a cDNA library from the transcript of particular tissue, or a genomic library.

Ligase. Enzyme used to join DNA molecules.

Ligation. Formation of phosphodiester bonds to link two nucleic acid molecules.

Linkage. Two loci situated close together on the same chromosome, the alleles at which are usually transmitted together in meiosis in gamete formation.

Linkage disequilibrium. The occurrence together of two or more alleles at closely linked loci more frequently than would be expected by chance.

Liposomes. Artificially prepared cell-like structures in which one or more bimolecular layers of phospholipid enclose one or more aqueous compartments, which can include proteins.

Localization sequences. Certain short amino acid sequences in newly synthesized proteins which result in their transport to specific cellular locations, e.g. the nucleus, or their secretion.

Location score. Diagrammatic representation of likelihood ratios used in multipoint linkage analysis.

Locus. The site of a gene on a chromosome.

Locus control region (LCR). A region near the β-like globin genes involved in the timing and tissue specificity of their expression in development.

Locus heterogeneity. The phenomenon of a disorder being due to mutations in more than one gene or locus.

Lod score. A mathematical score of the relative likelihood of two loci being linked.

Long interspersed nuclear elements (LINEs). 50 000–100 000 copies of a DNA sequence of approximately 6000 bp which occurs approximately once every 50 kb and encodes a reverse transcriptase.

Long terminal repeat (LTR). One of two long sections of double stranded DNA synthesized by reverse transcriptase from the RNA of a retrovirus involved in regulating viral expression.

Loss of constitutional heterozygosity (LOCH). Loss of an allele inherited from a parent frequently seen as evidence of a 'second hit' in tumorigenesis.

Loss-of-function mutation. Phenotypic features of a disorder due to reduced or absent activity of the gene.

Low resolution mapping. See *Chromosome mapping*.

Lymphokines. A group of glycoproteins released from T lymphocytes after contact with an antigen which act upon other cells of the host immune system.

Lyonization. The process of inactivation of one of the X chromosomes in females originally proposed by the geneticist Mary Lyon.

Major histocompatibility complex (MHC). A multigene locus which codes for the histocompatibility antigens involved in organ transplantation.

Malformation. A primary structural defect of an organ or part of an organ which results from an inherent abnormality in development.

Manifesting heterozygote or **carrier.** The phenomenon of a female carrier for an X-linked disorder having symptoms or signs of that disorder due to non-random X-inactivation, e.g. muscular weakness in a carrier for Duchenne muscular dystrophy.

Map unit. See *CentiMorgan*.

Marker. A loose term used for a blood group, biochemical or DNA polymorphism which, if shown to be linked to a disease locus of interest, can be used in presymptomatic diagnosis, determining carrier status and prenatal diagnosis.

Marker chromosome. A small extra structurally abnormal chromosome.

Maternal (matrilineal) inheritance. Transmission of a disorder through females.

Matrilineal inheritance. See *Maternal inheritance*.

Maturity onset diabetes of the young (MODY). Diabetes which is similar to type 2 but has an earlier age of onset.

Maximum likelihood method. The calculation of the Lod score for various values of the recombination fraction θ to determine the best estimate of the recombination fraction.

Meconium ileus. Blockage of the small bowel in the newborn period due to inspissated meconium, a presenting feature of cystic fibrosis.

Meiosis. The type of cell division which occurs in gamete formation with halving of the somatic number of chromosomes with the result that each gamete is haploid.

Meiotic drive. Preferential transmission of one of a pair of alleles during meiosis.

Mendelian inheritance. Inheritance which follows the laws of segregation and independent assortment as proposed by Mendel.

Merlin. The protein product of the neurofibromatosis type II gene.

Messenger RNA (mRNA). A single stranded molecule complementary to one of the strands of double stranded DNA which is synthesized during transcription and transmits the genetic information in the DNA to the ribosomes for protein synthesis.

Metabolic disorder. An inherited disorder involving a biochemical pathway, i.e. an inborn error of metabolism.

Metacentric. Term used to describe chromosomes in which the centromere is central with both arms being of approximately equal length.

Metaphase. The stage of cell division when the chromosomes line up on the equatorial plate and the nuclear membrane disappears.

Metaphase spreads. The preparation of chromosomes during the metaphase stage of mitosis in which they are condensed.

Methaemoglobin. A haemoglobin molecule in which the iron is oxidized.

Microdeletion. A small chromosomal deletion detectable by high resolution prometaphase chromosomal analysis or FISH.

Microdeletion syndrome. The pattern of abnormalities caused by a chromosome microdeletion.

Microsatellite DNA. Polymorphic variation in DNA sequences due to a variable number of tandem repeats of the dinucleotide CA, tri- or tetranucleotides.

Microsatellite instability. The alteration of the size of microsatellite polymorphic markers compared to the constitutional markers of an individual with hereditary non-polyposis colorectal cancer due to mutations in the genes for the mismatch repair enzymes.

Microtubules. Long cylindrical tubes composed of bundles of small filaments which are an important part of the cytoskeleton.

Minichromosomes. Artificially constructed chromosomes which contain centromeric and telomeric elements that allow replication of foreign DNA as a separate entity.

Minidystrophin. A modified dystrophin gene in which a large amount of the gene has been deleted but which still has relatively normal function.

Minigene. A construct of a gene with the majority of the sequence removed which still remains functional, e.g. a dystrophin minigene.

Minisatellite. Polymorphic variation in DNA sequences due to a variable number of tandem repeats of a short DNA sequence.

Mismatch repair genes. Genes for the DNA proof-reading enzymes, mutations in which cause hereditary non-polyposis colorectal cancer.

Missense mutation. A point mutation which results in a change in an amino acid-specifying codon.

Mitochondria. Minute structures situated within the cytoplasm which are concerned with cell respiration.

Mitochondrial DNA (mtDNA). Mitochondria possess their own genetic material which codes for enzymes involved in energy-yielding reactions, mutations of which are associated with certain diseases in humans.

Mitochondrial inheritance. Transmission of a mitochondrial trait exclusively through maternal relatives.

Mitosis. The type of cell division which occurs in replication of somatic cells.

Mixoploidy. The presence of cell lines with a different genetic constitution in an individual.

Modifier gene. Phenotypic variability due to the consequence of interactions with other genes.

Monosomy. Loss of one member of a homologous pair of chromosomes so that there is one less than the diploid number of chromosomes ($2N - 1$).

Monozygotic twins (= identical). Type of twins derived from a single fertilized ovum.

Morphogen. A chemical or substance which determines a developmental process.

Morphogenesis. The evolution and development of form and shape.

Morula. The 12–16 cell stage of the early embryo at 3 days post conception.

Mosaic. An individual with two different cell lines derived from a single zygote.

mRNA splicing. The excision of intervening non-coding sequences or introns in the primary mRNA resulting in the non-contiguous exons being spliced together to form a shorter mature mRNA before its transportation to the ribosomes in the cytoplasm for translation.

Mucoviscidosis. An older term used for cystic fibrosis.

Multifactorial inheritance. Inheritance controlled by many genes with small additive effects (polygenic) plus the effects of the environment.

Multigene families. Genes with functional and/or sequence similarity.

Multiple alleles. The existence of more than two alleles at à particular locus in a population.

Multiple myeoloma. A cancer of antibody-producing B cells which leads to the production of a single species of an antibody in large quantities.

Multipoint linkage analysis. Analysis of the segregation of alleles at a number of closely adjacent loci.

Mutagen. Natural or artificial ionizing radiation, chemical or physical agents which can induce alterations in DNA.

Mutant. A gene which has undergone a change or mutation.

Mutated in colorectal carcinoma (MCC). A gene involved in colorectal cancer as evidenced by loss of constitutional heterozygosity at 5q21.

Mutation. A change in genetic material, either of a single gene, or in the number or structure of the chromosomes. A mutation which occurs in the gametes is inherited, a mutation which occurs in the somatic cells (somatic mutation) is not inherited.

Mutation rate. The number of mutations at any one particular locus which occur per gamete per generation.

Mutational heterogeneity. The occurrence of more than one mutation in a particular single gene disorder.

Mutator genes. The equivalent in yeast to the DNA proof-reading enzymes which cause hereditary non-polyposis colorectal cancer.

Myeloma. A tumour of the plasma or antibody-producing cells.

Natural killer cells. Large granular lymphocytes which have carbohydrate binding receptors on their cell surface which recognize high molecular weight glycoproteins expressed on the cell surface of the infected cell as a result of the virus taking over the cellular replicative functions.

Neurofibromin. The protein product of the neurofibromatosis type I gene.

Neutral gene. A gene which appears to have no obvious effect on the likelihood of an individual's ability to survive.

New mutation. The occurrence of a change in a gene arising as a new event.

Non-conservative substitution. A mutation which codes for an amino acid which is chemically dissimilar, e.g. a different charge, will result in a protein the structure of which will be altered.

Non-disjunction. The failure of two members of a homologous chromosome pair to separate during cell division so that both pass to the same daughter cell.

Non-identical twins. See *Dizygotic twins*.

Non-insulin-dependent diabetes mellitus. Diabetes which can usually be treated with diet and/or oral medication, also known as type 2 diabetes.

Non-paternity. The biological father is not as stated or believed.

Non-penetrance. The occurrence of an individual being heterozygous for an autosomal dominant gene but showing no signs of it.

Non-random mating. See *Assortative mating*.

Nonsense mutation. A mutation which results in one of the termination codons, which leads to premature termination of translation of a protein.

Non-synonymous mutation. A mutation which leads to an alteration in the encoded polypeptide.

Northern blotting. Electrophoretic separation of mRNA with subsequent transfer to a filter which can be localized with a radiolabelled probe.

Nuclear envelope. The membrane surrounding the nucleus separating it from the cytoplasm.

Nuclear pores. The gaps in the nuclear envelope which allows substances to pass from the nucleus to the cytoplasm and vice versa.

Nucleolus. A structure within the nucleus which contains high levels of RNA.

Nucleosome. DNA–histone subunit of a chromosome.

Nucleotide. Nucleic acid is made up of many nucleotides, each of which consists of a nitrogenous base, a pentose sugar and a phosphate group.

Nucleus. A structure within the cell which contains the chromosomes and nucleolus.

Null allele. See *Amorph*.

Nullisomy. Loss of both members of a homologous pair of chromosomes.

Obligate carrier. An individual who, by pedigree analysis, must carry a particular gene, e.g. parents of a child with an autosomal recessive disorder.

Oligogene. One of a relatively small number of genes which contribute to a disease phenotype.

Oligonucleotide. A chain of, literally, a few nucleotides.

Oncogene. A gene affecting cell growth or development which can cause cancer.

Oncogenic. Literally, 'cancer causing'.

Opsonization. The 'making ready' of an infectious agent in the production of an immune response.

Origins of replication. The points at which DNA replication commences.

Orthologous. Conserved genes or sequences between species.

Ova. Mature haploid female gametes.

Oz. The group of genetic variants of the λ light chain immunoglobulins.

P1-derived artificial chromosomes (PACs). Combination of the P1 and F-factor systems to incorporate foreign DNA inserts up to 150 kb.

Pachytene quadrivalent. The arrangement which the two pairs of chromosomes involved in a reciprocal translocation adopt in meiosis I when undergoing segregation.

Packaging cell line. A cell line which has been infected with a retrovirus in which the provirus is genetically engineered to lack the packaging sequence of the proviral DNA necessary to produce infectious viruses.

Packaging sequence. The DNA sequence of the proviral DNA of a retrovirus necessary for packaging of the retroviral RNA into an infectious virus.

Paint. Use of fluorescent labelled probes derived from a chromosome or region of a chromosome to hybridize with a chromosome in a metaphase spread.

Pair-rule mutant. Developmental genes identified in *Drosophila* which cause pattern deletions in alternating segments.

Panmixis. See *Random mating*.

Paracentric inversion. A chromosomal inversion which does not include the centromere.

Paralogous. Close resemblance of genes from different clusters, e.g. *HOXA13* and *HOXD13*.

Parthenogenesis. The development of an organism from an unfertilized oocyte.

Partial sex-linkage. A term used to describe genes on the homologous or pseudoautosomal portion of the X and Y chromosomes.

Penetrance. The proportion of heterozygotes for a dominant gene who express a trait, even if mildly.

Peptide. An amino acid, a portion of a protein.

Pericentric inversion. A chromosomal inversion which includes the centromere.

Permissible dose. An arbitrary safety limit which is probably very much less than that which would cause any significant effect on the frequency of harmful mutations within the population.

Phage. Abbreviation for *Bacteriophage*.

Pharmacogenetics. The study of genetically determined variation in drug metabolism.

Phase. Assignment of the chromosome on which a particular allele is in relation to alleles at other closely linked marker loci.

Phenocopy. A condition which is due to environmental factors but resembles one which is genetic.

Phenol enhanced reassociation technique (pERT). Use of the chemical phenol to facilitate rehybridization of slightly differing sources of double stranded DNA to enable isolation of sequences which are absent from one of the two sources.

355

Phenotype. The appearance (physical, biochemical and physiological) of an individual which results from the interaction of the environment and the genotype.

Pink-eyed dilution. Human homologue to mouse pink-eye gene for albinism.

Plasma cells. Mature antibody producing B lymphocytes.

Plasmid. Small, circular DNA duplex capable of autonomous replication within a bacterium.

Platelet-derived growth factor (PDGF). A substance derived from platelets which stimulates growth of certain cell types.

Pleiotropy. The multiple effects of a gene.

Point mutation. A single base pair change.

Polar body. The daughter cell of gamete division in the female in meiosis I and II which does not go on to become a mature gamete.

Poly(A) tail. A sequence of 20–200 adenylic acid residues which is added to the 3'-end of most eukaryotic mRNAs, increasing its stability by making it resistant to nuclease digestion.

Polygenes. Genes which make a small additive contribution to a polygenic trait.

Polygenic inheritance. A term used to describe the genetic contribution to the aetiology of disorders in which there are both environmental and genetic causative factors.

Polymerase chain reaction (PCR). The repeated serial reaction involving the use of oligonucleotide primers and DNA polymerase which is used to amplify a particular DNA sequence of interest.

Polymorphic information content (PIC). The amount of variation at a particular site in the DNA.

Polymorphism. The occurrence in a population of two or more genetically determined forms in such frequencies that the rarest of them could not be maintained by mutation alone.

Polypeptide. An organic compound consisting of three or more amino acids.

Polyploid. Any multiple of the haploid number of chromosomes (e.g. $3N$, $4N$, etc.).

Polyribosome. See *Polysome*.

Polysome (= polyribosome). A group of ribosomes associated with the same molecule of mRNA.

Population genetics. The study of the distribution of alleles in populations.

Positional candidate gene. A gene which by virtue of its position to which a disorder maps becomes a possible gene responsible for the disorder.

Positional cloning. The mapping of a disorder to a particular region of a chromosome which then leads to the identification of the gene responsible.

Posterior information. Information available for risk calculation from the results of tests or analysis of offspring in pedigrees.

Posterior probability. The joint probability for a particular event divided by the sum of all possible joint probabilities.

Post-genomic genomics. See *Functional genomics*.

Post-translational processing. Various modifications of protein which occur after their synthesis, e.g. the addition of carbohydrate moieties.

Predictive testing. Presymptomatic testing, often used in relation to testing of persons at risk for Huntington's disease.

Preimplantation genetic diagnosis. The ability to detect the presence of an inherited disorder in an in vitro fertilized conceptus before reimplantation.

Premutation. The existence of a gene in an unstable form which can undergo a further mutational event to cause a disease.

Prenatal diagnosis. The use of tests during a pregnancy to determine whether an unborn child is affected with a particular disorder.

Presymptomatic diagnosis. The use of tests to determine whether a person has inherited a gene for a disorder before he/she has any symptoms or signs.

Prevalence. At a point in time, the proportion of persons in a given population with a disorder or trait.

Primary response. The response to an infectious agent with an initial production of IgM, then subsequently IgG.

Prion. A proteinaceous infectious particle implicated in the cause of several rare neurodegenerative diseases.

Prior probability. The initial probability of an event.

Probability. The proportion of times an outcome occurs in a large series of events.

Proband (= index case). An affected individual (irrespective of sex) through whom a family comes to the attention of an investigator. *Propositus* if male; *proposita* if female.

Probe. A labelled, single stranded DNA fragment which hybridizes with, and thereby detects and locates, complementary sequences among DNA fragments on, for example, a nitrocellulose filter.

Processing. Alterations of mRNA which occur during transcription including splicing, capping and polyadenylation.

Progress zone. The area of growth beneath the apical ectodermal ridge in the developing limb bud.

Prokaryotes. Lower organisms with no well-defined nucleus, e.g. bacteria.

Prometaphase. The stage of cell division when the nuclear membrane begins to disintegrate, allowing the chromosomes to spread with each chromosome attached at its centromere to a microtubule of the mitotic spindle.

Promoter. Recognition sequence for the binding of RNA polymerase.

Promoter elements. DNA sequences which include the GGGCGGG *consensus sequence*, the AT-rich *TATA* or *Hogness box*, and the *CAAT box* which are in a 100–300 bp region located 5' or upstream to the coding sequence of many structural genes in eukaryotic organisms and which control individual gene expression.

Pronuclei. The stage just after fertilization of the oocyte with the nucleus of the oocyte and sperm present.

Prophase. The first visible stage of cell division when the chromosomes are contracted.

Proposita. A female individual as the presenting person in a family.

Propositus. A male individual as the presenting person in a family.

Protein. A complex organic compound composed of hundreds or thousands of amino acids.

Protein truncation test. Using a special primer which contains a promoter and translation initiator sequence to make cDNA which is then translated in a specially designed transcription–translation system with the resulting protein product being analysed on a gel.

Proto-oncogene. DNA genomic sequences with homology to viral oncogenes, which are involved in regulating cell turnover.

Pseudoautosomal. A term used to describe genes which behave like autosomal genes as a result of being located on the homologous portions of the X and Y chromosomes.

Pseudodominance. The apparent dominant transmission of a disorder when an individual homozygous for a recessive gene has affected offspring through having children with an individual who is also a carrier.

Pseudogene. DNA sequence homologous with a known gene but is non-functional.

Pseudohermaphrodite. An individual with ambiguous genitalia or external genitalia opposite to the chromosomal sex in which there is gonadal tissue of only one type.

Pseudohypertrophy. Literally, false enlargement. Seen in the calf muscles of boys with Duchenne muscular dystrophy.

Pseudomosaicism. False mosaicism seen occasionally as an artefact with cells in culture.

Pulsed field gel electrophoresis (PFGE). A technique of DNA analysis using electrophoretic methods to separate large DNA fragments, up to 2 million base pairs in size, produced by digesting DNA with restriction enzymes with relatively long DNA recognition sequences which, as a consequence, cut DNA relatively infrequently.

Purine. A nitrogenous base with fused five- and six-member rings (adenine and guanine).

Pyrimidine. A nitrogenous base with a six-membered ring (cytosine, uracil, thymine).

Quantitative inheritance. See *Polygenic inheritance*.

Radiation absorbed dose (rad). A measure of the amount of any ionizing radiation which is absorbed by the tissues. 1 rad is equivalent to 100 erg of energy absorbed per gram of tissue.

Radiation hybrids. Cells exposed to radiation fragment their chromosomes which contain subchromosomal portions of a chromosome enabling assignment of a particular gene or DNA sequence to a specific region.

Random genetic drift. The chance variation of allele frequencies from one generation to the next.

Random mating (= panmixis). Selection of a spouse regardless of the spouse's genotype.

Reading frame. The order of the triplets of nucleotides in the codons of a gene which are translated into the amino acids of the protein.

Recessive. A trait which is expressed in individuals who are homozygous for a particular allele but not in those who are heterozygous.

Reciprocal translocation. A structural rearrangement of the chromosomes in which material is exchanged between one homologue of each of two pairs of chromosomes. The rearrangement is balanced if there is no loss or gain of chromosome material.

Recombinant DNA molecule. A union of two different DNA sequences from two different sources, e.g. a vector containing a 'foreign' DNA sequence.

Recombination. Cross-over between two linked loci.

Recombination fraction (θ). A measure of the distance separating two loci determined by the likelihood that a cross-over will occur between them.

Reduced penetrance. A dominant gene which does not manifest itself in a proportion of heterozygotes.

Relative probability. See *Posterior probability*.

Relative risk. How frequently a disease occurs in an individual with a specific marker compared to those without the marker in the general population.

Repetitive DNA. DNA sequences of variable length which are repeated up to 100 000 (middle repetitive) or over 100 000 (highly repetitive) copies per genome.

Replication. The process of copying the double stranded DNA of the chromosomes.

Replication bubble. The structure formed by coalescence of two adjacent replication forks in copying the DNA molecule of a chromosome.

Replication error. The phenomenon of microsatellite instability seen in hereditary non-polyposis colorectal cancer due to a mutation in one of the DNA proof-reading enzymes.

Replication fork. The structure formed at the site(s) of origin of replication of the double stranded DNA molecule of chromosomes.

Replication units. Clusters of 20–80 sites of origin of DNA replication.

Replicons. A generic term for DNA vectors such as plasmids, phages and cosmids, which replicate in host bacterial cells.

Repressor. The product of the regulator gene of an operon which inhibits the operator gene.

Repulsion. When a certain allele at a locus is on the homologous chromosome for a specific allele at a closely linked locus.

Response elements. Regulatory sequences in the DNA to which signalling molecules bind resulting in control of transcription.

Restriction endonucleases or **enzymes**. Group of enzymes each of which cleaves double stranded DNA at a specific nucleotide sequence and so produces fragments of DNA of different lengths.

Restriction fragment. DNA fragment produced by a restriction endonuclease.

Restriction fragment length polymorphism (RFLP). Polymorphism due to the presence or absence of a particular restriction site.

Restriction map. Linear arrangement of restriction enzyme sites.

Restriction site. Base sequence recognized by a restriction endonuclease.

Reticulocytes. Immature red blood cells which still contain messenger RNA.

Retrovirus. RNA virus which replicates via conversion into a DNA provirus.

Reverse genetics. The process of identifying a protein or enzyme through its gene product.

Reverse painting. Amplification using PCR of an unidentified portion of chromosomal material, such as a small duplication or marker chromosome, which is then used as a probe for hybridization to a normal metaphase spread to identify its source of origin.

Reverse transcriptase. An enzyme which catalyses the synthesis of DNA from RNA.

Reverse transriptase PCR (RT-PCR). Using a special primer which contains a promoter and translation initiator from mRNA (for PCR) to make cDNA.

Ribonucleic acid (RNA). See *RNA*.

Ribosomes. Minute spherical structures in the cytoplasm, rich in RNA; the location of protein synthesis.

Ring chromosome. An abnormal chromosome caused by a break in both arms of the chromosome, the ends of which unite leading to the formation of a ring.

RNA (= ribonucleic acid). The nucleic acid which is found mainly in the nucleolus and ribosomes. *Messenger RNA* transfers genetic information from the nucleus to the ribosomes in the cytoplasm and also acts as a template for the synthesis of polypeptides. *Transfer RNA* transfers activated amino acids from the cytoplasm to messenger RNA.

RNA-directed DNA synthesis. An exception to the central dogma, a process utilized by many RNA viruses to produce DNA which can integrate with the host genome.

Robertsonian translocation. A translocation between two acrocentric chromosomes with loss of satellite material from their short arms.

Roentgen equivalent for man (rem). The dose of any radiation which has the same biological effect as 1 rad of X-rays.

Satellite. A distal portion of the chromosome separated from the remainder of the chromosome by a narrowed segment or stalk.

Satellite DNA. A class of DNA sequences which separates out on density gradient centrifugation as a shoulder or 'satellite' to the main peak of DNA and corresponds to 10–15% of the DNA of the human genome consisting of short tandemly repeated DNA sequences which code for ribosomal and transfer RNAs.

Screening. The identification of persons from a population with a particular disorder, or who carry a gene for a particular disorder.

Secondary hypertension. Increased blood pressure which occurs as a result of another primary cause.

Secondary oocyte or **spermatocyte**. The intermediate stage of a female or male gamete in which the homologous duplicated chromosome pairs have separated.

Secondary response. The enhanced immune response seen after repeated exposure to an infectious organism or foreign antigen.

Secretor locus. A gene in humans which results in the secretion of the ABO blood group antigens in saliva and other body fluids.

Secretor status. The presence or absence of excretion of the ABO blood group antigens into various body fluids, e.g. saliva.

Segment polarity mutants. Developmental genes identified in *Drosophila* which cause pattern deletions in every segment.

Segmental. Limited area of involvement, e.g. a somatic mutation limited to one area of embryonic development.

Segregation. The separation of alleles during meiosis so that each gamete contains only one member of each pair of alleles.

Segregation analysis. Study of the way in which a disorder is transmitted in families to establish the mode of inheritance.

Segregation ratio. The proportion of affected to unaffected individuals in family studies.

Selection. The forces which affect biological fitness and therefore the frequency of a particular condition within a given population.

Selfish DNA. DNA sequences which appear to have little function and which, it has been proposed, preserve themselves as a result of selection within the genome.

Semi-conservative. The process in DNA replication in which only one strand of each resultant daughter molecule is newly synthesized.

Sense strand. Strand of genomic DNA to which the mRNA is identical.

Sensitivity. Refers to the proportion of cases which are detected. A measure of sensitivity can be made by determining the proportion of *false-negative* results, i.e. how many cases are missed.

Sequence. A stretch of DNA nucleotides. Also used in relation to birth defects or congenital abnormalities which occur as a consequence of a cascade of events intiated by a single primary factor, e.g. Potter's sequence which occurs as a consequence of renal agenesis.

Severe combined immunodeficiency. A genetically heterogeneous lethal form of inherited immunodeficiency with abnormal B and T cell function leading to increased susceptibility to both viral and bacterial infections.

Sex chromatin (= Barr body). A darkly staining mass situated at the periphery of the nucleus during interphase which represents a single, inactive, condensed X chromosome. The number of sex chromatin masses is one less than the number of X chromosomes (e.g. none in normal males and in 45,X females, one in normal females and XXY males, etc.)

Sex chromosomes. The chromosomes responsible for sex determination (XX in women, XY in men).

Sex-determining region of the Y (SRY). The part of the Y chromosome which contains the testis-determining gene.

Sex influence. When a genetic trait is expressed more frequently in one sex than another. In the extreme when only one sex is affected this is called *sex limitation*.

Sex limitation. When a trait is only manifest in individuals of one sex.

Sex-linkage. The pattern of inheritance shown by genes carried on the sex chromosomes. Since there are very few Mendelizing genes on the Y chromosome the term is often used synonymously for X-linkage.

Sex-linked inheritance. A disorder determined by a gene on one of the sex chromosomes.

Sex ratio. The number of male births divided by the number of female births.

Short interspersed nuclear elements (SINEs). 5% of the human genome consists of some 750 000 copies of DNA sequences of approximately 300 bp which have sequence similarity to a signal recognition particle involved in protein synthesis.

Siamese twins. Conjoined identical twins.

Sib (= sibling). Brother or sister.

Sickle-cell crisis. An acute haemolytic episode in persons with sickle-cell disease associated with a sudden onset of chest, back or limb pain, fever and dark urine due to the presence of free haemoglobin in the urine.

Sickle-cell disease. The homozygous state for haemoglobin S associated with anaemia and the risk of sickle-cell crises.

Sickle-cell trait. The heterozygous state for haemoglobin S which is not associated with any significant medical risks under ordinary conditions.

Sickling. The process of distortion of red blood cell morphology under low oxygenation conditions in persons with sickle-cell disease.

Sievert (Sv). Equivalent to 100 rem.

Signal transduction. A complex multistep pathway from the cell membrane, through the cytoplasm to the nucleus with positive and negative feedback loops for accurate cell proliferation and differentiation.

Silencers. A negative '*enhancer*', the normal action of which is to repress gene expression.

Silent mutation. A point mutation in a codon which, due to the degeneracy of the genetic code, still results in the same amino acid in the protein.

Single nucleotide polymorphisms (SNPs). Single nucleotide DNA sequence variation which is polymorphic occurring every 1/500 to 1/2000 base pairs.

Single stranded conformational polymorphism (SSCP). A mutation detection system in which differences in the three-dimensional structure of single stranded DNA result in differential gel electrophoresis mobility under special conditions.

Sister chromatids. Identical daughter chromatids derived from a single chromosome.

Sister chromatid exchange. Exchange (crossing-over) of genetic material between two chromatids of any particular chromosome in mitosis.

Site-directed mutagenesis. The ability to alter or modify DNA sequences or genes in a directed fashion by processes such as insertional mutagenesis or homologous recombination to determine the effect of these changes on their function.

Skeleton map. See *Framework map.*

Skewed X-inactivation. A non-random pattern of inactivation of one of the X chromosomes in a female which can arise through a variety of mechanisms, e.g. an X-autosome translocation.

Slipped strand mispairing. Incorrect pairing of the tandem repeats of the two complementary DNA strands during DNA replication which is thought to lead to variation in DNA microsatellite repeat number.

Small nuclear RNA molecules. RNA molecules involved in RNA splicing.

Soft markers. Minor structural ultrasound findings associated with the possibility of fetal abnormality.

Solenoid model. The complex model of the quarternary structure of chromosomes.

Somatic cells. The non-germ line cells of the body.

Somatic cell gene therapy. The alteration or replacement of a gene limited to the non-germ cells.

Somatic cell hybrid. A technique involving the fusion of cells from two different species which results in the loss of chromosomes from one of the cell types and which is used in assigning genes to particular chromosomes.

Somatic mosaicism. The occurrence of two different cell lines in a particular tissue or tissues which differ genetically.

Somatic mutation. A mutation limited to the non-germ cells.

Sonic hedgehog. One of three mammalian homologues of the segment polarity hedgehog genes.

Southern blot. Technique for transferring DNA fragments from an agarose gel to a nitrocellulose filter on which they can be hybridized to a radiolabelled single stranded complementary DNA sequence or probe.

Specific acquired or **adaptive immunity.** A tailor-made immune response which occurs after exposure to an infectious agent.

Specificity. The extent to which a test detects only affected individuals. If unaffected persons are detected, these are referred to as *false-positives*.

Spermatid. Mature haploid male gamete.

Spindle. A structure responsible for the movement of the chromosomes during cell division.

Splicing. The removal of the introns and joining of exons in RNA during transcription with introns being spliced out and exons being spliced together.

Splicing branch site. Intronic sequence involved in splicing of mRNA.

Splicing consensus sequences. DNA sequences surrounding splice sites.

Spontaneous mutation. A mutation which arises de novo, apparently not due to environmental factors such as mutagens.

Sporadic. When a disorder affects a single individual in a family.

SRY (sex-reversed Y). The sex-determining region of the Y chromosome which contains the testis-determining gene.

Stable mutation. A mutation which is transmitted unchanged.

Stop codons. One of three codons (UAG, UAA and UGA) which cause termination of protein synthesis.

Subchromosomal mapping. Mapping of a gene or DNA sequence of interest to a region of a chromosome.

Submetacentric. Term used to describe chromosomes in which the centromere is slightly off-centre.

Substitution. A single base pair replaced by another nucleotide.

Suppressor lymphocytes. A subclass of T lymphocytes which regulates immune responses, particularly suppressing an immune response to 'self'.

Switching. Change in the type of β- or α-like globin chains produced in embryonic and fetal development.

Synapsis. The pairing of homologous chromosomes during meiosis.

Synaptonemal complex. A complex protein structure which forms between two homologous chromosomes which pair during meiosis.

Syndrome. The complex of symptoms and signs which occur together in any particular disorder.

Synonymous mutation. See *Silent mutation.*

Syntenic genes. Two genes at different loci on the same chromosome.

T. Abbreviation for thymine.

TATA (Hogness) box. See *Hogness box*.

T cell surface antigen receptor. Antigenic receptor on the cell surface of T lymphocytes.

T lymphocytes. Lymphocytes involved in the cellular immune response, 'thymus'-derived.

Tandemly repeated DNA sequences. DNA which consists of blocks of tandem repeats of non-coding DNA which can be either highly dispersed or restricted in their location in the genome.

Target DNA. The carrier or vector DNA to which foreign DNA is incorporated or attached to produce recombinant DNA.

Telomere. The distal portion of a chromosome arm.

Telomeric DNA. The terminal portion of the telomeres of the chromosomes contains 10–15 kb of tandem repeats of a 6 base pair DNA sequence.

Telophase. The stage of cell division when the chromosomes have completely separated into two groups and each group has become invested in a nuclear membrane.

Template strand. The strand of the DNA double helix which is transcribed into mRNA.

Teratogen. An agent which causes congenital abnormalities in the developing embryo or fetus.

Teratogene. A gene which can mutate to form a developmental abnormality.

Terminator. A sequence of nucleotides in DNA which codes for the termination of translation of mRNA.

Tertiary trisomy. The outcome when 3 to 1 segregation of a balanced reciprocal translocation results in the presence of an additional derivative chromosome.

Tetraploidy. Twice the normal diploid number of chromosomes (4*N*).

Thalassaemia intermedia. A less severe form of β thalassaemia which requires less frequent transfusions.

Thalassaemia major. An inherited disorder of human haemoglobin which is due to underproduction of one of the globin chains.

Thalassaemia minor. See *Thalassaemia trait*.

Thalassaemia trait. The heterozygous state for β thalassaemia, associated with an asymptomatic mild microcytic, hypochromic anaemia.

Three-prime (3′) end. The end of a DNA or RNA strand with a free 3′ hydroxyl group.

Threshold. A concept used in disorders which exhibit multifactorial inheritance to explain a discontinuous phenotype in a process or trait which is continuous, e.g. cleft lip as a result of disturbances in the process of facial development.

Thymine. A pyrimidine base in DNA.

Tissue typing. Cellular, serological and DNA testing to determine histocompatibility for organ transplantation.

Trait. Any detectable phenotypic property or character.

***Trans*-acting.** Transcription factors which act on genes at a distance, usually on both copies of a gene on each chromosome.

Transcription. The process whereby genetic information is transmitted from the DNA in the chromosomes to messenger RNA.

Transcription factors. Genes which include the *Hox*, *Pax*, and zinc finger containing genes which control RNA transcription by binding to specific DNA regulatory sequences forming complexes which initiate transcription by RNA polymerase.

Transfection. The transformation of bacterial cells by infection with phage to produce infectious phage particles. Also the introduction of foreign DNA into eukaryotic cells in culture.

Transfer RNA. RNA molecule involved in transfer of amino acids in the process of translation.

Transformation. Genetic recombination in bacteria in which foreign DNA introduced into the bacterium is incorporated into the chromosome of the recipient bacteria. Also the change of a normal cell into a malignant cell, e.g. as results with infection of normal cells by oncogenic viruses.

Transgenic animal model. Use of techniques such as targeted gene replacement to introduce mutations into a particular gene in another animal species to study an inherited disorder in humans.

Transient polymorphism. Two different allelic variants present in a population whose relative frequencies are altering due to either selective advantage or disadvantage of one or the other.

Transition. A substitution involving replacement by the same type of nucleotide, i.e. a pyrimidine for a pyrimidine (C for T or vice versa) or a purine for a purine (A for a G or vice versa).

Translation. The process whereby genetic information from messenger RNA is translated into protein.

Translocation. The transfer of genetic material from one chromosome to another chromosome. If there is an exchange of genetic material between two chromosomes then this is referred to as a reciprocal translocation. A translocation between two acrocentric chromosomes by fusion at the centromeres is referred to as a *Robertsonian translocation*.

Transposon. Mobile genetic element able to replicate and insert a copy of itself at a new location in the genome.

Transversion. Substitution of a pyrimidine by a purine or vice versa.

Triple test. The test which gives a risk for having a fetus with Down's syndrome in mid-trimester as a function of age, serum α-fetoprotein, oestriol and human chorionic gonadotrophin levels.

Triplet amplification or **expansion**. Increase in the number of copies of triplet repeat sequences responsible for mutations in a number of single gene disorders.

Triplet code. A series of three bases in the DNA or RNA molecule which codes for a specific amino acid.

Triploid. A cell with three times the haploid number of chromosomes, i.e. 3*N*.

Trisomy. The presence of a chromosome additional to the normal complement (i.e. 2*N* + 1) so that in each somatic nucleus one particular chromosome is represented three times rather than twice.

Trophoblast. The outer cell mass of the early embryo which gives rise to the placenta.

Truncate ascertainment. See *Incomplete ascertainment*.

Tumour suppressor gene. A term to describe genes which appear to prevent the development of certain types of tumour.

Tyrosinase-negative albinism. Form of oculocutaneous albinsim with no melanin production which can be tested for in vitro.

Tyrosinase-positive albinism. Form of oculocutaneous albinism with some melanin production which can be tested for in vitro.

U. Abbreviation for uracil.

Ultrasound. Use of ultrasonic soundwaves to image objects at a distance, e.g. the developing fetus in utero.

Unbalanced translocation. A translocation in which there is an overall loss or gain of chromosomal material, e.g. partial monosomy of one of the portions involved and partial trisomy of the other portion involved.

Unifactorial (= Mendelizing). Inheritance controlled by a single locus.

Uniparental disomy. When an individual inherits both chromosomes of a homologous pair from one parent.

Uniparental heterodisomy. Uniparental disomy due to inheritance of the two different homologues from one parent.

Uniparental isodisomy. Uniparental disomy due to inheritance of two copies of a single chromosome of a homologous pair from one parent.

Unipolar illness. Affective depressive illness.

Universal donor. A person of blood group O, Rh-negative who can donate blood to any person irrespective of their blood group.

Universal recipient. A person of blood group AB, Rh-positive who can receive blood from any donor irrespective of their blood group.

Unstable mutation. Mutation which, when transmitted, is passed on in altered form, e.g. triplet repeat mutations.

Uracil. A pyrimidine base in RNA.

Utrophin. A gene on chromosome 6 with homology to the dystrophin gene.

Variable expressivity. The variation in the severity of phenotypic features seen in persons with autosomal dominant disorders, e.g. variable number of café-au-lait spots or neurofibromata in neurofibromatosis type I.

Variable region. The portion of the light and heavy chains of immunoglobulins which differs between molecules and which helps to determine antibody specificity.

Variants. Alleles which occur less frequently than in 1% of the population.

Vector. A plasmid, phage or cosmid into which foreign DNA can be inserted for cloning.

Virions. Infectious viral particles.

Virus. A protein-covered DNA- or RNA-containing organism which is only capable of replication within bacterial or eukaryotic cells.

Wingless. A group of morphogens produced by segment polarity genes.

X-chromatin. See *Barr body* or *Sex chromatin*.

X-inactivation. See *Lyonization*.

X-inactivation centre. The part of the X chromosome responsible for the process of X-inactivation.

X-linkage. Genes carried on the X chromosome.

X-linked dominant. Genes on the X chromosome which manifest in heterozygous females.

X-linked dominant lethals. Disorders which are seen only in females and not seen in males as they are thought to be incompatible with survival of the early embryo in hemizygous males, e.g. incontinentia pigmenti.

X-linked recessive. Genes which are carried by females and expressed in hemizygous males.

Xanthomata. Subcutaneous depositions of lipid, often around tendons; a physical sign associated with disordered lipid metabolism.

Yeast artificial chromosome (YAC). A plasmid-cloning vector which contains the DNA sequences for the centromere, telomere and autonomous chromosome replication sites that enable cloning of large DNA fragments up to 2–3 million base pairs in length.

Y-linked inheritance. See *Holandric inheritance*.

Zinc finger. A finger-like projection formed by amino acids positioned between two separated cysteine residues which form a complex with a zinc ion, found in genes which have important developmental regulatory roles.

Zona pellucida. Cellular layer surrounding the mature unfertilized oocyte.

Zone of polarizing activity. An area on the posterior margin of the developing limb bud which determines the antero-posterior axis.

Zoo blot. A Southern blot of DNA from a number of different species used to look for evidence of DNA sequences conserved during evolution.

Zygote. The fertilized ovum.

Index